UNIVERSITY OF IOWA

THE FAMILY PRACTICE HANDBOOK

NOTICE

Medicine is an ever-changing field. Standard safety precautions must be followed, but as new research and clinical experience broaden our knowledge, changes in treatment and drug therapy may become necessary or appropriate. Readers are advised to check the most current product information provided by the manufacturer of each drug to be administered to verify the recommended dose, the method and duration of administration, and contraindications. It is the responsibility of the treating physician, relying on experience and knowledge of the patient, to determine dosages and the best treatment for each individual patient. Neither the publisher nor the editor assumes any liability for any injury and/or damage to persons or property arising from this publication.

UNIVERSITY OF IOWA

THE FAMILY PRACTICE HANDBOOK

MARK A. GRABER, MD
Associate Professor of Family Medicine
and Emergency Medicine
Departments of Family Medicine and Emergency Medicine
University of Iowa College of Medicine
Iowa City, Iowa

MATTHEW L. LANTERNIER, MD
Assistant Clinical Professor of Family Medicine
Department of Family Medicine
University of Iowa College of Medicine
Iowa City, Iowa

FOURTH EDITION

a Mosby handbook

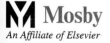

Mosby
An Affiliate of Elsevier

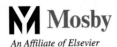
Mosby
An Affiliate of Elsevier

Acquisitions Editor: Elizabeth Fathman
Editorial Assistant: Paige Mosher Wilke
Project Manager: Pat Joiner
Production Editor: Rachel E. Dowell
Designer: Mark A. Oberkrom

Mosby
An Affiliate of Elsevier
11830 Westline Industrial Drive
St. Louis, Missouri 63146

Printed in the United States of America

Library of Congress Cataloging in Publication Data
The family practice handbook/[edited by] Mark A. Graber, Matthew L. Lanternier.
—4th ed.
    p.; cm.
  At head of title: University of Iowa.
  Includes bibliographical references and index.
  ISBN 0-323-01209-4 (alk. paper)
    1. Family medicine—Handbooks, manuals, etc.   I. Graber, Mark A., MD.
  II. Lanternier, Matthew L.   III. University of Iowa.
    [DNLM: 1. Family practice—Handbooks. WB 39 F1985 2001]
  RC55 .F25 2001
  616—dc21   2001030389

    04   05   TG/FF   9   8   7   6   5   4

CONTRIBUTORS

Alison C. Abreu, MD
Resident Physician, Departments of
Psychiatry and Family Medicine,
University of Iowa Hospitals and Clinics,
Iowa City, Iowa

Jatinder P. S. Ahluwalia, MD
Associate, Division of Gastroenterology
and Hepatology, Department of Internal
Medicine, University of Iowa College
of Medicine; Staff Physician, Division
of Gastroenterlogy and Hepatology,
University of Iowa Hospitals and Clinics,
Iowa City, Iowa

*Karen Brannon, MD
Private Practice, Muscatine, Iowa

Ke Chen, MD, PhD
Staff Physician, Immediate Care Center,
Iowa Health Physicians, Cedar Rapids,
Iowa

Kevin C. Doerschug, MD
Associate Fellow, Division of
Pulmonology, Department of Internal
Medicine, University of Iowa College of
Medicine, University of Iowa, Iowa City,
Iowa

Julie Kay Filips, MD
Resident Physician, Department of
Psychiatry, University of Iowa Hospitals
and Clinics, Iowa City, Iowa

James M. Fox, MD
Fellow, Division of Cardiology,
Department of Internal Medicine,
University of Iowa College of Medicine,
Iowa City, Iowa

Mark A. Graber, MD
Associate Professor of Family Medicine
and Emergency Medicine, Departments
of Family Medicine and Emergency
Medicine, University of Iowa College of
Medicine, Iowa City, Iowa

Rosanna Yuk-Kuen Kao, MD, PhD
Resident, Department of Family
Medicine, University of Iowa Hospitals
and Clinics, Iowa City, Iowa

Michael W. Kelly, PharmD, MS
Associate Professor, University of Iowa
College of Pharmacy, Iowa City, Iowa

Teresa Bailey Klepser, PharmD
Assistant Professor, Division of Clinical
and Administrative Pharmacy,
University of Iowa College of Pharmacy,
Iowa City, Iowa

Heidi Koch
Chief Resident, Department of
Pediatrics, University of Iowa College of
Medicine, Iowa City, Iowa

*Rudolf J. Kotula, MD
Physician, Private Practice in Infectious
Diseases, Methodist Hospital, Omaha,
Nebraska

David C. Krupp, MD
Resident Physician, Department of
Family Medicine, University of Iowa
Hospitals and Clinics, Iowa City, Iowa

Matthew L. Lanternier, MD
Assistant Clinical Professor of Family
Medicine, Department of Family
Medicine, University of Iowa College of
Medicine, Iowa City, Iowa

Sara Mackenzie, MD
Assistant Professor of Family Medicine,
Department of Family Medicine,
University of Iowa College of Medicine,
Iowa City, Iowa

Coleman O. Martin, MD
Fellow, Department of Neurology,
University of Iowa College of Medicine,
Iowa City, Iowa

Philip M. Polgreen, MD
Resident, Department of Internal
Medicine, University of Iowa Hospitals
and Clinics, Iowa City, Iowa

Sudha Rajavel, MD
Resident, Department of Family
Medicine, University of Iowa College of
Medicine, Iowa City, Iowa

*Formerly with the University of Iowa, Iowa City, Iowa.

William B. Silverman, MD
Associate Professor of Medicine, Division
of Gastroenterlogy and Hepatology,
Department of Internal Medicine,
University of Iowa College of Medicine,
Iowa City, Iowa

*Sarah Thomas, MD
Private Practice, Iowa City, Iowa

Alicia M. Weissman, MD
Assistant Professor, Department of
Family Medicine, University of Iowa
College of Medicine; Attending Physician,
University of Iowa Hospitals and Clinics,
Iowa City, Iowa

To my parents and siblings, Stanley, Selma, Jay, Alyssa, and Shari.

Also, thanks to some of my friends, David Kopaska-Merkel, Mark Joseph Grygier, Sarah Rogers, and Christine Saalbach.
MAG

To my loving wife, Natalie Lanternier, M.D., whose strength I admire, and to my first-born child, John Michael, who has brought immeasurable joy to my life. Also, a sincere thanks to my high school teachers, Linda Michael and Russell Byer, who inspired me to be not only a good student but also a caring person. Special thanks to Concepcion Flores for helping me develop the patience to listen to my elderly patients.
MLL

PREFACE

How many times have you heard "You're too smart to go into Family Practice?" or "Why would you want to do Family Practice?"

Well, I have news for our colleagues. Family Practice can be one of the most difficult, challenging, intellectually stimulating, and rewarding fields in medicine. You not only need to have the knowledge base specific to family medicine, you also have to be a competent internist and pediatrician among other skills.

It is with this scope of family medicine in mind that we have created the fourth edition of the *University of Iowa Family Practice Handbook*. Each concise and authoritative chapter has been written or reviewed by a Family Practice resident or fellow to make sure that the information is relevant to your practice. Several new topics have been added since the last edition, and all of the therapeutics have been updated. We have included evidence-based information about herbal medications, including side effects and drug interactions. This edition has also been reorganized to make information easier to find.

This edition should also be quite useful for medical students, physician assistants, and nurse practitioners. It covers a broad spectrum of both outpatient and inpatient medicine yet can still easily fit in a pocket.

As always, we are open to feedback both positive and negative (although *this* never happens!). Feel free to write me at mark-graber@uiowa.edu or from our web site at www.uiowa.edu/~famprac. We take your comments seriously and incorporate your ideas into each new edition. Enjoy.

Mark A. Graber

ACKNOWLEDGMENTS

The editors would like to thank the authors of this edition who made working on this book a pleasure. We would also like to thank Trenton Thomas Hoogerwerf. Even though he is only several months old, he has been diligently sitting at the keyboard typing away at the manuscript (he is a bit slow, though, since he can still only hunt and peck!).

Matt would like to thank Natalie and John for their patience.

Mark would like to thank, as always, Hetty, Rachel, and Abe. Finally, thanks to the *Who* and the *Kinks* (not to mention *They Might Be Giants*) for keeping me awake with loud noise in the wee hours of the morning.

CONTENTS

9   Neurology, 337
Coleman O. Martin

10   Infectious Diseases, 391
Philip M. Polgreen

ABBREVIATIONS

A/a	alveolar-arterial oxygen gradient
ABCs	airway, breathing, circulation
ABG	arterial blood gas
AC	before meals (ante cibum)
AC	acromioclavicular
ACE	angiotensin-converting enzyme
aCL	anticardiolipin (antibody)
ACLS	Advanced Cardiac Life Support
ACOG	American College of Obstetrics and Gynecology
ACTH	adrenocorticotropic hormone
AD	Alzheimer's dementia or disease
A Fib	atrial fibrillation
AFB	acid-fast bacilli
AFP	alpha-fetoprotein
AFV	amniotic fluid volume
AGCUS	atypical glandular cells of undetermined significance
AI	amnioinfusion
AIDS	acquired immunodeficiency syndrome
ALT	alanine aminotransferase
ANA	antinuclear antibody
ANCA	antineutrophil cytoplasmic antibody
AP	anteroposterior
APS	antiphospholipid syndrome
APSAC	anistreplase, anisoylated plasminogen-streptokinase activator complex
APTT	activated partial thromboplastin
ARC	AIDS-related complex
ARDS	adult respiratory distress syndrome
ARF	acute renal failure
ASA	acetylsalicylic acid
ASAP	as soon as possible
ASCUS	atypical squamous cells of undetermined significance
ASO	antistreptolysin O antibody
AST	aspartate aminotransferase
Atg	anti-human thymocyte globulin
ATN	acute tubular necrosis
AV	arteriovenous; atrioventricular
AZT	zidovudine (Azidothymidine)
B_{12}	vitamin B_{12}
BAER	brainstem auditory evoked responses
BBT	basal body temperature
BCG	bacille Calmette-Guérin
BCP	birth control pill
BHCG	beta human chorionic gonadotropin
BID	twice a day (bis in die)
BiPAP	bilevel positive airway pressure
BOOP	bronchiolitis obliterans-organizing pneumonia
BP	blood pressure
BPAD	bipolar affective disorder
bpm	beats per minute
BPP	biophysical profile
BPPV	benign paroxysmal positional vertigo
BSA	body surface area

BUN	blood urea nitrogen
BV	bacterial vaginosis
BVM	bag valve mask
C&S	culture and sensitivity
C-peptide	insulin chain C-peptide
C-section	cesarean section
C-spine	cervical spine
CABG	coronary artery bypass graft
CACl$_2$	calcium chloride
CAD	coronary artery disease
cap	capsule
c-ANCA	central antineutrophil cytoplasmic antibody
CBC	complete blood cell count
cc	cubic centimeter (for solids and gases but **ml** for liquids)
CD4+	helper T cell (cluster of differentiation no. 4+)
CDC	Centers for Disease Control and Prevention, Atlanta, Ga.
CEA	carcinoembryonic antigen
CFU	colony-forming unit
CHF	congestive heart failure
Chol	cholesterol
CIN	cervical intraepithelial neoplasia (1 to 3: mild to severe)
CK	creatine kinase
CLL	chronic lymphocytic leukemia
cm	centimeter
CMV	cytomegalovirus
CNS	central nervous system
CO$_2$	carbon dioxide
COPD	chronic obstructive pulmonary disease
CPAP	continuous positive airway pressure
CPD	cephalopelvic disproportion
CPK	creatine phosphokinase
CPPD	calcium pyrophosphate dihydrate (crystals) (pseudogout)
CPR	cardiopulmonary resuscitation
Cr	creatinine
CRF	chronic renal failure
CRP	C-reactive protein
CSF	cerebrospinal fluid
CST	contraction stress fluid
CT	computerized tomography
CVA	cerebrovascular accident
CVAT	costovertebral-angle tenderness
CVD	cerebrovascular disease
CVN	central venous nutrition
CVP	central venous pressure
CVS	cardiovascular system
c/w	consistent with
CXR	chest x-ray film or radiograph
D&C	dilatation and curettage
DBP	diastolic blood pressure
DDAVP	1-deamino-8-D-arginine vasopressin
DDC, ddC	dideoxycytidine, zalcitabine, Hivid
DDI, ddI	dideoxyinosine, didanosine
D$_5$W	5% dextrose in water
D4T	stavudine
DHE	dihydroergotamine
DHT	dihydrotestosterone
DIC	disseminated intravascular coagulation

DIP	distal interphalangeal joint
DKA	diabetic ketoacidosis
dl	deciliter
DM	diabetes mellitus
DPL	diagnostic peritoneal lavage
DPT	diphtheria-pertussis-tetanus (vaccine)
DS	double strength
DSM	Diagnostic and Statistical Manual (of Mental Disorders)
dsDNA	double-stranded deoxyribonucleic acid
DTR	deep tendon reflexes
DTs	delirium tremens
DVT	deep venous thrombosis
D/W	dextrose in water
EBV	Epstein-Barr virus
ECF	extracellular fluid
ECG	electrocardiogram
ECMO	extracorporeal membrane oxygenation
ED	emergency department
EDC	estimated date of confinement
EEG	electroencephalogram
EES	erythromycin ethylsuccinate
EGD	esophagogastroduodenoscopy
EIA	enzyme immunoassay
ELISA	enzyme-linked immunosorbent assay
EM	erythema multiforme
EMG	electromyogram
ENG	electronystagmography
ENT	ear, nose, throat
ER	emergency room
ERCP	endoscopic retrograde cholangiopancreatography
ESR	erythrocyte sedimentation rate
ET	endotracheal tube
FB	foreign body
FDA	U.S. Food and Drug Administration
Fe	iron
FE$_{Na}$	fractional excretion of sodium
FEF	forced expiratory flow
FEV$_1$	forced expiratory volume at 1 second
FFP	fresh frozen plasma
FH	family history
FHR	fetal heart rate
FSH	follicle-stimulating hormone
FTA	fluorescent treponemal antibody
FTA-ABS	fluorescent treponemal antibody absorption (test)
5-FU	5-fluorouracil
F/U	follow-up (study, exam, test, care)
FUO	fever of unknown origin
G	gauge
G6PD	glucose-6-phosphate dehydrogenase
GBS	group B *Streptococcus* bacteria, or group B streptococcal infection
GC	gonococcus
GCS	Glasgow Coma Scale
GCT	glucose challenge test
GDM	gestational diabetes mellitus
GE	gastroesophageal
GFR	glomerular filtration rate

GI	gastrointestinal
g	gram
GM-CSF	granulocyte-macrophage colony-stimulating factor
GN	glomerulonephritis
GnRH	gonadotropin-releasing hormone
GODM	gestational onset diabetes mellitus
gtt	drops (guttae)
GTT	glucose tolerance test
GU	genitourinary
GXT	graded exercise stress test
GYN	gynecologic
h, hr	hour
H&P	history and physical examination
HA	headache
Hb	hemoglobin
HC/AC	head circumference-to-abdominal circumference (ratio)
HCG	human chorionic gonadotropin
HCT	hematocrit
HCTZ	hydrochlorothiazide
HDL	high-density lipoprotein
HELLP	hemolysis, elevated liver enzymes, and low platelet count (syndrome)
HepBsAg	hepatitis B surface antigen
HGE	human granulocytic ehrlichiosis
HIV	human immunodeficiency virus
HME	human monocytic erlichiosis
HMG	human menopausal gonadotropin
h/o	history of
HPF	high-power field
HRT	hormone replacement therapy
HS	at bedtime (hora somni)
HSV	herpes simplex virus
ht, Ht	height
HTN	hypertension
HUS	hemolytic uremic syndrome
HZV	herpes zoster virus
I&D	incision and drainage
I&O	intake and output
ICF	intracellular fluid
ICP	intracranial pressure
ICU	intensive care unit
ID	infectious disease
IDDM	insulin-dependent diabetes mellitus
IFA	immunofluorescence assay
IgG	immunoglobulin G
IHSS	idiopathic hypertrophic aortic stenosis
IM	intramuscular
IMV	intermittent mandatory ventilation
IN	intranasally
INH	isoniazid, isonicotinc acid hydrazide
INR	International Normalized Ratio
IO	intraosseous
IPPV	intermittent positive-pressure ventilation
ISA	intrinsic stimulating activity
ITP	idiopathic thrombocytopenia purpura
IU	International Unit
IUD	intrauterine device

IUFD	intrauterine fetal demise
IUGR	intrauterine growth retardation
IUP	intrauterine pregnancy
IV	intravenous
IVDA	intravenous drug abuser
IVP	intravenous pyelogram
JRA	juvenile rheumatoid arthritis
JVD	jugular venous distension
kg	kilogram
K, K⁺	potassium
KOH	potassium hydroxide
KS	Kaposi's sarcoma
LA	lupus anticoagulant
LAT	preparation of lidocaine, epinephrine (adrenaline), tetracaine
LBBB	left bundle branch block
LDH	lactate dehydrogenase
LDL	low-density lipoprotein
LE	lupus erythematosus
LES	lower esophageal sphincter
LFT	liver function tests
LGI	lower GI (gastrointestinal)
LH	luteinizing hormone
LLQ	left lower quadrant
LMP	last menstrual period
LMW	low molecular weight
LOC	loss of consciousness
LP	lumbar puncture
LR	lactated Ringer's solution
L/S	lecithin-to-sphingomyelin (ratio)
LSIL	low-grade squamous intraepithelial lesion
LUQ	left upper quadrant
LV	left ventricular
MAI/MAC	*Mycobacterium avium-intracellulare/M. avium* complex
MAO	monoamine oxidase
MAOI	monoamine oxidase inhibitors
MAST	military antishock trousers
MCP	metacarpophalangeal joint
MCV	mean corpuscular volume
MDD	major depressive disorder
MDI	metered dose inhaler
MEE	middle ear effusion
mEq	milliequivalent
mg	milligram
μg	microgram
MI	myocardial infarction
min	minute
mm Hg	millimeters of mercury
mmol	millimole
MMPI	Minnesota Multiphasic Personality Inventory
MMR	measles-mumps-rubella (vaccine)
MMSE	Mini-Mental State examination
mOsm	milliosmole
MR	measles and rubella (vaccine)
MRI	magnetic resonance imaging
MS	multiple sclerosis
MTP	metatarsophalangeal joint
MVP	mitral valve prolaspe

N&V	nausea and vomiting
NCV	nerve conduction velocity
NG	nasogastric
NHL	non-Hodgkin's lymphoma
NIDDM	non-insulin dependent diabetes mellitus
NPH	neutral protamine Hagedorn
NPO	nothing by mouth (nulla per os)
NS	normal saline solution
NSAID	nonsteroidal anti-inflammatory drug
NST	nonstress test
NSVD	normal spontaneous vaginal delivery
NTD	neural tube defect
NTG	nitroglycerin
O&P	ova and parasites
OA	osteoarthritis
OCD	obsessive-compulsive disorder
OCP	oral contraceptive pill
17-OHS	17-hydroxysteroid (that is, 17-hydroxycorticosteroid)
OM	otitis media
OPV	oral poliovirus
ORS	WHO oral rehydration solution
osm, Osm	osmole; osmolality
OTC	over the counter
PA	posteroanterior
PAC	premature atrial contraction
PALS	Pediatric Advanced Life Support
Pap	Papanicolaou test or smear
PAS	para-aminosalicylic acid
PCA	patient-controlled analgesia
PCN	penicillin
PCOD	polycystic ovarian disease
PCP	*Pneumocystis* pneumonia
PCR	polymerase chain reaction
PCWP	pulmonary capillary wedge pressure
PD	Parkinson's disease
PDA	patent ductus arteriosus
PE	physical examination
PE	pulmonary embolism
PEEP	positive end-expiratory pressure
PEFR	peak expiratory flow rate
PET	positron emission tomography
PFTs	pulmonary function tests
PG	phosphatidylglycerol
pH	hydrogen-ion concentration; pH 7, normal; less is acidic; more is alkaline (or basic)
PID	pelvic inflammatory disease
PIH	pregnancy-induced hypertension
PIP	proximal interphalangeal joint
plt	platelet
PMNs	polymorphonuclear lymphocytes
PMR	polymyalgia rheumatica
PMS	premenstrual syndrome
PO	per mouth (per os)
POD	postoperative day
PPD	protein purified derivative
PR	per rectum
PRN	as needed (pro re nata)

PROM	premature rupture of membranes
PSA	prostate specific antigen
PSVT	paroxysmal supraventricular tachycardia
PT	prothrombin time
PTCA	percutaneous transluminal coronary angioplasty
PTL	premature labor
PTSD	post-traumatic stress disorder
PTT	partial thromboplastin time
PTU	propylthiouracil
PUD	peptic ulcer disease
PVC	premature ventricular contraction
QD	every day (quaque die)
QHS	properly "every hour of sleep," but usually "at every bedtime" (quaque hora somni)
QID	four times per day (quater in die)
QOD	every other day (tertio quoque die)
RA	rheumatoid arthritis
RBC	red blood cell
RCA	right coronary artery
REM	rapid eye movement
RF	renal failure
RFI	renal failure index
RIA	radioimmunoassay
RIND	reversible ischemic neurologic deficit
RLQ	right lower quadrant
RMSF	Rocky Mountain spotted fever
R/O, r/o	rule out
ROM	rupture of membranes; range-of-motion (exercise)
RPR	rapid plasma reagin
RSI	rapid-sequence intubation
RSV	respiratory syncytial virus
rt-PA	tissue-type plasminogen activator (recombinant) (Alteplase, Recombinant)
RUQ	right upper quadrant
RVMI	right ventricular myocardial infarction
SAARD	slow-acting antirheumatic drug(s)
SAH	subarachnoid hemorrhage
SBP	systolic blood pressure
SCIWORA	spinal cord injury without radiologic abnormality
SGA	small for gestational age
SGOT	See AST
SGPT	See ALT
SIL	squamous intraepithelial lesions
SK	streptokinase
SL	sublingual
SLE	systemic lupus erythematosus
SLR	straight-leg raising (test)
SOB	shortness of breath
sp. gr.	specific gravity
SPECT	single-photon emission computerized tomography
SQ	subcutaneous
SR	slow release
SROM	spontaneous rupture of membrane
SS	single strength
SSKI	saturated solution of potassium iodide
SSRI	selective serotonin reuptake inhibitors
STD	sexually transmitted disease

T_3	triiodothyronine
T_4	thyroxine
TAC	preparation of tetracycline, epinephrine (adrenaline), cocaine
Tb, TB	tuberculosis
TBG	thyroxine-binding globulin
TBSA	total body surface area
TBW	total body water
3TC	lamivudine
TCA	tricyclic antidepressant
TEDS	thromboembolic disease support (stockings, hose)
TEE	transesophageal echocardiography
TENS	transcutaneous electrical nerve stimulation
TFT	thyroid function test
TG	triglycerides
TIA	transient ischemic attack
TIBC	total iron-binding capacity
TM	tympanic membrane
TMJ	temporomandibular joint
TMP/SMX	trimethoprim-sulfamethoxazole (complex)
TORCHS	toxoplasmosis, rubella, cytomegalovirus, herpes simplex, syphilis (infection)
TPA	tissue plasminogen activator
TPN	total parenteral nutrition
TRH	thyrotropin-releasing hormone
TSH	thyroid-stimulating hormone
TTP	thrombotic thrombocytopenic purpura
TURP	transurethral prostatectomy
TWAR	Taiwan acute respiratory disease
U	unit
UA	urinalysis
UC	ulcerative colitis
UGI	upper gastrointestinal (tract)
U/P	urine-to-plasma ratio
URI	upper respiratory infection
U/S	ultrasound, ultrasonogram, ultrasonography
UTI	urinary tract infection
UV	ultraviolet (radiation); B refers to the shorter-wave, more damaging range
V Fib	ventricular fibrillation
V Tach	ventricular tachycardia
VBAC	vaginal birth after cesarean section
VCUG	voiding cystourethrogram
VDRL	Venereal Disease Research Laboratories (test)
V/Q	ventilation-perfusion ratio
VSD	ventricular septal defect
Vt	tidal volume
VT	vestibular training
vWF	von Willebrand's factor
WBC	white blood cell (count)
wt, Wt	weight

UNIVERSITY OF IOWA

THE FAMILY PRACTICE HANDBOOK

RESUSCITATION, AIRWAY MANAGEMENT, AND ACUTE ARRHYTHMIAS

Mark A. Graber

AIRWAY MANAGEMENT AND RAPID SEQUENCE INTUBATION

AIRWAY MANAGEMENT

A. **Adequate anesthesia** is critical for intubation in the awake patient.
   1. If you have time, lidocaine 4% at 5 ml by hand-held nebulizer facilitates intubation by blocking the gag reflex and providing excellent topical anesthesia.
   2. In nasal intubation, cetacaine/lidocaine spray and lidocaine jelly are helpful.

B. **Nasal intubation.**
   1. Simple to do blindly. Putting 5 cc of air in the ET balloon once it is in the posterior pharynx can facilitate a difficult intubation.
   2. Contraindicated in bleeding disorders, when you might want to use thrombolytics and in those with a basilar skull fracture or midface trauma.
   3. The patient must be breathing to use this technique.
   4. Almost all patients intubated nasally develop a sinusitis and should be given antibiotics if prolonged intubation is required.

BOX 1-1

RAPID SEQUENCE INTUBATION

Patient will not be able to maintain an airway or breathe after paralysis. Use this technique only if you are comfortable with intubation.

BEFORE PARALYSIS:

- Preoxygenate, IV lines, monitor, oximetry, equipment including that for emergency surgical airway control.
- Lidocaine 1 mg/kg (100 mg*).†
- Atropine 0.01 mg/kg (0.5 mg, minimum of 0.1 mg*).‡
- Vecuronium 0.01 mg/kg (1 mg*)§ prevents fasciculation **IF** using succinylcholine (no need with rocuronium or vecuronium).
- Begin Sellick maneuver (cricothyroid pressure to prevent vomiting and aspiration).

PARALYSIS:

- Midazolam 0.1 mg/kg (7 mg*)‖ **OR** Etomidate 0.3mg/kg IV (duration 3-5 minutes) **THEN** Succinylcholine 1.5 mg/kg (100 mg*)¶ **OR** Rocuronium 0.6-1.2 mg/kg IV **OR** Vecuronium 0.10 mg/kg (10 mg*)

INTUBATION WHEN RELAXED:

- Assess tube placement.
- Check patient's temperature 8 minutes after intubation if succinylcholine used.

*Usual adult dosage.
†May be omitted in non–head injury cases.
‡May be omitted in adults if no preexistent bradycardia.
§May use pancuronium (same dose). This step is optional.
‖May use thiopental 3 to 5 mg/kg (300 mg*).
¶Dose in children is 1.5 to 2 mg/kg.

TABLE 1-1

ENDOTRACHEAL TUBE SIZES FOR CHILDREN

Age	Endotracheal Tube Size
Premature	2.5, 3.0 uncuffed
Newborn	3.0, 3.5 uncuffed
6 months	3.5 uncuffed
12 to 18 months	4.0, 4.5 uncuffed
2 years	4.5, 5.0 uncuffed
4 years	5.0, 5.5 uncuffed
6 years	5.5 uncuffed
8 years	6.0 cuffed or uncuffed
10 years	6.5 cuffed
12 years	7.0 cuffed
>12 years	7.0-8.0 cuffed

To calculate: Approximate tube size = (Age/4) + 4.

RAPID SEQUENCE INTUBATION (RSI)

Before you try RSI, be sure that you are able to control the airway, since the patient will be paralyzed and unable to breathe. Always assess tube placement by auscultation, radiograph, oxygen saturation, and end-title CO_2, which will be low in esophageal intubation.

A. **Indications.** Respiratory failure, acute intracranial lesions, some overdoses, status epilepticus, combative trauma patients where behavior threatens life, possible cervical spine fracture where immobilization not possible because of delirium, etc.

B. **Drugs.**
  1. Succinylcholine.
     a. May cause bradycardia, increased intraocular and intracranial pressure, increased gastric pressure and emesis.
     b. Contraindicated in penetrating globe trauma.
     c. Rarely causes malignant hyperthermia, hyperkalemia.
     d. May cause fatal hyperkalemia in those with risk factors in particular time frames: (1) *Burns:* 24 hours to 2 years after burn; (2) *Denervation* (e.g., stroke, spinal cord injury): 1 week to 6 months after injury, always in MS, ALS; (3) *Crushed muscle:* 7 days to 90 days after injury. **Do not use succinylcholine in these patients.**
  2. Vecuronium: rapid onset (1 minute, maximal 3-5 minutes, duration 25-40 minutes), nondepolarizing, no cardiac toxicity.
  3. Rocuronium: rapid onset (<2 minutes, maximal 3 minutes, duration 31 minutes average), nondepolarizing, no cardiac toxicity.

C. RSI (**Box 1-1** and **Table 1-1**).

CRITICAL CARDIAC LIFE SUPPORT

The cardiac life support algorithms on the following pages are consistent with the new 2000 ACLS guidelines, which are licensed for publication by the American Heart Association.

GENERAL

The ABCs common to all emergency situations:

A Airway, including relieving obstruction, positioning.

B Breathing, including 100% O2 by bag-valve-mask or preferably intubation.

C Circulation, CPR.

D Drugs. **Lidocaine, atropine, naloxone, and epinephrine may be given via endotracheal tube.** Give 10 ml of sterile water (best) or saline after drug.

SPECIFIC RHYTHMS AND THEIR TREATMENT

I. Specific Rhythms and their Treatment are found in Figures 1-1 to 1-7.

II. For adult drug doses, see Table 1-2 and specific algorithms.

1

RESUSCITATION, AIRWAY MANAGEMENT, AND ACUTE ARRHYTHMIAS

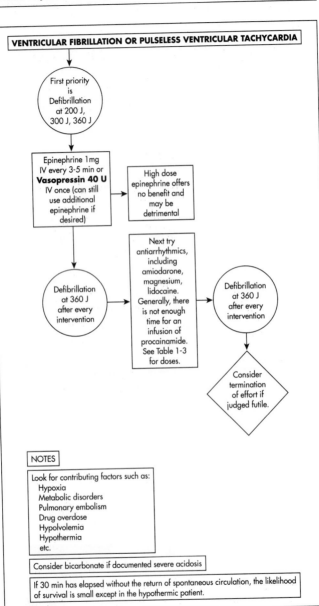

VENTRICULAR FIBRILLATION OR PULSELESS VENTRICULAR TACHYCARDIA

First priority is Defibrillation at 200 J, 300 J, 360 J

Epinephrine 1mg IV every 3-5 min or **Vasopressin 40 U** IV once (can still use additional epinephrine if desired)

High dose epinephrine offers no benefit and may be detrimental

Defibrillation at 360 J after every intervention

Next try antiarrhythmics, including amiodarone, magnesium, lidocaine. Generally, there is not enough time for an infusion of procainamide. See Table 1-3 for doses.

Defibrillation at 360 J after every intervention

Consider termination of effort if judged futile.

NOTES

Look for contributing factors such as:
Hypoxia
Metabolic disorders
Pulmonary embolism
Drug overdose
Hypolvolemia
Hypothermia
etc.

Consider bicarbonate if documented severe acidosis

If 30 min has elapsed without the return of spontaneous circulation, the likelihood of survival is small except in the hypothermic patient.

FIGURE 1-1

Torsade de pointes (polymorphic ventricular tachycardia)

Caused by digitalis toxicity, erythromycin, lidocaine, tricyclic antidepressants, quinidine, procainamide, mexiletine, tocainide, amiodarone, nifedipine, cisapride, antipsychotics, and others. Also, hypothermia and toxins, including arsenic and organophosphate poisoning. Other causes include hypocalcemia, hypomagnesemia, hypokalemia, and neurologic processes, including stroke and subarachnoid bleeding.
Avoid drugs that may prolong the QT interval further such as quinidine, lidocaine, and disopyramide.

TREATMENT

Magnesium is probably the best pharmocologic approach, although may get recurrence. Give 2 g bolus of $MgSO_4$ (10 ml of a 20% solution) over 1 to 2 minutes (can push if not perfusing). May follow with a second or third bolus if necessary at 5 to 15 minutes. Infusions of 3 to 20 mg/min for 7 to 48 hours or until the QT interval has decreased to less than 0.50 second. Magnesium toxicity is heralded by areflexia, bradycardia, coma, respiratory depression but should not be a problem in doses noted above. Magnesium is relatively contraindicated in renal failure.

Temporary overdrive pacing at 90-120 beats per minute.

Phenytoin 250 mg IV in normal saline over 10 minutes followed by 100 mg IV Q5 min as needed. Most will respond to 250 mg. Maximum loading dose of phenytoin is 10 to 15 mg/kg in adults. Do not infuse at a rate exceeding 50 mg/min.

Lidocaine is usually ineffective but can be tried.

Isoproterenol is a poor alternative to overdrive pacing and is no longer on the market in the United States.

FIGURE 1-1—cont'd

1

RESUSCITATION, AIRWAY MANAGEMENT, AND ACUTE ARRHYTHMIAS

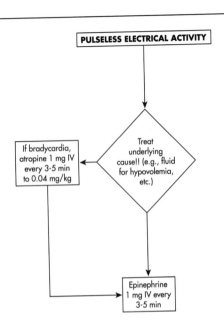

PULSELESS ELECTRICAL ACTIVITY

Treat underlying cause!! (e.g., fluid for hypovolemia, etc.)

If bradycardia, atropine 1 mg IV every 3-5 min to 0.04 mg/kg

Epinephrine 1 mg IV every 3-5 min

NOTES

Defined as absence of a pulse despite organized complexes at an adequate rate.

Consider underlying causes including hypothermia, hypovolemia, cardiac tamponade, pulmonary embolism, hypoxia, tension pneumothorax, acidosis, massive infarction, hyperkalemia, hypokalemia, overdose (beta-blockers, calcium channel blockers etc.)

If sure there is massive pulmonary embolism, may try thrombolytics if other measures fail (see Chapter 4)

FIGURE 1-2

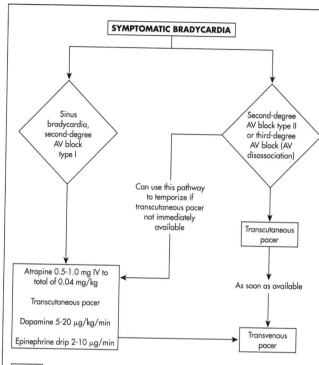

SYMPTOMATIC BRADYCARDIA

Sinus bradycardia, second-degree AV block type I

Second-degree AV block type II or third-degree AV block (AV disassociation)

Can use this pathway to temporize if transcutaneous pacer not immediately available

Transcutaneous pacer

Atropine 0.5-1.0 mg IV to total of 0.04 mg/kg

Transcutaneous pacer

Dopamine 5-20 μg/kg/min

Epinephrine drip 2-10 μg/min

As soon as available

Transvenous pacer

NOTES

Bradycardia is a pulse <60 or a pulse that is lower than expected for the clinical situation (e.g., a pulse of 70 in a patient with hypovolemia)

Symptomatic = hypotension, poor perfusion (e.g., CNS changes), weakness, etc.

Types of heart block:
  I. First-degree AV block with fixed PR interval >0.20 second.
  II. Second-degree AV block.
      a. Mobitz type I (Wenckebach). Progressive prolongation of PR interval until there is a nonconducted P wave.
      b. Mobitz type II. Fixed PR interval with dropped beats (may require a pacer).
  III. Third-degree AV block: no consistent relationship between P waves and QRS complexes.

For calcium channel blocker overdose, use calcium chloride 0.5 g to 1 g IV slow push.
For beta-blocker overdose, consider glucogon 5-10 mg IV followed by a drip of 1-5 mg/hr.

FIGURE 1-3

RESUSCITATION, AIRWAY MANAGEMENT, AND ACUTE ARRHYTHMIAS

1

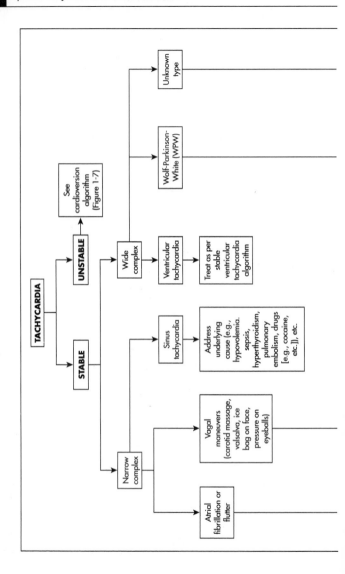

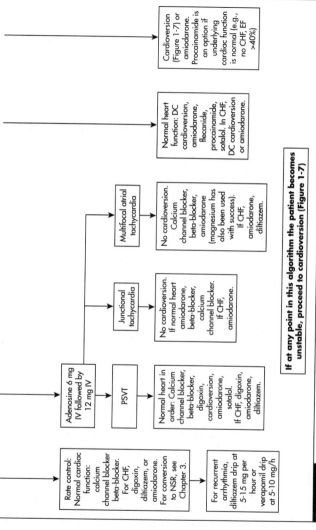

1

RESUSCITATION, AIRWAY MANAGEMENT, AND ACUTE ARRHYTHMIAS

FIGURE 1-4

NOTES

1. CHF for purposes of this algorithm means clinical CHF or EF <40%.
2. Unstable means hypotension, poor perfusion, cardiac ischemia, etc., related to rate.
3. Stable means good perfusion, no cardiac ischemia, stable, adequate blood pressure, etc.
4. **No DC cardioversion of narrow complex tachycardia** with EF <40% or CHF unless patient becomes unstable.
5. Can pretreat with calcium chloride, 3.3 cc IV before using calcium channel blockers. This mitigates hypotension without affecting antiarrhythmic properties.
6. Digoxin will not convert a-fib but may facilitate conversion by improving cardiac function. 50% will spontaneously convert to NSR.
7. Carotid massage has <0.28% complication rate and most of these are transitory (e.g., TIA).
8. Start appropriate oral medications as indicated (e.g., verapamil to prevent recurrent PSVT).

FIGURE 1-4—cont'd

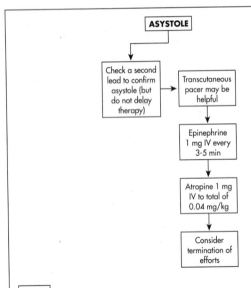

ASYSTOLE

Check a second lead to confirm asystole (but do not delay therapy)

Transcutaneous pacer may be helpful

Epinephrine 1 mg IV every 3-5 min

Atropine 1 mg IV to total of 0.04 mg/kg

Consider termination of efforts

NOTES

Recovery from true asystole is rare.

Consider defibrillation if fine V-fib is a possibility (about 9%) but not routinely recommended.

Aminophylline 250 mg IV has been successful in **uncontrolled** human trials but showed no benefit in swine trials. It is not standard of care but can be tried if conventional therapy has failed.

FIGURE 1-5

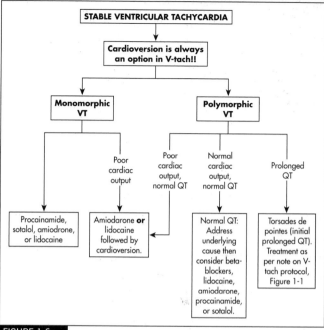

FIGURE 1-6

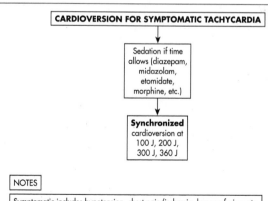

FIGURE 1-7

TABLE 1-2	
ADULT CARDIAC DRUG DOSES (see also specific algorithms)	
Drug	**Dose**
Adenosine	6 mg IV bolus followed by 12 mg IV
	Follow with 30 cc saline flush
Amiodarone	**Pulseless V-tach/V-fib:** 300 mg IV push, may repeat with 150 mg
	Perfusing rhythm: 150 mg IV slowly
Atropine	0.5-1 mg IV total of 0.04 mg/kg
Diltiazem	0.25 mg/kg IV over 2 minutes followed by 0.35 mg/kg. Drip at 5-15 mg/hr. See note under verapamil.
Epinephrine	1 mg IV push q 3-5 minutes (maximum of 0.02 mg/kg but high dose is of questionable benefit and may increase mortality)
Isoproterenol	2-8 μg/min for overdrive pacing of torsades de pointes
Lidocaine	**Pulseless V-tach/V-fib:** 1.5 mg/kg IV push, repeat in 3-5 minutes to total of 3 mg/kg
	Perfusing rhythm: 1-1.5 mg/kg slowly and then 0.5-0.75 mg/kg IV in 5-10 minutes to total of 3 mg/kg
	Drip: 2-4 mg/min
Magnesium	1-2 g IV push or over 5 min if patient has perfusing rhythm
Metoprolol	5 mg IV slowly with 5 mg every 5 minutes to total of 15 mg. Can titrate to effect.
Procainamide	17 mg/kg IV, maximum rate of 30 mg/min.
	Drip 1-4 mg/min.
Sodium bicarbonate	1 mEq/kg
Sotalol	1.0 to 1.5 mg/kg infused at 10 mg/min. Do not use if poor perfusion. Negative inotrope.
Vasopressin	40 U IV single dose only
Verapamil	2.5-5 mg IV and repeat with 5-10 mg. Maximum 20 mg. Note: Can pretreat with 3.3 cc of CaCl to mitigate hypotension. Drip at 5-10 mg/hr.

CRITICAL PEDIATRIC LIFE SUPPORT

The following critical pediatric life support algorithms are consistent with the new 2000 ACLS guidelines, which are licensed for publication by the American Heart Association.

I. **Critical Pediatric Life Support**

A. **Breathing** (remember positioning, suctioning, airway).

   1. Pediatric cardiac arrest almost always secondary to respiratory insult.

   2. Treat any signs of respiratory distress such as tachypnea, retractions, or stridor immediately. (See sections on asthma in Chapter 2 and stridor in Chapter 12 for differential.)

   3. Immediately provide humidified oxygen in highest concentration possible.

   4. For suspected epiglottitis, do not move patient or apply oxygen. Any agitation to the child may precipitate airway obstruction. See Chapter 12 for a discussion of epiglottitis.

   5. Aspiration of a foreign body is especially prevalent in those less than 5 years of age.

     a. **Present with** sudden-onset dyspnea, stridor, gagging.

     b. **Treatment:** Observe as long as moving air well and coughing. If there is increased respiratory difficulty or cough is ineffective, can try Heimlich maneuver or direct visualization of cords and removal of foreign body if necessary.

     c. **Bag-valve-mask with 100% O2 usually adequate even in situations such as epiglottitis.**

   6. If must intubate, see section on RSI (Box 1-1) and Table 1-1 for ET tube size.

B. **Cardiac assessment** (Figures 1-8 to 1-11).

   1. Tachycardia is usual response to stress.

   2. Bradycardia is evidence of impending cardiac arrest.

   3. Blood pressure may remain normal until cardiopulmonary arrest imminent (see Chapter 23 for normal blood pressure).

   4. Observe level of consciousness, urine output, capillary refill, color as gauge of end-organ perfusion.

   5. For fluid resuscitation: 20 ml/kg IV bolus of NS or LR. May repeat twice or more if needed.

   6. The efficacy of high-dose epinephrine (0.1 mg/kg) is unclear. It may actually worsen outcomes but is still standard of care.

   7. Drugs for pediatric resuscitation (Table 1-3).

1

RESUSCITATION, AIRWAY MANAGEMENT, AND ACUTE ARRHYTHMIAS

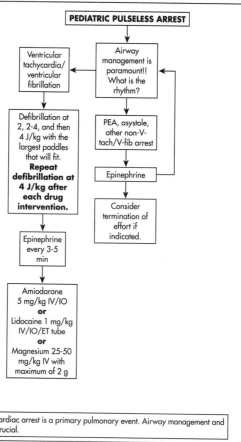

PEDIATRIC PULSELESS ARREST

Airway management is paramount!! What is the rhythm?

Ventricular tachycardia/ ventricular fibrillation

PEA, asystole, other non-V-tach/V-fib arrest

Defibrillation at 2, 2-4, and then 4 J/kg with the largest paddles that will fit. **Repeat defibrillation at 4 J/kg after each drug intervention.**

Epinephrine

Consider termination of effort if indicated.

Epinephrine every 3-5 min

Amiodarone 5 mg/kg IV/IO **or** Lidocaine 1 mg/kg IV/IO/ET tube **or** Magnesium 25-50 mg/kg IV with maximum of 2 g

NOTES

Most pediatric cardiac arrest is a primary pulmonary event. Airway management and oxygenation is crucial.

Consider underlying causes, including hypothermia, hypovolemia, cardiac tamponade, pulmonary embolism, hypoxia, tension pneumothorax, acidosis, massive infarction, hyperkalemia, hypokalemia, overdose (beta-blockers, calcium channel blockers, etc.), etc.

Epinephrine dose: IV/IO 0.01 mg/kg (1:10,000, 0.1 ml/kg)
By ET tube: 0.1 mg/kg (1:1000, 0.1 ml/kg)
Can use higher dose after first dose.

IV pressors (e.g., dopamine) as needed. Bicarbonate as needed if documented acidosis.

FIGURE 1-8

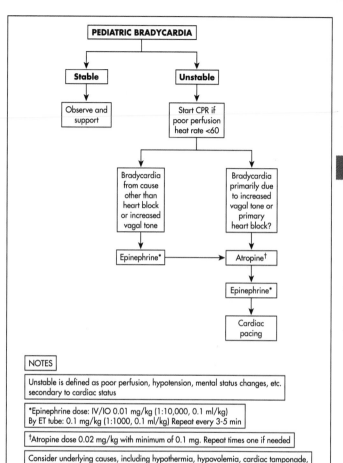

PEDIATRIC BRADYCARDIA

Stable → Observe and support

Unstable → Start CPR if poor perfusion heat rate <60

Bradycardia from cause other than heart block or increased vagal tone → Epinephrine*

Bradycardia primarily due to increased vagal tone or primary heart block? → Atropine† → Epinephrine* → Cardiac pacing

NOTES

Unstable is defined as poor perfusion, hypotension, mental status changes, etc. secondary to cardiac status

*Epinephrine dose: IV/IO 0.01 mg/kg (1:10,000, 0.1 ml/kg)
By ET tube: 0.1 mg/kg (1:1000, 0.1 ml/kg) Repeat every 3-5 min

†Atropine dose 0.02 mg/kg with minimum of 0.1 mg. Repeat times one if needed

Consider underlying causes, including hypothermia, hypovolemia, cardiac tamponade, hypoxia, head injury, overdose (beta-blockers, calcium channel blockers, digoxin, etc.) head injury, etc.

FIGURE 1-9

RESUSCITATION, AIRWAY MANAGEMENT, AND ACUTE ARRHYTHMIAS

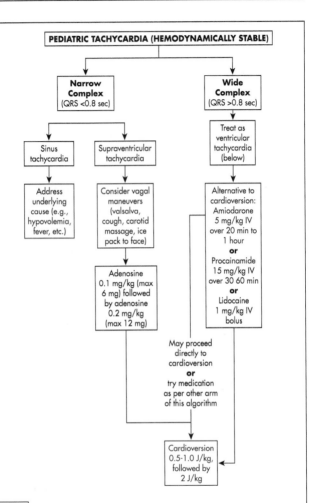

PEDIATRIC TACHYCARDIA (HEMODYNAMICALLY STABLE)

Narrow Complex (QRS <0.8 sec)

Wide Complex (QRS >0.8 sec)

Sinus tachycardia

Supraventricular tachycardia

Treat as ventricular tachycardia (below)

Address underlying cause (e.g., hypovolemia, fever, etc.)

Consider vagal maneuvers (valsalva, cough, carotid massage, ice pack to face)

Alternative to cardioversion: Amiodarone 5 mg/kg IV over 20 min to 1 hour **or** Procainamide 15 mg/kg IV over 30 60 min **or** Lidocaine 1 mg/kg IV bolus

Adenosine 0.1 mg/kg (max 6 mg) followed by adenosine 0.2 mg/kg (max 12 mg)

May proceed directly to cardioversion **or** try medication as per other arm of this algorithm

Cardioversion 0.5-1.0 J/kg, followed by 2 J/kg

NOTES

Stable means no signs or symptoms of hypoperfusion such as mental status changes, cyanosis, hypotension, etc.

Consider underlying causes including hypothermia, hypovolemia, cardiac tamponade, pulmonary embolism, hypoxia, tension pneumothorax, acidosis, massive infarction, hyperkalemia, hypokalemia, overdose (beta-blockers, calcium channel blockers, etc.), etc.

Consultation with pediatric cardiology is suggested before cardioversion.

FIGURE 1-10

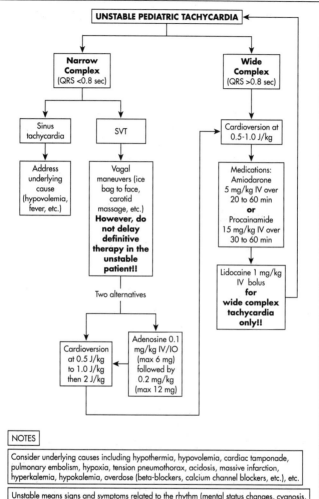

UNSTABLE PEDIATRIC TACHYCARDIA

Narrow Complex (QRS <0.8 sec)

Wide Complex (QRS >0.8 sec)

Sinus tachycardia

SVT

Cardioversion at 0.5-1.0 J/kg

Address underlying cause (hypovolemia, fever, etc.)

Vagal maneuvers (ice bag to face, carotid massage, etc.). **However, do not delay definitive therapy in the unstable patient!!**

Medications: Amiodarone 5 mg/kg IV over 20 to 60 min **or** Procainamide 15 mg/kg IV over 30 to 60 min

Lidocaine 1 mg/kg IV bolus **for wide complex tachycardia only!!**

Two alternatives

Cardioversion at 0.5 J/kg to 1.0 J/kg then 2 J/kg

Adenosine 0.1 mg/kg IV/IO (max 6 mg) followed by 0.2 mg/kg (max 12 mg)

NOTES

Consider underlying causes including hypothermia, hypovolemia, cardiac tamponade, pulmonary embolism, hypoxia, tension pneumothorax, acidosis, massive infarction, hyperkalemia, hypokalemia, overdose (beta-blockers, calcium channel blockers, etc.), etc.

Unstable means signs and symptoms related to the rhythm (mental status changes, cyanosis, hypotension etc.)

Generally, amiodarone and procainamide should not be used together.

FIGURE 1-11

RESUSCITATION, AIRWAY MANAGEMENT, AND ACUTE ARRHYTHMIAS

1

TABLE 1-3

DRUG DOSES FOR PEDIATRIC RESUSCITATION

Drug	Dose	Remarks
Adenosine	0.1 to 0.2 mg/kg Maximum single dose: 12 mg	Rapid IV bolus.
Atropine sulfate	0.02 mg/kg per dose	Minimum dose: 0.1 mg. Maximum single dose: 0.5 mg in child, 1.0 mg in adolescent.
Bretylium toslyate	5 mg/kg; may be increased to 10 mg/kg	Rapid IV.
Calcium chloride 10%	20 mg/kg per dose	Give slowly.
Dobutamine hydrochloride*	2-20 mg/kg/min	Titrate to desired effect.
Dopamine hydrochloride*	2-20 μg/kg/min	Adrenergic action dominates at $\geq$15-20 μg/kg/min.
Epinephrine for bradycardia	IV/IO: 0.01 mg/kg (1:10 000) = *0.1 ml/kg of 1:10,000* ET: 0.1 mg/kg (1:1000) = *0.1 ml/kg of 1:1000*	Be aware of effective dose of preservatives administered (if preservatives are present in epinephrine preparation) when high doses are used.
Epinephrine for asystolic or pulseless arrest	*First dose:* IV/IO: 0.01 mg/kg (1:10,000) = *0.1 ml/kg of 1:10,000* ET: 0.1 mg/kg (1:1000) = *0.1 ml/kg of 1:1000* Doses as high as 0.2 mg/kg may be effective. *Subsequent doses:* IV/IO/ET: 0.1 mg/kg (1:1000) = *0.1 ml/kg of 1:1000* Doses as high as 0.2 mg/kg may be effective.	Be aware of effective dose of preservative administered (if preservatives present in epinephrine preparation) when high doses are used.
Epinephrine infusion	Initial at 0.1 μg/kg/min Higher infusion dose used if asystole present.	Titrate to desired effect (0.1-1.0 μg/kg/min).
Lidocaine	1 mg/kg per dose	
Lidocaine infusion	20-50 μg/kg/min	
Sodium bicarbonate	1 mEq/kg per dose or 0.3 $\times$ kg $\times$ base deficit	Infuse slowly and only if ventilation is adequate.

From *JAMA* 268:16, October 28, 1992.

IV, Intravenous, *IO,* intraosseous, *ET,* endotracheal.

*Run these drugs in rapidly at first to clear the line and ensure drug delivery. When note clinical response (increase in heart rate, blood pressure), decrease drip rate to desired infusion rate.

Defibrillation: Energy dose = 2 J/kg. If this not effective, use 4 /kg = 2.

Dilutions: For dopamine and dobutamine: 6 $\times$ body weight (kg) = # of mg in 100 ml D$_5$W then 1 ml/hr = 1.0 μg/kg/min.

CRITICAL NEONATAL RESUSCITATION

I.   Apgar score at 1 minute of >5 indicates intrapartum asphyxia, 5 to 7, mild asphyxia, and <8 is normal. Reassess every 5 minutes until <7.
II. Figure 1-12 is an algorithm for neonatal resuscitation.
III. See Table 1-4 for medications for neonatal resuscitation.

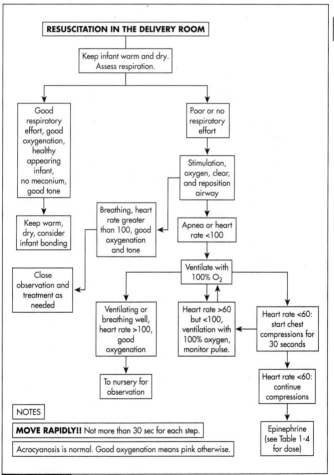

RESUSCITATION IN THE DELIVERY ROOM

Keep infant warm and dry. Assess respiration.

Good respiratory effort, good oxygenation, healthy appearing infant, no meconium, good tone

Poor or no respiratory effort

Stimulation, oxygen, clear, and reposition airway

Keep warm, dry, consider infant bonding

Breathing, heart rate greater than 100, good oxygenation and tone

Apnea or heart rate <100

Close observation and treatment as needed

Ventilate with 100% O$_2$

Ventilating or breathing well, heart rate >100, good oxygenation

Heart rate >60 but <100, ventilation with 100% oxygen, monitor pulse.

Heart rate <60: start chest compressions for 30 seconds

To nursery for observation

Heart rate <60: continue compressions

NOTES

MOVE RAPIDLY!! Not more than 30 sec for each step.

Acrocyanosis is normal. Good oxygenation means pink otherwise.

Epinephrine (see Table 1-4 for dose)

FIGURE 1-12

RESUSCITATION, AIRWAY MANAGEMENT, AND ACUTE ARRHYTHMIAS

1

TABLE 1-4
MEDICATIONS FOR NEONATAL RESUSCITATION

Medication	Concentration to Administer	Preparation	Dosage/Route		Total Dose/infant		Rate/Precautions
				Weight	**Total ml**		
Epinephrine	1:10 000	1 ml	0.1-0.3 ml/kg IV or ET	1 kg	0.1-0.3 ml		Give rapidly
				2 kg	0.2-0.6 ml		May dilute with normal saline to 1-2 ml if giving ET
				3 kg	0.3-0.9 ml		
				4 kg	0.4-1.2 ml		
				Weight	**Total ml**		
Volume expanders	Whole blood 5% Albumin-saline Normal saline Lactated Ringer's	40 ml	10 ml/kg IV	1 kg	10 ml		Give over 5-10 minutes
				2 kg	20 ml		
				3 kg	30 ml		
				4 kg	40 ml		
				Weight	**Total dose**	**Total ml**	
Sodium bicarbonate	0.5 mEq/ml (4.2% solution)	20 ml or two 10 ml prefilled syringes	2 mEq/kg IV	1 kg	2 mEq	4 ml	Give *slowly*, over at least 2 minutes give only if infant is being effectively ventilated
				2 kg	4 mEq	8 ml	
				3 kg	6 mEq	12 ml	
				4 kg	8 mEq	16 ml	

Drug	Concentration	Volume	Dose	Weight	Total dose	Total ml	Notes
Naloxone hydrochloride	0.4 mg/ml	1 ml	0.1 mg/kg (0.25 ml/kg) IV, ET, IM, SQ	1 kg	0.1 mg	0.25 ml	Give rapidly IV, ET preferred IM, SQ acceptable
				2 kg	0.2 mg	0.50 ml	
				3 kg	0.3 mg	0.75 ml	
				4 kg	0.4 mg	1.00 ml	
	1.0 mg/m	1 ml	0.1 ml/kg (0.1 ml/kg) IV, ET, IM, SQ	1 kg	0.1 mg	0.1 ml	
				2 kg	0.2 mg	0.2 ml	
				3 kg	0.3 mg	0.3 ml	
				4 kg	0.4 mg	0.4 ml	

Drug			Dose	Weight		Total µg/min	Notes
Dopamine			Begin at 5 µg/kg/min (may increase to 20 µg/kg/min if necessary) IV	1 kg		5-20 µg/min	Give as a continuous infusion using an infusion pump
				2 kg		10-40 µg/min	Monitor heart rate and blood pressure closely
				3 kg		15-60 µg/min	Seek consultation
				4 kg		20-80 µg/min	

$$\frac{\text{Weight (kg)} \times \text{Desired dose } \mu g/kg/min}{\text{Desired fluid (ml/h)}} = \text{mg of dopamine per 100 ml of solution}$$

ET, Endotracheal; *IM*, intramuscular; *IV*, intravenous; *SQ*, subcutaneous.

RESUSCITATION, AIRWAY MANAGEMENT, AND ACUTE ARRHYTHMIAS

1

BIBLIOGRAPHY

2000 Handbook of Emergency Cardiovascular Care for Healthcare Providers, 2000, American Heart Association.

EMERGENCY MEDICINE

Mark A. Graber

THE MANAGEMENT OF ACUTE CHEST PAIN IN THE EMERGENCY DEPARTMENT SETTING

I. Approach To Acute Chest Pain

A. See Table 2-1 for a partial differential diagnosis of chest pain.

B. **Obtain** an ECG, CXR, CBC, cardiac enzymes (e.g., CPK, CPK-MB troponin T or I or myoglobin depending on your institutional standard), and electrolytes as indicated. A systemic cause for angina (e.g., increased metabolic demand) may be found such as anemia or pneumonia. Do not withhold treatment until laboratory results are available. If anemic, consider transfusions as necessary.

C. **The character of the pain may help you decide if the patient has cardiac disease but cannot absolutely rule out cardiac disease (Box 2-1).** Age, smoking, family history of cardiac disease, diabetes, and hypertension are poor predictors of who has cardiac disease and should not influence your decision making. They may change prior probability, but even "low-risk" patients may have cardiac disease.

D. Administer oxygen to all patients with suspected angina.

II. **For Cardiac Pain**

A. **Nitrates,** either SL nitroglycerin 0.4 mg or IV nitroglycerin 10 to 300 μg/min, should be administered. Start IV NTG at 20μg/min and increase by 20 μg/min every 5 minutes until pain is relieved or the blood pressure begins to be unacceptably low. Occasionally a patient will get hypotensive after the SL administration of NTG so prior establishment of an IV dose is prudent though not mandatory. Hypotension related to nitrate use will respond to fluids and is self-limited. This is not a contraindication to the judicial use of IV NTG. Prolonged or severe hypotension related to the use of nitrates should be suggestive of a right ventricular infarction, which is often associated with an inferior wall MI and can be diagnosed by the use of right chest leads (see Chapter 3). Other processes that affect right ventricular function (e.g., pulmonary embolism, pericardial tamponade) can also cause nitrate-related hypotension. Tolerance to nitrates may develop within 24 hours.

B. **Aspirin** 325 mg (nonenteric coated) should be administered to any patient with possible angina who does not have a contraindication such as active bleeding.

C. **Morphine** given in 2 to 4 mg aliquots IV can be helpful in relieving chest pain and cardiac ischemia. The total dose should usually not exceed 12 to 14 mg.

D. **Heparin** is helpful in the patient with unstable angina and can be used in addition to aspirin in the patient without contraindications. Weight based dosing is preferred for heparin. Start with a bolus of 80 U/kg followed by a drip of 18 U/kg/hr. Enoxaparin (1mg/kg SQ Q12h) and other

2

TABLE 2-1

PARTIAL DIFFERENTIAL DIAGNOSIS OF ACUTE CHEST PAIN

Diagnosis	Cardinal Symptoms	Diagnosed By	Treated By	Commonly Mistaken For	Pitfalls and Comments
AMI	Substantial pressure with radiation to arms, neck, jaw, dyspnea, diaphoresis; occurs with exertion	History and ECG may show evidence of ischemia but may be normal in up to 50% with AMI	See text	Multiple illnesses, including gastric pain, musculoskeletal pain, etc	Pain may be of any type;. sharp or burning pain does not exclude cardiac ischemia (Box 2-1) Diabetics and elderly often have atypical presentation with only dyspnea or epigastric pain. May have right-sided chest pain, etc
Anxiety and hyperventilation	May feel chest pain, shortness of breath, feeling as though will die May have associated circumoral and acral paresthesias	Diagnosis of exclusion Generally have increased stress, history of similar episodes	Reassurance, diazepam IV	Cardiac disease	May have syncope secondary to CNS vasospasm May be associated carpal and pedal spasms
Esophageal spasm	May mimic MI or angina May respond to nitrates or calcium-channel blockers	Barium swallow or manometry	See Chapter 5	Cardiac disease	Need to rule out cardiac causes, since can mimic well

Condition	Symptoms/Signs	Diagnosis	Treatment	Comments
Gastritis/esophagitis	Burning chest pain	Endoscopy, upper GI, clinically	See text	May be relieved by "GI cocktail" (e.g., Maalox 30 ml, lidocaine 2% 15 ml) but not diagnostic, since some of those with cardiac disease will also have pain relief
Musculoskeletal including costochondritis, muscle strain, intercostal strain, rib fracture	Usually tender over specific point that reproduces pain; May be history of injury; may be respirophasic (pleuritic in nature)	History, physical exam Pain may be increased on motion		Presence of musculoskeletal disease does not rule out other causes of chest pain; 15% of those with AMI will have chest wall tenderness. Cardiac disease and vice versa
Pericarditis	Pleuritic, radiates to shoulder, worse when lying down, better sitting up May have a rub	ECG shows diffuse ST elevation, but 20% are false negative	See Chapter 3	May be viral, associated with renal failure, TB, or may be carcinomatous from breast or lung cancer
Pleurisy	Respirophasic (pleuritic) chest pain generally sharp in nature	Diagnosis of exclusion	Anti-inflammatory such as indomethacin	May be viral or associated with pulmonary embolism, pericarditis, pneumonia, etc. Must rule out "serious" cause
Pneumonia	Generally have associated cough, fever	CXR, CBC, clinical picture	Antibiotics (see Chapter 4)	May have associated abdominal pain, nausea, vomiting

AMI, Angina-Myocardial Infarction; PE, pulmonary embolism.

Continued

2

EMERGENCY MEDICINE

TABLE 2-1

PARTIAL DIFFERENTIAL DIAGNOSIS OF ACUTE CHEST PAIN—cont'd

Diagnosis	Cardinal Symptoms	Diagnosed By	Treated By	Commonly Mistaken For	Pitfalls and Comments
Pulmonary embolism	Sudden onset, respirophasic (pleuritic in nature), dyspnea (see Chapter 4)	Tachycardia, hypoxia, tachypnea May have normal O₂, however Need V/Q scan, angiogram, or spiral CT	See Chapter 4		Keep high clinical suspicion, since any symptom or sign may be absent (see Chapter 4)
Spontaneous pneumo-mediastinum	Sudden onset, severe pleuritic pain	CXR	Observation		May be with Valsalva maneuver, especially with smoking crack, marijuana from bong
Spontaneous pneumothorax	Sudden-onset severe pain (pleuritic in nature), dyspnea	CXR (expiratory)	Chest tube (see text) Oxygen may hasten resolution	Pulmonary embolism, substernal catch, pneumonia, PE	May be spontaneous to bleb rupture or secondary to trauma
Thoracic aortic aneurysm	Sudden-onset tearing pain radiating to back, arms, jaw, neck	Angiogram, CT, or transesophageal echocardiography	See text	MI, gastritis, esophageal spasm, etc.	May have unequal pulses and BP in upper extremities, but this may be absent

AMI, Angina-Myocardial Infarction; *PE,* pulmonary embolism.

> **BOX 2-1**
>
> **CHARACTERISTICS OF CHEST PAIN AND PROBABILITY OF CARDIAC DISEASE**
>
> Chest pain radiation to left: LR: 2
>
> Chest pain radiation to right: LR 3
>
> Chest pain radiation to both: LR 7
>
> Pressure, squeezing, aching: LR <2
>
> Pleuritic, sharp, stabbing, positional, reproducible pain on palpation: LR 0.2-0.4
>
> Normal ECG: LR 0.1-0.3
>
> Hypotension: LR 3
>
> Chest pain (squeezing, pressure): LR 1 (does not help differentiate cardiac from noncardiac disease)
>
> *LR,* Likelihood ratio.

   low molecular weight heparins may be marginally superior to standard heparin in this setting but long term data are not yet available. (See Chapter 6 for anticoagulation guidelines.)

E. **Beta-blockers, such as metoprolol** 15 mg IV in 5 mg aliquots every 5 minutes, can be helpful in patients without failure and a hyperdynamic state. Contraindications include heart block, COPD, bradycardia, and hypotension among others.

F. **Calcium-channel blockers.** Diltiazem: Recent evidence indicates that IV diltiazem 25 mg over 2 minutes followed by a drip at 5 mg/hr may be useful for refractory angina; this is not standard of care, however. IV diltiazem should be used cautiously in combination with IV beta-blockers. May cause AV conduction disturbances.

G. **Thrombolytics** may be indicated in the event of an MI. See section on myocardial infarction, in Chapter 3 for management details.

H. **Patients should be admitted for unstable angina as well as for r/o or actual MI.** The decision should be based on the history and a clinical gestalt, since the initial ECG may not reflect an AMI in 50% of those with an acute MI. Enzymes are also not helpful in deciding who to admit, since the CPK and troponin-T may not be elevated for up to 6 hours after an infarction. (CPK is more sensitive than troponin at 4-8 hours (84% vs 74%) and at 8-12 hours (94% vs. 88%). Troponin essentially 100% at 12 hours while the CPK sensitivity falls off.

SEIZURES

I. Febrile Seizures

A. Salient features.
   1. Generalized, nonfocal seizure with an autosomal dominant transmission. Patients are usually 6 months to 5 years of age.
   2. **Always self-limited,** generally after 4 to 5 minutes but may last up to 15 minutes.
   3. **Little postictal phase** with prompt return of baseline mental status. If postictal, drowsy, or more than one seizure, see "grand mal" below.

4. **2% to 5% will develop a chronic seizure disorder.** 48% under 15 months of age will have a recurrent febrile seizure in the future as will 30% of those over 15 months, and 45% of those with a first-degree relative with history of febrile seizures.
5. The American Academy of Pediatrics recommends against routine CT scanning, blood work, or EEG of patients with febrile seizures. Consider an LP for children under 18 months of age, and perform LP on those less than 12 months of age.
6. **Admission and work-up (CT/MRI or EEG) are indicated** if there are focal signs or altered mental status since by definition these patients do not have simple febrile seizures. A metabolic workup and workup for meningitis should be done if appropriate. Finger-stick glucose should be done unless the patient is clinically normal.

B. **Therapy.**
1. **No specific therapy for seizure** (but see grand mal below if seizure is protracted); treat underlying cause of fever. Always evaluate patient clinically for meningitis, or other bacterial infection. It is not necessary to do a lumbar puncture in simple febrile seizures unless otherwise indicated.
2. The American Academy of Pediatrics does not recommend seizure prophylaxis for patients with one or more febrile seizures.
3. **Long-term treatment.** Chronic phenobarbital therapy prevents recurrence but may adversely affect learning. Valproic acid is as effective as phenobarbital with less behavioral effects (but with other drawbacks such as liver toxicity, etc.). Neither carbamazepine nor phenytoin are effective in preventing recurrent febrile seizures.
4. **Prevention.** Diazepam 0.33 mg/kg PO Q8h starting at onset of fever and continuing for 24 hours after the fever reduced febrile seizures by 82% in those treated (intention to treat analysis equaled decrease of 44%). Oral diazepam may also be used. Acetaminophen and ibuprofen at the onset of a fever do not prevent febrile seizures.

II. **Grand Mal Seizures and Status Epilepticus**
A. **Salient features.**
1. **Prolonged** >15 minutes (if still seizing by time reach emergency department, by definition the patient has a grand mal seizure if transport time is included).
2. **May have focal signs or symptoms** and a prolonged postictal state.
3. May have the presence of a fever, but this is not a simple febrile seizure.

B. **Etiology.**
1. **Metabolic.** Check electrolytes, glucose, Ca^{++}, Mg^{++}, CBC.
2. **Toxins.** Look for pinpoint pupils, dilated pupils, excess salivation, etc. (See section on overdosage and toxidromes). Get drug (prescription and illegal usage) history from family or drug screen.
3. **Hypoxia.** Check respiratory status.
4. **Infection.** If clinically indicated, perform LP.

a. Do CT to rule out mass lesion (abscess) before doing LP in those with HIV (because of risk of toxoplasmosis) and those with localizing signs/symptoms **but do not withhold antibiotics to do a CT.**

5. **Space-occupying lesions** (e.g., subdural hematoma, subarachnoid bleed, tumor). Evaluate with non-contrast CT.

6. **Poor compliance with medications.**

C. **Target the work-up as indicated by history.** It is not necessary to repeat all labs on a patient with a known seizure disorder with a simple exacerbation caused by poor compliance. Watch for a change in type or frequency of seizure to guide your work-up. Drug levels are indicated in any patient using antiepileptics, theophylline, or other seizure-inducing agent.

D. **Treatment.** Because of the short half-life of benzodiazepines, patients will usually need a longer acting agent (e.g., phenytoin or phenobarbital) once the initial seizure resolves. Make sure to get levels in those already taking drugs.

1. **Be prepared to manage the airway:** Seizures may cause hypoxia and treatment (benzodiazepines, phenobarbital) may cause apnea.

2. Correct the underlying metabolic problem if one is present.

STEP 1 MEDICATIONS FOR TREATING ONGOING SEIZURES

3. **Treatment of choice.** Lorazepam (Ativan): Adults: 0.03 to 0.05 mg/kg IV (2 to 4 mg, 1-2 mg aliquots. Children: 0.05-0.1mg/kg IV maximum 4 mg) or double this rectally if IV access not possible.
   - Advantage over diazepam is longer clinical half-life (hours of seizure suppression versus minutes) with less respiratory depression and need for intubation.

4. Alternative is **diazepam** (Valium) 0.1 to 0.3 mg/kg IV (5 to 10 mg in adult but may need 20 to 30 mg) or double this rectally if no IV access. If above does not work, try the medications below.

STEP 2 MEDICATIONS FOR TREATING ONGOING SEIZURES

5. **Phenobarbital** 15-20 mg/kg IV (maximum 25-30mg/kg) at 25 to 50 mg/min. May give IM.
   - Respiratory depression is additive to that of benzodiazepines so patient may need intubation.

6. **Phenytoin** (Dilantin) 15 mg/kg IV (1 mg/kg/min IV not to exceed 50 mg/min). Do not exceed 1 g in adults; mix with NS (50 ml/500 mg in adults); use in-line filter.
   a. Monitor for QT prolongation and stop infusion if increases by >50% (risk of torsades de pointes).
   b. An alternative to phenytoin is fosphenytoin (Cerebryx), a pro-drug that requires metabolism to the active form. There is little advantage to fosphenytoin; cardiotoxicity, local irritation, and so on are comparable. However, fosphenytoin is absorbed IM and can be administered rapidly. Fosphenytoin should be infused at ≥100 to 150 mg/min; subtherapeutic levels may occur if infused slowly. Therapeutic blood levels occur in 30 minutes if drug is rapidly in-

fused. Dosing is the same as for phenytoin. The fosphenytoin dose is expressed as the phenytoin equivalent. Use in those with hepatic and renal disease is problematic because of their slower than normal metabolism to active drug and should be avoided.

STEP 3 MEDICATIONS FOR TREATING ONGOING SEIZURES

If above does not work (lidocaine and midazolam are not approved for these indications but are well tested):

7. **Lidocaine.** 1.5 to 2 mg/kg IV over 2 minutes and repeated in 5 minutes if necessary with a drip at 3 to 4 mg/min. Same class of drugs as phenytoin and an excellent membrane stabilizer.

8. **Midazolam** has been found to be useful in those unresponsive to full loading doses of lorazepam, phenobarbital, and phenytoin. Give midazolam bolus of 170 to 220 μg/kg followed by maximal infusion rates of 0.9 to 11 μg/kg/min. Can also give IM 0.07-0.3mg/kg. This may control seizures a bit faster but cannot titrate dose.

9. **Pyridoxine.** A very rare patient (generally children or those with an isoniazid overdose) will be pyridoxine responsive, and if no other measures work, consider pyridoxine (vitamin B_6) 100 mg IV. If suspect isoniazid overdose, give 4 g IV and then 1 g IV Q30 minutes until equal to amount INH ingested; may give IV push if patient seizing. For children with INH overdose give 40 mg/kg IV. Most vitamin B_6 responsive seizures occur in infants, but they have rarely been reported de novo in older children.

STEP 4 MEDICATIONS FOR TREATING ONGOING SEIZURES

10. Barbiturate coma. Call anesthesia department.

E. **Disposition:** Patients with a first seizure should be considered for admission, as should those with a prolonged seizure (although admission is not mandatory if patient is back to baseline). A patient with a seizure disorder who has a breakthrough seizure need not be admitted. Approximately 50% of patients with one seizure will have another within 2 years if not treated long term as will 24% of those treated. Whether or not to start anticonvulsants after a first seizure is controversial. An EEG should be performed 3 weeks after the initial seizure (it will be abnormal immediately after a seizure and therefore does not give you any information on an underlying seizure focus).

III. Neonatal Seizures

A. **May be atypical in physical presentation** because of CNS immaturity.

1. Grand mal may present with sequential clonic-tonic movements of extremities or only focal symptoms.

2. **Autonomic seizures** noted by changes in respirations, heart rate, and pupils.

3. **Myoclonic seizures.** Single clonic motions throughout day.

B. It is important to pursue a cause, since frequently there is a specific treatment available.

1. In ED, check electrolytes, calcium, glucose, magnesium, CBC, blood culture, and LP.
2. EEG, CT, skull radiograph, long bone radiograph, as indicated.
3. Bilirubin, ABG, urine amino acids as indicated.

C. **Treatment** for neonatal seizures in this order and in absence of known correctable cause.
   1. **Glucose** 2 ml/kg of D_{25}
   2. **Pyridoxine** (vitamin B6) 50-100mg IV push
   3. **Calcium gluconate** (10%)- 30 to 60 mg/kg (1-2 ml/kg of 10% solution, maximum 10ml), slow IV on monitor.
   4. **Magnesium sulfate** 50% solution, 0.2 ml/kg IM or IV
   5. **Phenobarbital.** Premature infant 10 to 20 mg/kg IM or IV; term infant 10 to 15 mg/kg IM or IV. Infuse no faster than 30 mg/min.
   6. **Phenytoin** 10 to 15 mg/kg IV. Infuse no faster than 1 mg/kg/min.
   7. **Lorazepam** 0.05 to 0.15 mg/kg IV.
   8. **Diazepam** 0.2 mg/kg repeat twice. Maximum dose 5 mg age <5 years, 10 mg if age :10 years.
      • Diazepam and lorazepam will increase hyperbilirubinemia by uncoupling albumin-bilirubin complex. Therefore be careful in children with jaundice.

ASTHMA/COPD/DYSPNEA (SEE ALSO CHAPTER 4)

I. **Causes of Dyspnea** (See appropriate chapters for in-depth discussions.)
A. **Upper airway disease/obstruction/foreign body aspiration.** As a general rule: Inspiratory stridor is above the cords, inspiratory and expiratory stridor is in the trachea, wheezing is below the trachea.
   1. **Aspiration:** Usually triphasic history—1/3 are not witnessed or not remembered by caregiver. Initial cough, choking, gagging; FB then passes in to smaller airways and have silent phase. Finally, recurrent pneumonia, wheezing
      a. Can take x-ray of lung with wheezing side down (trapped air will not leave), have mediastinal shift away from affected lung on expiration and affected lung will not deflate.
      b. Diagnosis only made 60% of time preoperatively so think of it and proceed to elective bronchoscopy (rarely an emergent procedure).
      c. Think of epiglottitis (in adults as well), croup, retropharyngeal abscess, angioedema. See the section on stridor in Chapter 12.
   2. **Pneumothorax** (see chest trauma section).
   3. **CHF, "cardiac asthma."** Look for basilar rales, peripheral edema, JVD, frothy sputum (see Chapter 3).
   4. **Pulmonary embolism** (see Chapter 4).
   5. **Pneumonia.** Fever, chills, purulent sputum, infiltrate or localized rales (see Chapter 4).
   6. **COPD.** Generally have prior history (see Chapter 4).

2

EMERGENCY MEDICINE

    7. **Central hyperventilation and metabolic acidosis.** Lungs clear, ABG reflects metabolic acidosis or primary respiratory alkalosis. (See Chapter 6 for a discussion of acid-base disturbance.)

    8. **Anemia** (see Chapter 6).

    9. **Wegener's and other connective tissue disorders** (see Chapter 4).

  10. **Hypersensitivity pneumonitis** (see Chapter 4).

II. Acute Asthma

A. Diagnose by history and physical examination.

    1. **History:** Important elements of the history are onset; trigger of current exacerbation; severity of symptoms, including limitation of exercise tolerance, interference with sleep, medications, prior hospitalizations and ED visits; severe exacerbations in past requiring ICU admissions or intubation; any other chronic medical conditions.

    2. **Physical examination.**

       a. **Document severity** of respiratory compromise: speech difficulty, use of accessory muscles of respiration, inability to lie supine, pulsus paradoxus (>12 mm Hg fall in systolic BP during inspiration see section on cardiac tamponade for procedure to determine pulsus paradoxus), tachycardia, tachypnea, cyanosis, level of alertness, air movement, wheezing.

       b. Complications of severe asthma include pneumothorax, pneumomediastinum.

       c. **Wheezing can be an unreliable guide** to the degree of obstruction; severe obstruction may be associated with a "silent chest" because of little or no air movement.

       d. **Beware if patient seems too calm.** This may represent CO_2 retention and narcosis.

       e. **Functional assessment.** Monitor peak flow (see Table 23-9 for normals) or FEV_1. Check pulse oximetry. Infants become hypoxemic earlier than adults, and physical assessment of respiratory status in children is less reliable. Check O_2 saturations on all infants and children by pulse oximetry. Room air saturation should be >95%. A room air saturation <93% in infants usually is predictive of the need for hospitalization. Check an arterial or capillary blood gas level on infants with O_2 saturation <90% or as needed.

B. **Lab tests. Do not withhold oxygen or delay treatment waiting for lab tests and radiographs.** After initial stabilization, consider the following:

    1. CBC if patient has fever or purulent sputum.

    2. CXR if suspect complication such as pneumonia or pneumothorax (no need for CXR in routine asthma exacerbations).

    3. Serum theophylline concentration in all patients taking theophylline.

    4. ABG in patients with severe distress, poor response to treatment, or abnormal pulse oximetry.

C. **High-risk patients.** Those at high risk of asthma-related death or life-threatening deterioration include those with:
  1. **Prior intubation for asthma** or prior ICU admission, two or more hospitalizations for asthma in past year, three or more ED visits in past year, hospitalization or ED visit in past month.
  2. **Using or withdrawing from systemic corticosteroids,** history of syncope or seizure related to hypoxia from asthma, poor social situation or psychiatric disease.
  3. **Infant** <1 year old.
  4. **<10% improvement** in PEFR or FEV_1 in ED; PEFR or FEV_1 <25% predicted.
  5. **PCO_2 40 mm Hg or more.** A normal PCO_2 is abnormal in the setting of asthma exacerbations where the patient should be hyperventilating, resulting in a low PCO_2. A normal PCO_2 may herald impending respiratory failure.
D. Treatment for asthma or COPD.
  1. **Oxygen may be needed to support patient and should not be withheld even to do an** ABG.
  2. Hydration is without benefit if the patient is euvolemic, and aggressive IV hydration may precipitate CHF.
  3. If severe asthma, consider cardiac monitoring.
  4. **Beta-agonists are the mainstay of treatment. Albuterol is generally more effective in asthma while ipratropium is generally more effective in COPD.**
    a. **Albuterol.** 2.5 mg in 3 ml of NS by nebulizer (adults). May give up to 4 treatments per hour. Some studies suggest that continuously nebulized albuterol works better. IV albuterol has been used but has little advantage over inhaled.
      (1) **In children,** can use **albuterol** 0.15 to 0.3 mg/kg by nebulizer every hour (ideally divided every 20 minutes or given continuously over 1 hour). The 0.3 mg/kg dosing is significantly better in moderate to severe asthma. Can use nebulized albuterol continuously if needed in children as well.
      (2) Tachycardia does not increase further after first several doses and since tachycardia is usually hypoxia driven, the pulse rate may drop with treatment.
      (3) May cause hypokalemia by shifting K+ intracellularly.
      (4) Metered-dose inhaler by means of a spacer is just as good as nebulizer if you give about 6 to 8 activations by a spacer, which is equal to one nebulized treatment.
    b. **Epinephrine-** 1:1000, 0.01mg/kg SQ, maximum 0.3-0.4mg can **be used in** those too sick to use a nebulizer (use 0.1cc/10kg). **For those facing intubation, IV epinephrine may be used (but reserve for these severe patients!).** The dose is 2 to 10 ml of a **1:10,000** solution (0.1ml/kg of a **1:10,000** solution, maximum 1mg) ad-

ministered over 5 minutes. This can be repeated with an infusion at 1 to 20 mg/min if there is improvement.

5. **Steroids.**
   a. Reduces return visits, admission rates. More effective in asthma than in COPD but do help in acute COPD exacerbations.
   b. Should be used in most patients: always in those already receiving steroids and in most of those who fail to clear after one nebulizer treatment.
   c. **Methylprednisolone.** For adults 125 mg IV and 40 mg IV Q6h. For children 1 to 2 mg/kg IV followed by 2 mg/kg/24 hours divided into Q6h doses.
   d. **Prednisone.** For adults 60 mg PO. For children 0.5 to 2.0 mg/kg Q24h for 3 to 7 days.
      (1) All evidence indicates that steroids given orally are just as effective as IV in acute exacerbations of asthma.
      (2) There is no need for a steroid taper in those not previously receiving steroids **if** only for a 5- to 7-day course. There is no increase in relapse without taper and no adrenal suppression with a 1-week course.
      (3) Dose of steroids varies depending on author.

6. **Anticholinergics** work better in COPD than asthma but do have some bronchodilating effect and are effective in the most severe asthmatics. They will not add anything to beta-agonists in those with mild or moderate disease, however. Both can be mixed in the same nebulizer with albuterol.
   a. **Ipratropium** can be used by metered-dose inhaler or nebulizer. The dose is 0.5 mg by nebulizer and can be given twice in the first hour of therapy. This is preferred over atropine, since there is little systemic effect.
   b. If ipratropium not available: **Atropine** 0.4 to 2 mg (adult 0.025 mg/kg) **by nebulizer.** May increase heart rate and cause pupils to dilate from contact with mist.

7. **Theophylline-aminophylline.** There no evidence that adding theophylline-aminophylline to maximized beta-adrenergic therapy is helpful in the treatment of acute asthma. **It is arrhythmogenic and has as a very low therapeutic index; always check a drug level if you feel compelled to use this drug.**
   a. Although frequent, optimal doses of beta agonists are more effective, if you choose to use aminophylline, use a 6 mg/kg loading dose to maximum of 350 mg over 30 to 45 minutes followed by a drip at 0.6 mg/kg/hr not to exceed 50 to 60 mg/hr. Levels should be checked. Maintenance dose dependent on patient's smoking status, presence of cor pulmonale, and age.

8. **Magnesium sulfate** may produce transient improvement in asthma for 60-90 minutes.
   a. Reasonable if patient has failed conventional therapy; less toxic than theophylline.

b. Dose: In adults 2 g IV over 15 to 20 minutes (may mix in 50 ml of normal saline). Very safe but do not use in renal failure. May get flushing, transient hypotension but rare.

c. Magnesium sulfate has been successfully used in children. The dose is 25 mg/kg.

9. **Heliox** (helium/oxygen mixture) may help in the severe patient. Intubation and nasal CPAP (continuous positive-pressure ventilation) are a last resort and may not work well in the asthmatic patient.

E. **Disposition.** Admit if persistent respiratory distress, O_2 saturation <94% after treatment (children), peak expiratory flow of <60% of predicated value in children or failure to increase by 15% above baseline or absolute value of 200 L/min in adults, failure of FEV_1 to increase by 500 cc or produce a total of <1.6 L (adults), hypercapnia (retaining CO_2 over baseline value), or pneumothorax. Additionally, clinical judgment is important. If the patient does not look well or still feels dyspneic, consider admission to hospital.

COMA

I. **What To Do First In Coma**

A. **ABCs** including cervical spine immobilization if **any** possibility of trauma.
   1. If patient has hypertension with associated bradycardia, consider increased intracranial pressure.
   2. Intubate to protect airway if no gag reflex or if otherwise indicated.

B. **Check finger-stick glucose** (if available) and rapidly administer:
   1. **Thiamine** 100 mg IV prevents Wernicke-Korsakoff encephalopathy.
      a. Do not withhold glucose if thiamine not available. A single dose of glucose will not induce Wernicke-Korsakoff encephalopathy.
   2. **Glucose** 25 to 50 g IV treats hypoglycemia.
   3. **Naloxone** 2 to 4 ampules of 0.4 mg treats narcotic overdose.
      a. Some will start with 2 mg and then 4 mg if no response.
      b. Make sure to restrain the patient if suspect will precipitate narcotic withdrawal.
   4. If suspect benzodiazepine overdose (diazepam, alprazolam, and others).
      • **Flumazenil** (Romazicon) 0.2 mg up to 5 mg IV. **Do not** use flumazenil if suspect **any other overdose,** concurrent tricyclic overdose or chronic benzodiazepine use. **It may precipitate status epilepticus and is contraindicated! This should not be routinely administered to the unconscious patient unless there is a clear indication and no contraindication. Intubation and supportive care is generally preferred for benzodiazepine overdose.**

II. **Differential Diagnosis of Coma**

A. **Coma with no localizing CNS signs** can be caused by the following:
   1. **Metabolic insults** including hypoglycemia, uremia, nonketotic hyperosmolar coma, Addison disease, diabetic ketoacidosis, hypothyroidism, hepatic coma, etc.
      • Children and young adults will often get hypoglycemic and may present with coma after alcohol ingestion including mouthwash.

2. **Respiratory** including hypoxia, hypercapnia.
3. **Intoxication** including barbiturates, alcohol, opiates, carbon monoxide poisoning and benzodiazepines.
4. **Infections** (severe systemic) including sepsis, pneumonia, typhoid fever.
5. **Shock** including hypovolemic, cardiogenic, septic, and anaphylactic.
6. **Epilepsy** including atonic seizures (no obvious abnormal motor activity).
7. **Hypertensive encephalopathy.**
8. **Environmental:** Hyperthermia (heat stroke), hypothermia.

B. **Coma with meningeal irritation without localizing signs** can be caused by meningitis, subarachnoid hemorrhage from ruptured aneurysm, AV malformation.

C. If focal brainstem or lateralizing signs, consider pontine hemorrhage, CVA, brain abscess, subdural-epidural hemorrhage.

D. **If patient appears awake but is unresponsive:**
   1. **Abulic state.** Frontal lobe function is depressed and so may take several minutes for the patient to answer a question.
   2. **Locked-in syndrome.** Destruction of pontine motor tracts. Upward gaze is preserved.
   3. **Psychogenic state.** Consider psychiatric disease

III. **Pathophysiology of Coma**

A. Coma can be caused only by:
   1. Bilateral cortical disease.
   2. Reticular activating system compromise.

IV. **To Differentiate Between Cortical and Brainstem Lesions**

A. **Use calorics**—ice water in each ear. Nystagmus refers to the fast return phase. **Four possible responses:**
   1. Both eyes deviate toward side cold water instilled and have good nystagmus (e.g., eyes return to center). Patient not comatose.
   2. Both eyes deviate toward cold water; no fast return phase. Brainstem function intact. Coma is caused by bilateral cortical problem.
   3. No eye movement despite cold stimuli to both sides. No brainstem function (same as absent oculocephalic reflex, or "doll's eyes").
      • Not necessarily a permanent lesion; may be caused by severe hypothermia or drug overdose.
   4. Movement of only one eye ipsilateral to stimulus indicates an intranuclear lesion, which almost always indicates brainstem damage and demands rapid evaluation to determine if a correctable lesion is present.

B. **Pupils.**
   1. Generally resistant to metabolic insult.
   2. Remember that a dilated eye may be secondary to topical or systemic drugs.
   3. A dilated pupil in an alert person is not secondary to impending herniation; these patients are always unconscious. **However, a**

unilateral dilated pupil in an unconscious patient may herald imminent uncal herniation.
4. Propoxyphene (Darvon and others) can cause coma without pinpoint
   pupils.
5. Eyes will deviate toward side of physiologically inactive lesion (CVA)
   and away from an active lesion (seizure).
6. 5% of the normal population will have anisocoria (asymmetric
   pupils).

V. Laboratory Work-up of Coma

A. CBC, electrolytes, BUN, creatinine, glucose, calcium, magnesium, arterial blood gas, toxic screen, carboxyhemoglobin, liver enzymes, serum
ammonia, etc. as indicated by clinical presentation.

B. CT scan and LP.
   • If suspect meningitis, do not withhold antibiotics while waiting to do
     an LP. Antibiotics should be started before the patient goes to the CT
     scanner. Your culture results will not be affected.

HEAD TRAUMA

See also evaluation of coma.

I. **Glasgow Coma Scale** (Table 2-2). Useful in a general sense, but 18% of
those with a GCS score of 15 have an abnormal CT scan, and 5% of
those with a GCS score of 15 require neurosurgical intervention. The
GCS score is especially unreliable in children.

TABLE 2-2

GLASGOW COMA SCALE

Parameter	Response	Score
Eye opening	Spontaneous	4
	To voice	3
	To pain	2
Verbal response	None	1
	Oriented	5
	Confused	4
	Inappropriate	3
	Incomprehensible sounds	2
	None	1
Motor response	Obeys command	6
	Localizes pain	5
	Withdraws to pain	4
	Flexion response to pain	3
	Extension response to pain	2
	None	1

Coma score is most useful in triage and in following status. Initial score of <7 indicates a poor prognosis if a cause other than trauma cannot be found and corrected quickly. Assessment should be
done frequently and recorded accurately on a flow sheet with times documented.

II. **Classification of Head Injuries and Treatment**
A. Frequently associated with other severe trauma.
   1. **ABCs take priority.** Saving only the head will not save the patient.
   2. Hypotension in adults is never caused by an isolated head injury except near death. Look for other injuries including cord injuries.
   3. Physical exam includes complete neurologic exam as well as inspection for evidence of basilar skull fracture (CSF rhinorrhea, Battle's sign, raccoon eyes, hemotympanum), etc.

B. **Low-risk injuries.**
   1. **Criteria.**
     a. Minor trauma, scalp wounds.
     b. No signs of intracranial injury, no loss of consciousness or loss of consciousness for less than 1 minute, no amnesia. May have up to 3 episodes of vomiting, GCS 15.
     c. Patient has returned to baseline functioning.
   2. **Treatment.** Observation for any sign or symptom of brain injury. CT optional. Obtain at your discretion but especially for those who are intoxicated, have a significant mechanism of injury, children, etc. (it never hurts to err on the side of caution)!! Must discharge to a reliable observer who will continue observation at home.

C. **Moderate-risk injuries.**
   1. **Criteria.**
     a. Symptoms consistent with intracranial injury including protracted vomiting (>3 episodes), LOC for >1 minute, severe headache, post-traumatic seizures, amnesia, evidence of basilar skull fracture (CSF rhinorrhea, Battle's sign, raccoon eyes, hemotympanum).
     b. **Nonfocal neurologic exam.**
   2. **Treatment.** Observation and "neuro checks," obtain CT.
   3. **Admit** for observation and monitoring.

D. **High-risk injuries.**
   1. Criteria. Depressed level of consciousness, focal neurologic signs, penetrating injury of skull or palpable depressed skull fractures.
   2. **Approach.** Immediate CT, neurosurgical consultation.
   3. **Support and treatment of increased intracranial pressure** while awaiting definitive neurosurgical care: There is little evidence to support most of these measures but they are still standard of care.
     a. **Intubation.** Pretreatment with lidocaine 1 mg/kg IV may prevent rise in intracranial pressure (ICP). See also section on RSI in Chapter 1 and resuscitation.
     b. **Hyperventilation** to maintain PO_2 >90 torrs, PCO_2 25 to 30 torrs.
       (1) PEEP relatively contraindicated because reduces cerebral blood flow.
       (2) Avoid tight cervical collars. Any pressure on the external jugular veins will increase the ICP.
       (3) **Hyperventilation may actually increase ischemia in at risk brain tissue if PCO2 <25 torr by causing excessive vasocon-**

striction and is falling out of favor. Prophylactic hyperventilation for those without increased ICP is contraindicated and worsens outcomes.

   c. **Maintain normal cardiac output.**
     (1) If hypotensive from other cause such as multi-trauma, treat shock as usual. Normal saline is preferred over LR since LR is slightly hypotonic. Hypertonic saline (3% or 7.5%; see section on shock, below) can be used but there is no clear evidence that it improves neurologic outcome.
     (2) If markedly hypertensive, consider labetalol or nitroprusside. Vasodilator, such as nitroprusside, increases cerebral blood flow and ICP (see section on hypertensive emergencies for dosing). **Avoid lowering the blood pressure unless diastolic blood pressure is >120 mm Hg.**
   d. **Mannitol 1 g/kg** IV over 20 minutes induces osmotic diuresis. (Controversial if patient not herniating. Consult your neurosurgeon.) Avoid if hypotensive or have CHF/renal failure.
   e. Some suggest **furosemide** (Lasix and others) 20 mg IV. Avoid if hypotensive.
   f. **Elevate head of bed 30 degrees** (if not hypotensive).
   g. **Steroids** are ineffective in controlling ICP in the trauma setting.
   h. **Seizure prophylaxis:** Phenytoin will reduce seizures in the first week after injury but does not change the overall outcome.

E. **Skull radiographs.**
  1. Generally not indicated in adults unless one suspects depressed fracture and cannot palpate skull because of hematoma, etc. Can have intracranial injury without a skull fracture and vice versa. If suspect head trauma with skull fracture, a head CT with bone windows is the preferred imaging study.
  2. Plain radiographs may be useful in those up to 7 years of age because a skull fracture can lead to nonunion because of rapid head growth and for documentation of abuse. Use clinical judgment as to severity of injury.

III. **Concussion:** Box 2-2 contains a summary of recommendations for returning to normal activities after concussion.

IV. **Post-concussive syndrome.**

A. **May occur with minor trauma and is characterized by** headache, depression, memory difficulty, attention deficit, personality changes, vertigo and light-headedness and a negative CT (may represent disruption of axonal support structures, axonal stretching).

B. Patients may have abnormal findings on formal neuropsychologic testing. 15% still have symptoms at 1 year even after minor brain injury.

C. Treat headache with nonnarcotic analgesics (e.g., NSAIDS) and depression as per Chapter 19.

2

EMERGENCY MEDICINE

BOX 2-2

RETURNING TO NORMAL ACTIVITIES AFTER CONCUSSION

SUMMARY OF RECOMMENDATIONS FOR MANAGEMENT OF CONCUSSION IN SPORTS

A concussion is defined as head-trauma–induced alteration in mental status that may or may not involve loss of consciousness. Concussions are graded in three categories. Definitions and treatment recommendations for each category are presented below.

GRADE 1 CONCUSSION

- Definition: Transient confusion, no loss of consciousness, and a duration of mental status abnormalities of <15 minutes.
- Management: The athlete should be removed from sports activity, examined immediately and at 5-minute intervals, and allowed to return that day to the sports activity only if post-concussive symptoms resolve within 15 minutes. Any athlete who incurs a second Grade 1 concussion on the same day should be removed from sports activity until asymptomatic for 1 week.

GRADE 2 CONCUSSION

- Definition: Transient confusion, no loss of consciousness, and a duration of mental status abnormalities of >15 minutes.
- Management: The athlete should be removed from sports activity and examined frequently to assess the evolution of symptoms, with more extensive diagnostic evaluation if the symptoms worsen or persist for >1 week. The athlete should return to sports activity only after asymptomatic for 1 full week. Any athlete who incurs a grade 2 concussion subsequent to a grade 1 concussion on the same day should be removed from sports activity until asymptomatic for 2 weeks.

GRADE 3 CONCUSSION

- Definition: Loss of consciousness, either brief (seconds) or prolonged (minutes or longer).
- Management: The athlete should be removed from sports activity for 1 full week without symptoms if the loss of consciousness is brief or 2 full weeks without symptoms if the loss of consciousness is prolonged. If still unconscious or if abnormal neurologic signs are present at the time of initial evaluation, the athlete should be transported by ambulance to the nearest hospital emergency department. An athlete who suffers a second Grade 3 concussion should be removed from sports activity until asymptomatic for 1 month. Any athlete with an abnormality on computed tomography or magnetic resonance imaging brain scan consistent with brain swelling, contusion, or other intracranial pathology should be removed from sports activities for the season and discouraged from future return to participation in contact sports.

From *MMWR* 46:10, March 14, 1997.

TRAUMA
MULTIPLE TRAUMA AND GENERAL PRINCIPLES
I. Stabilization and Primary Survey

Remember ABCDE:

Airway

Breathing

Circulation

Drugs/Disability/Allergies

Eating/Exposure

Keep patient warm! Hypothermia contributes to mortality.

A. **Airway.** If depressed level of consciousness or upper airway bleeding, intubate **without moving neck.**
   1. Intubation is safe even with neck fracture, but avoid Sellick maneuver.
   2. Confirm placement with a radiograph, by auscultation, oxygen saturation, and with end-title CO_2 (low in esophageal intubation).
B. **Breathing.** Ventilate with 100% O_2.
   • Check breath sounds and place chest tubes as needed for hemothorax, pneumothorax, tension pneumothorax.
C. **Circulation.** For "all" multiple trauma victims:
   1. Stop obvious bleeding with pressure. **Consider the chest and abdomen to be sites of potential blood loss in the hypotensive patient.**
   2. Two large-bore peripheral IV lines (14 to 16 gauge). The short catheters allow more rapid volume replacement than longer central lines.
   3. Run NS or LR wide open if tachycardic or hypotensive. Using warmed fluids will decrease mortality and help preserve hemostatic mechanisms.
      a. As a rule of thumb, if more than 2 liters of isotonic fluid are needed in the trauma setting, the patient will need blood.
      b. Can also use 3% or 7.5% saline (250 ml over 1 to 5 minutes) if unable to infuse large volumes.
      c. **For children,** use NS 20 ml/kg IV as a bolus and repeat to a total of 60 ml/kg. Consider blood at this point if child still hypotensive from hypovolemia.
      d. There is no advantage to colloids in this setting.
      e. Not all people in shock are tachycardic and hypotension may be a late finding. This is especially true in children. Use clinical judgment.
      f. Hypotension is not caused by isolated brain injury in adults except near death.
D. **Drugs, allergies, disability.** Document functional status for a baseline examination.
E. **Eating and exposure.** Time of last meal. Uncover the patient including visualizing the back.
F. **A Foley catheter** should be inserted after ruling out GU trauma (see section on urologic trauma). Urine output is a good indication of adequate

perfusion. Try to maintain output at 30 to 60 ml/hour in adults or 0.5 to 1 ml/kg/hour in children.

II. **Laboratory and X-ray Evaluation of the Multiple Trauma Patient**

A. CBC, electrolytes, BUN, creatinine, glucose, coagulation studies, liver enzymes, amylase, lipase, urinalysis, pregnancy test, ABG. Not all patients need all tests; use clinical judgment. (CBC often indicates an anemia with acute blood loss but may not reflect the true magnitude of the problem until blood equilibrates with infused fluids, generally 15 minutes.)

B. If patient known to be hypotensive in the field, get two units of type O-negative blood ready.

C. **Radiographs.** C-spine (AP, lateral, odontoid), CXR, AP pelvis. Cervical spine films should be done in the radiology suite as long as patient is maintained in immobilization. Cross table films are frequently inadequate.

D. Remember antibiotics, tetanus prophylaxis and CT scan as indicated. Obtain a full spine series when the patient is stable.

III. **Secondary Survey to Set Further Priorities**

A. **Stabilize patient first.**

B. Complete head-to-toe examination.

C. Pass NG tube if no contraindication such as basilar skull fracture or midface trauma. Can pass oral gastric tube if midface trauma, etc.

D. Identify possible internal injuries. See specific sections below. Any head-injured, unconscious, multi-trauma patient should have the abdomen evaluated by CT, ultrasound or DPL (diagnostic peritoneal lavage) because of an inability to report pain accurately.

E. Splint bones, etc.

F. A comment on MAST (military antishock trousers, pneumatic antishock garment). They are contraindicated in penetrating cardiac trauma, cardiogenic shock, impaled objects/evisceration, and diaphragmatic injury. Head injury is **not** a contraindication. May help stem intraabdominal bleeding from the spleen and aorta. Overall benefit probably less than previously believed; MAST trousers are falling out of favor. Useful when stabilizing pelvic and femur fractures.

NECK TRAUMA

I. General

A. **Initial treatment:** Must immobilize neck **and restrain chest** to immobilize C-spine. If C-spine injury is strongly suspected and unable to restrain patient, consider paralysis (see **RSI**).

   1. Neutral position differs in adults and children: Children <8 years old may require elevation of shoulders and back to approximate a neutral position. Adults and older children may require padding under the head to approximate a neutral position. **Most important, however, is maintaining immobilization.**

   2. Prolonged immobilization (even <30 minutes) on a backboard will cause most individuals to have occipital headache and lumbar/sacral pain regardless of underlying trauma.

> ## BOX 2-3
>
> ### CRITERIA FOR RULING OUT CERVICAL SPINE FRACTURES ON A CLINICAL BASIS
>
> Patient does not complain of neck pain when asked **and**
>
> Patient does not have neck tenderness on palpation **and**
>
> Patient does not have any history of loss of consciousness **and**
>
> Patient does not have any mental status changes resulting from trauma, alcohol, drugs, etc. **and**
>
> Patient has no symptoms referable to a neck injury, such as paralysis, sensory changes (including transitory symptoms now resolved), and so on, **and**
>
> Patient has no other distracting painful injuries, such as fractured ankle, fractured ribs, and so on.

2

EMERGENCY MEDICINE

B. **Blunt injury** including falls and motor vehicle accidents: can rule out cervical spine injury on a clinical basis

II. **Clearing the Cervical Spine**

A. To clinically clear the C-spine, all of the criteria in Box 2-3 must be met. These criteria have not been adequately tested in children. All other patients require clearance of the C-spine by radiograph.

B. **X-Ray approach**

1. Need 3 views including lateral film showing all 7 cervical vertebrae and the C7-T1 interspace, a PA and an odontoid view to effectively rule out a C-spine fracture. **The most common cause of missed C-spine injuries is an inadequate C-spine series.** If radiographs are inadequate or there is a questionable fracture, CT scanning may be helpful.

2. Flexion/extension films can be done to rule out ligamentous injury in the patient with persistent neck pain once cervical spine fractures have been ruled out by radiograph. Do not force flexion or extension; let the patient control head movement

3. **Those with one spinal fracture have about a 10% chance of having another, noncontiguous, spine fracture and should have a full spine series.**

C. Parameters of normal C-spines and types of fractures (Table 2-3).

D. **Table 2-4 lists common C-spine injuries.**

III. **Cord Injuries:** in transection

A. Look for paralysis, other signs of cord injury including priapism, urinary retention, fecal incontinence, paralytic ileus, and immediate loss of all sensation and reflex activity below the level of the injury.

B. Spinal neurogenic shock leads to vasomotor instability from loss of autonomic tone and may lead to hypotension and/or temperature instability. This will respond to adrenergics.

C. May get hypoxia and hypoventilation if above C-5: **consider intubation.**

TABLE 2-3

MEASURABLE PARAMETERS OF NORMAL C-SPINE

	Adults	Children
Predental space	3 mm	4-5 mm
C2/C3 pseudosubluxation	3 mm	4-5 mm
Retropharyngeal space	<7 mm (5 mm by some sources	1/2-2/3 vertebral body distance AP
Cord dimension	10-13 mm	Adult size, age 6

Notes
- 40% of children younger than 7 years old and 20% of those 16 years old have anterior displacement of C2 on C3. 14% of children to age 8 yrs have C3/C4 subluxation.
- 60-70% of fractures in children occur in C1/C2.
- 16% of adult fractures occur at C1/C2.
- 20% of young children have increased space between dens and anterior arch of C1.

D. **Neurologic symptoms frequently occur in children without associated C-spine fractures** (spinal cord injury without radiologic abnormality [SCIWORA] syndrome). This may be responsible for up to 70% of cord injuries in children and is especially common in children under 8 years old. Presentation of the neurologic deficit may be delayed up to 4 days. MRI can demonstrate the cord injury. Those with delayed presentation and an intact cord generally recover function.
E. **Any person with a spinal cord injury (including SCIWORA) should receive methylprednisolone—30mg/kg over one hour followed by 5.4 mg/kg/hr IV over the next 23 hours. This should be started within 8 hours of the injury.**
IV. **Penetrating Neck Trauma**
A. Although management still controversial, "all" should be explored in the OR if there is penetration of the platysma.
B. Do NOT remove foreign body until patient in OR.
C. **Consider CT/angiography if foreign body close to arterial blood supply**
V. **Airway Injuries**
A. **Clinical signs** include stridor, hoarseness, dyspnea, and subcutaneous emphysema.
B. **Management:** ENT consult, **early oral intubation** if possible and indicated. Expanding hematoma may rapidly compromise the airway and make intubation progressively more difficult. **Avoid causing further trauma.**

CHEST TRAUMA
I. Types of Injury and Treatment
A. **Flail chest.** Paradoxical chest wall motion secondary to multiple fractured ribs.
   1. **Treatment** by intubation if respiration is compromised. Positive-pressure ventilation may lead to a tension pneumothorax. Prophylactic placement of a chest tube should be considered.

TABLE 2-4
COMMON C-SPINE INJURIES

Level	Name	Stable or Unstable	Mechanism/Clinical Setting	Radiologic Findings
C1	Jefferson fracture	Moderately unstable	Burst fracture. Occurs with axial load or vertebral compression	Displaced lateral aspects C1 on odontoid view. Predental space >3 mm.
	Atlantoaxial subluxation	Highly unstable	Found in Down syndrome, RA, other destructive processes	Asymmetric lateral bodies on odontoid view. Increased predental space.
C2	Odontoid fracture	Highly unstable	Mechanism poorly understood	May be difficult to see on plain film. High clinical suspicion requires CT.
	Hangman's fracture	Unstable	Occurs with sudden deceleration (hanging) and with hyperextension as in MVA	Bilateral pedicle fracture of C2 with or without anterior subluxation. Look on lateral film.
Any level	Flexion teardrop injury	Highly unstable	Sudden and forceful flexion	Large wedge off anterior aspect of effected vertebra. Ligamentous instability causes alignment abnormalities.

From Graber MA, Kathol M: *Am Fam Physician* 59(2): 331-341, 1999.

Continued

2

EMERGENCY MEDICINE

TABLE 2-4

COMMON C-SPINE INJURIES—cont'd

Level	Name	Stable or Unstable	Mechanism/Clinical Setting	Radiologic Findings
Any level—cont'd	Bilateral facet dislocations	Highly unstable	Flexion or combined flexion/rotation	Anterior displacement of 50% or more of one cervical vertebrae on lateral.
	Unilateral facet dislocations	Unstable	Flexion or combined flexion/rotation	Anterior dislocation 25%-33% of one cervical vertebrae on lateral. An abrupt transition in rotation so that lateral view of effected vertebrae rotated. Lateral displacement of spinous process on AP view.
Lower cervical or upper thoracic	Clay shoveler's fracture	Very stable	Flexion, such as picking up and throwing heavy loads (e.g., snow or clay)	Avulsion of posterior aspect of spinous process. Frequently an incidental finding.

From Graber MA, Kathol M: *Am Fam Physician* 59(2): 331-341, 1999.

B. **Tension pneumothorax.** Air under pressure in the pleural space.
  1. Decreased breath sounds, shifted heart sounds, dyspnea, trachea shift from midline, hyperresonance on percussion, distended neck veins, chest pain, hypotension.
  2. **Treatment.** Needle thoracostomy in the second intercostal space, mid-clavicular line, followed by a chest tube.
C. **Simple pneumothorax-hemothorax** from deceleration or penetrating trauma (pneumothorax may also occur spontaneously).
  1. Symptoms as above but without midline shift, may have hypotension from blood loss in hemothorax.
  2. Expiratory films are more sensitive than are a normal chest radiograph. CT scanning is more sensitive, but the clinical significance of pneumothorax-hemothorax found only on CT scan is unknown. Some suggest the placing of a chest tube if the patient has rib fractures and is going to have positive-pressure ventilation.
  3. **Treatment.** Tube thoracostomy (chest tube) (see Chapter 21).
     • If small pneumothorax (<15%), observe and administer oxygen, which will hasten resolution of pneumothorax 4-fold.
D. **Cardiac tamponade.**
  1. **Clinically:** Note hypotension, jugular venous distension, muffled heart sounds, pulsus paradoxus.
     • Pulsus paradoxus. Normally, systolic pressure drops less than 10 mm Hg on inspiration. Decide on systolic pressure when patient has exhaled. Next have the patient inhale and determine the difference between the two systolic pressures. If this number is >10, pulsus paradoxus is present.
  2. **Treatment** is rapid fluid infusion, pericardiocentesis.
E. **Myocardial contusion** defined as blunt trauma to the heart.
  1. 33% to 88% will have abnormal ECG. Many have normal CPK-MB, and there is no correlation between the CPK-MB and the degree of injury. Best diagnostic tests are echocardiography, first-pass biventricular angiography.
  2. Best approach is to simply monitor the hemodynamically stable patient. Specific intervention is seldom needed, and the stable patient does not require diagnostic imaging studies to "prove" the presence of cardiac contusion. Usually the only clinical problem is episodes of PSVT or self-limited ventricular tachycardia. In the patient with pre-existing cardiac disease, myocardial contusion can be manifest as CHF.
F. **Aortic disruption** from deceleration injury.
  1. **Look for widened mediastinum** (85% sensitive) on chest radiograph. Blurred and enlarged aortic knob, esophageal deviation to right (look at NG tube), apical cap (blood collected at the upper apex of the lungs) are present in less than 25% of aortic injuries. Thus, absence of radiographic signs does not guarantee an intact aorta. Definitive diagnosis by CT, transesophageal echocardiogram or angiogram depending on your institution's protocol.

2

EMERGENCY MEDICINE

2. **Open emergency thoracotomy is not indicated for blunt chest trauma.** It is almost never successful. A stab wound to the heart or aorta may be amenable to emergency department intervention. Do this only if trained in the technique and with the blessing of the surgeon who will manage the case in the OR unless patient is obviously terminal if not treated immediately.

ABDOMINAL TRAUMA IN THE MAJOR TRAUMA VICTIM

(including assault and abuse in children)

I. Diagnosis

Possible intraabdominal injury indicated by:

A. Systolic blood pressure less than 100 or hematocrit <29. No criterion is absolute, and physical examination is only about 65% accurate; **use clinical judgment.**

B. "Lap-belt ecchymosis" in children is associated with hollow organ injury, lumbar spine fracture, solid organ (liver/spleen) injury. May portend severe injury in adults as well.

C. Elevated ALT and AST may indicate liver injury.

D. Patients with severe chest injuries or pelvic fractures are more likely to have intra-abdominal injury.

II. Penetrating Trauma of Abdomen

A. Requires exploration if penetrates the peritoneum.

B. Some centers are doing CT only but this is not yet universally accepted as the standard of care.

III. Blunt Trauma of the Abdomen

A. If hemodynamically **unstable** and have an acute abdomen, need laparotomy. Do not wait for CT, ultrasound, or diagnostic peritoneal lavage (DPL) before consulting surgery.

B. If hemodynamically **stable** and patient complains of abdominal pain or is intoxicated or has head injury, proceed with CT, ultrasound, or DPL. Both CT and DPL have strengths and weaknesses. Ultrasound is rapidly available at the bedside; however, it is less sensitive than CT.

EXTREMITY TRAUMA

See Chapter 16 for fracture and dislocation management. These are the lowest priority injuries early on unless there is a threat to a limb.

I. Arterial Injury

A. Can be caused by blunt or sharp injury. **Blunt may be more dangerous because less obvious.**

B. **Absolute indications for arteriogram.** Pain, pallor, paralysis, paresthesia, pulselessness, hemorrhage, expanding hematoma, bruits. **20% of arterial injuries will have a pulse distal to the injury.**

C. Penetrating trauma in proximity to a vessel is not necessarily an indication for arteriogram.

1. **Arterial pressure index** (arterial pressure in injured limb divided by arterial pressure in unaffected limb). Good screening: if >0.90, can safely observe in the absence of other indications for arteriography.

2. **Shotgun injuries** are a high-risk category and should be studied with arteriography.

II. **Compartment Syndrome**

A. **Caused especially by** crush injuries, electrical burns, circumferential scars, tight casts, hematoma in compartment, snake bites, and anything else that can increase pressure in a compartment.

B. Can result in muscle, nerve, and vessel necrosis from hypoperfusion.

C. **Clinical presentation.**

1. Severe, constant pain in affected limb, pain on muscle palpation, passive stretch, and active contraction, paresthesia and loss of distal pulses are late signs and herald poor outcome.

2. Compartment may be tense, but a normal turgor does not rule out compartment syndrome. Can diagnose by manometry:

a. Normal tissue pressure less than 10 mm Hg.

b. Capillary blood flow compromised at 20 mm Hg.

c. At risk for ischemic necrosis above 30 mm Hg.

D. **Treatment** is by fasciotomy and requires immediate surgical consultation.

III. **Amputations**

A. Control bleeding with direct pressure. Avoid clamping vessels. Place severed part in saline-soaked gauze, place in plastic bag, and put in cooler with ice. **Avoid freezing part.** Refer to plastic or orthopedic surgery.

UROLOGIC TRAUMA

I. **Kidney Trauma**

A. **Blunt.**

1. Serious injury **rare (but does occur)** with microscopic hematuria <30 RBC per HPF **if** the patient is hemodynamically stable **and there are no other significant intraabdominal injuries.**

a. IVP or CT is not required in these patients unless have other another indication (such as multiple trauma) or indications of urologic trauma, such as pelvic fractures, lower rib fractures, or localized hematoma, since it is unlikely there will be a surgically correctable lesion.

b. Management. Frequent monitoring of vital signs and repeat urinalysis at about 4 hours.

2. In those with >30 RBC/HPF, gross hematuria, or <30 RBC/HPF and shock **or** intraabdominal injury, IVP or CT is indicated.

a. CT scanning has replaced IVP in evaluating renal injury in most settings since it can also help define other intraabdominal trauma.

b. IVP has a 30% false-negative rate in those with renal pedicle injuries, which represent 2% of all renal injuries. 36% of those with pedicle injuries will **not** have hematuria. However, they will usually have a deceleration mechanism suggestive of this injury and other associated injuries. IVP will show a nonfunctioning kidney.

c. Most renal contusions, tears, and hematomas can be managed conservatively.

      d. Renal pelvis rupture is rare and will present with high fever, increasing abdominal pain and tenderness. Diagnosed by retrograde pyelogram.

B. **Penetrating.** All penetrating trauma to the kidney warrants investigation including IVP or CT. Some would argue for surgical exploration in all of these patients.

II. **Urethral Trauma**

A. Heralded by blood at the meatus, a high-riding prostate in males. This requires retrograde urethrogram **before** catheterization or other manipulation of the urethra. Obtain urology consultation. In an emergency, a temporary urostomy can be preformed by using the Seldinger technique and placing a central line into the distended bladder transabdominally.

III. **Bladder Trauma**

A. Bladder trauma is usually related to pelvic fracture. A cystogram will show extravasation of urine into abdomen. Exploration of the abdomen and surgical repair is indicated.

HYPERTENSIVE CRISIS

I. Clinically, a Hypertensive Emergency is defined by having end-organ damage or dysfunction including CHF, renal failure, hypertensive encephalopathy, hematuria, retinal hemorrhage, etc. It is not based on the absolute level of blood pressure.

A. Goal is to reduce blood pressure by 30% in 30 minutes. Individuals with chronic hypertension may not tolerate a "normal" blood pressure so be judicious when lowering blood pressure.

B. **Drugs**

    1. **Nitroprusside.** Mix 50 mg of Nipride in 500 ml D5W (100 μg/ml) and start infusion at 0.5 μg/kg/min. Titrate until desired blood pressure reduction is obtained. Average dose is 0.5 to 10 μg/kg/min.

      a. Very potent arterial and venous dilator.

      b. Can be used in all hypertensive emergencies though it is not the drug of choice for preeclampsia (see Chapter 14, obstetrics).

      c. Its use with clonidine has caused MIs.

    2. **Nitroglycerin.** Mix 25 mg in 250 ml and start infusion at 10 μg/min (6 ml/hr). Titrate by 10 to 20 μg/min until desired effect is obtained. Nitroglycerin is a venous and arterial dilator with maximum affect on capacitance vessels.

    3. **Labetalol** (Normodyne, Trandate). Give by bolus, 20 to 40 mg IV. May repeat in 10 minutes. Usual effective dose is 50 to 200 mg. May also administer as a continuous infusion of 2 mg/min (mix 200 mg in 160 ml D_5W = 200 ml = 2 ml/min. Stop the infusion when blood pressure control is achieved. Could combine by giving initial bolus and then infusion.

      a. Combined alpha-blocker and beta-blocker though primarily a beta-blocker. It does not change cerebral blood flow and is probably the drug of choice in hypertension secondary to increased intracranial pressure.

b. It is especially useful in catecholamine-mediated hypertension such as a pheochromocytoma, discontinuation of clonidine and avoids the reflex tachycardia seen with nitroglycerin and nitroprusside.

c. The onset is in 5 minutes, maximum response in 10 minutes. Duration about 8 hours.

Note: The use of oral or sublingual medications in hypertensive emergencies is not indicated.

II. **Hypertensive Urgency includes diastolic pressure of greater than 115 mm Hg without evidence of end-organ damage.**

A. Goal is to reduce blood pressure to "normal" within 24 to 48 hours. If possible, start the patient on a drug that he or she will be able to continue to use as part of an antihypertensive regimen.

B. There is no evidence that an elevated diastolic pressure of 115 or less is a risk factor for an acute event (stroke, MI) unless there is evidence of end-organ damage (see above). It is clearly a long-term risk factor and requires follow-up care but does not require emergency treatment.

C. **Never** make the diagnosis of new-onset, mild hypertension in an emergency department setting. The BP elevation may be attributable to pain or may be situational.

D. **Treatment.**

1. In most patients, simple observation and time is **as effective as** pharmacologic intervention.

2. Some options for treatment include:

a. Captopril 25 mg PO or SL. Is absorbed in 30 minutes SL with peak effect 50 to 90 minutes.

b. Labetalol 200 mg PO.

c. Another antihypertensive of your choice.

d. **Avoid SL Nifedipine.** Although rare, it can cause complications such as stroke or MI.

AORTIC DISSECTION (THORACIC)

A. **Characterized by** a severe tearing pain in the chest, back, epigastrium, and flanks. Have a high index of suspicion in those with unexplainable chest pain. **Pain is generally of short duration and very intense.** Pain may migrate from the chest downwards as the dissection progresses.

B. **Clinical findings.** Only 16% have loss of peripheral pulses and only 50% have unequal upper extremity pulses. Only 50% have a new aortic regurgitation murmur. Up to 40% have EKG changes suggestive of ischemia. Rarely have DIC or microangiopathic changes on blood smear.

C. **Diagnosis is by:**

1. **No finding on a plain radiograph is sensitive enough to rule out aortic dissection by its absence.** Radiograph **may** demonstrate a wide mediastinum, blurred and enlarged aortic knob, esophageal deviation

to right (look at NG tube), apical cap (blood collected at the upper apex of the lungs). There may be extension of blood beyond the calcific boarder of the aortic wall. **However, none of these may be present on the plain radiograph of a patient with aortic dissection.**

2. **Suspicion requires testing.** Transesophageal ultrasonography and CT are gaining in popularity but aortogram remains the gold standard.

D. **Treatment.**

1. **Control blood** pressure with a combination of

   a. **Nitroprusside** (see previous section, hypertensive emergencies for dose) **and a beta-blocker** to prevent shear forces caused by reflex tachycardia.

   b. **Propranolol** (Inderal): 0.5 to 1 mg IV Q2-5 min (maximum 15mg) to control heart rate (60-80 beats per minute).

   or

   c. **Esmolol:** Mix 5 mg in 500 ml to give concentration of 10 mg/ml. Give loading dose of 500 µg/kg (0.5 mg/kg) over 1 minute and start infusion of 50 µg/kg/min for 4 minutes. If no response, reinfuse bolus and increase drip to 100 µg/kg/min for 4 minutes. Continue this procedure increasing the drip by 50 µg/kg/min until have achieved desired results or get a total of 200 µg/kg/min, since will not get added benefit. Esmolol has the advantage of a short, 9-minute, half-life.

   or

   d. **Metoprolol**: 5mg IV Q5 min for a total of 15 mg or more to control pulse

   or

   e. **Labetalol**: See hypertensive crisis (above) for dosing.

   f. **Surgical consultation** is mandatory for consideration of repair. Recently, stents have been used as a temporizing measure. This will vary depending on your institution.

ABDOMINAL AORTIC ANEURYSM

I. Characterized by **colicky or constant, severe abdominal or back pain which may radiate to groin, hips or lower extremities. May mimic urolithiasis including hematuria and vomiting.**

II. Exam may show **a pulsatile mass (sensitivity between 44% to 97%)** but exam is not adequate to rule out a AAA if you have a clinical suspicion of AAA. **May also have a tender and possibly distended abdomen, and signs of shock depending on how much hemorrhage has occurred. Distal pulses are often maintained and are an unreliable sign!**

III. Immediate imaging is indicated. Treatment **as per thoracic dissection above. Stents are being used for unruptured aneurysms but surprisingly there is no difference in perioperative mortality or complications. Additionally, the grafts tend to migrate over time (1 to 3 years out).**

IV. Appropriate follow-up of the patient with an **asymptomatic AAA** found on routine exam:

A. Risk of rupture is essentially 0% for aneurysms <4cm, 1% annually for aneurysms 4- 5.0cm and 11% for those greater than 5.0cm. Surgical mortality is higher the than risk of rupture in those <5.0-5.5 cm and outcome in those with <5.0cm is the same at 6 years with observation as it is with surgery.

B. The best strategy is annual ultrasound of those aneurysms <4cm and twice yearly ultrasound of those aneurysms >4cm with repair at 5.0-5.5 cm.

SHOCK

I. **Characterized by Inadequate Tissue Perfusion and Cellular Hypofunction/Hypoxia**

II. **Classified by Etiology**

A. **Hypovolemic shock** from volume loss (e.g., dehydration, blood loss, burns)

B. **Distributive shock** based on loss of vascular tone (e.g., anaphylactic, septic, toxic shock).

C. **Cardiogenic shock** based on pump failure.

D. **Dissociative shock** based on inability of RBC to deliver oxygen (e.g., methemoglobinemia, carbon monoxide poisoning).

III. **Diagnosis**

A. **Hypotension. Blood pressure drop is a late finding.** Orthostatic vital signs may be normal in hypovolemic individuals, or normal individuals may exhibit orthostatic changes; so use clinical judgment and base treatment on symptoms. Additionally, alcohol ingestion, a meal, increased age, antihypertensives, etc. may cause orthostatic changes in BP and pulse in the absence of hypovolemia.

    1. An orthostatic systolic decrease of 10 to 20 mm Hg or increase in pulse of 15 beats/min is considered "significant."

    2. Take orthostatic vital signs recumbent and after standing for 1 to 2 minutes.

B. **Tachycardia** usually present but may not be, especially in the presence of diaphragmatic irritation, which causes vagal stimulation.

C. **Hypoperfusion** including decreased urine output, decreased mentation, cool extremities, mottling, etc.

    • Goal of resuscitation is to maintain urine output between 30 and 60 ml/hr.

IV. **Treatment**

Remember to keep patient warm and in Trendelenburg position if appropriate (contraindicated in CHF, though). Remember the ABCs.

A. **Hypovolemic shock.** See trauma section.

B. **Septic shock:** See Chapter 10.

C. **Anaphylactic shock** (applies also to acute urticaria).

    1. Systemic allergic reaction characterized by urticaria, itching, angioedema, dyspnea/cough/wheezing, and hypotension/syncope. May have vomiting or diarrhea, diffuse erythroderma. Caused by IgE-mediated hypersensitivity.

2

EMERGENCY MEDICINE

2. Anaphylactic shock has about a 3% mortality.
3. Common causes include foods, insect venoms especially Hymenoptera stings, drugs including aspirin and penicillins, radio-contrast materials (about 5% of patients are allergic).
4. Seafood allergy is protein related and not related to iodine. Therefore, these patients can have IVP dye. Penicillin allergic patients can almost always tolerate 3rd generation cephalosporins.
5. **Differentiate from scombroid fish poisoning,** which occurs after eating dark meat fish such as tuna (including canned), mackerel, swordfish, etc. Fish may taste metallic, peppery or bitter. Onset in 20-30 minutes of skin flushing, vomiting, urticaria, wheezing, dyspnea, headache, and palpitations. Caused by histamine and is self limited (usually <3 hours). Treat like anaphylaxis.
6. **Management of anaphylaxis.**
   a. **Epinephrine.**
      (1) **If stable:** Epinephrine 0.3 to 0.5 ml of 1:1000 subcutaneous (0.01 ml/kg in children). May repeat Q10-15 min × 3.
      (2) **If hypotensive or unstable:** Epinephrine 0.1-0.5 mg IV in boluses or can infuse at 1 to 4 μg/min (in adults) or 0.1 μg/kg/min in children.

All patients should also get:

   b. **Diphenhydramine** 25 to 50 mg PO for mild or up to 2 mg/kg IV for serious reactions (1 to 1.5 mg/kg/dose in children Q6h). This is a histamine$_1$-blocker.

AND

   c. **Cimetidine** 300 mg IV (5 to 10 mg/kg Q6-12h in children, maximum 300 mg/dose), or Ranitidine 50 mg IV (0.33 to 0.66 mg/kg IV Q8h in children, maximum 50 mg/dose).
      (1) Is an H-2 blocker, has been shown to be more effective than diphenhydramine with less sedation and should be used concurrently with diphenhydramine.
   d. **Corticosteroids** will not help stabilize the patient with anaphylactic shock. They are useful in preventing recurrences and in blocking late-phase reactants. Administer hydrocortisone succinate 100 mg IV to block late-phase reactants. Other options are methylprednisolone 60 to 125 mg IV (1 to 2 mg/kg in children) or oral prednisone.
   e. **For wheezing:** Nebulized albuterol ± epinephrine (SQ/IV) as per asthma section depending on clinical picture.
   f. **For discharge.** Because anaphylaxis can be biphasic with recurrence within 48 hours, continue diphenhydramine or hydroxyzine 25 to 50 mg PO Q6h and cimetidine 400 mg BID or ranitidine 150 mg PO BID for 48-72 hours. Can also continue on prednisone 40 mg QD if desired for 5 to 7 days. This will reduce itching and urticaria.

D. **Staphylococcal and Streptococcal Toxic Shock Syndrome (TSS)** (see MMWR 46(RR10): 1-55, 1997.)
   1. **Case definitions** for staphylococcal TSS: include fever 102° F (38.9° C), diffuse macular rash, desquamation 1-2 weeks after on-set of illness, hypotension, multisystem involvement, including myalgia (elevated CPK), mucous membrane hyperemia, renal, hepatic, CNS, or hematologic abnormality (platelets <100,000). Differentiate from Kawasaki's disease (see Chapter 12), Rocky Mountain spotted fever, etc.
   2. **Case definitions** for streptococcal TSS: hypotension, multiorgan involvement including renal, hematologic (DIC or platelets <100,000), liver, respiratory, generalized erythematous rash, or soft tissue necrosis (e.g., necrotizing fasciitis, myositis, gangrene).
   3. **Toxic shock is associated with** tampon use but 20% are related to other staphylococcal infections including postoperative infections, ingrown nails, abrasions, etc. Streptococcal TSS often due to skin infection (such as after varicella).
   4. **Treatment** includes antibiotics (a beta-lactamase–resistant penicillin, such as nafcillin or a first-generation cephalosporin or vancomycin or clindamycin), fluids, and pressors as noted in septic shock (see Chapter 10).
E. **Cardiogenic shock.** See Chapter 3, section on acute pulmonary edema.

OVERDOSE AND TOXIDROMES

I. **General Approach**
A. Remember ABCs.
B. Remember to decontaminate gut, clothing, skin, and environment.
C. If unconscious, remember glucose, thiamine, naloxone.
D. Determine to the best of your ability what was ingested. All overdose patients should have serum acetaminophen levels drawn (see acetaminophen below).
E. Contact your closest poison control center for further information about the particular toxin in question.
F. Poisoning (especially recurrent) in a child may indicate neglect but can also be associated with pica and lead toxicity.

II. **Gut Decontamination**
A. **Ipecac** is not useful, is fraught with untoward effects (e.g., delayed charcoal administration, aspiration, prolonged vomiting), and can no longer be recommended.
B. **Gastric lavage.**
   1. It is not generally effective or recommended beyond 1 to 1½ hours after ingestion but may want to try in severely ill patients. Lavage alone is not adequate and must be combined with charcoal.
   2. Use orogastric tube or largest NG tube available.
   3. Patient should have airway protection (patient should be alert or intubated). Many complications of overdose therapy are related to gastric lavage.

2

EMERGENCY MEDICINE

4. Instill 300 ml aliquots of saline and remove until clear or have irrigated with 5 liters of fluid.

C. **Activated charcoal.**
   1. Treatment of choice in most ingestions. Best if used within the first hour post ingestion of overdose. **Does not work for metals such as iron and lithium.**
   2. Administer activated charcoal 10 to 25 g in children, 50 to 100 g in adults (1 g/kg). A sorbitol mixture reduces transit times but should be used only with the first dose if are going to use multiple doses of charcoal. There is no evidence that cathartics reduce absorption or toxicity, however.
   3. Have the patient drink the charcoal or administer it by NG tube. 30% will vomit the charcoal but you can re-administer it if needed.
   4. Multiple-dose charcoal still controversial. May be indicated for theophylline, tricyclics, phenobarbital, phenytoin, and digitalis.
   5. However, recent data suggests that a charcoal-deferoxamine slurry of 3:1 (8gm deferoxamine to 25 gm charcoal) by weight will reduce absorption of iron. For lithium, cation exchange resins such as sodium polystyrene sulfonate (Kayexelate) can reduce lithium absorption.

D. **Whole bowel irrigation (WBI).**
   1. May be useful after the ingestion of enteric-coated and time-release medications (e.g., verapamil). May also be useful in "body packers," etc. Reduces bowel transit time. **Use in other ingestions may be helpful, but data are sparse.** Do not delay charcoal administration to use WBI.
   2. Use polyethylene glycol (Go-Litely) 1 to 2 L/hr in adults, 500 ml/hr in children to a total of 3 to 8 liters.

III. **Toxidromes:** symptom complexes associated with a toxin.

A. **Cholinergics.**
   1. **Cholinergics include** organophosphates, carbamates, pilocarpine, and some mushrooms.
   2. **Toxidrome includes** diaphoresis, salivation, lacrimation, defecation, urination, miosis, mental status changes, and weakness (blind as a mole, moist as a slug, weak as a kitten). Can check for serum cholinesterase activity.
      a. Mostly farmers and other industrial workers.
      b. Manifestations include nausea, sweating, diarrhea, salivation, headache, fatigue, convulsions, muscle weakness, and cardiovascular collapse. Death usually occurs from respiratory muscle depression and excessive secretions or bronchospasm.
   3. **Treatment.**
      a. **Decontaminate.** Decontamination includes washing the skin with alkaline soap and then ethanol. Decontaminate GI tract if needed with lavage and multiple-dose charcoal.
      b. **Atropine** 2 mg IV every 5 minutes to dry secretions and may require up to 200-500 mg in first hour; endpoint is drying of secre-

tions or signs of toxicity. For children use dose of 0.05 mg/kg. Atropine will treat the muscarinic effects only. Overabundant secretions are a cause of early mortality. Watch for ileus secondary to atropine.

    c. **Pralidoxime (2-PAM).** Adults 1-2 g IV over 15 to 20 minutes, children 20 to 40 mg/kg over 15 to 20 minutes. Can repeat in 1 to 2 hours. Follow serum cholinesterase levels.

        (1) 2-PAM regenerates acetylcholine esterase. Should be reserved for those who are symptomatic. Needs to be used early because the organophosphate-enzyme complex becomes irreversible after 24 to 36 hours.

    d. Morphine and aminophylline are contraindicated.

  4. **Sequelae.**

    a. **An intermediate syndrome occurs 24 to 96 hours after treatment** of initial insult and presents with rapidly developing respiratory failure, cranial nerve palsy, and proximal upper limb girdle weakness. Treatment is supportive only and does not respond to pharmacologic therapy.

    b. **Long-term sequelae** include impairment of auditory attention, visual memory, visuomotor speed, sequencing, and problem solving, motor steadiness, reaction time, and dexterity. No increase in depression, other psychologic problems.

    c. **May also have a delayed peripheral neuropathy** starting at 1 to 5 weeks that may progress for 3 months but will eventually resolve.

B. **Anticholinergics.**

  1. **Anticholinergics.** Atropine, scopolamine, belladonna alkaloids, antihistamines, antipsychotics, plants (Jimsonweed and others), tricyclics, mushrooms (*Amanita* species).

  2. **Toxidrome.** "Dry as a bone, red as a beet, mad as a hatter." Mydriasis, dry mucous membranes, urinary retention, cutaneous flushing, mental status changes.

  3. **Treatment.** Conservative therapy with decontamination. Treat seizures, arrhythmias (avoid class Ia agents), hyperpyrexia, and hypertension as in any other patient. Treat agitation with benzodiazepines (avoid phenothiazines that have anticholinergic properties). Physostigmine 0.5 to 2 mg IV in adults and 0.02 mg/kg in children may be used if severe symptoms that cannot be controlled otherwise (malignant hypertension, coma with respiratory depression, seizures unresponsive to conventional therapy, for example). **Reserve for severe problems: may induce seizures and arrhythmias. Do not use in tricyclic overdose!**

C. **Opiate poisoning.**

  1. By heroin, morphine, clonidine, codeine, diphenoxylate (Lomotil), others.

  2. **Toxidrome.** Sedation, hypotension, bradycardia, respiratory depression, usually pinpoint pupils (may not be present with mixed overdose or propoxyphene [Darvon and others]).

3. **Treatment.** Use these drugs with caution in those who are narcotic addicts. May precipitate acute opiate withdrawal. Can intubate and support until narcotic wears off if this is a concern. **Always observe the patient until there is no chance of further respiratory depression. This is especially important with naloxone, which has a relatively short half-life.**

   a. **Naloxone** 0.4 to 2 mg in adults up to 10 mg and may repeat if needed. Short acting; half-life is 1.1 hours. **May have recurrent narcotization when naloxone wears off.**

   b. **Nalmefene.** Long acting, half-life is 10.8 hours. However, the patient should still be observed until there is no possibility of recurrent sedation. Methadone has a longer half-life. **For nonopiate dependent patients** start with 0.5 mg/70 kg and follow with another 1.0 mg/70 kg in 2 to 5 minutes. If total dose of 1.5 mg/70 kg does not work, no further drug is indicated. **For opiate-dependent patients,** use a test dose of 0.1 mg/70 kg, and if there is no withdrawal in 3 to 5 minutes, follow above guidelines.

IV. **Specific Ingestions:** Read general guidelines for decontamination first.

A. **Petroleum distillates** (gasoline, fuel oil, airplane glue).

   1. Main toxicity is pulmonary from inhalation.
   2. Do not perform lavage or induce vomiting if swallowed.
   3. CXR (ARDS, infiltrates), ABG, and follow clinical course.
   4. If no symptoms within 6 hours, no need for further observation.

B. **Tricyclic antidepressants.**

   1. **Main toxicity.** Cardiac arrhythmias, anticholinergic effects (see toxidrome above), vomiting, hypotension, confusion, seizures.
   2. **Avoid emesis!** The patient may aspirate. Charcoal/lavage (see above) mainstay of decontamination.
   3. The patient may appear fine and rapidly deteriorate so admit to a monitored unit. **Be prepared to intubate the patient.** If the patient is totally asymptomatic 6 hours after ingestion, no need to admit to monitored bed but may require psychiatric admission.
   4. **Cardiac complications.** Prolonged QRS, QT interval, torsade, other arrhythmias.

      a. **Sodium bicarbonate** to maintain blood pH above 7.45 (1 to 2 mEq/kg bolus until QRS <100 msec narrows, QT shortens, 2 amps in 1 liter of D_5W as a drip to maintain alkalinization). Helps prevent the development of arrhythmias. Recent data indicates that hyperventilation and saline may also be effective but are not standard of care.

      b. **IV magnesium sulfate** can be used to control torsade de pointes or a prolonged QT interval: 2 g of magnesium sulfate IV over 5 to

10 minutes depending on acuity (see Chapter 1, resuscitation).

    c. **Lidocaine** can be used for arrhythmias as well. Avoid class IA and IC antiarrhythmics, beta-blockers, calcium-channel blockers, phenytoin.

  5. **Neurologic complications.** Agitation, seizures.

    a. **Diazepam** 5 to 10 mg or lorazepam 1-2 mg IV titrating to control agitation.

    b. **Seizures** are usually brief and self-limited. Treat as per seizure section with first-line drug being lorazepam 1-2mg IV. Avoid phenytoin!

  6. **Hypotension.** Treat initially with fluids and sodium bicarbonate IV (see above). Norepinephrine is the vasopressor of choice. Dopamine may give a paradoxical hypotension.

  7. Physostigmine, the mainstay of therapy in the past, is now controversial (see anticholinergic toxidrome) and should not be used.

C. **Salicylates (aspirin).**

  1. **Main toxicity.** Tinnitus, nausea, vomiting, combined respiratory alkalosis (from central hyperventilation) and metabolic acidosis, fever, hypokalemia, hypoglycemia, seizures, and coma.

    a. Many are misdiagnosed as sepsis or gastroenteritis on initial presentation (fever, acidosis, vomiting, etc.). This misdiagnosis is particularly common in the elderly.

  2. **Toxic dose:** 150 mg/kg with 300 mg/kg being very toxic.

  3. **Treatment.**

    a. **IV normal saline to maintain BP.**

    b. **Urine alkalinization** (promotes excretion of salicylates). Use IV sodium bicarbonate (1 to 2 mEq/kg bolus, 2 amps in 1 liter of D_5W as drip). Must have adequate K^+ otherwise will get potassium reabsorption in exchange for hydrogen ions. Therefore will not alkalinize the urine.

    c. **Hemodialysis** for severe toxicity.

  4. Follow clinically and with serum salicylate levels. The Dome nomogram is not accurate unless there was only a single ingestion without previous ingestion in the last 24 hours and no enteric-coated ASA.

C. **Acetaminophen (Tylenol and others).**

  1. **Main toxicity** is hepatic, which occurs 24 to 72 hours after ingestion. May also manifest vomiting, nausea.

  2. **If patient is vomiting and unable to keep down charcoal,** consider metoclopramide. Ondansetron has also been particularly effective. Toxic ingestion is 140 mg/kg or 10 g in adults. In alcoholics the toxic dose is often much less, even as little as 4 g/day.

  3. **Check acetaminophen level at least 4 hours after ingestion. For extended release acetaminophen or if there is a co-ingestion (including food), recheck a level at 8-12 hours unless acetaminophen is

undetectable at 4 hours. Just checking a 4 hour level does not guarantee patient safety.
4. Compare to Rumack-Matthew nomogram to determine risk (Fig. 2-1).
5. If in toxic range, treat with N-acetylcysteine 140 mg/kg orally or by

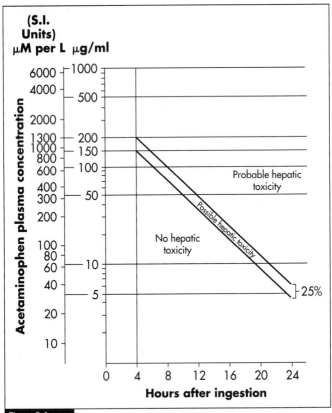

Figure 2-1

Rumack-Matthew nomogram for the single acute acetaminophen poisoning. Semilogarithmic plot of plasma acetaminophen levels versus time. Caution s for use of this chart: (1) The time coordinates refer to time of ingestion. (2) Serum levels drawn before 4 hours may not represent peak levels. (3) The graph should be used only in relation to a single acute ingestion. (4) The lower solid line 25% below the standard nomogram is included to allow for possible errors in acetaminophen plasma assays and estimated time from ingestion of an overdose. *(Adapted from Rumack BH, Matthew H: Pediatrics 55:871-876, 1975.)*

NG tube or IV (same preparation can be used both orally and IV) and then 17 doses of 70 mg/kg every 4 hours. **IV use is not approved in the United States but is safe and effective.** IV use may be associated with an anaphylactoid-type reaction that responds to diphenhydramine and inhaled albuterol (for wheezing). **This generally does not preclude further IV use of N-acetylcysteine. Wait one hour and if patient is asymptomatic it is safe to restart the infusion.**

6. **Repeat any doses vomited within 1 hour of administration.** Do not withhold N-acetylcysteine even if 24 to 26 hours from ingestion. Late N-acetylcysteine, though not so effective as early, still reduces mortality.

7. Charcoal use is indicated in acetaminophen overdose and only minimally interferes with N-acetylcysteine. Additionally, charcoal should be given early and N-acetylcysteine at least 4 hours later.

D. **Caustic ingestion** including alkaline (drain cleaner), industrial bleach, battery acid, etc. **Household bleach relatively is nontoxic** (unless inhaled) and rarely causes any difficulties when ingested.

   1. **Main toxicity.** Local tissue necrosis of esophagus with alkali and of stomach with acids; respiratory distress. May have obvious facial, oral burns and emesis. Have hoarseness and stridor reflecting epiglottic edema. This especially true in acids. Frequently have dyspnea and infiltrates if inhaled and may progress to ARDS.

   2. **Treatment.** Do not induce emesis or lavage patient. Charcoal is not indicated. If have visible burns, there is a 50% chance of lower burns of significance. However, the absence of visible lesions does not rule out significant injury (10% to 30% will have burns beyond the mucosa), and all ingestions need to have EGD. **For household bleach: If the patient is asymptomatic,** no further treatment or workup is required. For dyspnea, administer oxygen, obtain CXR and ABG as indicated.

E. **Digoxin.**

   1. **Main toxicity.** Any cardiac arrhythmia is possible with digoxin intoxication. Hypokalemia predisposes to digoxin toxicity (but digoxin toxicity causes hyperkalemia).

   2. **Manifested by** anorexia, nausea, vomiting, confusion, blurred vision, altered color perception (yellow tinge but occurs only in a minority).

   3. **Laboratory.** Hyperkalemia, elevated serum digoxin level.

   4. **Treatment.**

      a. **Treat arrhythmias as in Chapter 1,** resuscitation (magnesium sulfate particularly effective for digoxin-induced arrhythmias).

      b. **Treat hyperkalemia.** Avoid calcium because will increase digoxin binding to the heart.

      c. **Digoxin-specific antibody fragments** (Digibind) indicated for:

         (1) **Adults:** Hyperkalemia 5-5.5, ; life-threatening arrhythmias; ingestion of 10 mg in adults with signs of toxicity,

(2) **Children:** 0.1 mg/kg in children; serum level 5 mg/dl with signs of toxicity, potassium >6.0.

(3) **To treat:** Calculate Fab dose: 1 vial of Fab (40 mg) will bind 0.6 mg of digoxin. Calculate total body digoxin load: Total body dose dig = (Serum dig level × 5.6 L/kg × Wt in kg)/1000 × 0.8 (bioavailability). Vials Fab needed = Total body dig/0.6. **If dose unknown** and cannot get digoxin level, give 10 to 20 vials. If more likely a chronic toxicity, give 4 or 5 vials to start.

(4) Serum digoxin levels are useless after digoxin Fab given since will measure both bound and unbound digoxin. Serum digoxin level may increase tenfold to twentyfold after digoxin Fab. **Watch for hypokalemia** from reversing digoxin-induced hyperkalemia.

F. **Carbon monoxide.**

1. **Main toxicity.** Central nervous system including confusion, coma, seizures, headache, fatigue, nausea. May have arrhythmias, cardiac ischemia and rhabdomyolysis. Consider carbon monoxide poisoning in a cluster of "flu" cases in the wrong season (fatigue, muscle aches, nausea, etc.).

2. **Diagnosis** is by clinical background including a clustering of cases, exposure to furnace or car exhaust (especially in children in the back of pickup trucks, etc.), carboxyhemoglobin level. A venous carboxyhemoglobin level just as good as arterial. Pulse oximetry will generally be normal even in severe carbon monoxide poisoning. Obtain EKG and serum CPK levels.

3. **Treatment.** Administration of 100% oxygen (displaces carbon monoxide from hemoglobin). Hyperbaric oxygen (HBO) is recommended for any patient with evidence of myocardial ischemia, carboxyhemoglobin level of 30% (some say >18%) at exposure time zero, any impairment of CNS function. All pregnant women should have HBO. Recent data questions the effectiveness of HBO. However, it is still the standard of care.

H. **Cocaine and methamphetamines.**

1. **Major toxicity.** Seizures, hypertension, tachycardia, paranoid behavior or other alteration in mentation, rhabdomyolysis, myocardial infarction, CVA.

2. **Treatment.** Cocaine has a relatively short half-life, and so most symptoms are self-limited. Methamphetamines have a longer half-life and may require treatment.

   a. Beta-blockade (esmolol, propranolol, others) **is contraindicated** in the treatment of cocaine and methamphetamine-induced hypertension, tachycardia, and coronary spasm **unless already have given an alpha-blocker.** Unopposed alpha-adrenergic affects may worsen problems.

      b. For coronary vasospasm, hypertension, or tachycardia, observation is probably adequate, since cocaine has short half-life. For amphetamines treatment may be required.

      c. If treatment is urgent, phentolamine 5 to 10 mg IV is the drug of choice. Once have alpha-blockade can gently use beta-blockers to control arrhythmias.

         (1) Treat as would any MI; thrombolytics are safe. MI and CVA may occur up to 72 hours after cocaine use. Concurrent use of alcohol increases the likelihood of cardiac vasospasm with cocaine use. All chest pain is not MI. Think of pneumomediastinum in crack use, bronchospasm.

      d. Seizures. Generally self-limited but will respond to normal seizure treatment (see section on seizures, above).

      e. CNS symptoms such as agitation and paranoia can be treated by diazepam or lorazepam.

BITES

I. Animal Bites

The main morbidity from animal bites is infection or scarring. Rabies must be considered in any warm-blooded animal bite but is almost nonexistent in the domestic animal population of the United States. It is present in the wild, mainly in bats, raccoons, skunks, or dogs from Mexico or Latin America, Asia, or Africa. Rabies is very rarely found in rodents (such as squirrels, rats, or mice) and almost never in lagomorphs (rabbits).

A. Gather data on what species of animal was involved and whether it has a current vaccination, whether the attack was provoked or unprovoked, the extent of wounds, and whether the animal is available for examination.

B. **Management.**

    1. Cleanse the wounds thoroughly with soap and water.

    2. Contact the local police. Domestic, unvaccinated animals should be observed by a veterinarian for 10 days or killed and the heads refrigerated and sent to an appropriate lab for testing, generally the state lab. All wild animals captured or killed should have the head sent for testing.

    3. Check tetanus status and give booster if >5 years.

    4. Treat wound like any other wound with irrigation and debridement. Do not close puncture wounds or human bites because of high incidence of infection. Consider consultation for extensive damage or facial wound. Dog bites especially cause a lot of soft-tissue damage with pain and surrounding bruising.

    5. Antibiotics for bites:

      a. **Human bites.** Antibiotics should be given prophylactically for all human bites: amoxicillin/clavulanate 20 to 40 mg/kg/day divided TID; cefixime is an alternative. Consider IV antibiotics if infection has already occurred, especially on the hand. If a joint may be in-

2

EMERGENCY MEDICINE

volved (e.g., MP joint after an altercation), surgical exploration is indicated.

b. **Cat bites.** Antibiotics are routinely given for cat bites. The drug of choice is amoxicillin/clavulanate 20 to 40 mg/kg/day divided TID × 7 days. Doxycycline or ceftriaxone are acceptable alternatives.

c. **Dog bites.** Only 5% become infected (the same rate as most wounds), and routine prophylaxis is not recommended. If need to treat, amoxicillin/clavulanate is the drug of choice with clindamycin, plus a fluoroquinolone or TMP/SMX, being good alternatives. Wounds can be closed if not extensive and not a lot of tissue crushed.

6. **Rabies prophylaxis** should be instituted for all wild carnivore bites (such as skunk, fox, raccoon, cat, dog, or bat) unless animal available for study.

   a. Rabies immunoglobulin in persons not previously immunized 20 IU/kg. It should all be infiltrated around the wound if feasible. Otherwise, give as much as possible infiltrated around the wound and the rest IM.

   b. Human diploid cell rabies vaccine, 1.0 ml IM on days 0, 3, 7, 14, and 28.

   c. **For bats: Transmission without a bite is exceedingly rare. The CDC recommends:** "Postexposure prophylaxis should be considered when direct contact between a human and a bat has occurred, unless the exposed person can be certain a bite, scratch, or mucous membrane exposure did not occur. In instances in which a bat is found indoors and there is no history of bat-human contact, the likely effectiveness of postexposure prophylaxis must be balanced against the low risk such exposures appear to present. In this setting, postexposure prophylaxis can be **considered** for persons who were in the same room as the bat **and who might be unaware that a bite or direct contact had occurred** (e.g., a sleeping person awakens to find a bat in the room or an adult witnesses a bat in the room with a previously unattended child, mentally disabled person, or intoxicated person) and rabies cannot be ruled out by testing the bat. Postexposure prophylaxis would not be warranted for other household members. (*MMWR* 48 (RR-1): 1998.)

II. Tick Bites

Tick bites can be from a variety of different species, the deer tick *Ixodes dammini* (Lyme disease carrier) and wood tick and dog tick, which are carriers of Rocky Mountain spotted fever, are most well known. Tick bites can also cause tick paralysis, an ascending motor paralysis caused by a neurotoxin secreted in the tick's saliva.

A. Ticks should be looked for especially on ankles or scalp after any exposure to woods or tall grass. Removal is accomplished by steady traction with forceps grasping tick as close to skin as possible to avoid leaving the head behind. Do not use hot matches or other home remedies because they often kill the tick leaving the head embedded and may cause the tick to regurgitate, increasing the risk of infection.

B. **Prevention** is best accomplished with covering exposed skin and wearing insect repellent when exposed to tick-infested areas. Prompt removal of ticks can prevent transmission of disease. Transmission after a bite in endemic areas is only about 0.6%. According to the CDC, **"In most circumstances, treating persons who only have a tick bite is not recommended."** [www.cdc.gov/ncidod/dvbid/lymeprevent.html (June 1999)]

C. See Chapter 10 for information on Rocky Mountain spotted fever, Lyme disease, and other tick-borne illnesses.

III. **Spider Bites.**
Spider bites are usually not serious unless there is an allergic reaction. Treatment with ice, cleansing, and acetaminophen is usually adequate. Black widow and brown recluse spiders can cause more severe reactions and occasionally death. Antivenom is available for black widow spider bites but should only be used if the reaction is severe and is unable to be controlled with opiates and benzodiazepines. Specific discussion is beyond the scope of this manual.

ENVIRONMENTAL ILLNESS AND BURNS

I. **Sunburn** occurs after exposure to sun and presents within 24 hours of sun exposure. Generally peaks at 72 hours and may have erythema, blistering, and pain.

A. Best therapy is prevention by wearing of clothing or sun block and avoiding sun exposure at peak day (10:00 AM to 3:00 PM). **Cool compresses** and pain medications may produce symptomatic relief. Topical steroids (such as betamethasone) and **oral NSAIDs** (such as indomethacin) may be beneficial and seem to be additive. **Oral prednisone** 20 to 30 mg/day in adults may decrease symptoms.

II. **Hyperthermia.** Hyperthermia results from an imbalance in heat production, dissipation. Predisposing factors include dehydration, chronic illness, old age, alcohol, alteration in skin function (scleroderma etc.), drugs including anticholinergics, phenothiazines, tricyclic antidepressants, MAO inhibitors, amphetamines, and succinylcholine. Think also of thyroid storm.

A. **Malignant hyperthermia.**
1. **Causes:** 1:20,000 in response to a muscle-relaxing agent (such as succinylcholine) or an inhaled anesthetic (such as halothane). Is hereditary. May also be secondary to physical or emotional stress.
2. **Characteristics.** Hyperthermia, muscle rigidity, tachycardia, acidosis, shock, coma, rhabdomyolysis.
3. **Treatment** includes IV dantrolene 1 to 10 mg/kg IV titrated to effect, management of acidosis and shock, peripheral cooling (see management of heat stroke below).

B. **Neuroleptic malignant syndrome.**
1. **Cause.** Neuroleptics (phenothiazines, etc.)
2. **Characteristics.** Same symptoms as malignant hyperthermia but generally develops over days instead of minutes.
3. **Treatment.** As per malignant hyperthermia.

C. **Serotonin syndrome.**
1. **Cause.** Serotonin excess. Generally secondary to combination of MAO and SSRI or rarely to excess SSRI ingestion.
2. **Characteristics.** Rapid development of fever, hypertension, muscle rigidity, decreased mental status. Much more rapid onset than neuroleptic malignant syndrome.
3. **Treatment.** Treat like malignant hyperthermia (above). Cyproheptadine, a serotonin antagonist, 4-8mg has been effective in case reports. Also diazepam in 5 mg aliquots IV for muscle spasm, intubation as needed, cooling blankets, acetaminophen. Treat hypertension as per malignant hypertension.

D. **Heat cramps.**
1. **Cause.** Strenuous physical activity.
2. **Characteristics.** Skeletal muscle cramps, profuse sweating, hyponatremia secondary to free water intake, normal body temperature.
3. **Treatment.** Rest, oral or IV rehydration.

E. **Heat exhaustion.**
1. **Cause.** Secondary to sweating, volume depletion, tissue hypoperfusion.
2. **Characteristics.** Fatigue, light-headedness, nausea, vomiting, headache, tachycardia, hyperventilation, hypotension, normal or slightly elevated temperature, profuse sweating.
3. **Treatment.** Rest, rapid IV fluid replacement (1 to 2 liters of NS or more).

F. **Heat stroke.**
1. **Cause.** Volume depletion, sweating, etc.
2. **Characteristics.** Hyperpyrexia (often >40° C [106° F]), Patient may be sweating or may be dry, and have loss of consciousness or alteration in mental status (hallucinations, bizarre behavior, status epilepticus, other neurologic symptoms).
3. **Treatment. This is a true emergency.** Check and follow labs including electrolytes, CBC twice a day, liver enzymes, CPK (may develop rhabdomyolysis), and clotting studies. Remove clothing; apply water to skin and fan to promote evaporative heat loss. (Avoid inducing shivering and peripheral vasoconstriction with ice. Shivering can be controlled with diazepam IV or chlorpromazine or meperidine.) Treat with fluids (but many do not have significant fluid deficits; be cautious), cooling blankets.

BURNS, COLD, AND THERMAL INJURY

I. Assessment of Burns

A. **Surface area** (Figure 2-2).

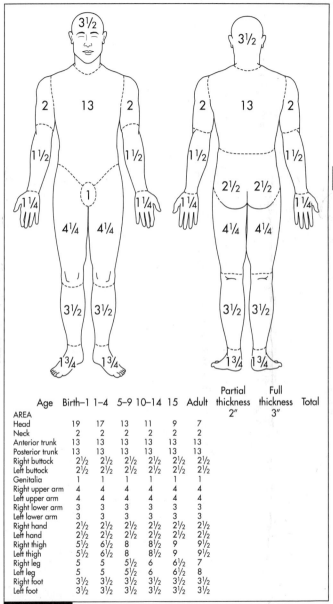

Age	Birth–1	1–4	5–9	10–14	15	Adult	Partial thickness 2"	Full thickness 3"	Total
AREA									
Head	19	17	13	11	9	7			
Neck	2	2	2	2	2	2			
Anterior trunk	13	13	13	13	13	13			
Posterior trunk	13	13	13	13	13	13			
Right buttock	2½	2½	2½	2½	2½	2½			
Left buttock	2½	2½	2½	2½	2½	2½			
Genitalia	1	1	1	1	1	1			
Right upper arm	4	4	4	4	4	4			
Left upper arm	4	4	4	4	4	4			
Right lower arm	3	3	3	3	3	3			
Left lower arm	3	3	3	3	3	3			
Right hand	2½	2½	2½	2½	2½	2½			
Left hand	2½	2½	2½	2½	2½	2½			
Right thigh	5½	6½	8	8½	9	9½			
Left thigh	5½	6½	8	8½	9	9½			
Right leg	5	5	5½	6	6½	7			
Left leg	5	5	5½	6	6½	8			
Right foot	3½	3½	3½	3½	3½	3½			
Left foot	3½	3½	3½	3½	3½	3½			

Figure 2-2

Estimating surface area in burns. *(Adapted from Nussbaum MS, editor: The Mont Reid Handbook, St Louis, 1987, Mosby.)*

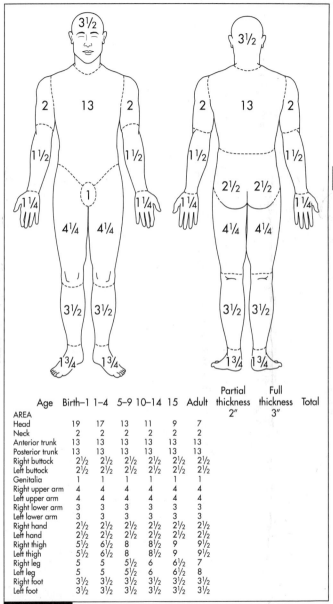

B. **Depth.** It is frequently impossible to tell the true depth of a burn at the initial evaluation. All burns should be serially examined over days and followed closely.
   1. **Superficial.** Epidermis only, painful and erythematous (previously first degree).
   2. **Superficial partial thickness.** Epidermis and outer half of dermis with sparing of hairs.
   3. **Deep partial thickness.** Epidermis and destruction of reticular dermis. Can easily convert to full thickness if secondary infection, mechanical trauma, or progressive thrombosis. (Previously second degree.)
   4. **Full thickness.** Dry, pearly white, charred, leathery. Heals by epithelial migration from the periphery and by contracture. May involve adipose, fascia, muscle, or bone. (The burn formerly known as third degree.)

C. **Severity**
   1. **Minor burn** defined as first degree and partial thickness <15% body surface area (BSA) in adults and <10% BSA in children <6 years of age; full thickness <2% BSA in adults.
   2. **Moderate burn** defined as partial-thickness 15% to 25% BSA in adults and 10% to 20% in children; full-thickness burns <10% BSA.
   3. **Major burn** (requiring burn unit or burn center care) defined as partial-thickness burns >20% to 25% BSA in adults and >20% in children; full-thickness burns >10% BSA; burns of hands, face, eyes, ears, feet, perineum; inhalation burns; electrical burns; burns complicated by fracture or major trauma; all burns in infants or elderly, patients at poor risk secondary to prior medical conditions.

D. **Causes of burns.**
   1. **Thermal.**
      a. Flame, especially with clothing, tends to be full thickness.
      b. Molten metal, tars, or melted synthetics lead to prolonged skin contact and should be cooled as rapidly as possible. See below for tar removal.
      c. Liquid burns should be cooled rapidly and any clothing in contact with the area rapidly removed to decrease the contact time.
   2. **Electrical.** Similar to crush injuries: get muscle necrosis, rhabdomyolysis, and myoglobinuria.
      a. Watch for cardiac arrhythmias. Cardiac monitoring essential for 24 hours if there is loss of consciousness, abnormal initial ECG or dysrhythmias. It is suggested for all others with significant exposure.
      b. Place in cervical collar; look for long bone fractures secondary to muscle contraction.
      c. **In children with lip burns from electrical cords,** watch for bleeding from the labial artery 3 or 4 days after injury.

 d. Follow CBC, electrolytes, ECG, urine myoglobin, CPK, cardiac enzymes, ABG.
 e. Can cause thrombosis of any vessel in the body. Injury usually much more than is visible on the skin. Be cautious and observe these patients closely. Consider admission.
3. **Chemical agents.**
 a. Strong acids are quickly neutralized or quickly absorbed. Rinse off skin and call Poison Control Center for specific instructions.
 b. Alkalis cause liquefaction necrosis and can penetrate deeply, leading to progressive necrosis up to several hours after contact.
4. **Radiation burns.**
 a. Initially appear hyperemic and may later resemble third-degree burns. Changes can extend deeply into the tissue.
 b. Sunburns are of this type and involve moderate superficial pain.

II. Treatment of Burns

Always watch for renal failure from rhabdomyolysis and sepsis in severe burns.

A. **Emergency department including thermal burns.** Cover wounds with normal saline-soaked gauze (which will help the pain to some degree) and use intravenous narcotics for pain. Tetanus immunization status should be checked and the patient treated accordingly.
 1. **Clean** with bland soap and water. Debride loose and foreign material. May leave blister intact if relatively small and patient is reliable. Rinse well with normal saline.
 2. **Wound-dressing choices:**
 a. Nonadherent inner layer of porous material followed by soft bulky absorbent gauze and covered with semielastic outer layer.
 b. Topical antibacterial agents such as 1% silver sulfadiazine or bacitracin are applied and then covered with gauze pads. See manufacturer's insert for contraindications.
 3. **Fluids.** Initiate if >15% to 20% body surface area burns in adults, >10% in children (see Figure 2-2).
 • Fluids in first 24 hours = 2 to 4 ml/kg $\times$ % of percentage of body surface area burned (Parkland formula).
 • Give ½ in first 8 hours and ½ in next 16 hours. Colloids are not indicated in this setting. Goal is to maintain urine output at 1 ml/kg/hr in children, 30 to 60 ml/hr in adults.
 4. Heterograft, allograft, or xerograft dressings can be used on an inpatient basis for partial-thickness wounds.
 5. **Chemical burns** should be washed with tap water at least 15 and preferably 30 minutes in duration **after powders are removed by brushing.** This should be started at the scene if possible. Alkali burns should be irrigated for 1 to 2 hours after injury. Chemical binding may be required for certain burns.
 6. **Tar burns** need cooling, gentle cleaning, and application of a petrolatum-based antibacterial ointment. Petroleum-based products,

EMERGENCY MEDICINE

2

household shortening or butter can be used to soften the tar for removal. Avoid chemical solvents, which may cause additional burns. After 24 hours the tar can be washed away and treated as a thermal burn.

B. **Follow-up care.**

1. Daily to twice-daily dressing changes should be performed. Mild soap can be used for cleaning. Necrotic debris and eschar require debridement and can be facilitated by tub soaks or whirlpool treatments. Absolute sterility is not mandatory (at home); however cleanliness and thorough cleaning of hands, sinks, tubs, and any instruments used must be emphasized. 0.25% acetic acid can be applied for pseudomonal prophylaxis.

2. **Contractures** may not be apparent for weeks to months. Therefore range-of-motion exercises should be started during the early healing period. If the hands are involved extensively, early excision and autografting may decrease the scarring of deep partial-thickness and full-thickness burns. Splinting and prolonged physical therapy may be required for rehabilitation. If the patient is prone to keloids, special garments may be used to reduce this scarring.

3. **Analgesics** should be given as needed and especially before dressing changes. Codeine or hydrocodone are normally adequate after the initial ED visit. If the dose is taken a half hour before the dressing change, it will facilitate cleaning and debridement.

4. All burns should be seen within 24 hours of initial treatment, and if any signs of infection develop, cultures should be performed and hospitalization considered.

5. **Prophylactic antibiotics** should rarely be required but may be considered for immunocompromised hosts, patients at high risk of endocarditis, or patients with artificial joints. Broad-spectrum coverage with first-generation cephalosporin or with a penicillinase-resistant penicillin plus an aminoglycoside may be used if necessary. Vancomycin may be needed depending on your institution.

6. In **circumferential burns,** extensive extremity burns, or electrical burns, watch for vascular or neurologic compromise, indicating a developing compartment syndrome. Immediate escharotomy is then required. Extremities should be elevated to minimize swelling.

7. In **extensive burns,** nutritional support is extremely important. Metabolic rate may be increased 100% to 200% above normal. Intravenous hyperalimentation may be required until the gastrointestinal tract is functioning.

III. Cold Injury

A. **Without tissue freezing.**

1. **Chilblain.** Peripheral cold injury without freezing of tissue.

a. **Cause.** Prolonged dry exposure at temperatures above freezing.

b. **Clinically.** Areas are pruritic, reddish-blue, maybe swollen, may have blisters or superficial ulcerations.

     c. **Treatment.** Rewarm as for frostbite below.

     d. Areas may be more temperature sensitive in future; no permanent injury. Pain medication should be provided.

  2. **Trench foot and immersion injury.**

     a. **Cause.** Prolonged wet exposure at temperatures above freezing.

     b. **Clinically** may have tissue destruction resembling partial-thickness burns including blisters, pain, hypersensitivity to cold. Temperature sensitivity may be permanent.

     c. **Treatment.** Rewarm as for frostbite below.

B. **With tissue freezing: frostbite.**

  1. **Cause.** Freezing of the tissue with ice crystal formation.

  2. **Classification.**

     a. **Frostnip.** Superficial, skin changes reversible.

       (1) **Clinically.** Skin blanched with loss of sensation.

       (2) **Treatment.** As below.

     b. Superficial frostbite tissue below skin pliable, soft.

       (1) **Clinically.** Blisters in 24 to 48 hours, fluid resorbs, develops hard, blackened eschar generally superficial, remains sensitive to heat, cold.

       (2) **Treatment.** As below. Treat conservatively. Generally resolves without surgical intervention in 3 to 4 weeks.

     c. Deep frostbite. Feels woody under skin; affects muscles, tendons, etc.

       (1) **Clinically.** Extremity cool, deep purple or red, with dark, hemorrhagic, blisters and loss of distal function.

       (2) **Treatment:** May take several months to determine extent of injury. Frozen tissue will eventually slough.

       (3) **Treatment: Rapid** rewarming of part by immersion in 42° C water. Do not rub. **Slow rewarming is not as good!** If in the field, do not thaw extremity until assured it will not refreeze.

         (a) Pruritus and burning sensation increase with rewarming. May require narcotic analgesia for severe injury. NSAIDs and topical aloe may help minimize tissue injury.

         (b) Debridement of clear blisters.

         (c) Local wound care, whirlpools, topical antibiotics and debridement as indicated (see burns above). Delay surgical intervention. Generally looks much worse than it is.

IV. **Hypothermia**

A. **Defined** as core temperature less than 35° C (95° F). Need to use a hypothermia thermometer to diagnose, since most thermometers will not read low enough.

B. **Risks.** Chronic illness, altered state of consciousness, elderly, neonates, drugs such as alcohol and barbiturates. Endocrinologic illness (Addison's disease, hypothyroidism, hypopituitarism, hypoglycemia), CNS dysfunction, sepsis

C. **Causes.** Exposure to cold, metabolic abnormalities.

2

EMERGENCY MEDICINE

D. **Clinically.** All changes are progressive and more pronounced with a greater degree of hypothermia.
   1. **Presentation** is of progressive decrease in mental status including confusion, lethargy, coma with areflexia, shivering or may have loss of shivering reflex, bradycardia, hypotension; have cold diuresis; may be hypovolemic.
   2. **Cardiac irritability.** Usually progressed from bradycardia to ventricular fibrillation. Do not roughly handle the hypothermic patient. This may induce arrhythmias. ECG may show J wave (Osborne wave).
E. **Treatment.**
   1. **Remove wet clothing and move to a warm environment.**
   2. **Examine the patient for a full minute** (or have on monitor) before beginning CPR, since pulse may be very difficult to detect in the bradycardic or hypothermic patient.
   3. **For rewarming:** Use blankets, heating blankets, warm-water immersion, radiant heat, heated IV fluids; warm, humidified, oxygen. For severe hypothermia, use heated gastric and colonic lavage, heated bladder irrigation, peritoneal or pleural lavage, mediastinal irrigation, heated hemodialysis and/or cardiopulmonary bypass.
   4. **Peripheral rewarming can be associated with shock,** acidosis and hyperkalemia when cold, acidotic peripheral blood is returned centrally. Central body rewarming is preferred with the extremities left for last.
F. No one is dead unless that person is warm and dead.
   1. If have ventricular fibrillation, defibrillate twice and then continue CPR and rewarm to 30° C. The heart is relatively resistant to drug therapy when cold. Try defibrillation periodically during rewarming.
   2. Based on the clinical situation, consider administration of thiamine 100 mg IV, glucose 50 ml of $D_{50}W$, hydrocortisone succinate 100 mg IV, thyroid hormone replacement.
V. **Cold Water Drowning**
A. Diving reflex is protective.
B. May survive intact after 40 minutes of cold water drowning. However this is the exception rather than the rule. Warm patient to at least 86° or 90° F before abandoning resuscitation.

RHABDOMYOLYSIS

Rhabdomyolysis refers to the breakdown of muscle tissue leading to systemic problems including renal failure. Renal failure may progress over a number of days so BUN and creatinine should be checked daily for 72 hours if suspect rhabdomyolysis. Also watch for developing hyperkalemia (see hyperkalemia for treatment).
A. **Causes of rhabdomyolysis include:**
   1. **Environmental** causes including heat stroke and severe frostbite, some snake bites and scorpion bites.

2. **Injuries** including burns and electrical burns, crush injuries, compartment syndrome, muscle infarction from ischemia.
3. **Toxins** including cocaine, narcotics, amphetamines, gemfibrozil plus an HmG CoA reductase inhibitor (very rare), amphotericin B,
4. **Overexertion/exercise/metabolic** abnormalities including prolonged seizures, malignant hyperthermia, serotonin syndrome, thyroid storm, hypokalemia.
5. **Viral** causes such as influenza, Epstein-Barr virus.

B. **Signs, symptoms, systemic effects**
   1. **Muscle aches and cramps,** dark colored/smoky colored urine from myoglobin, renal failure.
   2. **Laboratory/Diagnosis:** Myoglobin in urine (positive dipstick for hemoglobin with a negative microscopic exam). Elevated serum CPK, aldolase, serum potassium, elevated creatinine and BUN from secondary renal failure. Common laboratory abnormalities also include hyperphosphatemia, hypocalcemia followed later in the course by hypercalcemia.

C. **Treatment** is aimed at maintaining a good urine output (200-300ml/hr) and correcting the underlying abnormality.
   1. **Treat with normal saline or lactated Ringers** solution as soon as possible. Maintain urine output at 200-300ml/h. May require up to 20 liters per day. Check electrolytes frequently.
   2. **One approach is to use mannitol** to maintain urine output. Generally give about 12.5-25 g (0.5-2.5 g/kg) repeated in ½ hour if there is no diuresis. Maintain urine output with repeated boluses of mannitol and saline as needed. However, if there is no response to the first two boluses, do not give more. Mannitol will cause plasma volume expansion and may precipitate CHF.
   3. Others have used a solution of sodium chloride and sodium bicarbonate (sodium chloride 110 mmol/L; chloride 70 mmol/L; bicarbonate 40 mmol/L) in 5% glucose solution to which 10 g of mannitol per liter is added. This is administered at a rate of approximately 12 L/day (in a young 75 kg adult) to maintain urine output in normal range.
   4. **Alkalinization** of the urine is also important to prevent myoglobin from precipitating in the kidney (see salicylate toxicity section for technique).

2

EMERGENCY MEDICINE

BIBLIOGRAPHY

Ariano RE et al: Comparison of sedative recovery time after midazolam versus diazepam administration, *Crit Care Med* 22(9):1492, 1994.

Bailey B et al: Management of Anaphylactoid reactions to intravenous N-acetylcysteine, *Ann Emer Med* 1998 31(6): 710-15

Bakker AJ et al: Troponin T And myoglobin at admission: value of early diagnosis of acute myocardial infarction, *Heart J* 15(1):45, 1994.

Baraff L et al: Orthostatic vital signs: variation with age, specificity, and sensitivity in detecting a 450 ml blood loss, *Am J Emerg Med* 10(2):99, 1992.

Better OS et al: Early management of shock and prophylaxis of acute renal failure in traumatic rhabdomyolysis, *N Engl J Med* 322(12):825, 1990.

Bizovi K: Late increase in acetaminophen concentration after overdose of tylenol extended relief *Ann Emer Med* 28(5):549, November 1996

Buckley N et al: Slow-release verapamil poisoning: use of polyethylene glycol whole-bowel lavage and high-dose calcium, *Med J Aust* 158(3):202, 1993.

Hetland O et al: Cardiac markers in the early hours of acute myocardial infarction: clinical performance of creatine kinase, creatine kinase mb isoenzyme (activity and mass concentration), creatine kinase mm and mb subform ratios, myoglobin and cardiac troponin t, *Scand J Clin Lab Invest* 56(8):701, December 1996,

Cohen M et al: A comparison of low-molecular-weight heparin with unfractionated heparin for unstable coronary artery disease, *N Engl J Med* 337(7):447, August 14, 1997

Committee on Drugs: Reappraisal of lytic cocktail/Demerol, Phenergan, and Thorazine (DPT) for the sedation of children, *Pediatrics* 95(4):598, 1995.

De Bleecker J et al: The intermediate syndrome in organophosphate poisoning: presentation of a case and review of the literature, *Clin Toxicol* 30(3):321, 1992.

Dolan DL: Intravenous calcium before verapamil to prevent hypotension, *Ann Emerg Med* 20(5):588, 1991.

Perry HE et al: Efficacy of oral versus intravenous N-acetylcysteine in acetaminophen overdose: results of an open-label clinical trial, *J Pediatr* 132(1):149, January 1998.

Fabian TC et al: Prospective study of blunt aortic injury: multicenter trial of the American Association for the Surgery of Trauma, *J Trauma* 42(3):374, March 1997.

Graber MA, Hoehns B, Perry P: Sertraline-Phenelzine drug interaction: a serotonin syndrome reaction, *Ann Pharmacother* 28(6):732-735, 1994.

Graudins A et al: Treatment of the serotonin syndrome with cyproheptadine, *J Emerg Med* 16(4):615, June 1998.

Harley EH et al: Liquid household bleach ingestion in children: a retrospective review, *Laryngoscope* 107(1):122, January 1997.

Haude M et al: Sublingual administration of captopril inpatients with acute myocardial ischemia, *Clin Cardiol* 14(6):463, 1991.

Henry JA; Hoffman JR: Continuing controversy on gut decontamination, 352: 420-421, 1998.

Hetland O et al: Cardiac markers in the early hours of acute myocardial infarction: clinical performance of creatine kinase, creatine kinase mb isoenzyme (activity and mass concentration), creatine kinase mm and mb subform ratios, myoglobin and cardiac troponin t, *Scand J Clin Lab Invest* 56(8):701, December 1996.

Hoffman RS et al: The poisoned patient with altered consciousness: controversies in the use of a "coma cocktail," *JAMA* 274(7):562, 1995.

Holland RW et al: Grand mal seizures temporally related to cocaine use: clinical and diagnostic features, *Ann Emerg Med* 21(7):772, 1992.

Joint Working Group of the Research Unit of the Royal College of Physicians and the British Paediatric Association: Guidelines for the management of convulsions with fever: *Br Med J* 303(6803):634, 1991.

Katz RW et al: Safety of continuous nebulized albuterol for bronchospasm in infants and children, *Pediatrics* 92(5):666, 1993.

Lange RA et al: Potentiation of cocaine-induced coronary vasoconstriction by beta-adrenergic blockade, *Ann Intern Med* 112(2):897, 1990.

Lederle FA et al: Does this patient have abdominal aortic aneurysm? *JAMA* 281(1):77, January 6, 1999.

Moore WS et al: Abdominal aortic aneurysm: a 6-year comparison of endovascular versus transabdominal repair, *Ann Surg* 230:298-308, 1999.

Nypaver M et al: Neutral cervical spine positioning in children, *Ann Emerg Med* 23(2):208, 1994.

Pang D et al: Spinal cord injury without radiographic abnormality in children—the SCIWORA syndrome, *J Trauma* 29(5):654, 1989.

Panju AA et al: Is this patient having a myocardial infarction? *JAMA* 280(14):1256, October 14, 1998.

Pollack CV et al: Outpatient management of acute urticaria: the role of prednisone, *Ann Emerg Med* 26(5):547, 1995.

Reed MD et al: Ondansetron for treating nausea and vomiting in the poisoned patient, *Ann Pharmacother* 28(3):331, 1994.

Reed WW et al: Learning from the last ultrasound: a population-based study of patients with abdominal aortic aneurysm, *Arch Intern Med* 157:2064-2068, 1997.

Rosenstock L et al: Chronic central nervous system effects of acute organophosphate pesticide intoxication, *Lancet* 338:223-227, 1991.

Sacchetti A et al: Pediatric analgesia and sedation, *Ann Emerg Med* 23:237-250, 1994.

Scheinkenstel CD et al: Hyperbaric or normobaric oxygen for acute carbon monoxide poisoning: a randomised controlled clinical trial, *Med J Australia* 170:203, 1999.

Schneider SM: Neuroleptic malignant syndrome: controversies in treatment, *Am J Emerg Med* 9(4):360, 1991.

Sinert R et al: Exercise-induced rhabdomyolysis, *Am J Emerg Med* 23(6):1301, 1994.

Snyder HS: Lack of tachycardiac response to hypotension with ruptured ectopic pregnancy, *Am J Emerg Med* 8(1):23, 1990.

Tenenbein M, Shannon M: The poisoned patient: is gastrointestinal decontamination all washed up? Two responses, *Ped Emerg Care* 14(5):380, 1998.

The UK Small Aneurysm Trial Participants: Mortality results for randomised controlled trial of early elective surgery or ultrasonographic surveillance for small abdominal aortic aneurysms, *Lancet* 352:1649-1655, 1998.

Tintinalli JE et al: *Emergency medicine, a comprehensive study guide,* New York, 1999, McGraw-Hill.

Touger M, Gallagher EJ, Tyrell J: Relationship between venous and arterial carboxyhemoglobin levels in patients with suspected carbon monoxide poisoning, *Ann Emerg Med* 25(4):481-483, 1995.

Verbeek PR et al: Nontapering versus tapering prednisone in acute exacerbations of asthma: a pilot trial, *J Emerg Med* 13(5):715, 1995.

2

EMERGENCY MEDICINE

CARDIOLOGY

James M. Fox

ACUTE CORONARY SYNDROMES

Angina pectoris is a symptom of myocardial ischemia or infarction caused by an imbalance between myocardial oxygen supply and demand.

I. **Etiology.** Ischemia is secondary to coronary artery disease in 95% of patients. A decreased oxygen supply from anemia, hypotension, vasospasm, or arrhythmias or an increase in oxygen demand secondary to exercise, emotional stress, CHF, hypertension, tachycardia, sepsis, etc., can lead to a worsening of symptoms. Ischemia can occur in patients with normal coronary arteries in the setting of LV hypertrophy, aortic stenosis or insufficiency, hypertrophic cardiomyopathy, coronary vasospasm, or cocaine abuse.

II. Types of Angina

A. **Stable.** Intensity, character, and frequency of episodes can be predicted, and angina occurs in response to a known amount of exercise or other stress.

B. **Unstable.** Intensity, frequency, or duration of episodes is changed and can no longer be predicted. Pain is precipitated by less exercise or is of longer duration. This includes angina at rest and new-onset angina.

C. **Variant.** Pain, which may occur at rest, is secondary to vasospasm of coronary arteries.

III. Diagnosis

A. **History.** Classically described as substernal chest pressure or heaviness radiating to the left shoulder and arm, neck, or jaw, associated with nausea, diaphoresis, and shortness of breath. It is usually brought on and exacerbated by exercise and stress and alleviated with rest or sublingual nitroglycerin. Typically, the pain lasts 2 to 10 minutes and rarely 30 minutes. Atypical presentations may include epigastric pain, indigestion, right arm pain, light-headedness, nausea, or shortness of breath (anginal equivalents (see also Box 2-1). In the elderly, symptoms such as confusion, pallor, fatigue or dyspnea may be suggestive of ischemia. Ambulatory ECG monitoring reveals that at least 25% of ischemic episodes are silent even in patients with a history of typical angina.

B. **Physical exam.** An S_4 gallop may be present during an episode. The patient may be dyspneic, diaphoretic, or have a new heart murmur. High-risk features of angina include heart failure and hypotension. A focused physical exam is crucial in making an assessment of risk.

C. Evaluation of patients with angina.

1. **Which test?** In a population of patients with symptomatic disease and no work-up bias, the sensitivity of a graded exercise test (GXT) is about 45% with a specificity of 85%. The sensitivity of SPECT scanning (thallium GXT) and stress echo are both about 86% with a specificity of 64% and 77%, respectively. Stress-echocardiogram is

more operator-dependent. In some patients it may be more cost effective to do cardiac angiography as a first step.

2. **ECG.** During an episode of pain, the ECG may show ST-segment depression or T-wave inversions, or it may be normal. The absence of ECG changes during an episode of angina does not rule out cardiac ischemia because the circumflex and posterolateral distributions can be electrically silent. Increasing use is being made of echocardiography and nuclear studies (see below) to evaluate patients with continuing symptoms in the absence of ECG changes. CAD is suggested if there is evidence of an old MI.

3. **GXT or treadmill test.** The predictive value of a positive test depends on the prevalence of disease in the population being tested. Specificity is high in particular groups of symptomatic individuals but is generally <50% in asymptomatic individuals. Compared with men, women (especially young women) have higher rates of false-positive GXT. Overall, the GXT is less sensitive for CAD than is a nuclear study or stress echocardiogram. An early positive GXT may be indicative of left main disease or three-vessel disease. Absolute contraindications to GXT include acute CHF, acute MI, active myocarditis, ongoing unstable angina, recent embolism, dissecting aneurysm, acute illness, thrombophlebitis, moderate-to-severe aortic stenosis, and an ECG that cannot be interpreted (e.g., LBBB). Relative contraindications include severe hypertension, mild-to-moderate aortic stenosis, hypertrophic obstructive cardiomyopathy, frequent ectopy, and many other conditions that may increase the risk of a GXT.

4. **Nuclear (thallium or technetium) chemical or exercise stress tests.** Nuclear scans can be useful for patients who cannot tolerate the physical demands of the GXT or in whom the diagnosis will be pursued even in the light of a negative GXT (e.g., those considered to have a high clinical risk of disease). During the test, tracer is taken up by viable, well-perfused myocardium. Areas of MI are indicated by fixed perfusion defects with no uptake during rest or exercise. During the nuclear-GXT, areas that are hypoperfused (i.e., ischemic) demonstrate thallium uptake only during the postexercise "resting" images. Adenosine, dipyridamole, and dobutamine may be used to augment the perfusion of normal myocardium and shunt blood flow away from areas of relative ischemia. These agents are used in patients who have a contraindication to exercise or are unlikely to attain target heart rates. More recently, administration of tracer to patients during episodes of angina has been shown to be a sensitive way to detect abnormalities of perfusion when compared to scans done once the patient is rendered pain free. This can be used as a screening method for the detection of previously undiagnosed coronary disease.

5. **Echocardiography.** The stress echocardiogram is a widely performed test used to assess patients for coronary disease. Baseline echocar-

diographic images are obtained at rest. These are used to evaluate left ventricular function and wall motion. Images are then acquired during peak stress (i.e., during a GXT or with dobutamine) and compared with those at rest. Regional wall-motion abnormalities with stress indicate areas of hypoperfusion or ischemia. Echocardiography is now used more commonly to assess CAD in women because of their high false-positive rate on GXT. It is also gaining increased usage among patients with an abnormal baseline ECG (e.g., LBBB), those receiving digoxin, and after CABG or PTCA.

6. **Coronary angiography.** Used to identify foci of coronary disease. It is the evaluation of choice in patients with angina that is (1) poorly responsive to medication or (2) unstable. It is also indicated in patients with test results consistent with a high risk for CAD.

IV. **Outpatient Treatment of Stable Angina**

A. **Medical.** May use two- or three-drug combination to maximize benefit while minimizing side effects.

1. **Aspirin.** Daily aspirin (325 mg) unless contraindicated to inhibit platelet aggregation. For those unable to tolerate aspirin an alternative is clopidogrel (75 mg QD).

2. **Beta-blockers.** Decrease myocardial oxygen demand by decreasing heart rate, systolic blood pressure, and contractility. Because they prolong diastole, beta-blockers also increase O_2 supply by increasing myocardial perfusion time. Some beta-blockers (those without intrinsic sympathomimetic activity [ISA] activity), especially lipophilic ones (timolol, metoprolol, and propranolol) prolong life when given for the first year after an MI. This benefit extends into subsequent years in those with a complicated course. They are also useful in patients whose angina is regularly provoked by exercise, although beta-blockers may limit exercise tolerance. Start with a low dose and increase until symptoms are controlled or the resting heart rate is 50 to 60 beats/min. Side effects can include bradycardia, bronchospasm, fatigue, GI upset, symptoms of LV failure, and orthostatic hypotension. Impotence, depression, and Raynaud's phenomenon can occur. Do not discontinue beta-blockers abruptly, since rebound tachycardia can occur. Diabetes and class I and II stable CHF are no longer considered to be contraindication to beta-blocker use.

3. **Calcium-channel blockers** (verapamil, diltiazem, amlodipine, and others). These drugs act by blocking the influx of calcium through slow channels into vascular smooth muscle and myocardial cells. They promote peripheral arterial vasodilatation, which decreases oxygen demand by decreasing afterload. Calcium-channel blockers also decrease coronary vasospasm and improve collateral flow. Diastolic relaxation of the LV is enhanced, and coronary perfusion is increased with those agents that slow heart rate. Verapamil and diltiazem decrease conduction through the AV node. Heart block or asystole can develop in patients with AV node or sinus node disease.

First-generation calcium-channel blockers have negative inotropic effects, which can lead to CHF in patients with impaired LV function. Other common side effects of calcium-channel blockers include headache, ankle swelling, GI upset, increased risk of GI bleeding and bleeding after surgery, and constipation. Diltiazem and verapamil are relatively contraindicated after MI in those with CHF and should be avoided. Nifedipine increases heart rate and may increase mortality in some patients. The incidence of these side effects is reported to be less with the newer agents (amlodipine, felodipine).

4. **Nitrates** (nitropaste, nitropatches, isosorbide dinitrate, others). Effects include venous and arteriolar vasodilatation, which decreases oxygen demand. The resulting coronary artery vasodilatation increases coronary oxygen supply. Tolerance can develop but can be overcome by providing an 8-hour nitrate-free interval each day. Preparations include oral, transdermal patches, ointment, sublingual tablets, or spray. A common side effect is headache, which usually responds to aspirin or acetaminophen and tends to improve with continued use. Sublingual nitroglycerin tablets (0.4 mg PRN) or spray are used for acute episodes of angina and may be repeated at 5-minute intervals for up to 3 doses. Patients should be instructed to go to the emergency department if angina is not relieved after 3 doses of nitroglycerin.

5. **ACE inhibitors.** Recently, ramipril has been shown to have a beneficial effect on the incidence of MI, congestive heart failure and stroke in patients with coronary artery disease and in those with diabetes and one other risk factor for CAD. This is likely to be a class specific effect of ACE inhibitors. It is unclear if this benefit is provided by angiotensin receptor blockers (ARB).

B. **Revascularization.**

1. **Coronary artery bypass grafting (CABG).** Primary indication is angina refractory to medical therapy or lesions that are more amenable to surgery than to angioplasty. CABG has been shown to prolong survival in patients with left main disease (50% luminal narrowing) and in three-vessel CAD with LV dysfunction (ejection fraction <50%). Surgery may prolong survival in three-vessel disease with normal LV function and in two-vessel disease with significant proximal stenosis of LAD (if not anatomically suited for PTCA). Surgical advances such as minimally invasive surgery, transcutaneous myocardial revascularization (TMR), and selected single vessel bypass have made surgical therapy an option for patients who previously would not have been considered surgical candidates secondary to significant co-morbidity or poor target vessels.

   a. **Contraindications to CABG.** Advanced age with pronounced debility, absence of ischemia, or ungraftable coronary arteries. Advanced age in and of itself is not a contraindication. In one sample of patients 80 years and older, coronary revascularization by either CABG or PTCA (see below) was associated with a high likelihood of attaining a good or excellent quality of life and of a patient being able to care for himself or herself subsequent to an MI.

2. **Intracoronary stenting.** The current standard for interventional cardiology involves the use of intracoronary stents combined with antiplatelet agents (aspirin and clopidogrel). The indications for the different therapeutic modalities in interventional cardiology are beyond the scope of this text. Choice of intervention versus surgery, type of intervention, and medical therapy should be made in consultation with a cardiologist. It has been recently established that the use of g2,3b platelet aggregation receptor inhibitors (abciximab, tirofiban) in conjunction with primary coronary intervention (PCI) is superior to medical therapy alone, or the use of such interventions without those inhibitors. Percutaneous transluminal coronary angioplasty (PTCA) still has uses and indications. Several controlled clinical trials have shown that PTCA can be used as an alternative to CABG in two- and three-vessel CAD when lesions are amenable to PTCA. There was general agreement among these trials that the procedures provide equal improvement in angina. **The PTCA groups generally have a higher frequency of antianginal use after 1 year and are more likely to require additional intervention (CABG or repeat PTCA) compared to patients who undergo CABG.** PTCA or stenting is an acceptable alternative to repeat CABG if lesions are amenable to dilatation (single-vessel stenosis, or easily accessible two-vessel stenoses). Diabetics have a worse long-term result with PTCA than does the non-diabetic population. Consequently, intracoronary stenting is preferred in these patients.

3. **Vascular endothelial growth factor (VEG-F)** has been used to increase the vascular supply of the heart in those who are not candidates for bypass or PTCA. Although short-term studies are favorable, long-term outcomes are not known.

4. **Transmyocardial revascularization** uses a laser to create channels through the myocardium. It clearly reduces anginal pain, but it is not clear if this is just a result of nerve destruction (i.e., the patient can no longer feel anginal pain) or because of revascularization. There are no long-term outcome studies and this is currently considered experimental.

INPATIENT TREATMENT OF ANGINA AND MI

See chapter 2 for treatment of acute chest pain. Inpatient treatment is indicated for (1) unstable angina, (2) prolonged anginal episode, which might represent an infarction, and (3) MI.

I. **Unstable Angina (USA)**

A. **Management.**

1. **The decision to admit** is based on the history, since 50% of patients with acute MI will have a nondiagnostic ECG changes and cardiac

enzymes will not be positive for up to 6 hours after an infarction. If ECG changes indicate MI, or if enzymes are positive, treat as per MI section below.

2. **Admit to monitored bed.** Bed rest with bedside commode, continuous cardiac monitoring, oxygen, and IV access. Obtain screening lab tests, including cardiac enzymes, CBC, glucose, BUN, creatinine, UA, serum electrolytes, including sodium, potassium, chloride, CO_2, and magnesium, PT/PTT/INR if planning to anticoagulate.

3. **Obtain serial cardiac enzyme levels.** Cardiac troponin I and T are proteins that are highly sensitive and specific for myocardial injury. These markers are now considered the standard. An alternative is creatine phosphokinase (CPK). Obtain an MB isoenzyme level if the total CPK is elevated since CPK can be the result of both cardiac and other muscle breakdown. The CPK is more sensitive than the troponin at hours 4-8 (84% versus 74%) and at 8-12 hours (94% versus 88%). The troponin is essentially 100% sensitive at 12 hours. The troponin may remain elevated for 4 to 7 days. Either troponin or CPK levels should be checked Q8h × 3 (although if the CPK and troponin are negative at 12 hours after pain resolves, an MI is effectively ruled out).

4. **Serial ECGs** with intervals depending on circumstances.

5. **Increase anti-anginals.** Topical, oral, or SL nitrates, calcium-channel blockers, or beta-blockers. May need IV nitroglycerin. Morphine (2 to 5 mg Q10-20min) may be given for analgesia, preload reduction, and anxiety. *Ongoing chest pain that does not respond to standard anti-ischemic regimens (aspirin, heparin, beta-blockers and IV nitroglycerin) is a cardiac emergency and should prompt consideration of referral to a center equipped with a catheterization laboratory.*

6. **Other medications.** Sedation may be beneficial in certain patients. Acetaminophen and a stool softener may be given for headache and preventing the need to strain, respectively.

7. **Aspirin.** With few exceptions, **aspirin should be given to anyone with unstable angina or an evolving MI** and will reduce the rate of MI and death. Aspirin should be continued indefinitely.

8. **Heparin.** Those patients who appear particularly unstable or who have recurrent ischemia are likely to benefit from adding heparin (APTT 1.5 to 2 times normal) to aspirin for the duration of the period of the unstable angina. See Chapter 6 for the details of heparin management. Recently, enoxaparin 1mg/kg SQ BID has been shown to be at least as good and perhaps superior to IV heparin for this indication. However, these data are preliminary and need to be confirmed.

9. **G2,3B platelet inhibitors.** Studies have shown benefit from treating the patient with eptifbatide (Integrelin) (180 μg/kg load then 2 μg/kg/min × 72 hours] or tirofiban (Aggrastat) [0.4 μg/kg/min × 30 min, then 0.1 μg/kg/min × 2-4 days as indicated) combined

with heparin (dosed to achieve PTT of 2 times control). These drugs are indicated in essentially all patients who are going for other intervention (e.g., PTCA or stent placement). There is still debate about the usefulness of these agents before planned bypass surgery and in those with unstable angina in whom no further intervention is planned. If coronary artery bypass surgery is planned, aspirin should be started preoperatively because it increases postoperative graft-patency rates.

10. **For patients not anticoagulated,** heparin 5000 units SQ Q12h should be given for DVT prophylaxis.

11. **If cardiac enzymes become positive,** treat the patient for MI. If the patient is ruled out for an MI, the patient will still need some assessment of myocardium at risk (such as GXT on increased medications, a thallium study, or cardiac catheterization).

II. Acute MI (AMI)

Modalities begun for acute angina should be continued (see Chapter 2). Thrombolysis should be used as if the patient meets ECG criteria and is within the first 12 hours by symptoms.

A. Defined by ECG changes or serum cardiac enzyme changes; 50% of patients with an acute MI will have a nondiagnostic initial ECG, and so the decision to admit should be made on the basis of the history.

1. **ECG patterns.**

   a. Ischemia is indicated by ST-segment depression, nonspecific ST-T-segment changes, and T-wave inversion. These may also accompany a non-Q wave infarction.

   b. Injury indicated by ST-segment elevation. Tall peaked T waves (10 mV) are suggestive of hyperacute injury.

   c. Infarct indicated by the development of Q waves.

2. Infarct location by ECG (Table 3-1).

TABLE 3-1

INFARCT LOCATION BY ECG

ECG Changes	Location of Injury	Coronary Artery
II, III, aV$_F$	Inferior wall (may be associated with RV injury, consider right precordial leads)	RCA or dominant distal left circumflex
V$_{1-3}$	Anteroseptal	LAD
V$_{3-5}$	Anterior wall	LAD
V$_6$, I, aV$_L$	Lateral	Marginal branch off circumflex or diagonal off LAD
ST depression in V$_{1-2}$ with large R wave.	Posterior	RCA

B. **Management. See acute management of chest pain in Chapter 2.**
   1. Orders similar to unstable angina. Unless contraindication, all patients should have aspirin.
   2. Hypokalemia and hypomagnesemia are risk factors for arrhythmias and should be corrected if present.
   3. Studies are currently underway to assess the efficacy of MAGIK (magnesium, glucose, insulin and potassium) in acute MI. At this point, these cannot be recommended for routine use.
   4. **Percutaneous coronary intervention (PCI).** In the era of intracoronary stents with antiplatelet agents, this has clearly become the preferred modality for the treatment of AMI. If care is rendered at a facility where PCI can be performed in a timely fashion, it is recommended that this be done. Otherwise, treat as per thrombolytics section.
   5. **Thrombolytics.** It is recommended that every patient with an evolving MI be **considered** for thrombolytic therapy, which reduces both in-hospital and 1-year mortality by 25%. Evolving MI is defined as at least 30 minutes of ischemic cardiac pain and at least 1 mm of ST-segment elevation in at least two adjacent limb leads or at least 1 to 2 mm of ST-segment elevation in at least two adjacent precordial leads. (These criteria indicate a high likelihood of evolving MI.) The presence of a new complete bundle branch block in addition to characteristic pain also indicates the patient will benefit from thrombolysis. Patients with only ST-segment depression or normal ECGs, even with symptoms, do not benefit. There is evidence that patients who receive thrombolytics from 6 to 12 hours after onset of acute MI may still benefit, although the benefit is less than that for patients who present less than 6 hours after onset of pain.
      a. **Absolute contraindications** to thrombolytic therapy include recent (<6 weeks) surgery or biopsy of a noncompressible site, recent stroke, **any history of hemorrhagic stroke,** intracranial neoplasm, recent head trauma, pregnancy, or prolonged or traumatic CPR, aortic dissection, acute pericarditis, active bleeding, and antibodies to streptokinase (substitute tissue-type plasminogen activator [TPA] if the patient has antibodies to streptokinase). If there has been a previous allergic reaction to streptokinase, use of TPA is indicated.
      b. **Dosing and administration.** TPA may provide a greater decrease in mortality than does streptokinase. In general, if there are no contraindications, streptokinase is preferred by some because of its lower cost.
         (1) **Streptokinase** 1.5 million IU given IV over 1 hour **or**
         (2) **TPA** 100 mg of single-chain preparation. The accelerated dose regimen is preferred and consists of giving 60 mg during the first half-hour and the second 40 mg over an additional hour. Concurrent heparin infusion to achieve PTT 2 times normal (see Chapter 6 for management of anticoagulation) **or**

(3) **Reteplase** 10.8 units over 2 minutes; repeat in 30 minutes. Concurrent heparin infusion.

6. **Heparin and aspirin.** It is recommended that every patient who receives thrombolytic therapy be considered for adjuvant anticoagulation therapy for approximately 48 hours (heparin to keep APTT 1.5 to 2 times control, see Chapter 6 for management of anticoagulation). **Discontinuing heparin after 72 hours or so may result in rebound angina because of a relatively hypercoagulable state from antithrombin III deficiency.** Long-term aspirin therapy (160 to 325 mg QD) should be considered for all patients unless specifically contraindicated.

7. **Beta-blockers** are indicated for most patients early (within 6 or 7 hours) during the evolution of an MI and those with persistent or recurrent pain or tachyarrhythmias. A beta-blocker such as metoprolol 15 mg can be given in 5 mg aliquots Q5min. This should be followed by oral beta-blocker therapy to reduce long-term mortality. Patients who are seen in the first 4 to 6 hours of onset of an MI or who present with hypertension or sinus tachycardia and are not in heart failure are considered to be good candidates for beta-blockade.

   a. **Some of the relative contraindications to beta-blocker use include:** lengthening of the PR interval 0.24 second, second- or third-degree AV block, bradycardia with pulse <50, systolic blood pressure <90 mm Hg, pulmonary artery wedge pressure greater than a range of 20 to 24 mm Hg, rales audible in greater than one-third of the lung fields, wheezing or history of asthma or bronchospasm, and recent use of IV calcium-channel blockers.

8. **Angiotensin-converting enzyme (ACE) inhibitors.** There are several large prospective controlled clinical trials demonstrating the efficacy of ACE inhibitors both acutely and chronically in patients who have sustained an MI. Starting an ACE inhibitor within 24 hours of an MI (enalapril 2.5 mg PO BID titrated to 10 mg PO BID) reduces mortality. Additionally, ACE inhibitors (captopril titrated to 50 mg PO TID or ramipril given at a dose of 5 mg PO BID) continued after an MI in those with CHF or an ejection fraction <45% will decrease mortality (including sudden death), increase exercise capacity, reduce CHF, enable ventricular remodeling, and control hypertension.

9. **Angiography.** Post-MI coronary angiography and revascularization are indicated for patients with continuing ischemia. Asymptomatic patients with uncomplicated MI and without any inducible angina generally do not require angiography.

10. **Ambulatory monitoring.** Ambulatory monitoring after an MI adds information and may be an alternative to stress testing in determining which patient continues to have asymptomatic ischemia.

3

CARDIOLOGY

11. **Prophylactic lidocaine** is no longer routinely used for patients with suspected acute MI but is still the drug of choice for the treatment of malignant ventricular arrhythmias. Many patients with ventricular tachycardias or ventricular fibrillation will not have a warning arrhythmia.

COMPLICATIONS OF ACUTE MI

I. **Left Ventricular Dysfunction.** See section on congestive failure for long term management of CHF.

A. The extent of LV dysfunction in the days after an acute MI provides prognostic information.

B. Treatment of LV dysfunction (CHF) depends on severity but may include: 1) Avoiding medications that exacerbate heart failure. 2) A low-sodium diet and a diuretic to prevent fluid overload (such as furosemide). 3) Increase FiO_2 and provide ventilatory support if required.

C. **If the patient is in cardiogenic shock,** IV inotropic agents such as dopamine 2 to 20 μg/kg/min or dobutamine 2.5 to 15 μg/kg/min may help to improve LV function. Hemodynamic monitoring and a urinary catheter maybe required to manage fluid status. A PCWP <10 mm Hg is suggestive of the need for additional fluid volume, whereas a PCWP 20-25 mm Hg is suggestive of fluid overload.

1. If the cardiogenic shock is secondary to ischemic "stunned" myocardium, intra-aortic balloon counterpulsation, cardiac catheterization, or emergency revascularization may be warranted.

II. **Right Ventricular Dysfunction**

A. Especially prominent with an inferior wall MI secondary to right ventricular infarction. Pronounced hypotension in response to nitrates should be suggestive of this diagnosis.

B. The triad of clear lung fields, hypotension, and jugular venous distension (JVD) in a patient with an inferior infarction is highly suggestive of a right ventricular infarction. JVD has a sensitivity of 88% and a specificity of 69% for right ventricular infarction. Kussmaul's venous sign (distension of the jugular vein during inspiration) is also highly suggestive. There may also be tricuspid regurgitation, right ventricular gallops, and atrioventricular dissociation.

C. An ECG with right-sided chest leads can confirm right ventricular MI (RVMI). A 1-mm ST-segment elevation in the right precordial lead CR4R is highly predictive for an RVMI (sensitivity 70%, specificity 100%). Other ECG findings include right bundle branch block and complete heart block.

D. Echocardiography may reveal right ventricular wall dyskinesia and dilatation. There may be abnormal interventricular septal motion because of a reversal in the transseptal pressure gradient secondary to increased right ventricular end-diastolic pressure.

E. In addition to conduction deficits, patients with RVMI may develop right ventricular mural thrombi (placing them at high risk for pulmonary embolism), tricuspid regurgitation, and pericarditis.

F. The following are important components of a treatment regimen for right ventricular infarction:
   1. Maintain right ventricular preload with volume loading as indicated. An infusion of IV normal saline frequently corrects hypotension and increases cardiac output. The use of nitrates, diuretics, and morphine sulfate are all relatively contraindicated, since these medications decrease preload.
   2. Reduce right ventricular afterload if there is concomitant left ventricular dysfunction (e.g., treat left-sided CHF).
   3. Initiate inotropic support with dobutamine if the patient is not stabilized hemodynamically with a saline infusion.
   4. Begin sequential atrioventricular pacing if the patient develops complete heart block.
   5. Initiate thrombolytic therapy or perform angioplasty as indicated.
G. Among patients who survive a right ventricular infarction, right ventricular function returns to nearly normal levels over time.

III. **Arrhythmias Complicating Acute MI**
A. **Premature ventricular complexes (PVCs).**
   1. Common in first 72 hours after an MI **and may not have an antecedent arrhythmias.**
   2. Usually do not require treatment unless they are:
      a. Frequent (10/min).
      b. Multiform.
      c. Occurring close to preceding T-wave (R-on-T phenomenon), or
      d. Occurring in pairs, triplets, or short runs.
   3. Usually treated with a lidocaine bolus followed by infusion. See ACLS protocol in Chapter 1.
B. **Ventricular tachycardia or fibrillation.** See protocol in Chapter 1.
C. **Supraventricular tachycardias including PSVT and atrial fibrillation or flutter.** See protocol in Chapter 1.
   1. Tachycardia increases O_2 demand; so treat promptly.
   2. Rule out reversible underlying causes (such as hypokalemia, hypomagnesemia and hypoxia).

IV. **Atrioventricular Block**
A. **Mobitz I (Wenckebach).**
   1. Common in acute inferior infarction.
   2. See ACLS protocol in Chapter 1.
   3. A permanent pacemaker is rarely required, since Wenckebach block usually resolves within days.
B. **Mobitz II.**
   1. Usually occurs in patients with acute anterior Mis.
   2. In the setting of an acute MI, with Mobitz II AV block, a temporary pacemaker should be placed. Often the block is permanent, and a permanent pacemaker should be placed if the block persists for 1 week or more.

3

CARDIOLOGY

C. **Third-degree AV block.**
   1. Third-degree AV block is often transient in the setting of an acute inferior MI.
   2. When associated with an anterior MI, it often represents necrosis of the conducting tissue below the AV node and may be permanent, requiring permanent pacemaker implantation.
D. **Bundle branch block.**
   1. A left bundle branch block is the most common bundle branch block seen with an MI. The combination of a right bundle branch block and a left anterior hemiblock is also frequently seen.
   2. When a bundle branch block occurs, the site of the infarction is usually anteroseptal, and the infarct is often large.
   3. If the patient is known to have an old bundle branch or fascicular block a temporary pacemaker is not necessarily indicated unless dictated by the patient's symptoms and hemodynamic status.
   4. If the patient has a **new** left bundle branch block or bifascicular block associated with an MI, a temporary pacemaker may be indicated. A bifascicular block is defined as the combination of a right BBB and a left anterior posterior hemiblock.
V. **Left Ventricular Aneurysm**
A. **Incidence** 7% to 15%, suggested by persistent ST elevations weeks to months after an MI.
B. **May lead to CHF,** systemic emboli (caused by mural thrombus formation), and recurrent arrhythmias.
C. **Can be demonstrated on echocardiogram** or radionuclide ventriculogram.
D. Some authors recommend long-term anticoagulation to reduce the risk of embolization. Surgical resection may be indicated for refractory LV failure, recurrent emboli despite anticoagulation, or medically refractory ventricular arrhythmias if electrophysiology studies indicate that the aneurysm maybe the focus of the arrhythmia.
VI. **Recurrent Chest Pain**
A. **Extension of MI.**
   1. Occurs in 10% to 15%.
   2. Characterized by reelevation of cardiac enzymes and additional ECG changes.
   3. Patients with non-Q wave infarcts are at higher risk of extension of infarct in the 12 months after an MI than patients with transmural infarcts.
B. **Angina.** For treatment and diagnosis, see section above. If post-MI angina is refractory to medical therapy, cardiac catheterization may be indicated to define anatomy and suitability for revascularization or to perform PTCA.
C. **Pericarditis.** May occur after an MI or as the result of a viral infection (especially coxsackie virus), or secondary to uremia. In the setting of an infarction, pericarditis usually occurs after a large transmural infarct.

1. **Physical exam** may reveal an audible friction rub.
2. **Pleuritic pain,** exacerbated by lying supine, relieved by sitting forward, may be present; tends to radiate to shoulder and be worse on inspiration.
3. **ECG may show** diffuse ST-segment elevations, and echocardiogram frequently reveals the presence of a pericardial effusion. However, the ECG may be false negative in up to 20%.
4. **Treatment.** NSAIDs, especially indomethacin. Steroids may be used for viral pericarditis but should be avoided in an acute MI. **Avoid** anticoagulation because of the risk of converting the effusion into a hemorrhagic one with risk of cardiac tamponade.

D. **Pulmonary embolism.** If not on IV heparin, post-MI patients should be maintained on prophylactic doses of SQ heparin (5000 units Q12h) until fully mobile. See Chapter 4 for the work-up and treatment of pulmonary embolism.

E. **Pneumonia.**

IV. **Dressler's Syndrome**

A. **Cause.** Pleuropericarditis occurring usually 2 to 4 weeks after an MI. Possibly represents an autoimmune inflammatory reaction.

B. **Symptoms.** Pericardial and pleural pain.

C. **Signs.** Fever, pericardial friction rub (may be intermittent), and perhaps decreased breath sounds at lung bases and a pleural rub. Chest radiograph may show enlarged cardiac silhouette because of pericardial effusion. ECG may show diffuse ST-segment elevations, decreased R-wave voltage, and occasionally electrical alternans. An echocardiogram may show pericardial effusion.

D. **Treatment.** Usually self-limited. NSAIDs; glucocorticoids if NSAIDs not effective. Avoid anticoagulation for reasons stated above.

CARDIAC ARRHYTHMIAS

For outpatient assessment, an "event monitor" worn for a prolonged period and activated when patient has symptoms is more sensitive than a 24- to 48-hour "Holter" monitor and is the preferred modality for intermittent or sporadic arrhythmias.

I. **Atrial fibrillation (A fib)** results in the loss of atrial contraction and an irregular ventricular rate. Clinically recognized by an irregularly irregular heart rate. Some causes include hypertension, hyperthyroidism, acute pulmonary embolism, CHF, valvular disease (especially mitral valve), acute alcohol use ("holiday heart"), and postoperative state, especially, thoracotomy.

A. **See protocol in Chapter 1 for acute management** of A fib with a rapid ventricular response.

B. **Rate control.** Long-term therapy must control ventricular rate with agents that increase the refractory period of the AV node (digoxin, verapamil, diltiazem, or beta-blockers). The ventricular rate should be decreased to a range of 80 to 100 beats/min. Generally, beta-blockers are

3

CARDIOLOGY

the drugs of choice. Digoxin is useful in rate control in those with CHF or at bed rest but may not be sufficient in those who are ambulatory. Additionally, digoxin is proarrhythmic.

C. **Long-term anticoagulation** with warfarin (INR 2.0 to 3.0) is indicated for those in A fib who are older than 60 years of age or have valvular disease, underlying heart disease, hypertension, diabetes, or previous evidence of embolism (CVA, TIA). Those with "lone" A fib (age less than <60, none of the above risk factors, and no cardiovascular disease) have a low incidence of complications and need not be anticoagulated. Aspirin is second best and should be reserved for those not able to take warfarin (e.g., because of high risk of falls).

D. Many of those with A fib will convert back to sinus rhythm spontaneously. May attempt to convert back to a sinus rhythm with either class III drugs (amiodarone or sotalol) or class I drugs (quinidine or procainamide), flecainide, or cardioversion. **However, these patients should be anticoagulated for 3 weeks before cardioversion if A fib has been present for more than 48 hours.** Anticoagulation should be continued for 2 weeks after conversion. Ibutilide has been used to convert atrial fibrillation but is falling out of favor.

II. **Paroxysmal supraventricular tachycardia.** Most commonly caused by atrioventricular node reentry with 1:1 atrioventricular conduction, although may also be caused by sinus node reentry, atrial ectopy, or an accessory pathway. Commonly associated with Wolff-Parkinson-White syndrome.

A. Must be distinguished from a ventricular tachycardia.

B. See protocol in Chapter 1 for acute management.

C. Chronically may be suppressed with calcium-channel blockers (verapamil and diltiazem). However, radioablation of the accessory pathway is both safe and effective.

III. **Ventricular tachycardia.** Ventricular rate is generally 150 to 180 beats/min. Rhythm tends to be regular, and AV dissociation is a common feature. By definition, it is characterized by three or more consecutive complexes arising inferior to the bifurcation of the bundle of His at a rate that exceeds 100 beats/min.

A. May be caused by heart disease, electrolyte imbalances, hypoxia, and drug toxicity. The most frequent cause of sustained ventricular tachycardia is reentry along the margin of old infarcted myocardium.

B. See protocol in Chapter 1 for acute treatment.

C. Since recurrence rates are high, long-term antiarrhythmic therapy or the implantation of a cardioverter-defibrillator may be indicated **for those with sustained or symptomatic ventricular tachycardia. Overall, implantable defibrillators seem to have the best outcomes.** Traditional antiarrhythmic agents (e.g., flecainide/encainide) actually increase mortality 2- to 3-fold. Sotalol and amiodarone are showing promise in the treatment of these patients. Beta-blockers (such as metoprolol, propranolol) also may be useful. Generally, a cardiology consult should be obtained to determine the best approach to chronic suppression of this arrhythmia.

IV. **Sick sinus syndrome.**
A. Episodes of bradycardia interspersed with episodic tachycardia from si-nus tachycardia or atrial fibrillation. May cause syncope.
B. Generally a disease of the elderly.
C. Treatment generally requires pacemaker to prevent bradycardia as well as medications such as digoxin or verapamil to control tachycardia.

VALVULAR HEART DISEASE

I. **General.** Can present with a spectrum of symptoms based on the valve involved, stenosis or regurgitation, right- or left-sided, and single valve or multivalvular disease. An echocardiogram is critical to the evaluation of a patient with a heart murmur to determine if the murmur is the result of a valve lesion. Table 3-2 summarizes valvular heart disease.

II. **Mitral Valve Prolapse (MVP).** May result from leaflet billowing, progres-sive expansion of the mitral annulus, or valve-leaflet myxomatous de-generation. Most patients with MVP are asymptomatic and will have a benign clinical course. Symptoms may include palpitations, fatigue, dyspnea, syncope, atypical chest pain, and episodes of supraventricular tachycardia. **However, these symptoms are as common in the general population as in those with MVP and many patients with MVP found incidentally on echocardiography do not have these symptoms.** A small proportion of patients experience strokes, TIAs, seizures, or episodes of amaurosis fugax, but whether this is related to the MVP is questionable (Freed LA et al: *NEJM* 341:1, 1999). Patients with severe myxomatous change and thickened leaflets are at greatest risk of embolic events.

A. **Examination.** MVP is associated with a midsystolic click, which may be intermittent. If there is mitral regurgitation, the aforementioned click will be followed by a midsystolic to late systolic murmur.

B. **Management and Treatment.** Diagnosis may be confirmed with the use of echocardiography. Antibiotic prophylaxis should be used for patients with MVP who have regurgitation or are symptomatic from their illness.

CONGESTIVE HEART FAILURE

I. **Causes.** Two-thirds caused by CAD. The second most common cause is dilated cardiomyopathy, which can be idiopathic or may result from tox-ins (alcohol, doxorubicin), infection (often viral), or collagen vascular disease. Other causes include chronic hypertension (diastolic dysfunc-tion), valvular heart disease, hypertrophic cardiomyopathy, and restric-tive cardiomyopathy (amyloidosis, sarcoidosis, and hemochromatosis).

II. **Evaluation.**
A. **History.** Typical symptoms include fatigue, dyspnea, orthopnea, paroxys-mal nocturnal dyspnea, nocturia, or chronic cough.
B. **Physical exam.** JVD, hepatojugular reflux, S_3 gallop, rales, and periph-eral edema. However, these are not present in all those with CHF.
C. **Studies.** Baseline CXR and ECG. An echocardiogram should always be done to evaluate LV and RV ejection fractions, movement of chamber

3

CARDIOLOGY

TABLE 3-2

COMMON VALVULAR LESIONS AND THEIR MANAGEMENT

Lesion	Etiology	Symptoms	Complications	Treatment	Endocarditis Prophylaxis?	Follow-up
Mitral stenosis	Rheumatic heart disease	CHF, dyspnea	A-fib, pulmonary hypertension, pulmonary fibrosis, or edema	Repair or replacement before symptoms are severe	Yes	Periodic echo (1-2 yrs)
Mitral regurgitation	CAD, endocarditis, connective tissue disorder, dilated cardiomyopathy	CHF, respiratory distress	A-fib	Treat for CHF, replace valve if unstable.	Yes	Periodic echo (1-2 yrs)
Mitral valve prolapse	See text	See text	See text	See text	See text	See text
Aortic stenosis	Congenital bicuspid valve, rheumatic heart disease, age-related valve sclerosis.	Angina, syncope, CHF		Repair or replace valve as soon as possible, if symptomatic. If CHF, patients survive less than 2 yrs.	Yes	Any symptomatic patient should have cardiac cath and consideration for valve replacement. If asymptomatic, echo every 12 mon.

Aortic regurgitation (chronic)	Rheumatic fever, myxomatous degeneration, Marfan's syndrome, syphilis, Reiter's disease, ankylosing spondylitis	CHF, PND, palpitations, chest, neck, back pain	Diuretics, digoxin, salt restriction. Not vasodilator therapy, though. Valve replacement before significant CHF. EF not <55%.	Yes	Echo every 6 mon to 1 yr with valve replacement while EF is not less than 55%.
Aortic regurgitation (acute)	Trauma, endocarditis, acute rheumatic fever, dissection	Sudden onset dyspnea, tachycardia, tachypnea, shock	Acute intervention for surgery		

EF, Ejection fraction.

walls and valves, and chamber sizes and to differentiate systolic from diastolic dysfunction. In systolic dysfunction, ejection fraction is decreased. Electrolytes, BUN, creatinine, ABG, CBC, and serum digoxin level if indicated. Patients should also be evaluated for obstructive sleep apnea, which can lead to CHF (see Chapter 4).

III. **Treatment of Acute CHF Secondary to Systolic Dysfunction**

A. **Precipitators of acute pulmonary edema** (in a previously compensated patient). Poor compliance with medical or diet therapy, increased metabolic demands (infection, especially pneumonia, pregnancy, anemia, hyperthyroidism), progression of underlying heart disease, arrhythmias (e.g., tachycardia), drug effect (beta-blockers, calcium-channel blockers, other negative inotropes), silent MI, pulmonary embolism.

B. **Diagnosis.** The diagnosis of pulmonary edema is usually made initially by physical exam and confirmed by CXR. Treatment may have to be started before one obtains a detailed history, etc. However, once the patient is stable, a careful work-up should be undertaken to determine underlying causes and precipitating factors.

　1. **History.** Past history of cardiac and pulmonary disease or hypertension. History of shortness of breath, orthopnea, dyspnea on exertion, faintness, chest pain. Recent weight gain, edema. Recent infection, exposure to toxic inhalants, smoke, possible aspiration. Current medication regimen, compliance with diet and medications. **However, PND and orthopnea are not specific for CHF.**

　2. **Physical exam.** Tachypnea, tachycardia, often BP is elevated. If patient has fever, suspect concurrent infection, which may increase metabolic demand and lead to CHF. Cyanosis, diaphoresis, retractions, use of accessory muscles of respiration, wheezing ("cardiac asthma"), and rales on lung auscultation. Cough may be productive of pink, frothy sputum. Listen for S3 gallop or murmurs. Peripheral edema and positive hepatojugular reflux are suggestive of CHF, and bruits may be a clue to underlying vascular disease.

C. **Diagnostic tests.**

　1. **Lab tests.** Electrolytes, BUN, creatinine, cardiac enzymes, serum protein and albumin, urinalysis, differential CBC count, and ABG.

　2. **CXR.** Initially will show interstitial edema as well as thickening and loss of definition of the shadows of pulmonary vasculature. Fluid in septal planes and interlobular fissures cause the characteristic appearance of Kerley A and B lines. Eventually, pleural effusions and perihilar alveolar edema may develop in the classic "butterfly" pattern. CXR findings may lag behind the clinical presentation by up to 12 hours and may take 4 days to clear after clinical improvement in the patient.

　3. **EKG.** Evaluate for evidence of MI and arrhythmia. The sudden onset of atrial fibrillation or PSVT may cause acute decompensation in previously stable chronic CHF. LVH may signal underlying aortic stenosis, hypertension, or cardiomyopathy.

4. **Echocardiography.** Not imperative acutely. In work-up for underlying cause, it is useful to evaluate for valvular disease, valvular vegetations, wall-motion abnormalities, LV function, and cardiomyopathy.

D. **Treatment**

1. **Oxygen.** By nasal cannula or mask. May require endotracheal intubation if unable to adequately oxygenate despite use of 100% oxygen by non-rebreather mask. Mask continuous positive airway pressure (CPAP) has been shown to reduce the need for intubation and is an excellent alternative.

2. **Other general measures.** Elevate head of bed 30 degrees. May need Swan-Ganz catheter for hemodynamic monitoring if the patient becomes hypotensive. However, Swan-Ganz catheters may have an adverse effect on mortality and should be used only after careful consideration. If indicated, place a Foley catheter for fluid management.

3. **Medications.**

a. **Vasodilators** are considered the first drug of choice in acute CHF and act by preload and afterload thereby decreasing LV work. May also reverse myocardial ischemia. **IV nitroglycerin** is commonly used, especially if there is concern that ischemia is an underlying or precipitating factor. Start at 10 to 20 μg/min and increase by increments of 10 to 20 μg/min Q5 min until the desired effect is achieved. **Sublingual nitroglycerin** 0.4 mg repeated Q5 min PRN can also be used acutely as can topical nitrates. However, topical nitrates may not be effective acutely with a maximal effect at 120 minutes. **Nitroprusside is an alternative** (start at 0.5 μg/kg/min and increase by 0.5 μg/kg/min Q5 min). Most patients respond to less than 10 μg/kg/min but titrate to effect. **Nitroprusside** is more likely to cause hypotension than is IV nitroglycerin. A fluid bolus may help to reverse nitrate-induced hypotension but should be used judiciously in those with CHF.

b. **Furosemide and other diuretics.** If the patient has never been treated with **furosemide** may start with 20 mg IV and observe response. Titrate dose upward until adequate diuresis is established. If the patient is receiving furosemide over a long-term give 1 to 2 times the usual daily dose by slow (over 1 to 2 minutes) IV bolus. Larger doses (up to 1 g) may be needed in those patients receiving large doses or with a history of renal disease. Alternatively, a furosemide drip can be established for higher doses. Give 20% of the dose as a bolus (that is, 200 mg) and infuse the rest over 8 hours. This has a greater efficacy than a single, large bolus does. Up to 2 g has been safely administered in this fashion. **Ethacrynic** acid 25 to 100 mg IV may be needed if the patient does not respond to furosemide. **Bumetanide** (0.5 to 1.0 mg IV) may also be used. Adding **metolazone** (5 to 20 mg) or **chlorothiazide** 500 mg IV to furosemide may generate additional diuresis. Some authors would consider phlebotomy if diuretics are ineffective and patient has a high HCT, but this is a high risk procedure.

c. **Morphine** acts as a venodilator and decreases anxiety. Start with 1 to 2 mg IV. Tritiate carefully in COPD and CHF, since narcotics can decrease respiratory drive.

d. **ACE inhibitors** can be used acutely in the management of CHF but are more common as chronic therapy. Captopril 12.5 to 25 mg SL or IV at 0.16 mg/min increased by 0.08 mg/min every 5 minutes until it has the desired effect. This is safe and effective and should can be used in patients unresponsive to oxygen, nitrates and diuretics.

e. **Dobutamine** (2.5 to 15 μg/kg/min) or dopamine (2 to 20 μg/kg/min) may be needed for pressure support or as a positive inotrope. These drugs are effective immediately; however, although dopamine increases renal perfusion, it may not increase GFR.

f. **Digoxin.** Check ECG, serum potassium, BUN, and creatinine first before loading with digoxin. After digoxin loading, it may be difficult to distinguish ischemic changes on ECG from digoxin effect. Inquire about previous use of digoxin and any adverse reactions. Determine if patient has any history of renal, pulmonary, liver, or thyroid disease. Be aware of other medications that the patient takes that might affect digoxin levels such as amiodarone, flecainide, quinidine, and verapamil. Decrease digoxin dose if the patient has renal disease. The aim is to achieve serum levels of 1.0 to 1.5 ng/ml.

4. **Surgery** may be indicated under rare conditions such as valvular heart disease or rupture of ventricular septum after an MI. In severe LV failure, an intra-aortic balloon pump may be beneficial as a temporizing measure.

IV. **Outpatient Treatment of CHF Secondary to Systolic Dysfunction**

A. **Nonpharmacologic therapy.** Avoid excessive physical stress, reduce dietary salt, consider compressive stockings if needed to reduce risk of DVT (consider SQ heparin if inpatient), and weight loss if obese. Work on walking and endurance training.

B. **Pharmacologic therapy.**

1. **Drugs that have been shown to reduce mortality in CHF:** ACE inhibitors, beta-blockers (e.g., metoprolol), spironolactone and the combination of hydralazine + isosorbide dinitrate.

2. **Diuretics.** Loop diuretics are usually recommended (e.g., furosemide). Some patients develop resistance to loop diuretics after chronic usage. A single dose of metolazone (5 to 20 mg QD) will often result in significant diuresis in such patients. Patients with heart failure who are receiving diuretics should have potassium and magnesium levels monitored. Supplementation should be provided if necessary, since hypokalemia and hypomagnesemia are risk factors for

the development of arrhythmias. **The use of spironolactone at low dose (25 mg QD) has recently been shown to reduce morbidity in patients even if already treated with a standard therapy, including loop diuretics (RALES trial).**

3. **ACE inhibitors.** These agents function primarily as afterload reducers and have been shown to reduce morbidity (CHF progression, MI, need for hospitalization) and mortality. ACE inhibitors also improve hemodynamics and increase exercise tolerance in heart failure. Up to now only captopril, enalapril, lisinopril, and ramipril have been shown to be efficacious in large controlled clinical trials however, it is likely a class specific effect. Begin therapy at low doses such as enalapril 2.5 mg PO BID and titrate to 10 mg PO BID gradually. Observe the patient for hypotension or persistent cough. Monitor electrolytes and renal function because ACE inhibitors can cause elevation of serum potassium and can cause a **reversible** decrease in renal function in some patients. Patients at high risk for adverse effects from ACE inhibitors include those with connective tissue diseases, preexisting renal insufficiency, or bilateral renal artery stenosis. Contraindications to their use include a history of hypersensitivity to ACE inhibitors, serum potassium greater than 5.5 mEq/L (consider evaluation for hypoaldosteronism or Addison's disease), or a previous episode of angioedema during their use. Relative contraindications include renal failure and hypotension. However, ACE inhibitors actually protect renal function in those with chronic renal failure (see Chapter 8 for details). In the latter two patient groups, ACE inhibitor therapy should be initiated at half the usual starting dose and titrated to desired effect.

4. **Beta-blockers.** The use of beta-blockers in patients with CHF caused by systolic dysfunction is now the standard of care. The initiation and titration of these medications should be undertaken with care. The studied agents that are recommended are carvedilol and metoprolol (specifically Toprol-XL). These agents appear to confer myocardial protection by inhibiting a variety of damaging neurohumoral effects activated by CHF.

5. **Angiotensin-receptor blockers** (ARBs) function by afterload reduction and have been shown to have an equivalent effect to ACE inhibitors. The limitations of ACE inhibitors (cough, angioedema) are not prevalent with these agents; however, their effects on renal function are still under investigation. They should not supplant ACE inhibitors but can be substituted for them for patients who are intolerant of ACE-I. The results of studies investigating the combined use of ARBs with ACE inhibitors are not yet known.

6. **Other vasodilators.** ACE-I therapy increases survival in heart failure more than the combination hydralazine and isosorbide therapy. However, in patients unable to tolerate ACE inhibitors or an ARB, a combination of hydralazine and isosorbide dinitrate may be used.

3

CARDIOLOGY

7. **Digoxin** is shown to improve **symptoms** in severe heart failure and in cases where atrial fibrillation is a complication of CHF. **However, digoxin has no effect on mortality because of a proarrhythmic effect and should be considered a measure for symptom control only.** Rapid digitalization is not necessary in patients with chronic CHF. The half-life of digoxin is 1½ to 2 days in patients with normal renal function. The usual starting dose is 0.25 mg/day. Decrease the dose in small or elderly patients and in those receiving other drugs (such as quinidine, amiodarone, and verapamil) that raise digoxin levels. Decrease the dose in patients with impaired renal function. Monitor levels, especially after dose adjustments or after changes in other medications that may affect digoxin levels (such as quinidine, verapamil, and oral azole antifungals). **Avoid digoxin in patients with idiopathic hypertrophic subaortic stenosis (IHSS) and those with diastolic dysfunction.** Watch potassium levels closely; hypokalemia renders the heart more sensitive to digoxin and will predispose to digoxin toxicity.

8. **Intermittent intravenous inotrope infusions. Dobutamine** is the parenteral inotropic agent of choice in severe, chronic CHF. Onset of action is immediate and stops quickly when the infusion is discontinued. It should not be used in patients with IHSS except in consultation with a cardiologist. May cause tachycardia, angina, and ventricular arrhythmias. Alternatively, **Milrinone** may be used to both improve contractile functions and cause some degree of vasodilation. May cause ventricular arrhythmias. Effect of these modalities on mortality is not yet known.

9. **Calcium-channel blockers.** Some calcium-channel blockers, especially verapamil and diltiazem, are relatively potent negative inotropic agents and should generally be avoided in patients with poor LV function. In patients with CHF and hypertension, amlodipine (a second-generation dihydropyridine calcium-channel blocker with no negative inotropic effect) has been shown to be efficacious.

10. **Antithrombotic therapy.** Patients with a previous history of embolism or A fib are at high risk for thromboembolic complications and should be considered for warfarin therapy unless a contraindication exists. Titrate the dose to an INR of 2.0 to 3.0 (prothrombin time not more than 1.5 times normal) to avoid increased risk of bleeding complications. If warfarin cannot be used, consider aspirin for the antiplatelet effect (80 to 300 mg/day).

11. **Ventricular Assist Devices** (VADs). These devices have been shown to improve morbidity and survival in selected patients waiting to undergo transplantation. The decision to implant such a device should be made only after careful evaluation by a surgeon trained in their insertion. Follow-up care involves close collaboration with transplant facility. VADs are being studied as stand-alone therapy for patients not considered candidates for transplantation.

V. **Follow-up.** Once the acute episode of pulmonary edema is under control, a careful search for the underlying cause must be undertaken. Further work-up might include echocardiography to evaluate valve function and chamber size, radionuclide studies to evaluate LV and RV ejection fraction and wall motion, and cardiac catheterization.

VI. **Idiopathic Hypertrophic Subaortic Stenosis (IHSS)** most commonly presents in young adults before the third decade.

A. **Etiology and Examination.** Caused by a thickened septum impinging on anterior mitral leaflet and creating a dynamic obstruction in the left ventricular outflow tract. It is an autosomal dominant mutation, 50% penetrance, male/female equal occurrence. Signs are commonly dyspnea, angina, syncope, and fatigue. Examination is notable for a laterally displaced apical impulse, rapid rise and biphasic carotid pulse, variably split S2 and loud S4, harsh crescendo-decrescendo murmur at the lower left sternal border and apex. The murmur classically increases and lengthens with Valsalva, decreases with handgrip.

B. **Management and treatment.** Aimed at reducing ventricular rate, allowing increased ventricular volume and outflow tract dimensions. Most commonly beta-blockers or calcium channel blockers. Do not use digitalis preparations. Avoiding strenuous physical activity, especially competitive sports. Some recommend AV sequential pacing. Surgical therapy may be helpful in selected cases, with left ventricular myomectomy or heart transplantation for cases with severe left ventricular failure.

DIASTOLIC DYSFUNCTION

I. **General.** Diastolic dysfunction refers to congestive heart failure with a normal or increased ejection fraction but decreased cardiac output caused by a stiff, noncompliant ventricle and small chamber size secondary to muscle hypertrophy. Depending on the population studied, diastolic dysfunction is found in up to 40% of the patients presenting with symptoms of congestive heart failure. Generally found in the elderly, those with long-standing hypertension and those on dialysis. May be secondary to cardiac fibrosis, hypertension, valvular disease, other underlying illness.

II. **Clinically.** May be indistinguishable from CHF secondary to systolic dysfunction. However, echocardiogram or gated pool study demonstrate good ejection fraction and hypertrophy of ventricle wall.

III. **Treatment.**

A. **Calcium-channel blockers** (except nifedipine, use diltiazem and verapamil) are useful in patients with IHSS and diastolic dysfunction (reduced ventricular compliance). Start low and increase slowly and only if you see the desired clinical effect and there is no evidence of increase in CHF.

B. **Beta-blockers** are indicated for the treatment of CHF induced by diastolic dysfunction. They do not promote myocardial relaxation. However, beta-blockers are believed to exert benefit by reducing myocardial oxygen demands, slowing the heart rate, controlling hypertension, and promoting the regression of left ventricular hypertrophy (thereby restoring

3

CARDIOLOGY

the ventricle's elasticity and normalizing end-diastolic pressure and volume). Again, start with a low dose.

C. **ACE inhibitors** may allow for left ventricular remodeling and may have a direct effect on myocardium that is beneficial in diastolic dysfunction.

D. **Digoxin and afterload reducers may be detrimental** in these patients and should be used with caution.

E. **Diuretics** may be helpful in acute dyspnea. Preload reduction may also reduce cardiac output, thus diuretics must be used with caution.

HYPERTENSION

I. **Overview.**

A. **Hypertension is defined** as a sustained systolic blood pressure (SBP) of greater than or equal to 140 mm Hg or a sustained diastolic blood pressure (DBP) of greater than or equal to 90 mm Hg. For patients with diabetes the goal is a SBP of 130 mm Hg and a DBP of 85 mm Hg. For patients with renal insufficiency (greater than 1 g of proteinuria in 24 hours) the goal is a SBP of 125 mm Hg and a DBP of 75 mm Hg.

B. Before diagnosing an individual as hypertensive, one should document an elevated blood pressure on at least three occasions over a 2-week period. The patient should be free of stress at the time of the exam including being free of pain and anxiety (such as white coat hypertension).

C. **Use a cuff of the proper size** (small size gives falsely elevated readings) and the arm should be resting comfortably on an armrest. If the results are still inconclusive, consider 24-hour ambulatory monitoring. Treatment of hypertension can reduce many of the complications such as CHF, nephropathy, and cerebrovascular events.

II. **Causes**

A. **Essential hypertension** is the most common form of hypertension in all age groups except children. The cause of essential hypertension is not completely understood.

B. **Secondary hypertension** is the result of some identifiable pathologic process, usually related to renal physiology. Causes of secondary hypertension include renal artery stenosis (or other cause of increased plasma renin), renal parenchymal disease (glomerulonephritis, diabetic neph-ropathy, polycystic disease, obstructive uropathy), drugs (oral contraceptives, steroids), increased levels of catecholamines (pheochromocytoma), glucocorticoids (Cushing's syndrome), or mineralocorticoids (hyperaldosteronism, which is manifested by hypokalemia, hypertension, and possibly edema).

III. **Evaluation**

A. **The initial evaluation** of the patient with newly detected mild to moderately elevated blood pressure (not yet defined as hypertension) should include the following:

1. **Thorough history** regarding diabetes, hypertension (HTN), and cardiovascular disease in the family; personal history of cardiovascular symptoms; drug and alcohol use; level of physical activity; and diet.

2. **A physical examination** to include weight, funduscopic exam for evidence of retinopathy, cardiac exam, auscultation of abdomen and neck for bruits, and palpation of kidneys.
3. **Laboratory evaluation** may be postponed until follow-up visits have established the diagnosis of HTN.
4. **Recommend salt restriction,** increased exercise, weight reduction if indicated, and follow-up exam in 2 to 4 weeks for blood pressure recheck.

B. **Once the formal diagnosis of hypertension is made,** the evaluation should consist of the following:
  1. Urinalysis and serum creatinine to evaluate for renal disease; ECG; cholesterol and triglycerides (as part of CAD risk factor assessment); electrolytes and uric acid as baseline for determining appropriate medications; and serum glucose to evaluate for diabetes.
  2. Other tests may be indicated by physical exam or laboratory results that indicate a possible cause of secondary hypertension. IVP, renal arteriography, captopril renal scan, renal ultrasound with doppler flow to each kidney and urinary catecholamine evaluation may be indicated in certain patients. Routine use of these studies is not suggested unless additional factors support the presence of a secondary cause.

IV. **Treatment**

A **Education.** All patients with HTN should be counseled regarding the nature of the disorder and the importance of long-term compliance with particular treatment regimens. Home blood pressure monitoring should be taught.

B. **Lifestyle interventions.** Exercise, salt restriction, and weight reduction are appropriate for many patients with HTN but may be of limited efficacy due to poor compliance. Smoking cessation should be encouraged. If the patient abuses alcohol or other substances, appropriate treatment should be encouraged and arranged. Increased intake of calcium and magnesium should be encouraged to help reduce blood pressure unless a contraindication is present.

C. **Medications.** Numerous medications are available for the pharmacologic treatment of HTN. The widely varying side-effects, costs, and dosing schedules allow tailoring of the medications to the particular needs of each patient. Pharmacologic intervention is indicated in the mildly to moderately hypertensive individual when the above-mentioned measures have not produced adequate control. A stepped-care regimen has been advocated in the past; however, some studies have suggested that monotherapy with more potent agents may be as or more effective in preventing sequelae of HTN. Individualized therapy is recommended with consideration for factors such as demographics (race and age, which may affect response to certain antihypertensive agents), quality of life (related to side effects), and concomitant medical disease and cardiovascular risk factors, which may influence choice of therapy. **In gen-**

3

CARDIOLOGY

eral, start with a diuretic or beta-blocker. A diuretic or long-acting di-hydropyridine followed by the beta-blockers are the best choices for isolated systolic hypertension.

1. **Diuretics.** Thiazide diuretics are effective alone and are useful in off-setting the fluid retention caused by other agents. Loop diuretics are more effective in patients with impaired renal function. Examples of thiazides are hydrochlorothiazide and chlorothiazide. The dosing range of HCTZ is 6.25 to 50 mg PO QD. **Advantages:** safe, inexpensive. **Disadvantages:** may result in hypokalemia, impaired glucose tolerance (usually not clinically significant); increased uric acid levels and risk of gout, and increased plasma lipids. Dyazide and Maxzide are combinations of HCTZ and triamterene and are potassium sparing. Long term, the potassium-sparing diuretics are less expensive since they do not require potassium monitoring and replacement. **Compared to thiazide diuretics alone, potassium-sparing combinations are associated with a lower risk of sudden cardiac death.**

2. **Beta-blockers** (nadolol, atenolol, metoprolol, propranolol, and others) reduce cardiac output (negative inotropic and chronotropic effects) but increase peripheral resistance. Also useful to treat angina and ar-rhythmias and as prophylaxis against migraines. Generally felt to be most effective in the younger patient with a "hyperdynamic" cardio-vascular system as evidenced by elevated resting pulse (high normal or tachycardic) and excessive response of blood pressure to exercise. **Advantages:** many are relatively inexpensive and effective. **Disadvantages:** may cause significant bradycardia or AV block, sedation, fatigue, bronchospasm in patients with asthma, erectile dysfunction, impaired glucose tolerance, possibly elevated uric acid and plasma lipids (except those with ISA activity). Should not be withdrawn abruptly, especially in patients with CAD, because rebound tachycardia and hypertension may occur. Labetalol is a unique agent that provides both alpha-blockade and (predominantly) beta-blockade. It tends to cause less bradycardia than other agents and has a direct peripheral vasodilating effect.

3. **Central sympatholytics.** Methyldopa, clonidine, guanabenz, and guanfacine. Sedation and fatigue may occur. A withdrawal syndrome may occur with abrupt cessation (especially clonidine).

4. **Alpha-blockers.** Prazosin and terazosin. Severe orthostatic hypotension may occur with first dose. Fluid retention may occur. Sedation and headache are commonly seen early during treatment but tend to diminish with time. These drugs are good choices in elderly men who have hypertension and benign prostatic hypertrophy. **However, recent data suggests less of a reduction in mortality when using this class of agents for hypertension.**

5. **Arterial vasodilators.** Hydralazine and minoxidil. Both are potent vasodilators and may cause reflex tachycardia and fluid retention. Should be used only with a diuretic and sympathetic inhibitor (such

as a beta-blocker). Should not be used in patients with angina. Minoxidil is usually reserved for severe hypertension. A lupus-like syndrome has been seen with hydralazine.

6. **Calcium-channel blockers.** Verapamil, diltiazem, nicardipine, nifedipine, amlodipine, and others. Verapamil and diltiazem both slow AV nodal conduction. Both also have some negative inotropic effect (especially verapamil) and peripheral vasodilatory effects. Calcium-channel blockers generally do not adversely affect glucose tolerance or plasma lipids. They may be especially appropriate in the patient who needs both antianginal and an antihypertensive drug. Mild edema and constipation are frequent side effects of calcium-channel blockers. Orthostatic hypotension and reflex tachycardia can occur, particularly with nifedipine. There is some concern that nifedipine may increase cardiac mortality.

7. **ACE inhibitors** (angiotensin-converting enzyme inhibitors). Captopril, enalapril, lisinopril, and others. All are effective for HTN and have been used in CHF. Captopril requires more frequent dosing. All may contribute to hyperkalemia and cause reversible decreased renal function. Side effects tend to be minimal with no significant sedation, fatigue, or exercise intolerance in most patients. Occasional patients may have trouble with persistent cough; aspirin 325 mg PO QD may decrease cough as may indomethacin or inhaled cromolyn. However, switching to another ACE inhibitor does not improve the cough caused by these agents. Angioedema occurs in a small subset of patients taking ACE inhibitors and may be life threatening. Patients should be warned about this possibility. Patients at high risk for adverse renal effects include those with connective tissue disease, bilateral renal artery stenosis, or preexisting renal insufficiency. ACE inhibitors may have a favorable effect in preserving renal function or in slowing the progression of proteinuria in chronic renal failure. They also facilitate cardiac remodeling.

8. **Angiotensin II type 1 receptor blockers (ARBs).** If ACE inhibitors are poorly tolerated by a patient, consideration should be given to losartan, irbesartan, or valsartan, etc, members of this new drug class. These drugs antagonize the action of angiotensin II by displacing it from its receptor. They thereby inhibit angiotensin II-induced vascular smooth muscle contraction, aldosterone release, and adrenal and presynaptic catecholamine release, among other effects. They do not stimulate cough and have been shown to be as effective as enalapril in controlling hypertension. They do not adversely affect lipid parameters or glucose levels. Because of the uricosuric activity they reduce serum uric acid levels.

D. **Follow-up study.** Initially patients should be scheduled for frequent office visits until blood pressure is adequately controlled and potential side-effects are evaluated. Thereafter, visits may be scheduled every 3 to 6 months. Laboratory evaluation should include those indicated by the medications they are using (such as K^+ level, if receiving diuretics).

3

CARDIOLOGY

SYNCOPE

I. **Definition.** Differentiate between near syncope and vertigo because the differential diagnosis is different. See Chapter 9 for work-up and differential of vertigo.

A. **Syncope** is a sudden, brief loss of consciousness (LOC) and, strictly speaking, is related to abrupt cerebral hypoperfusion. Only two CNS lesions can cause syncope: bilateral cortical dysfunction (e.g., from hypoperfusion, etc.) or reticular activating system injury.

B. **Near syncope** is a sense of impending LOC or weakness, occurs more frequently, and provides valuable diagnostic clues, since the patient usually has better recollection of the event.

C. **Frequency of causes.** 55% vasovagal, 10% cardiac, 10% neurologic, 5% metabolic or drug-induced, 5% "other," and 10% undiagnosed causes.

II. Causes of Syncope and Near Syncope

A. Cardiac and circulatory.

1. Cardioinhibitory (bradycardia, enhanced parasympathetics), neurocardiogenic (e.g., vasovagal), vasodepressor (decreased systemic vascular resistance) are the most common causes and tend to be familial. It occurs when a susceptible person is confronted with a stressful situation, etc. **Prodromal** symptoms: restlessness, pallor, weakness, sighing, yawning, diaphoresis, and nausea. These symptoms may be followed by light-headedness, blurred vision, collapse, and LOC. Occasionally, mild clonic seizures occur, but a seizure work-up is not indicated unless other signs point in this direction. Spells are brief in duration with prompt recovery on recumbency. These episodes may be recurrent.

2. **Orthostatic hypotension** is a fall in blood pressure when one is assuming an upright position. It is seen in a variety of settings.

   a. **Hypovolemia** (hemorrhage, vomiting, diarrhea, diuretics).

   b. **Interference with normal reflexes** (nitrates, vasodilators, beta-blockers, calcium-channel blockers, neuroleptics, etc.).

   c. **Autonomic failure.** Primary or secondary. Diabetes most common form of secondary autonomic neuropathy, whereas advanced age is a common cause of primary autonomic failure. Also consider Shy-Dragger syndrome (autonomic failure with CNS symptoms).

   d. **Postprandial syncope** in the elderly.

3. **Outflow obstruction.** IHSS, aortic stenosis, mitral stenosis, pulmonic stenosis, and subclavian steal syndrome. These patients may present with exertional syncope. Mechanical valve malfunction may also cause outflow obstruction.

4. **Myocardial ischemia or infarction.**

5. **Arrhythmias.**

   a. **Bradyarrhythmias:** sick sinus syndrome, AV-node blocks, etc.

   b. **Tachyarrhythmias:** PSVT, Wolf-Parkinson-White syndrome, ventricular tachycardia, etc.

6. **Carotid sinus hypersensitivity.** Syncope may occur with shaving or wearing a tight collar. Rarely the carotid sinus may be stimulated by tumor.

B. **Metabolic causes.** Episodes are usually amplified by exertion but may occur when patient is supine. The onset and resolution are usually prolonged.
   1. **Hypoxia,** as with shunting in congenital heart disease.
   2. **Hyperventilation.** Results in cerebral vasoconstriction with symptoms of breathlessness, anxiety, circumoral tingling, paresthesias of hands or feet, carpopedal spasm, and, occasionally, unilateral or bilateral chest pain. Patients can reproduce these spells by hyperventilating in a controlled environment.
   3. **Hypoglycemia.**
   4. **Alcohol** intoxication or other drug.

C. **Neurologic causes. Transient ischemic attacks (TIAs) rarely if ever cause syncope.** To do so the reticular activating system must be involved. When this occurs, there are almost always other neurologic manifestations such as cranial nerve abnormalities.
   1. **Migraine.** Second most common cause in adolescents. LOC is followed by headache.
   2. **Seizure.** Usually easily differentiated by aura, history of tonic-clonic movements, and postictal state.
   3. **Abrupt rise of intracranial pressure** as seen with subarachnoid hemorrhage or obstructive colloid cyst of the third ventricle.

D. **Reflex syncope** results from impaired right-sided heart filling and global cerebral hypoperfusion. The patient is usually standing upright before an episode because gravitational pooling of blood plays a causal role. Potential etiologies include pulmonary embolism or infarction, pericardial tamponade, pulmonary hypertension, a pregnant uterus as it compresses the inferior vena cava, and coughing, which decreases preload by increasing intrathoracic pressure.

E. **Miscellaneous.** Cough syncope, Postmicturition syncope, psychogenic, severe visceral or ligamentous pain, and subsequent to severe vertigo.

III. **Evaluation**

A. **History** is the most important part of evaluation. The patient and witnesses should be questioned as to precipitating circumstances, prodromal symptoms, time course of onset and recovery, and medication history.

B. **Physical exam.**
   1. Blood pressure and pulse supine and standing (however, orthostatic vital signs are neither sensitive nor specific for hypovolemia).
   2. Auscultation of subclavian and carotid arteries.
   3. Cardiac exam with attention to murmurs, extra heart sounds. Provocative maneuvers (Valsalva) as indicated.
   4. Careful neurologic exam.

3

CARDIOLOGY

C. **Laboratory studies** should be directed by history and physical exam. May include blood glucose, blood gases, electrolytes, and hematocrit.

D. **ECG/Holter Ambulatory Monitoring/Event monitor.** Event monitors that are worn for a month and activated when patient has a feeling of palpations or near syncope are more cost effective and sensitive than 24 to 48 hours of ambulatory monitoring but only if the patient is going to be able to activate the monitor in the presyncopal period.

E. **Signal-averaged ECG** may be helpful in patients suspected of having ventricular arrhythmias.

F. **Echocardiography.** Useful in evaluating valvular and myocardial disease.

G. **EEG.** Obtain if seizure disorder is suspected; however, may be falsely negative in 50% of cases. Nasopharyngeal leads, sleep deprivation, and hyperventilation may all increase yield.

H. **Electrophysiologic** invasive cardiac studies may be indicated in patients with structural heart disease and unexplained syncope, or a history that is suggestive of an arrhythmia.

I. **Tilt testing** helps in carefully selected patients but has a low specificity.

VI. **Treatment.** Depends on cause.

A. **Vasovagal** syncope usually responds to avoiding stimuli that trigger syncope. If it is clinically severe, beta-blockers, cardiac pacing, and SSRI antidepressants have all been used. However, the success rate is poor. The frequency of cough syncope might be reduced by antitussives.

B. **Medical.** See appropriate section based on diagnosis. Antiepileptics, antiarrhythmics, mineralocorticoids (for chronic orthostatic hypotension), support hose (to prevent blood pooling) or migraine prophylaxis will all be useful in selected cases. Midodrine, an alpha antagonist, has been used successfully for orthostatic syncope but may cause recumbent hypertension.

C. **Surgical.** For critical aortic stenosis, carotid artery disease, etc.

DYSLIPIDEMIAS

I. **Classification**

A. May be grouped on the basis of serum lipid concentrations and electrophoretic patterns, genotype, or by pathophysiologic features (Table 3-3). May be classified as primary, which includes familial hyperlipidemia, or secondary.

B. **Secondary causes.**

1. **Exogenous.** Alcohol, oral contraceptives, estrogens, androgens, corticosteroids, diuretics (thiazides), beta-blockers, obesity, and high-cholesterol diet.

2. **Endocrine and metabolic.** Diabetes, hypothyroidism, Cushing's or Addison's diseases, hepatic disease, nephrotic syndrome.

3. **Miscellaneous.** Pregnancy, pancreatitis, systemic lupus erythematosus (SLE).

II. **Evaluation and Initial Therapy.** Recommendations of the American Heart Association and the American College of Physicians differ. The American Heart Association proceeds in a stepwise fashion.

TABLE 3-3

CLASSIFICATION OF LIPOPROTEIN DISORDERS BY PHENOTYPES, GENOTYPES, AND CORRESPONDING CLINICAL MANIFESTATIONSTIONS

Phenotype	Plasma Lipid Levels		Genotype	Xanthomas	Other Clinical Manifestations
	Cholesterol	Triglyceride			
I	Normal or elevated	Elevated lipemia	Familial lipoprotein lipase deficiency, Apo C-II deficiency	Eruptive, tuberoeruptive	Recurrent abdominal pain, other gastrointestinal symptoms, hepatosplenomegaly
IIA	Normal	Elevated	FHC, familial combined hyperlipidemia—polygenic and sporadic hypercholesterolemia	Tendinous, xanthelasma, tuberous; planar (homozygous)	Premature CAD, arcus corneae, aortic stenosis (homozygous FHC), arthritic symptoms
IIB	Elevated	Elevated	Familial combined hyperlipidemia, FHC		
III	Elevated	Elevated	Familial dysbetalipoproteinemia	Planar (especially palmar), tuberous	Premature CAD and peripheral vascular disease; male > female, obesity, abnormal glucose tolerance, hyperuricemia, aggravated by hypothyroidism, good response to therapy
IV	Noraml or elevated	Elevated	Familial hypertriglyceridemia, familial combined hyperlipidemia, sporadic hypertriglyceridemia	Usually none; rarely eruptive or tuberoeruptive	CAD and peripheral vascular disease, obesity, abnormal glucose tolerance, hyperuricemia, arthritic symptoms, gall bladder disease
V	Normal or elevated	Elevated	Homozygous FHC	Eruptive, tuberoeruptive	Recurrent abdominal pain, other gastrointestinal symptoms, hepatosplenomegaly, peripheral paresthesia

CAD, Coronary artery disease; FHC, familial hypercholesterolemia; IDL, intermediate-density lipoprotein; LDL, low-density lipoprotein; VLDL, very-low-density lipoprotein.

3

CARDIOLOGY

A. **Step 1.** Initial classification is based on total cholesterol.
   1. <200 desirable, repeat every 5 years.
   2. 200 to 240 borderline.
   3. >240 high.
B. **Step 2.** If, on repeat testing, cholesterol is >240 **or** 200 to 240 **and** the patient has CHD **or** two CAD risk factors (table 3-4) **then** obtain full lipid profile after a 12 to 14-hour fast. When risk factors are being evaluated, if the patient has an HDL >60, one risk factor may be subtracted from the total.
C. **Step 3.** If total cholesterol on repeat testing is borderline and <2 risk factors, initiate step-1 diet.
D. **Step 4.** If total cholesterol on repeat is elevated fractionate and treat as below.
   1. **LDL calculation:** LDL = Total chol − (TG/5) − HDL
   2. **<130 desirable.** Repeat every 5 years.
   3. **If the patient has <2 risk factors and no CHD, then:**
      a. Step 1 diet if >160 mg/dl.
      b. Diet and medication if >190 mg/dl.
      c. The goal for these patients is an LDL <160 mg/dl. Repeat lipid profile annually to monitor LDL level.
   4. **If the patients has >2 risk factors and no CHD, then:**
      a. Diet if >130 mg/dl.
      b. Diet and medication if >160 mg/dl.
      c. The goal of therapy is an LDL <130 mg/dl.
   5. **If the patient has CAD (patients with angina, survivors of MI), then:**
      a. Diet if LDL >100 mg/dl.
      b. Diet and medication if LDL >130 mg/dl.
      c. The goal of therapy is LDL <100 mg/dl.
      d. In patients who do not reach target LDL level, may change drugs or add a second agent to regimen.
E. Initiation of step-1 diet. Reduce total fat to <30%, saturated fat to <10% of calories, reduce cholesterol to <300 mg/day.
F. *Check cholesterol in 6 weeks and 3 months.* If no improvement, refer to dietitian for retrial of step-1 diet, or advance to step-2 diet: Reduce saturated fat to <7%, reduce cholesterol to <200 mg/day.
G. Exercise, weight loss, and smoking cessation should also be part of the program. If no improvement, consider drug therapy.
H. **Triglyceride levels.** A triglyceride level of <250 mg/dl is desirable. The risk for CHD may begin to increase at >250 mg/dl. **Recent evidence suggests that in patients with low HDL cholesterol, the addition of gemfibrozil to the regimen reduces mortality, MI, CVA, etc.**
   1. If the triglyceride level is >250 mg/dl, then recommend weight loss, a low-fat diet (<10% fat), exercise, and reduced alcohol consumption.
   2. If the TG level is >1000, the patient has an increased risk of pancreatitis.

> **BOX 3-1**
>
> **RISK FACTORS FOR CAD VIS-À-VIS CHOLESTEROL MANAGEMENT**
>
> Age [men >45, women >55]
>
> Family history of premature CAD in first-degree relative [men <55, women <65]
>
> Premature menopause without estrogen replacement
>
> Smoking
>
> Hypertension
>
> HDL <35
>
> Diabetes
>
> Obesity
>
> History of cerebral or peripheral vascular disease

III. **American College of Physicians recommends the following as screening guidelines:**

A. Total cholesterol screening is not to be performed in men younger than 35 or women younger than 45 unless:

1. There is suspicion of a lipoprotein disorder by either history or physical examination.

2. The patient has at least two other CHD risk factors (Box 3-1).

3. Cholesterol screening for the primary prevention of CHD is appropriate for 35- to 65-year-old men and 45- to 65-year-old women.

   a. There is insufficient evidence to recommend or discourage screening for the primary prevention of CHD in patients 65 to 75 years of age.

   b. Screening is not recommended for patients >75 years of age.

   c. All patients with CHD or peripheral vascular or cerebrovascular disease should undergo periodic lipid evaluation.

IV. **Pharmacologic Therapy**

A. **Bile acid sequestrants and resins** (colestipol, cholestyramine) decrease total and LDL cholesterol by 20% to 40%. These are considered one of the drugs of choice for isolated LDL elevation because of low incidence of systemic side effects. Start at 4 g BID and increase to 16 to 24 g/day. Constipation and GI upset are frequent side effects, which may be alleviated somewhat by increasing dietary fiber and adding psyllium laxatives. Resins may increase TG and should be used with caution in patients with elevated TG. Often used with other agents such as niacin, lovastatin, or gemfibrozil. May affect the GI absorption of other drugs; other medications should be taken 1 to 2 hours before or 4 hours after resin dose. Levels of concurrent medications (such as digoxin or PT/INR for patients receiving warfarin) should be monitored.

B. **Nicotinic acid** (niacin) decreases both LDL and TG, increases HDL. Also lowers lipoprotein A blood levels. Common side effects include skin flushing, GI upset, elevation in serum glucose, elevated liver enzymes, and elevated uric acid. Rare side effects can include headaches, worsening of peptic ulcer disease, cardiac dysrhythmias, and elevations in serum muscle enzymes. Tolerance to minor side effects (flushing, nausea) can be improved if one starts with low doses (100 mg BID-TID) and takes with meals. The maximum dose is 3 g QD. Taking 325 mg of aspirin 30 to 60 minutes before niacin decreases flushing. The sustained-release preparations of niacin are hepatotoxic and should not be used.

C. **HMG CoA reductase inhibitors** (lovastatin, simvastatin, pravastatin, atorvastatin) inhibit HMG CoA reductase, which is the rate-limiting enzyme in the production of cholesterol by the liver. These agents reduce total cholesterol and LDL. A slight to moderate decrease in TG and an increase in HDL may occur, especially with atorvastatin. Side effects are rare and include elevated liver function test results, elevated muscle creatinine phosphokinase secondary to myopathy, and rarely rhabdomyolysis. The starting dose of simvastatin is 5 to 10 mg PO Q PM and can be titrated up to a maximum dose of 40 mg PO Q PM. Pravastatin is started at 10 to 20 mg PO QHS and can be titrated to 40 mg PO QHS. Repeat fasting serum lipid levels can be obtained at 4- to 6-week intervals until the desired adjustments are achieved.

D. **Fibric acid derivatives** (gemfibrozil, clofibrate). Use of clofibrate has declined because of one large trial showing an increase in GI cancers and increased overall mortality. Gemfibrozil is still used to decrease VLDL synthesis and lower fasting TG. It may increase HDL and has a variable effect on LDL. GI side effects common. Rare side effects: myalgias, increase in liver or muscle enzymes, headache, gallstones, arrhythmias, hypokalemia, anemia, and leukopenia. Can potentiate oral hypoglycemics and warfarin.

E. **Probucol.** Developed as an antioxidant; decreases total and LDL cholesterol and decreases HDL. Common cause of QT prolongation on ECG.

F. **Fish oils** (omega-3 fatty acids) decrease VLDL synthesis, may decrease chylomicrons (and therefore TG). May reduce risk of acute pancreatitis in patients with severe hypertriglyceridemia. Clinical trials underway regarding role of fish oils in slowing progression of CAD.

PROPHYLAXIS AGAINST BACTERIAL ENDOCARDITIS

I. **General Comments.** Endocarditis can occur from transient bacteremia. Because a variety of health care procedures can result in bacteremia, prophylaxis against bacteria that can adhere to endocardium is recommended, particularly in patients at high risk for endocarditis. The frequency of bacteremia is highest subsequent to oral and dental procedures (because of the abundant oral flora), intermediate for genitourinary procedures, and lowest for diagnostic procedures of the gastrointestinal tract. It is important to give prophylactic antibiotics before a procedure because bacterial adhesion can occur within minutes after bacteremia develops.

II. **Endocarditis Prophylaxis Recommended.**

A. Cardiac conditions.

1. **Prosthetic cardiac valves** (including bioprosthetic, homograft, and mechanical).

2. **Previous episode of bacterial endocarditis.**
3. **Most congenital cardiac defects** (especially cyanotic congenital heart disease, patent ductus arteriosus, ventricular septal defects, and surgically repaired intracardiac defects with residual hemodynamic abnormalities).
4. **Valvular heart disease** resulting from rheumatic or other disease (aortic regurgitation and stenosis, mitral regurgitation and stenosis).
5. **Hypertrophic cardiomyopathy.**
6. **Mitral valve prolapse with regurgitation.**

B. **Dental or surgical procedures.**
   1. Dental or surgical procedures that cause gingival or mucosal bleeding, including mechanical dental hygienic procedures.
   2. Tonsillectomy or adenoidectomy.
   3. Surgical procedures involving upper respiratory or gastrointestinal mucosa.
   4. Rigid bronchoscopy.
   5. Sclerotherapy of esophageal varices.
   6. Esophageal dilatation.
   7. Transesophageal echocardiography
   8. Gallbladder surgery
   9. Urethral catheterization or urinary tract surgery if infection present
   10. Prostate surgery
   11. I & D of infected tissue
   12. Vaginal hysterectomy
   13. Vaginal delivery in the presence of infection (chorioamnionitis, etc.)

III. **Endocarditis Prophylaxis Not Recommended**

A. **Cardiac conditions.**
   1. **Previous coronary artery bypass surgery.**
   2. **Mitral valve prolapse without regurgitation.** (If MPV is associated with thickening or redundancy of valve leaflets, may have increased risk of endocarditis, especially in men >45 years of age).
   3. **Functional or innocuous heart murmurs.**
   4. **Cardiac pacemakers** and implantable defibrillators.
   5. **Isolated secundum** atrial septal defect.
   6. **6 months or more status postsurgical** repair of PDA, VSD without residua.
   7. Previous rheumatic heart disease or Kawasaki disease without valve dysfunction.

B. **Dental or surgical procedures.**
   1. Dental procedures not likely to cause gingival bleeding such as fillings above the gum line, adjustment of orthodontic appliances.
   2. Injection of intraoral anesthetics.
   3. Shedding of primary teeth.
   4. Tympanostomy tube insertion.
   5. Endotracheal intubation, flexible bronchoscopy with or without biopsy specimens.
   6. Cardiac catheterization.

3

CARDIOLOGY

7. Endoscopy with or without biopsy.
8. In absence of infection, urethral catheterization, D&C, uncomplicated vaginal delivery, abortion, sterilization procedures, insertion or removal of an IUD, or laparoscopy.

IV. **Standard Regimens**

A. **Dental, oral, upper respiratory tract.** (Total children's dose should not exceed adult dose).
   1. **For adults.** Amoxicillin 2 g (children, 50 mg/kg) PO 1 hour before procedure.
   2. **In penicillin-allergic patients.** Clindamycin 600 mg (children, 20 mg/kg) PO *OR* Cephalexin or Cefadroxil 2.0 g (children, 50 mg/kg) PO *OR* Azithromycin or Clarithromycin 500 mg (children, 15 mg/kg) PO 1 hour before procedure
   3. **If unable to take oral medications.** Ampicillin 2.0 g (children 20 mg/kg) IV or IM 30 minutes before procedure. Alternative: clindamycin 600 mg (children 20 mg/kg) IV 30 minutes before procedure.
   4. **In the high-risk, penicillin-allergic patient.** Vancomycin 1.0 g IV over 1 hour, starting 1 hour before surgery. A repeat dose is not necessary.

B. **GI or GU procedures.** (Total children's dose should not exceed adult dose).
   1. **High risk.** Ampicillin 2.0 g IV (children, 50 mg/kg) + Gentamicin 1.5 mg/kg IV (for adults and children, not to exceed 120 mg) 30 minutes before procedure, then amoxicillin 1.0 g (children, 25 mg/kg) PO 6 hours later, or ampicillin 1.0 g (children, 25 mg/kg) IV 6 hours after first dose.
   2. **High-risk, penicillin allergic.** Vancomycin 1.0 g (children, 20 mg/kg) IV (over 1 hour) starting 1 hour before procedure + Gentamicin 1.5 mg/kg IV (both adults and children, not to exceed 120 mg) 1 hour before. Complete infusion 30 minutes before procedure.
   3. **Moderate or low-risk.** Amoxicillin 2.0 g (children, 50 mg/kg) PO 1 hour before procedure. Or, Ampicillin 2.0 g (children 50 mg/kg) IM or IV 30 minutes before procedure.
   4. **Moderate or Low-risk, penicillin allergic.** Vancomycin 1.0 g (children, 20 mg/kg) over 1 hour. Complete infusion 30 minutes before starting procedure.

BIBLIOGRAPHY

Acute Infarction Ramipril Efficacy (AIRE) Study Investigators: Effect of ramipril on mortality and morbidity of survivors of acute myocardial infarction with clinical evidence of heart failure, *Lancet* 342:821, 1993.

Advisory Statements of the International Liaison Committee on Resuscitation, *Circulation* 95:2172-2173, 1997.

Bonow RO et al: ACC/AHA Guidelines for the management of patients with valvular heart disease: a report of the American College of Cardiology/American Heart Association Task Force on Practice Guidelines (Committee on Management of patients with valvular heart disease), *J Am Coll Cardiol* 32:1486-1588, 1998

Brener SJ et al: Randomized, placebo-controlled trial of platelet glycoprotein IIb/IIIa blockade with primary angioplasty for acute myocardial infarction, *Circulation* 98:734-741, 1998.

Cairns JA et al: Antithrombotic agents in coronary artery disease, *Chest* 114(5):611-633S, 1998.

Cairns JA et al: Coronary thrombolysis, *Chest* 114(5):634-657S, 1998.

Cannegieter SC et al: Optimal oral anticoagulant therapy in patients with mechanical heart valves, *N Engl J Med* 333:11, 1995.

Carabello BA, Crawford F: Valvular heart disease, *N Engl J Med* 337(1):32,1997.

Chun SH et al: Long-term efficacy of amiodarone for the maintenance of normal sinus rhythm in patients with refractory atrial fibrillation or flutter, *Am J Cardiol* 76(16):47, 1995.

Dejani, AS et al: Prevention of bacterial endocarditis. Recommendations by the American Heart Association, *JAMA* 277(22):1794-1801, 1997.

Diagnosis and Management of Infective Endocarditis and Its Complications. Ad Hoc Writing Group of the Committee on Rheumatic Fever, Endocarditis, and Kawasaki Disease, American Heart Association, *Circulation* 98:2936-2948, 1998.

Durack DT: Prevention of infective endocarditis, *N Engl J Med* 332:38, 1995.

Erwin III JP et al: Dual chamber pacing for patients with hypertrophic obstructive cardiomyopathy: A clinical perspective in 2000, *Mayo Clin Proc* 75(2):173-180, 2000.

EPIC Investigators. Use of monoclonal antibody directed against the platelet glycoprotein IIb/IIIa receptor in high-risk coronary angioplasty, *N Engl J Med* 330:956-961, 1994.

EPILOG Investigators. Platelet glycoprotein IIb/IIIA receptor blockade and low dose heparin during percutaneous coronary revascularization, *N Engl J Med* 336:1689-1696, 1997

EPISTENT Investigators. Randomized placebo controlled and balloon-angioplasty-controlled trail to assess safety of coronary stenting with the use of platelet glycoprotein-IIb/IIIa blockade. Evaluation of Platelet IIb/IIIa Inhibitor for Stenting, *Lancet* 352:87-92, 1998.

Fletcher GF et al: Exercise standards. A statement for health-care professionals from the American Heart Association Writing Group, *Circulation* 91:580-615, 1995.

Fuster V, Pearson TA: Twenty-seventh Bethesda Conference: Matching the intensity of risk factor management with the hazard for coronary disease events, *J Am Coll Cardiol* 27:957-1047, 1996.

Gheorghiade M, Pitt B: Digitalis Investigation Group (DIG) trial: a stimulus for further research, *Am Heart J* 134(1):3-12, 1997.

Gregoratus G et al: ACC/AHA guidelines for implantation of cardiac pacemakers and antiarrhythmia devices: a report of the American College of Cardiology/American Heart Association Task Force on Practice Guidelines (Committee on Pacemaker Implantation), *J Am Coll Cardiol* 31:1175-1209, 1998.

Grimes CL et al: Coronary angioplasty with or without stent implantation for acute myocardial infarction. Stent Primary Angioplasty in Myocardial Infarction Study Group, *N Engl J Med* 341(26):1946-1956, 1999.

Goldstein S: Beta blockers in hypertensive and coronary heart disease, *Arch Intern Med* 156(12):1267-76, 1996.

Goodfriend TL, Elliott ME, Catt KJ: Angiotensin receptors and their antagonists, *N Engl J Med* 334(25):1649-1654, 1996.

Guidelines for the Management of Patients with Acute Myocardial Infarction. Report of the American College of Cardiology/American Heart Association Task Force on Practice Guidelines (Committee on Management of Acute Myocardial Infarction), *J Am Coll Cardiol* 28:5;1328-428, 1999.

Guidelines for the Management of Patients with Chronic Stable Angina. Report of the American College of Cardiology/American Heart Association Task Force on Practice Guidelines (Committee on Management of Patients with Chronic Stable Angina), *Circulation.* 99:2829-2848, 1999.

Haffner SM et al: Mortality from coronary heart disease in subjects with type 2 diabetes and in nondiabetic subjects with and without prior myocardial infarction, *N Engl J Med* 339(2):229-234, 1998.

3

CARDIOLOGY

Hansson L et al for the HOT Study Group: Effects of intensive blood-pressure lowering and low-dose aspirin in patients with hypertension: principle results of the Hypertension Optimal Treatment (HOT) randomized trial, *Lancet* 351:1755-1762, 1998.

Heart disease: *A textbook of cardiovascular medicine.* In Braunwald E, editor: ed 5, Philadelphia, 1997, WB Saunders.

Heart Outcomes Prevention Evaluation Study Investigators: Effects of an Angiotensin-converting-enzyme inhibitor, Ramipril, on Cardiovascular events in high-risk patients, *N Engl J Med* 342(3), 145-153, 2000.

Heart Outcomes Prevention Evaluation Study Investigators: Vitamin E supplementation and cardiovascular events in high-risk patients, *N Engl J Med* 342(3), 154-160, 2000.

Heller GV et al: Clinical value of acute rest technutiom-99m tetrofosmin tomographic myocardial perfusion imaging in patients with acute chest pain and non-diagnostic electrocardiograms, *J Am Card Cardiol* 31(5):1011-1017, 1998.

Hopson JR, Kienzle MG: Evaluation of patients with syncope, *Postgrad Med* 91:5, 1992.

ISIS-4 Collaborative Group: ISIS-4: a randomized factorial trial assessing early oral captopril, oral mononitrate, and intravenous magnesium sulphate in 58,050 patients with suspected acute myocardial infarction, *Lancet* 345:669, 1995.

Kaplan NM: Do calcium antagonists cause myocardial infarction? *Am J Cardiol* 77(1):81-82, 1996.

Karon BL: Diagnosis and outpatient management of congestive heart failure, *Mayo Clin Proc* 70:1080, 1995.

Kendall MJ et al: Beta-blockers and sudden cardiac death, *Ann Intern Med* 123(5):358, 1995.

Kinch JW, Ryan TJ: Right ventricular infarction, *N Engl J Med* 330:1211, 1994.

King SB et al: A randomized trial comparing coronary angioplasty with coronary bypass surgery, *N Engl J Med* 331:1044-1050, 1994.

Kudenchuk PJ et al: Amiodarone for resuscitation after out-of-hospital cardiac arrest due to ventricular fibrillation, *N Engl J Med* 341(12):871-879, 1999.

Laupacis A et al: Antithrombotic therapy in atrial fibrillation, *Chest* 114(5):579-589S, 1998.

Lechat P et al: Clinical effects of β-adrenergic blockade in chronic heart failure. A meta-analysis of double-blind, placebo-controlled, randomized trails, *Circulation* 98:1184-1191, 1998.

Mark DB et al: Cost effectiveness of thrombolytic therapy with tissue plasminogen activator as compared with streptokinase for acute myocardial infarction, *N Engl J Med* 332:1418, 1995.

Molitreno DJ et al: Coronary-artery vasoconstriction induced by cocaine, cigarette smoking or both, *N Engl J Med* 330:454-459, 1994.

Naccarelli GV et al: Amiodarone: What have we learned from clinical trials? *Clin Cardiol* 23:73-83, 2000.

Packer M. The neurohormonal hypothesis: a theory to explain the mechanism of disease progression in heart failure, *J Am Card Cardiol* 20:248-254, 1992.

PARAGON Investigators. An international randomized controlled trial of lamifiban (a platelet glycoprotein IIb/IIIa inhibitor), heparin or both in unstable angina, *Circulation* 97:2386-95, 1998.

Pedersen TR, Kjekshus J, Berg K, et al: Randomized trial of cholesterol lowering in 4444 patients with coronary heart disease: The Scandinavian Simvastatin Survival Study (4S), *Lancet* 344:1383-1389, 1994.

Pitt B et al: Pravastatin limitation of atherosclerosis in the coronary arteries (PLAC 1): reduction in atherosclerosis progression and clinical events, *J Am Card Cardiol* 26:1133-1139, 1995.

Pitt B, Waters D, Brown WV, et al: Aggressive lipid-lowering therapy compared with angioplasty in stable coronary artery disease. Atorvastatin versus Revascularization Treatment Investigators, *N Engl J Med.* 341(1):70-76, 1999.

Pitt B et al: The effect of spironolactone on morbidity and mortality in patients with severe heart failure, *N Engl J Med* 341(10): 709-718, 1999.

Platelet Receptor Inhibition in Ischemic Syndrome Management in Patients Limited by Unstable Signs and Symptoms (PRISM) Study Investigators. A comparison of aspirin plus tirofiban with aspirin plus heparin for unstable angina, *N Engl J Med* 338:1498-505, 1998.

Platelet Receptor Inhibition in Ischemic Syndrome Management in Patients Limited by Unstable Signs and Symptoms (PRISM-PLUS) Study Investigators. Inhibition of the platelet glycoprotein IIb/IIIa receptor with tirofiban in unstable angina and non-Q-wave myocardial infarction, *N Engl J Med* 338:1488-1497, 1998.

PURSUIT Trial Investigators. Inhibition of platelet glycoprotein IIb/IIIa with eptifibatide in patients with acute coronary syndromes, *N Engl J Med* 339:436-43, 1998.

Pylora et al: Cholesterol lowering with simvastatin improves prognosis of diabetic patients with coronary heart disease: A subgroup analysis of the Scandinavian Survival Study (4S), *Diabetes Care* 20:614-620, 1997.

Radensky PW et al: Potential cost effectiveness of initial myocardial perfusion imaging for assessment of emergency department patients with chest pain, *Am J Cardiol* 79(5):595-599, 1997.

Rubins HB, Robins SJ, Collins D, et al: Gemfibrozil for the secondary prevention of coronary heart disease in men with low levels of high density lipoprotein cholesterol, Veterans Affairs High Density Lipoprotein Cholesterol Invention Trial Study Group, *N Engl J Med*. 341:6:410-418,1999.

Roden DM: Risks and benefits of antiarrhythmic therapy, *N Engl J Med* 331:785, 1994.

Sackner-Bernstein JD, Mancini DM: Rationale for treatment of patients with chronic heart failure with adrenergic blockade, *JAMA* 274:1462, 1995.

Sacks FM, Pfeffer MA, Moye LA, et al: The effect of pravastatin on coronary events after myocardial infarction in patients with average cholesterol levels. Cholesterol and Recurrent Events trial investigators, *N Engl J Med* 335:1001-1009, 1996.

Sanford JP et al: *Guide to antimicrobial therapy,* Dallas, 1999, Antimicrobial Therapy, Inc.

Speigler EJ: Implementation of an acute myocardial imaging program for patients with chest pain and non-diagnostic electrocardiograms: the St. Agnes experience. The strategy of Chest Pain Units (in Emergency Departments) in the war against heart attacks: Proc First Maryland Chest Pain Center Res Conf, *Maryland Med J* 46(10): 33-35S, 1997.

Serneri GG et al: Randomized comparison of subcutaneous heparin, intravenous heparin, and aspirin in unstable angina, *Lancet* 345(8959):1201-1209, 1995.

Shepherd J, Cobbe SM, Ford I, et al: Prevention of coronary heart disease with pravastatin in men with hypercholesterolemia. West of Scotland Coronary Prevention Study Group, *N Engl J Med* 333:1301-1307, 1995.

Sigurdsson E et al: Unrecognized myocardial infarction: epidemiology, clinical characteristics, and the prognostic role of angina pectoris, *Ann Intern Med* 122:96, 1995.

Sixth Report of the Joint National Committee on Detection, Evaluation and Treatment of High Blood Pressure, *Arch Intern Med* 157:2413-2446, 1997.

Stein PD, et al: Antithrombotic therapy in patients with mechanical and biological prosthetic heart valves, *Chest* 114(5):602-610S, 1998.

Stone GW et al: Prospective, multicenter study of the safety and feasibility of primary stenting in acute myocardial infarction: In-hospital and 30-day results of the PAMI stent pilot trial, *J Am Card Cardiol* 31:23-30, 1998.

Topol EJ, editor: *Textbook of cardiovascular medicine,* Philadelphia, 1998, Lippincott-Raven.

Wilson PWF, D'Agostino RB, Levy D, et al: Prediction of coronary heart disease using risk factor categories, *Circulation* 97:1837-1847, 1998.

Yamamoto K et al: Left ventricular diastolic dysfunction in patients with hypertension and preserved systolic function, *Mayo Clin Proc* 75(2):148-155, 2000.

Yeghiazarians Y, Braunstein JB, Askari A, et al: Unstable angina pectoris, *N Engl J Med* 342(2):101-114, 2000.

3

CARDIOLOGY

PULMONARY MEDICINE

Kevin C. Doerschug

PULMONARY EMBOLISM AND DEEP VENOUS THROMBOSIS

I. Deep Venous Thrombosis (DVT)

A. **Lower extremity DVT** is characterized by unilateral swelling and tenderness of the calf and thigh, which may be erythematous and warm. These physical findings are present in only 23% to 50% of patients with a DVT, however.

B. **Upper extremity DVT** may occur especially in active individuals with repetitive upper arm motion or sports activities. These may present clinically up to several weeks out from clot formation.

C. **Superficial thrombophlebitis** is characterized by tenderness, erythema, and edema in the area of a superficial vein. **However, these may propagate into the deep veins in up to 40%. Additionally, isolated saphenous vein thrombi may embolize** (*J Vasc Surg* 30:1113-1115, 1999). However, it is not clear if anticoagulation is routinely indicated for these clots.

D. **Embolization.** DVTs in the calf rarely embolize *although they may;* those in the thigh and pelvis do. Serial Doppler studies should be done to follow a calf DVT for propagation into the thigh or pelvis. Alternatively, the patient can be anticoagulated.

E. **DVT predisposed to by:**

1. Smoking, prior DVT, recent lower extremity surgery or trauma, stasis, such as with prolonged bed rest and trips, even as short as 2 hours.

2. Hypercoagulable states including protein C and protein S deficiency, protein C activation resistance, antithrombin III deficiency, Factor V Leiden, prothrombin gene rearrangement, estrogen use, cancer, anticardiolipin antibodies (e.g. with lupus), nephrotic syndrome, elevated factor VIII levels, etc.

3. One third of patients with homocystinuria will develop deep venous thrombosis, and elevated levels of homocysteine have been linked to an increased risk of DVT in the elderly. Folate and B-12 supplementation can minimize this risk.

F. **Diagnosis.**

1. **Physical exam,** including Homan's sign, does not reliably predict the presence or absence of DVT (but can change prior probability). Therefore, if DVT is considered, further testing is indicated.

2. **Venogram** is the gold standard but is painful, requires a dye load, and may induce DVT formation in a normal extremity.

3. Venous Doppler

   a. **Performs well** (e.g., is sensitive and specific) in:
      (1) Symptomatic patients (e.g., those with a swollen leg).
      (2) For clots above the knee

4

  b. **Does not perform well** (e.g., is not sensitive or specific):
    (1) As a screening test in those without symptoms (e.g., postoperative patients or in those with suspected PE but no swollen leg).
    (2) For clots below the knee.
    (3) For clots in the pelvis.
    (4) **Preliminary** evidence suggests that **isolated** noncompressible femoral veins are frequently false positive with only a 17% conformation of clot on venogram (*Arch Intern Med* 160(3):309-313, 2000). There is a high rate of pelvic malignancies in these patients.
  c. **A DVT cannot be ruled out by a single Doppler exam.** A second study should be done 1 week after the first. This is the protocol that the literature would suggest is prudent. A Doppler is not likely to be positive in a patient without a DVT (e.g., a few false positives).
4. **Impedance plethysmography** is not sensitive for DVT and should not be used.
5. **D-dimer.** See discussion under pulmonary embolism. Preliminary data indicates that a negative d-dimer ELISA plus a negative Doppler effectively rules out a DVT and obviates the need for a follow-up Doppler at 1 week. However, this is not yet standard of care.

G. **Treatment of DVT.**
1. **Anticoagulate.** See Chapter 6 for a complete discussion of anticoagulation. **Patients should be anticoagulated for 6 months after a first episode and for life after a second.**
2. **Subcutaneous low-molecular-weight** (LMW) **heparins** are marginally safer and marginally more effective than IV heparin and are generally preferable. They do not affect the PTT, and lab monitoring is not required. There is also a lower incidence of bleeding and thrombocytopenia than with unfractionated heparin. The best studied LMW heparin is enoxaparin, which is dosed at 1 mg/kg SQ Q12h for anticoagulation for DVT or PE. Although not standard of care, recent evidence indicates that the subcutaneous administration of enoxaparin at home for DVT may be both safe and effective and may preclude the need for hospitalization in the otherwise healthy patient.
3. **Postthrombotic syndrome** consists of chronic leg swelling secondary to venous obstruction or incompetence, leg pain and ulcer formation. **Compression stockings** can help prevent postthrombotic syndrome and should be used in most patients after a first episode of DVT. Horse chestnut extract has been used in a double-blind study for the same indication with positive results.
4. **Consider work-up for predisposing conditions** if there is no identifiable cause (such as prolonged travel). However, tests for clotting disorders may not be reliable in the acute setting or while patient is on

warfarin. Testing may be completed after prescribed therapy is completed and may have genetic implications for the family.

H. **DVT prophylaxis after surgery** (see Chapter 15.)

II. **Pulmonary Embolism (PE)**

A. **Characterized** by dyspnea (78%), pleuritic chest pain (59%), cough (43%), tachycardia (30%), tachypnea (73%), rales (55%), syncope (13%), and hypoxia (80%). These symptoms and signs are relatively nonspecific for PE but can help to raise your level of suspicion. Any sign or symptom may be missing in a patient and the absence of one or more symptoms or signs cannot be used to rule out PE.

B. **Look for predisposing factors** for DVT, which increase likelihood of PE.

C. **Look for ventilation-perfusion mismatch** by calculating the alveolar (A)-arterial (a) gradient. An elevated A/a gradient is present in 80% to 90% of those with PE **but is normal in 10% to 20%.**

$$\text{A-a gradient} = PaO_2 \text{ (alveolar)} - PaO_2 \text{ (arterial)}$$
$$PAO_2 \text{ (alveolar)} = 150 - 1.2(PaCO_2), \text{ assuming patient breathing room air } (FiO_2 \text{ } 21\%).$$
Normal A-a gradient is 5-20 and increases with age.

D. **Testing for PE.**

1. **Angiography** is the gold standard and is safe.
2. **A chest radiograph and ECG** should be done to rule out other causes of dyspnea and tachypnea but are not sensitive or specific enough to diagnose or exclude PE.
3. **O_2 saturation and ABG** may be normal in up to 15% of patients with a PE and cannot be used to differentiate between those with or without PE, although they do change your pretest probability.
4. **Ventilation-perfusion scanning** (V/Q scanning).
   a. Must interpret with caution. Scans are read as "normal," "low," "medium," or "high-probability" of PE. The overall likelihood of the presence of PE is determined with both the scan interpretation and pre-test clinical suspicion.
   b. Table 4-1 includes possible V/Q scan outcomes and interpretations.
5. **Spiral CT** may demonstrate central PE but the role of this test is unclear. The sensitivity for segmental PE may be as low as 60%. There is significant inter-institutional variability in interpretation and methods are not standardized. Thus, if the test is positive, it is helpful. If it is negative, additional evaluation is done (e.g., angiogram).
6. **Doppler** can be helpful if a patient has swollen leg and symptoms are suggestive of PE. However, 50% of patients with PE proven by angiography will not have an obvious source on Doppler scanning and venogram. **Doppler need not be done if the legs are clinically normal; it is expensive and has a low yield.**
7. **D-dimer,** a marker for thrombosis and fibrinolysis, can be useful in the exclusion of PE. In those with non–high probability scans and a

TABLE 4-1			

INTERPRETATION OF V/Q SCAN

Interpretation	Clinical Suspicion	Approximate Probability of PE	Interpretation
High probability	High or intermediate	96%+	Treat for PE
Medium probability	Low	12%	*Need further evaluation
Medium probability	Intermediate	33%	*Need further evaluation
Low probability	High	16%	*Need further evaluation
Low probability	Low	4%<	No PE
Normal	Low	2%	No PE

NOTE: Any other combination of results is not helpful and patients should have other testing.
*Start with Doppler of a **swollen leg** and then angiography if Doppler is negative.

history suggestive of PE, a normal D-dimer done by ELISA suggests less than a 3% likelihood of PE. **However, use of the D-dimer in the diagnosis of PE is not yet the standard of care. The technique used to determine the D-dimer is critical.** ELISA is the only test that is sensitive enough to be helpful. The sensitivity of latex agglutination is not sufficient to rule out PE (30% with PE will have normal D-dimer). The whole-blood assay has an intermediate sensitivity (15% with PE will have a normal D-dimer). Contact your lab about their cutoff value. Specificity of D-dimer is low. Most people with an elevated D-dimer do not have PE. Specific conditions that will give positive D-dimer tests include trauma, postoperative state, and malignancies.

E. **Treatment.**
  1. **Treat as for any respiratory distress** including O_2, monitoring, hospitalization, fluid resuscitation for secondary right-sided heart failure, dopamine, etc. (See Chapter 2 for treatment of shock.)
  2. **Anticoagulate** (see Chapter 5).
  3. **Thrombolysis** is indicated if PE is **confirmed** with angiogram (or high-probability V/Q in some opinions) and there is evidence of right heart failure (hypotension, JVD, EKG showing right heart strain) unresponsive to standard therapy. Thrombolysis may be considered in the setting of respiratory failure from PE, but the benefits are less well established.
     a. Regimens approved by FDA include the following:
        (1) **Streptokinase** 250,000 IU over 30 minutes followed by 100,000 IU/hr for 24 to 72 hours.
        (2) **TPA** 100 mg as continuous infusion over 2 hours.
        (3) **Catheter-directed** thrombolysis has the same rate of systemic bleeding as IV thrombolysis and is rarely used.

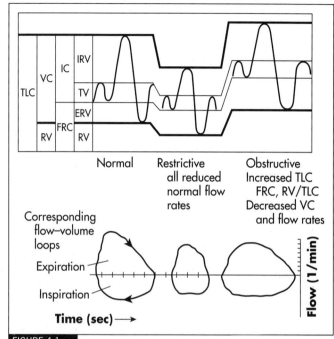

Normal

Restrictive
all reduced
normal flow
rates

Obstructive
Increased TLC
FRC, RV/TLC
Decreased VC
and flow rates

Corresponding
flow–volume
loops

Expiration

Inspiration

Flow (1/min)

Time (sec) ⟶

4

PULMONARY MEDICINE

FIGURE 4-1

Pulmonary function tests.

(4) Patients still require heparin anticoagulation after thrombolysis. LMW heparin, although not approved for this indication, may be more effective than unfractionated heparin. See treatment of DVT above.

(5) Menstruation is not a contraindication to the use of thrombolytics or heparin if they are needed to treat PE. Data are anecdotal, but there have been no bleeding problems to date.

4. Continue using anticoagulation (warfarin) for at least 6 months.

5. If anticoagulation is contraindicated or ineffective, consider vena cava interruption with a filter such as the Greenfield filter. **Vena cava filters are less effective than anticoagulation and may lead to increased rates of DVT and may not protect against PE** (same PE and death rates as conrols). Their use should only be considered when patients have contraindications to anticoagulation.

PULMONARY FUNCTION TESTS (Figure 4-1)

I. **Spirometry** (Figure 4-2)

A. **Forced vital capacity (FVC)** is the maximum volume of gas that can be expired forcefully after a maximum inspiration.

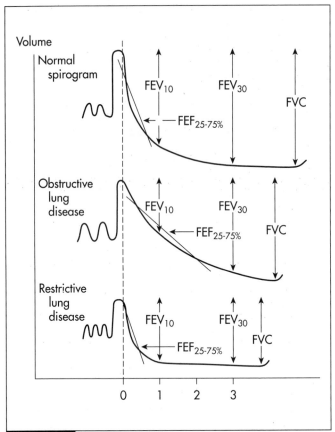

FIGURE 4-2
Spirometry.

B. **Forced expiratory volume in 1 second (FEV$_1$)** is the volume of gas expired during the first second of an FVC maneuver.

C. **Forced expiratory flow (FEF)** 25% to 75% in middle of forced expiration.

II. **Lung Volumes**

A. **Total lung capacity (TLC):** The volume in lungs at maximum inspiration.

B. **Vital capacity (VC):** The maximum volume expired after a maximum inspiration.

C. **Tidal volume (TV):** The volume inspired and expired during normal reathing.

D. **Residual volume (RV):** The volume left in the lungs after maximal expiration.

III. **Diffusion Capacity (DLCO).**
A. DLCO measures the diffusion of carbon monoxide across the alveolar surface.
B. Decreased by interstitial thickening (fibrosis) or decrease in alveolar surface area (emphysema, pneumonectomy, and consolidation).
C. May be increased with significant pulmonary hemorrhage.

IV. **Average Values.**
A. **VC** (predicted):
- Women = $(21.78 - [0.101 \times$ age in years$]) \times$ height in cm.
- Men = $(27.63 - [0.112 \times$ age in years$]) \times$ height in cm.

B. **TV**
- Child: 7.5 ml/kg.
- Adult Female: 6.6 ml/kg.
- Adult Male: 7.8 ml/kg.

V. **Interpreting Patterns of Abnormal PFTs**
A. **Obstructive Disorders.**
1. Defined by an FEV_1/FVC of less than 0.8. Differential diagnosis includes emphysema, chronic bronchitis, and asthma.
2. With bullous disease and air trapping, the RV and TLC will be increased, with a normal-to-decreased VC and TV.

B. **Restrictive Disorders.**
1. *Suggested* by a decrease in both FEV_1 and FVC, but with an FEV_1/FVC ratio of 0.8 or greater. However, restrictive disease is defined by a decrease in TLC.
2. Differential diagnosis includes interstitial lung diseases (sarcoidosis, environmental disease, pneumoconiosis, interstitial pneumonias, connective tissue disorders, pulmonary vascular diseases), fibrosis, and obesity. Also, kyphoscoliosis, status postsurgery, paralysis, ascites, pleuritis and pleural effusion.

VENTILATORS AND OXYGEN THERAPY

I. **General.** Respiratory failure is defined as the inability of the lungs to meet the metabolic demands of the body. This can involve failure of tissue oxygenation or failure of CO_2 homeostasis, or both. Acute respiratory failure is a medical emergency requiring prompt diagnosis and management and should be suspected when a patient breathing room air has a PO_2 <60 mm Hg or a PCO_2 >50 mm Hg with a pH <7.3.

II. **Oxygen Therapy**
A. Oxygen-delivery systems (Table 4-2).
B. Complications of oxygen therapy.
1. **Pulmonary oxygen toxicity** including mucosal drying, mucociliary dysfunction, atelectasis, interstitial and alveolar edema, and alveolar hemorrhage.
2. **Decreased respiratory drive,** carbon dioxide retention, and respiratory failure in patients with chronic hypoxemia, who have a respiratory drive based on hypoxia (as in those with COPD).

4

PULMONARY MEDICINE

TABLE 4-2
OXYGEN-DELIVERY SYSTEMS

Type	O_2 Flow (L/min)	% O_2 Delivered	Comments
LOW-FLOW SYSTEMS			
1. Nasal cannula	0.25 to 8	22 to 45	Precise regulation of FiO_2 not possible
			Comfortable but limited to low flow rate <4 L/min
			Nasal mucosa drying common
2. Simple mask	6 to 10	35 to 55	Offers little over nasal cannula
			Less comfortable, hot; skin irritation
			Not low enough FiO_2 for COPD
			O_2 rates must be at least 5 L/min to clear CO_2
3. Reservoir masks			
a. Nonrebreathing	12 to 15	90 to 95	High FiO_2 delivered; reservoir fills during expiration, which provides increased volume of O_2
b. Partial rebreathing	8 to 12	50 to 80	Flow must be sufficient to keep reservoir bag from deflating on inspiration
HIGH-FLOW SYSTEMS			
1. Venturi mask	4 to 12	21 to 100	Exact FiO_2 can be delivered
			Poor humidification
			Uncomfortable
2. Nebulizer with:			
a. Aerosol mask, face tent	0 to 12	30 to 100	Used to deliver precise FiO_2 or aerosol, or both
			Can provide controlled temperature of gas
			May need 2 or 3 setups to meet inspirational flows for FiO_2 >0.5
			Aerosol may induce bronchospasm, fluid overload, overmobilization of secretions, or contamination
b. Mask CPAP and BiPAP	0 to 12	Up to 100	Useful in COPD and CHF but less so in asthma
			May prevent intubation and decrease hospital stays
c. T-tube	0 to 12	30 to 100	For spontaneous breathing through endotracheal tube
			Flow rates should be 2 or 3 times minute ventilation

   3. **Retrolental fibroplasia** in neonates of low birth weight or gestational age <34 weeks.
   4. **Bronchopulmonary dysplasia** in infants who require mechanical ventilation after birth.
   5. **Risk of fire and explosion.**
III. **Ventilators.** Note: Initiate ventilation at 10 ml/kg tidal volume, FiO_2 of 100%, and a rate of approximately 14.
A. Indications for mechanical ventilation.
   1. **Hypercapnia.** Increased PCO_2 with inability to maintain adequate alveolar ventilation. Seek treatable causes (such as narcotics). Some patients with chronic lung disease will tolerate an increased $PACO_2$, remaining awake and comfortable. However, an arterial pH below 7.1 is considered an indication for mechanical ventilation.
   2. **Raised intracranial pressure.** However, hyperventilation may actually cause increased CNS ischemia and worsen brain injury.
   3. **Hypoxemia.** PAO_2 will usually be improved by IPPV. Specific criteria for instituting mechanical ventilation are the following
      a. PAO_2 <40 torr on maximal inspired O_2
      b. Increasing obtundation,
      c. Rapidly progressing respiratory disease,
      d. Increased work of breathing (as with intercostal retractions during inspiration),
      e. Elevation of $PACO_2$.
B. Modes of mechanical ventilation.
   1. **Volume-cycled ventilation.** A tidal volume is set, with airway pressures being increased until a set volume is delivered. Examples of volume-cycled ventilation include controlled mandatory ventilation (a fixed rate and volume are delivered), assist control (fixed minimum rate and volume are delivered with the patients respirations triggering additional breaths), and volume support. In volume-cycled ventilation, the minute ventilation is guaranteed assuring gas exchange, but the airway pressures are variable, allowing for dangerous generations of high pressures and risk of barotrauma (pneumothorax). Pressures needed depend on chest wall and lung compliance.
   2. **Pressure-cycled ventilation.** An inspiratory pressure is set, with the tidal volume dependent on pressure and patient compliance. Examples include pressure-control and pressure-support ventilation. The minute ventilation can change since delivery of a set volume is not guaranteed. Hence, gas exchange can vary, making dangerous hypercapnia or alkalosis possible. However, since inspiratory pressures are controlled, the risk of barotrauma is less. Since ventilator-associated pneumothorax may be instantly life-threatening, pressure-cycled ventilation may be preferred in patients with variable compliance (pneumonia, ARDS).

4

PULMONARY MEDICINE

IV. **Ventilator Management.**

A. **Oxygenation.** Arterial oxygen content should be maintained at 60 mm Hg or higher, or saturations at 90% or higher. Generally, initiate mechanical ventilation with an FiO_2 of 100%, then taper 10% every 10 to 15 minutes to find the lowest FiO_2 necessary to maintain adequate oxygenation. An FiO_2 of greater than 60% for over 24 hours has been associated with lung injury. PEEP may be added to decrease the A-a gradient, allowing a lower FiO_2 while maintaining oxygenation (see below).

B. **Ventilation.** Measured by minute ventilation (= tidal volume × respiratory rate) and is reflected in the PCO_2. Increases in minute ventilation will cause a decrease of PCO_2. Goals of ventilations should be to maintain a pH (as determined by PCO_2 and underlying diseases) of 7.3-7.4.

C. **Permissive hypercapnia.** In certain situations (e.g., ARDS) it may be permissible to allow the PCO_2 to rise (permissive hypercapnia) to decrease injury from ventilation as long as the patient maintains hemodynamic stability and oxygenation. This has been shown to decrease mortality in some cases (e.g., ARDS).

D. **Minute ventilation** is the product of tidal volume and rate; it is approximately 5 to 10 L/min or 100 ml/kg/min.

E. **Tidal volume** (Vt). Initial volume is 8 to 10 ml/kg. A large Vt improves gas exchange and prevents atelectasis. However, it may decrease venous return higher volumes may increase risk of barotrauma. A smaller Vt may be required if PEEP is added.

F. **Inspiratory time and flow.** Adjust inspired flow rate to maintain a ratio of inhalation time to exhalation time of 1 to 1.5 in most patients. Patients with airway obstruction (asthma, COPD) may require additional time for exhalation. This can be accomplished by decreasing inspiratory time, or by decreasing respiratory rate.

G. **Positive end-expiratory pressure** (PEEP) may increase compliance and decrease the work of breathing by preventing atelectasis, and thereby decreasing shunting. It is usually begun at 3 to 5 cm H_2O and increased in small increments. High levels may result in decreased venous return and severe hemodynamic compromise. Other negative consequences include overventilation, barotraumas, and elevated intracranial pressure. Cardiac output should be measured if there is an indication of problems because it may increase or decrease with increased PEEP.

H. **Peak airway pressure** reflects the pressure required to overcome airway resistance and is the peak pressure during the inspiratory cycle. The alarm limit should be set 10 cm H_2O above this. If the peak inspiratory pressure increases, you need to consider obstruction in the ET tube, bronchospasm, decreased lung compliance, or a pneumothorax from barotrauma.

I. **Sedation and neuromuscular paralysis** allow the patient to rest, decrease anxiety, and ensure better compliance with the ventilator. However, periodic interruption of sedation (if tolerated) reduces the total number of days on a ventilator.

1. **Initial therapy includes** midazolam, diazepam, lorazepam and propofol. Dosages should be titrated to desired effect, with monitoring of hemodynamic and respiratory status.

2. **Neuromuscular paralysis** is occasionally necessary if sedation fails, **but patients should still be sedated.** Monitoring alarms must be functioning because ventilator malfunction is rapidly fatal if the patient is paralyzed. Immediate, short-term paralysis (3 to 7 minutes) can be achieved with succinylcholine 1 mg/kg IV. For long-term paralysis use non-depolarizing agents such as pancuronium, vecuronium, or *cis*-atracurium. If repeated dosing or continuous drips are necessary, consider nerve-stimulation testing to avoid over-medication. Prolonged use of these agents, especially in continuous infusions, is associated with prolonged (days to months) muscle weakness and ventilatory dependence. Use of nerve-stimulators can decrease the dose of paralyzing agents while maintaining adequate control. If necessary, a neostigmine-atropine combination can be used to reverse the non-depolarizing agents.

V. **Prevention of Respirator-Associated Complications.**

A. **Continuous subglottic aspiration** of secretions reduces the incidence of nosocomial pneumonia. A semirecumbent position in bed also will minimize the risk of ventilator-associated pneumonia. A bacteriologic diagnosis should be aggressively pursued in ventilator-associated pneumonia and will reduce mortality.

B. **Stress ulcer prophylaxis.** Sucralfate, H2 blockers, and proton-pump inhibitors have all been shown to be effective. However, sucralfate may be associated with a lower rate of ventilator associated pneumonia.

C. **DVT prophylaxis.** Heparin 5000 U SQ Q12h or LMW heparins (enoxaparin 40 mg SQ QD or 30 mg SQ Q12h) are preferred, unless contraindicated (coagulopathy, thrombocytopenia, active bleeding, recent or future surgery). Compression stockings and intermittent pneumatic devices (TEDS and Kendals) are also effective.

VI. **Withdrawal of Mechanical Ventilation.**

A. **Guidelines** for weaning from mechanical ventilation:

1. An awake, alert patient.
2. PO_2 >60 torrs, with an FiO_2 <50%.
3. PCO_2 acceptable and a pH in normal range.
4. PEEP <8 cm H_2O.
5. Minute ventilation less than 10 L/min.
6. Patient is able to generate maximum voluntary ventilation without retractions.
7. Patient is able to generate a peak negative inspiratory pressure of at least 20 cm H_2O.

B. **Weaning from the ventilator:**

1. Explain the process to the patient and encourage cooperation.
2. Begin during the daytime; allow the patient to rest at night and between trials of weaning.

3. Place the patient in an upright position.
4. Causes of weaning failure include poor respiratory or cardiac function, underlying infection, high metabolic demands, poor nutrition and energy stores, and inadequate rest.
5. Discontinue weaning if:
   a. pH <7.3, PCO_2 >50 torrs, PO_2 <60 torrs.
   b. The patient becomes anxious, fatigued, demonstrates increasing respiratory distress, or develops significant arrhythmias or hemodynamic deterioration.
6. **Methods of weaning from ventilator**
   a. Of the following three common methods, the pressure-support and T-tube methods have similar rates of success. Intermittent (IMV) has resulted in increased time to wean in some studies. However, most patients will wean successfully with any method.
   b. **Pressure-support method.** Switch from an assisted mode of breathing to pressure support, setting pressures to generate Vt similar to the assisted volumes with a ventilation rate less than 20. Gradually decrease the inspiratory pressure until 8-10 cm H_2O above expiratory pressure. If patient can maintain adequate volumes with a ventilation rate of less than 20 for 30-60 minutes, consider extubation.
   c. **T-tube method.** (A T-tube allows the patient to breathe through an endotracheal tube without assistance from the ventilator.) Have the patient use a T-tube with humidified oxygen. If the patient tolerates this for 1 to 4 hours without deterioration, discontinue mechanical ventilation. If the patient fails the attempt, resume mechanical ventilation and consider IMV method (below) for weaning.
   d. IMV method. Gradually decrease the number of assisted respirations in 1 or 2 breath increments over 30- to 90-minute intervals. Monitor ABGs and vital signs. When an assisted rate of <4 breaths/min is achieved, consider a brief T-tube trial. If the patient remains stable, discontinue mechanical ventilation. If the trial fails, increase assisted rate until patient stabilizes. Repeat attempt the following day with a more gradual decrease in the rate of assisted breaths.

CHRONIC OBSTRUCTIVE PULMONARY DISEASE (COPD)

I. **Definition.** A generalized increased resistance to airflow during expiration that includes chronic bronchitis, emphysema, chronic asthma, and bronchiolitis. Patients rarely have pure emphysema or chronic bronchitis. Most patients will have both processes present. COPD occurs in 10% to 15% of cigarette smokers.

II. **Chronic Bronchitis**

A. **Characterized** by chronic cough productive of mucus for at least 3 months in each of last 2 years with inflammatory changes in the bronchial mucosa.

B. **Results from** prolonged exposure to pulmonary irritants including cigarettes, allergens, pollution, and recurrent infections.

III. **Emphysema**

A. **Characterized by** destruction of the lung parenchyma beyond the terminal bronchioles with coalescence of alveoli.

B. **Divided into:**
   1. **Panlobular,** which is the result of alpha1-antitrypsinase deficiency.
   2. **Centrilobular,** which is the result of smoking and of chronic bronchitis.

IV. **Diagnosis**

A. **Diagnose with pulmonary function tests,** including spirometry (before and after bronchodilators), lung volumes, and DLCO.

B. **Spirometry** shows obstructive airflow patterns, generally nonreversible (see section on PFTs). Although degree of decrease in FEV_1 does not correlate with symptoms, it a strong prognostic factor. When FEV_1 is less than 1 L, 5-year survival is 50%.

C. **Diffusion capacity** is decreased in emphysema; may be normal or low in chronic bronchitis.

D. **Lung volumes** may show hyperinflation (increased TLC) and air trapping (increased RV).

E. **CXR may be normal,** show evidence of bullous disease, hyperinflation, or increased interstitial markings from chronic airway inflammation.

F. **Blood gases** can show hypoxia and/or compensated hypercapnia (normal pH) in late stages.

G. **Laboratory data**
   1. **With acute exacerbations,** CBC, ABG, CXR, and ECG may be indicated, depending on the clinical situation.
   2. **Hypercapnia with acidosis** is suggestive of acute decompensation.
   3. **A high CO_2 level with a normal pH** is suggestive of a compensated chronic state.
   4. **ECG** may show multifocal atrial tachycardia, and if it is present, one should be aware of the possibility of theophylline toxicity.
   5. **Bedside peak flows** can document response to treatment.

V. **Cor pulmonale** can result from long-standing COPD. Essentially, vascular tone in the lungs increases leading to right heart failure. Patients present with leg edema, JVD, and possibly a palpable liver with elevated liver enzymes. This may respond to long-term oxygen therapy.

VI. **Acute Treatment of COPD**

A. **See Chapter 2 for acute treatment of COPD.**

B. **Treat any underlying infection.** (See section on pneumonia later.)

C. **Hospitalize** if clinically indicated (worsening tachypnea, falling O_2, acidosis, increasing CO_2.)

D. **Beware if the patient seems too calm.** It may indicate CO_2 retention with CO_2 narcosis. This can occur as the result of giving high-flow O_2 to a patient with chronic COPD. **However, do not withhold oxygen from a symptomatic, hypoxic patient even if it means the need for intubation.**

4

PULMONARY MEDICINE

VII. Long-term Management of COPD

A. **Immunization.** All patients with COPD should have an annual flu shot and Pneumovax every 5 years.

B. **Patients should be educated** about their disease and taught that if they start having difficulties with breathing, they should contact their health care professional.

C. **Pulmonary rehabilitation,** including conditioning and breathing techniques, improves lifestyle.

D. **Low-flow O_2** has been shown to be useful in reducing pulmonary arterial resistance, which if uncontrolled, leads to cor pulmonale.

1. **Use continuous oxygen** in those with either a PO_2 <55 mm Hg, an O_2 saturation of <89%, or a PO_2 <59 mm Hg with evidence of cor pulmonale (peripheral edema, HCT >55, P pulmonale on ECG).

2. **O_2 saturation should be kept above 90%** (PO_2 of 60 to 80 mm Hg). This usually can be accomplished with 2 L/min O_2 but titrate to patient's needs.

3. **Survival significantly enhanced with oxygen** use 24 hours a day. Patients should be encouraged to use oxygen at least 15 hours a day.

E. **Inhaled bronchodilators.** The use of these medications is predicated on instruction of the patient in their proper use. A spacer should be used with most metered dose inhalers. Additionally patients should be given instructions about what to do if they notice a need for increased amounts of medication to remain symptom free or if their symptoms persist despite the use of normal doses of bronchodilators. Since response varies over time, even those with a poor response on post-bronchodilator PFTs should be given a long-term trial of inhaled bronchodilators.

1. **Beta-adrenergic agonists** (such as albuterol, metaproterenol) to be used PRN for symptoms.

   a. Many of those with COPD are resistant to beta-agonists and will respond better to inhaled anticholinergics (below).

   b. **Dose.** One nebulizer of albuterol (2.5 mg) is equal to about 6 to 8 puffs of an MDI via spacer. Patients can use 4 to 8 puffs every 3 to 4 hours as needed but should be instructed on what to do (such as start steroids by mouth) if their need for albuterol increases.

   c. **Long-acting beta-agonists,** such as salmeterol, may be used to prevent nocturnal symptoms and to control symptoms during the day. However, salmeterol is not useful for the control of acute symptoms. Formoterol is an alternative.

2. **An anticholinergic agent** (such as ipratropium) is the bronchodilator of choice in COPD. Besides bronchodilation, it also limits secretions, which can cause mucous plugging. The normal dose is 2 puffs every 6 hours. It is also available for nebulization in higher doses. The equivalence of MDI versus nebulization is not as well worked out as it is for beta-agonists. However, it probably similar and higher doses of an MDI may be helpful. Anticholinergics have an effect that is additive to the inhaled beta-agonists. Combined beta-agonist/

anticholinergic inhalers are available (Combivent). Tiotropium, a QD anticholinergic, will soon be available in the United States.

3. **Inhaled steroids** (such as beclomethasone) should be used in patients that show some degree of reversibility to beta-agonists. Only about 15% of patients with COPD will respond to inhaled steroids. Generally, those who are responsive to inhaled beta-agonists and have acute attacks of dyspnea will be responsive to steroids.

4. **Oral steroids** (such as prednisone) are helpful in the subset of COPD patients with reversible disease (see above) but have many side effects and should be reserved for acute exacerbations and for those who do not respond to inhaled steroids.

5. **Leukotriene inhibitors** have no role in COPD.

6. **Theophylline** has an extremely limited role in COPD due to it's low benefit and high potential for complications in an elderly patient population (heart disease, drug-drug interactions, increased drug clearance).

7. **Long-term antibiotics are not helpful** but should be used to treat acute purulent exacerbations. For patients with recurrent purulent exacerbations, antibiotics for 7 days each month may prevent need for hospitalization. Amoxicillin or amoxicillin/clavulanate 500 mg TID, trimethoprim-sulfamethoxazole (Septra DS) 1 PO BID, or doxycycline 100 mg PO BID are recommended.

8. **Lung reduction surgery** may be appropriate for some patients (under age 75, no longer smoking, no cor pulmonale) and improves FEV_1 and symptoms. Randomized trials of survival are currently underway.

ASTHMA

I. **Definition.**

A. Asthma is an inflammatory disease of the airways characterized by reversible airway obstruction. Asthma, nasal polyps, and aspirin sensitivity make a common clinical triad.

II. **Diagnosis.**

A. **History.**

1. **Symptoms** include wheezing, cough, chest tightness, shortness of breath.

2. **Exacerbating factors** include sinusitis, reflux esophagitis, viral URI, and allergens (including dust and cockroach exposure).

3. **Episodic bronchospasm may be secondary** to exacerbating factors such as exercise, cold, exposure to smoke or workplace chemicals, etc.

B. **Physical Exam.** The physical exam may be normal between exacerbations. Wheezing, prolonged expirations, depressed diaphragms (hyperinflation) may be present especially with acute exacerbations. Look for signs of sinusitis, nasal polyps, and GE reflux.

C. **Additional testing.**

1. **Pulmonary function testing** is the mainstay of asthma diagnosis. Spirometry shows airway obstruction, which reverses by 12% or

4

PULMONARY MEDICINE

greater after inhaled bronchodilators. However, spirometry may be normal between exacerbations. Chronic asthma may lead to fibrosis and irreversible airflow obstruction.

2. **Serial peak flow readings** taken at home (e.g. before and after work or school) may show airflow variability.

3. **Bronchoprovocation** with methacholine or histamine may help establish the diagnosis.

4. **Skin testing** for common allergens may be indicated for those with moderate, persistent asthma since immunotherapy may be useful.

5. **Specific testing** for sinusitis (rhinoscopy) or reflux (pH probe) to identify contributing factors may be indicated.

III. **Chronic Disease Severity.** The National Asthma Education Program (and National Heart Lung and Blood Institute) classify chronic disease severity into four levels. Patients are classified according to the most severe class in which they have any features. Additionally, patients at any level of severity can have mild, moderate, or severe exacerbations.

A. **Mild intermittent asthma.** Symptoms occur fewer than 3 times/week, nocturnal symptoms fewer than 3 times per month, with normal FEV_1, and peak flows that vary less than 20%.

B. **Mild persistent asthma.** Symptoms occur 3-6 times/week, nocturnal symptoms 3-4 times month, with normal FEV_1, and peak flow varies 20%-30%.

C. **Moderate persistent asthma.** Daily symptoms, nocturnal symptoms 5 or more times per month, with FEV_1 60% to 80% predicted, and peak flow varies 30% or more.

D. **Severe persistent asthma.** Continual symptoms, frequent nocturnal symptoms, FEV_1 less than 60% predicted, and peak flow varies 30% or more.

IV. **Management**

A. **General Principles of Management.** Anti-inflammatory medications should be considered the mainstay of asthma therapy. Medications used for maintenance and rescue therapy are different.

B. **Written Plan. All patients should have a written plan for dealing with exacerbations** (e.g. start oral steroids, increase beta-agonists, and parameters for calling their health care provider).

C. **Inhalers.** All hand-held inhalers should be administered via the use of a spacer, or by holding the inhaler 1 inch from the patient's lips. Inhalers require initial training and periodic review of technique in order to provide adequate treatment and minimize side-effects.

D. **Monitoring.** Signs and symptoms of asthma are quite subjective. Therefore disease monitoring for those with more than mild asthma (both chronic and acute) should include objective measurement of airflow obstruction. This includes home peak flow meters, as well as intermittent formal spirometry depending on the severity of disease. See Tables 22-9 and 22-10 for normals.

E. **Indicators of control.** Indicators of poor asthma control include nocturnal symptoms, urgent care visits, and increased need for rescue inhaled beta 2-agonists (daily use for a week or more than one canister per month)

V. **Chronic Medications**

A. **Antiinflammatory drugs** are the mainstay of asthma therapy.

  1. **Inhaled corticosteroids.** Indicated for all severities of asthma with the exception of mild intermittent asthma. Different formulations have different potencies; beclomethasone <triamcinolone <fluticasone. However, clinically, the effectiveness is equal in equipotent doses.

  2. **Cromolyn and nedocromil.** May be used as monotherapy in children <5 years old with mild persistent asthma. However in adults, and children with moderate or severe asthma, these drugs should be an adjunct to inhaled corticosteroids to assure adequate antiinflammatory activity.

  3. **Leukotriene inhibitors.** The role of leukotriene inhibitors is not well-defined, but they are not recommended for first-line use. They are no more effective than inhaled steroids but have more potential toxicity, including Churg-Strauss syndrome (also known as "allergic granulomatosis and angiitis"). Churg-Strauss syndrome is a necrotizing angiitis. It occurs in those with preexisting asthma or allergies. Manifestations include pulmonary nodules with an abnormal CXR (25%), skin purpura and nodules, and a mononeuritis multiplex. Renal involvement is rare. Patients usually have a peripheral eosinophilia and a positive p-ANCA. The illness responds to steroids and the prognosis is good. Leukotriene inhibitors are not recommended at all for children less than 12 years of age (although montelukast can be used in those as young as 6 years old). Examples include zafirlukast (Accolate) and zileuton (Zyflo).

  4. **Oral corticosteroids.** With adequate dosing of above antiinflammatory agents, chronic systemic steroids are rarely needed. If used, attempt to wean to minimum dose or alternate day dosing to limit side effects.

B. **Long-acting beta$_2$-agonists.** Examples include salmeterol (inhaled) and extended release albuterol (systemic), as well as famoterol. May be particularly useful for nocturnal symptoms. Salmeterol has been shown to decrease the needed dose of inhaled corticosteroids, but in most cases should not be used as a replacement for steroid inhalers. Also important to instruct patients that long-acting agents should not be used for rescue therapy.

C. **Short-acting beta$_2$-agonists.** Scheduled use of short-acting bronchodilators is generally not recommended. Control with scheduled use of beta-agonists is not as good as that achieved with PRN use. Short-acting beta$_2$-agonists (e.g., albuterol, terbutaline, pirbuterol) should be used PRN for wheezing and symptom exacerbation, before exercise, etc. There is no advantage to levalbuterol, which is the L isomer of albuterol.

4

PULMONARY MEDICINE

The same clinical results can be obtained at a lower cost by increasing the dose of albuterol.

D. **Theophylline.** May add additional long-term control, but due to significant side-effects and low therapeutic window, theophylline is a third-line agent behind inhaled corticosteroids and long-acting beta$_2$-agonists. If used, serum drug levels should be monitored regularly and maintained at 10 to 15 μg/ml.

VI. **Quick Relief (Rescue) Medications.** See Chapter 2 for in-hospital treatment of asthma exacerbations.

A. **Short-acting beta$_2$-agonists.** Inhaled albuterol, terbutaline, pirbuterol; available as both metered dose inhalers, as well as nebulized solutions. Inhaled bronchodilators, such as metaproterenol or epinephrine (available over the counter), should be discouraged due to potential for excessive cardiac stimulation from nonselective adrenergic properties. Patients can safely use up to 6 or 8 puffs every 2 hours but should contact their health care practitioner if increasing doses are needed.

B. **Anticholinergics. Ipratropium bromide.** Produces bronchodilation by reducing vagal tone to airways. May be particularly helpful in conjunction with beta-agonists.

C. **Methylxanthines.** Theophylline and aminophylline are not recommended for rescue medications; they provide no additional benefit over inhaled beta- agonists, and may produce adverse effects.

BRONCHIECTASIS

I. **Definition.** Bronchiectasis is a chronic dilatation and inflammation of medium-sized bronchi. Clinically it looks similar to chronic bronchitis with chronic mucopurulent sputum production. However, sputum production is often copious and may contain *Pseudomonas* organisms. Occurs mostly in the left lower lobe followed by the lingula and the right middle lobe with hemoptysis and recurrent pneumonia in a single lobe.

II. **Predisposed** to by recurrent pneumonia, granulomatous disease, carcinoma, or any process that can lead to a sequestered lobe.

A. **CT scanning** will demonstrate areas of bronchiectasis (enlarged peripheral airways with thickened airway walls).

B. **Treat as for COPD.** A 6-month course of antibiotics (e.g., amoxicillin/clavulanate or doxycycline) initially may help eradicate underlying infections. Patients with bronchiectasis may benefit from a course of antibiotics for the first 10 days of every month (such as TMP/SMX or doxycycline).

C. **Surgical resection** of affected lobe is alternative treatment if antibiotics fail.

PNEUMONIA

I. **General.** An infection of the lower respiratory tract, including bacterial, viral, or fungal etiologies. Clinical manifestations include fevers, cough with or without sputum production, shortness of breath, and pleuritic chest pain. Physical exam may reveal crackles (rales) in the lungs with dullness to percussion and egophony. Infiltrates with or without pleural effusions may be seen on CXR. Patients may have few of these findings, particularly the very young or old, or those with other chronic illnesses. Additionally, these findings are nonspecific, and other diagnoses deserve consideration. **In children, tachypnea is the most sensitive physical finding and warrants an x-ray even in the absence of rales, etc.** The differential diagnosis includes heart failure, malignancy, pulmonary embolism, pulmonary vasculitis, eosinophilic pneumonia, and inflammatory lung diseases, etc.

II. **Diagnosis**

A. **Diagnosis is based** on physical exam, CXR (PA and lateral), and clinical scenario (see below for differential diagnosis of pulmonary infiltrates). However, the clinical exam for pneumonia is imprecise (even among pulmonologists) and a CXR should be done if there is any question. **The appearance on CXR (lobar versus diffuse) does not reliably differentiate between typical and atypical pneumonia. Base treatment on age, etc (see below), and not on appearance.** CBC with WBC differential may be helpful. Arterial O_2 saturation should be obtained by pulse oximetry. Send a blood gas to assess for adequacy of ventilation in those who have a low O_2 saturation or appear particularly dyspneic, cyanotic, etc.

B. **For outpatients,** attempts at microbiologic diagnosis are not time nor cost effective.

C. **For inpatients,** most feel attempts at defining the etiology are warranted, but a specific pathogen is identified in only 50% of patients even with extensive evaluation. Treatment should not be delayed awaiting results. Gram stain of sputum analysis may be helpful, but be aware of significant false negatives and false positives (especially for *Streptococcus pneumoniae*). Sputum cultures are similarly imprecise. Blood cultures should be obtained and are frequently positive in pneumococcal pneumonia. A diagnostic thoracentesis should be done if effusion is present. *Legionella* urinary antigen, *Mycoplasma* antibodies, and other pathogen-specific tests might be helpful.

D. **Immunosuppressed** patients have a high incidence of atypical pathogens not covered by standard regimens, and early bronchoscopic lavage or biopsy should be considered (see Chapter 11).

III. **Management**

A. **Antimicrobial therapy** is based upon culture results when possible. Empiric therapy is based upon patient population and regional variances. Specific populations are discussed below.

B. **Viral influenza,** type A or B, is a common cause of pneumonia, especially in winter months. See viral respiratory infections for management.

C. **Bacterial pneumonia.** Treatment should continue for 7-21 days, depending on severity and etiology. Intravenous antibiotics may be switched to oral agents 24-48 hours after defervescence.

4

PULMONARY MEDICINE

D. **Course.** Patients may continue to be febrile 3 days into treatment, but up to 7 days for gram-negative infections and in patients with comorbid conditions. Therefore treatment changes are not indicated as long as the patient is not worsening.

E. **The chest x-ray may lag** behind clinical symptoms, but a change in therapy is not indicated if the patient is stable. X-ray resolution will be evident in 73% at 6 weeks and 94% at 24 weeks. Most patients should be followed radiographically to assure resolution.

IV. **Management of Patients Who Do Not Respond to Initial Therapy**

A. **If the patient deteriorates,** or fails to resolve, consider further testing and change in treatment.

1. **Consider resistant organisms,** such as *Staphylococcus aureus, Haemophilus influenzae,* atypical agents *(Legionella, Chlamydia).* Also viral pneumonia (influenza A and B).

2. **Consider unusual pathogens.** Histoplasmosis in Midwest/Ohio river valley, *Coccidioidomycosis* in southwestern US, psittacosis with bird exposure, Q fever with various farm animal exposures, tuberculosis, etc. (see also Chapter 11).

3. **Consider noninfectious diagnoses** such as the following:

   a. **Unifocal infiltrates.** Pulmonary contusion, pulmonary embolism, alveolar cell carcinoma, pulmonary hemorrhage, lymphoma, radiation pneumonitis, lipoid pneumonia, rarely lobe torsion, foreign body.

   b. **Multifocal infiltrates.** Hypersensitivity pneumonitis (see below), tuberculosis, fungal infections, alveolar cell carcinoma, Hodgkin's lymphoma, eosinophilic pneumonia, allergic granulomatosis and angiitis, collagen-vascular diseases (e.g rheumatoid arthritis, lupus, scleroderma), Wegner's granulomatosis, silicosis, black lung disease, amyloidosis, sarcoidosis.

   c. **Other illness.** This list is not inclusive.

4. **Re-image chest,** particularly looking for effusions, abscess, tumor causing a post obstructive pneumonia. Further testing with CT, bronchoscopy, or open lung biopsy may be useful.

V. **Resistant Organisms**

A. *S. pneumoniae.* Penicillin-resistant *S. pneumoniae* (PRSP) is becoming more prevalent, but this depends on the region. Be sure to differentiate between intermediate resistance (MIC <4) and high resistance, as most beta-lactam antibiotics achieve high levels in the lung. Studies have shown that even in the face of intermediate resistance, outcomes are still good in patients treated with beta-lactam antibiotics. In cases of known high resistance or endemic areas, consider vancomycin or extended spectrum fluoroquinolone until sensitivities return.

B. *H. influenza.* Chronic colonizer in smokers. Most have beta-lactamase, therefore beta-lactamase inhibitors needed such as clavulanate or sulbactam. Also resistant to erythromycin, but clarithromycin and azithromycin give good coverage.

C. *Staphylococcus aureus.* Resistant to most beta-lactams, except synthetics like methicillin and nafcillin, or those with a beta-lactamase inhibitors. Where methicillin-resistant *Staphylococcus aureus* (MRSA) is prevalent, consider vancomycin.

VI. **Empiric Treatment Based on Patient Population**

A. **Neonates <5 days old.** Caused by maternal vaginal flora, including Group A and B *Streptococcus, E. coli, Chlamydia, Treponema.* Treat with ampicillin and gentamicin or third-generation cephalosporin.

B. **Neonates (5 days to 1 month).** Group A or B *Streptococcus, S. aureus, E. coli, Chlamydia.* Treat with penicillinase-resistant penicillin (nafcillin). Consider vancomycin if MRSA is prevalent. For cough and infiltrates without a fever, consider *Chlamydia trachomatis* even in the absence of conjunctivitis. These children should be treated with a macrolide.

C. **Children (1 month to 5 years).** 80% of mild-to-moderate cases are viral. Bacterial causes include pneumococcus, *H. influenzae,* also chlamydia or *Mycoplasma.* Treat with extended spectrum macrolide for outpatients (e.g., clarithromycin, azithromycin). Consider third-generation cephalosporin ± aminoglycoside for inpatients.

D. **Children over 5 years.** Same as adults without comorbid factors.

E. **Adult outpatients without comorbid factors.** Most common agents are pneumococcus, *Mycoplasma, Chlamydia pneumoniae.* Treat with macrolide (tetracycline if intolerant). Must also cover *H. influenzae* in smokers, so use extended spectrum macrolide (azithromycin or clarithromycin).

F. **Adult outpatients with comorbid factors** (smoking, age >60, diabetes, emphysema, heart disease, etc). If multiple comorbid factors, consider inpatient treatment. Common etiologies same as those without comorbid factors, but increased prevalence of gram-negative rods and Moraxella. Treat with TMP/SMX + macrolide or Augmentin + macrolide. Extended spectrum macrolide or extended spectrum fluoroquinolone (e.g., levofloxacin) may be used as monotherapy.

G. **Adult inpatients not requiring ICU.** Similar organisms but increased incidence of *Legionella* and gram-negative rods. Treat with third-generation cephalosporin + macrolide, beta-lactam with inhibitor + macrolide. Consider monotherapy with extended spectrum macrolide (azithromycin IV) or extended spectrum fluoroquinolone (e.g., levofloxacin).

H. **Adult inpatients requiring ICU.** Most common agents are pneumococcus, gram-negative rods, and *Legionella. Mycoplasma* in elderly. Therapy includes a macrolide plus a third-generation cephalosporin. Consider adding an aminoglycoside to cover gram-negative rods especially if the patient is hypotensive.

I. **Adult, hospital-acquired pneumonia.** As patients remain in the hospital, the oropharynx become increasingly colonized with gram-negative rods

4

PULMONARY MEDICINE

and MRSA. Therefore, for hospital acquired pneumonias that develop within the first 2-5 days after admission, treat with a third-generation cephalosporin or fluoroquinolone. After this, aggressive gram-negative rods are common so treat with two anti-pseudomonal agents (aminoglycoside or ciprofloxacin + antipseudomonal beta-lactam like piperacillin, piperacillin-tazobactam, imipenem), consider adding vancomycin for MRSA.

VII. **Atypical Pneumonia Syndrome**

A. Cough may be nonproductive and often have associated pleuritic pain, URI symptoms, fever, headache, and myalgias. Symptoms are usually milder than with bacterial pneumonia. See also section under pneumonia for other possible diagnoses. Common in school-age children and young adults.

B. **Organisms.** Usually *Mycoplasma,* others can include TWAR *(Chlamydia pneumoniae),* Q fever, *Chlamydia psittaci* (especially in bird owners), influenza A and B, adenovirus, RSV, Legionnaire's disease, *Pneumocystis carinii* pneumonia (PCP) in the immunocompromised, etc (Table 4-3). See also Chapter 11, as well as differential diagnosis of infiltrates in previous pneumonia section.

C. **Treatment.** As for all pneumonia above. However, if bacteriologic diagnosis is available, treat as per Table 4-3.

HYPERSENSITIVITY PNEUMONITIS

I. Epidemiology

A. **Occurs** in up to 8.6% of farmers. Also responsible for "sick building" syndrome.

B. **Etiology.** There are various etiologies of hypersensitivity pneumonitis (Table 4-4). In farmers it is caused by inhalation of *Actinomyces* spores, which are present in moldy hay, silage and moldy grain.

C. **Onset of illness** may range from weeks to years after first exposure to antigen.

D. **Clinical differentiation.** Not all individuals exposed at a work site will develop hypersensitivity pneumonitis. This is in contrast with **toxic organic dust syndrome,** which results from inhalation of gram-negative endotoxin and affects all workers at a site. Additionally, the CXR is normal in toxic organic dust syndrome.

II. Clinically

A. Acute form

    1. Fever, chills, cough, dyspnea, malaise, fever which occurs 4-8 hours after exposure to the inciting antigen; it does not occur right after exposure such as might occur with asthma. If no further exposure, symptoms will resolve spontaneously in 2-5 days spontaneously.

    2. **Chronic exposure.** May have a prolonged flu like illness if exposures occur daily.

    3. **Bronchoalveolar lavage** reveals lymphocytosis.

    4. **CXR** reveals a reticulonodular pattern.

TABLE 4-3

COMMON ATYPICAL PNEUMONIAS

Organism	Clinical Presentation	Diagnosis Made by Treatment
Chlamydia pneumonia (TWAR)	10% of all pneumonias in US, hoarseness may be present, clinically similar to *Mycoplasma* pneumonia without neurologic and GI symptoms May also cause bronchitis and asthma	WBC usually normal, IgG antibody test available, self-limited but may use tetracycline or macrolide.
Fungal pneumonias (coccidioidomycosis/ blastomycosis/ histoplasmosis)	Occur in a geographic distribution: *Coccidioidomycosis*: southwestern US/California *Blastomycosis*: southeast/south central US *Histoplasmosis*: eastern US (to midwestern US) All cause an influenza-like illness with pneumonia	*Coccidioidomycosis*: find spores in sputum; + skin test; IgG antibody Prescribe fluconazole, itraconazole, or amphotericin B *Blastomycosis*: culture from sputum (4 wks!); KOH of sputum Prescribe itraconazole, ketoconazole, amphotericin-B *Histoplasmosis*: organism culture; skin test (not specific); identification of polysaccharide in urine and blood (with disseminated disease) Prescribe itraconazole but amphotericin B if moderately or severely ill

Continued

4

PULMONARY MEDICINE

TABLE 4-3

COMMON ATYPICAL PNEUMONIAS—cont'd

Organism	Clinical Presentation	Diagnosis Made by Treatment
Hantavirus	Mice and rats are vectors Occurs throughout the US (most common: southwest) Myalgias, fever, headache, abdominal pain, cough, rapid onset of respiratory failure, ARDS	Hemoconcentration, thrombocytopenia, hypoxia IgM and IgG antibody tests available Ribavirin may be useful, contact the CDC
Legionnaires' disease (*Legionella pneumophila*)	1-2 day prodrome of headache, myalgias then fever, chills, tachypnea, dry cough May become obtunded; associated vomiting, diarrhea	WBC mildly elevated (8000 to 10,000); cold agglutinins negative; sputum immunofluorescent antibody available; look for *Legionella* antigen in urine (90% sensitive but only for one serotype); serum antibody titers available Treatment is erythromycin (500 mg Q6h), clarithromycin, or azithromycin
Pneumocystis (PCP)	See Chapter 11	See Chapter 11
Mycoplasma pneumonia	Occurs in epidemics Associated pharyngitis, fever, headache, dry cough May have clear exam but infiltrate on x-ray May have cold agglutinin-mediated hemolysis, meningeal signs, cranial nerve deficits, nausea, vomiting, diarrhea	WBC usually normal (<25% elevated 10 to 20,000) Cold agglutinin titer 1:128 (other pneumonias may have lower titers) IgG and IgM antibodies PCR testing available Treat with erythromycin, azithromycin, clarithromycin

Psittacosis (Chlamydia psittaci)	Especially in bird owners	WBC usually normal but may be up or down
	Headache, high fever, dry cough, myalgias, chest pain, perhaps vomiting and diarrhea	Antibody titers diagnostic
		Treat with doxycycline 100 mg BID
	Splenomegaly common and suggests the diagnosis, hepatomegaly, myocarditis, perhaps	X-ray may not clear for 6 wks
Q-fever (Coxiella burnetii)	Especially in dairy and abattoir workers and those with livestock contact	Antibody titers against "chlamydia burnetii" diagnostic
	Fever, cough, headache, malaise, hepatitis, endo-carditis	Treat with tetracycline 500 mg Q6h
Tularemia (Francisella tularensis)	From rabbits (are nonpulmonary variants as well)	Antibody titers and culture to diagnose
	Tracheitis, pneumonia, cough, dyspnea, hemoptysis	Treatment is streptomycin
Viral disease (influenza, para-influenza, RSV, adenovirus)	Varies by virus	Generally normal WBC unless secondary infection

4

PULMONARY MEDICINE

TABLE 4-4

COMMON CAUSES OF HYPERSENSITIVITY PNEUMONITIS

Source	Antigen	Disease
Hay, straw	Thermophilic bacteria	Farmer's lung
Heater water (e.g., humidifiers including in the home)	Thermophilic bacteria	Humidifier lung
Sugar cane	Thermophilic bacteria	Bagassosis
Parrots, pigeons, ducks, chickens, etc	Animal protein and excreta	Bird breeder's lung
Many other sources, including industrial solvents, rubber, cork, plastics, etc	Various	Detergent workers lung, chemical workers lung, and so on

    5. **Biopsy** (if done) shows interstitial inflammation and granuloma formation.
B. **Chronic form:** No systemic symptoms but may present with cough and symptoms suggestive of a chronic interstitial lung disease. Up to 50% will deny having a primary illness. 50% have bronchiolitis obliterans but see chronic exposure above.

III. **Diagnostic criteria**
A. **Exposure to antigen** with presence of antigen specific antibodies in blood.
B. **Symptoms** appearing within several hours after exposures.
C. **If CXR is normal,** the patient must have a positive biopsy in order to make the diagnosis of hypersensitivity pneumonitis.
D. **Minor criteria include** rales, decreased diffusion capacity, decrease O_2 sat, positive provocation test.
E. **Differential includes** asthma (absent systemic symptoms), atypical pneumonia (not recurrent), toxic organic dusts syndrome (discussed above).

IV. **Ancillary testing**
A. **X-ray:** Acute may have diffuse pulmonary infiltrates, which are generally nonlobular. However, may be normal. In chronic disease have reticulo-nodular pattern, fibrosis. High-resolution chest CT shows typical "ground glass" appearance.
B. **Lab:** Will generally have antibodies against *Actinomyces* but only indicates exposure and does not make diagnosis of Farmer's lung. Up to 50% of asymptomatic pigeon breeders have antibodies.

V. **Management**
A. Minimize exposure (increase ventilation, wear respirator).
B. Store only dried materials, wet surface before moving materials.
C. Removal from exposure will frequently lead to spontaneous resolution of symptoms.

D. Steroids are indicated for acute disease if there are severe systemic symptoms and/or gas exchange abnormalities. Must remove from source if going to use steroids. Inhaled steroids are ineffective.

E. Once fibrosis begins it may not resolve and the patient may have progressive disease even if steroids used. Follow antibody levels as indication of exposure.

VIRAL RESPIRATORY TRACT INFECTIONS

I. **General.** Approximately 80% of acute respiratory illnesses result from viral infections. These are usually self-limited syndromes caused by a variety of viruses: rhinovirus, adenovirus, echovirus, coxsackievirus, influenza, and parainfluenza viruses. Occasionally, pneumonia may complicate these infections, either primary viral pneumonia, or secondary bacterial pneumonia. In the compromised host less common pathogens, such as varicella virus, measles virus (paramyxovirus), CMV, and HSV can result in life-threatening infections.

II. **The Common Cold**

A. **Causes.** Rhinovirus, adenovirus, echovirus, and coxsackievirus, respiratory syncytial virus (RSV).

B. **Clinical presentation.** Chief complaints include congestion, sneezing, clear to mucopurulent nasal discharge, dry sore throat, low-grade fever, and cough. Physical exam reveals erythematous nasal and oropharyngeal mucosa, and there is a normal chest exam.

C. **Management.** Treatment is primarily symptomatic. Rest, hydration, decongestants, such as pseudoephedrine for comfort, acetaminophen for analgesia and fever. Antihistamines have no proven benefit but those with anticholinergic properties may dry the nasal mucosa.

D. **Ipratropium nasal spray** is available for symptomatic treatment. Use the 0.06% spray, 2 puffs per nostril BID or TID.

E. Zinc gluconate lozenges and ecchinacea may have some minimal benefit if started early but this is controversial.

F. Educate patients about hand washing and that antibiotics do not work.

III. **Influenza**

A. **Overview.** Influenza is a systemic illness resulting from infection with an influenza virus, which are orthomyxovirus types A, B, or rarely C. These viruses can change their envelope proteins as their host population develops immunity, thereby maintaining the ability to cause recurrent infection in a single host population. Influenza vaccinations for the predicted virulent strains are available in the fall months and are generally effective in preventing or decreasing the intensity and duration of infection. However, response to vaccine wanes with increasing age so that of the nursing home population, only 50% will mount a significant response.

B. **Clinical presentation.** There is usually an abrupt onset of high fever, chills, dry cough, headache, myalgia, and prostration. Physical exam is usually unremarkable with the exception of basilar rales in some pa-

4

PULMONARY MEDICINE

tients. Chest radiograph is usually normal. Occasionally, perihilar promi-nence and increased markings can be present. The development of infil-trates is suggestive of a complicating pneumonia, either viral or bacte-rial. Nasal swabs can confirm the diagnosis.

C. **Management.** The illness is usually self-limited, lasting 4 to 7 days. Rest, hydration, and acetaminophen are recommended. For influenza type A, amantadine hydrochloride 100 mg PO BID for 10 days started within 48 hours of symptom onset can shorten the course and can be used for prophylaxis in compromised close contacts of infected individu-als (also give vaccine if not already done). Rimantadine 100 mg PO BID may also be used and has a lower incidence of side effects. Reduce dosage of both drugs for renal or liver impairment, for the elderly, and in the presence of a seizure disorder. These agents should be continued for 5 days or 24-48 hours after symptoms resolve. Zanamivir (Relenza) and Oseltamivir (Tamiflu) are neuraminidase inhibitors that cover both in-fluenza A and B. However, they are expensive, and influenza B is un-usual in the US. They have no significant advantage over rimantadine in most cases. Consider prophylaxis in appropriate population.

D. **Complications.** Myocarditis, myositis (including rhabdomyolysis), peri-carditis, Reye's syndrome, and Guillain-Barré syndrome have been re-ported as complications of influenza. Additionally, secondary bacterial pneumonia may occur. This should be considered if a patient is getting better and develops worsening symptoms of cough, dyspnea, fever.

IV. **Bronchitis**

A. **Characterized by** cough with purulent sputum, rhonchi, and sometimes fever. Mostly viral in cause, but also consider *H. influenzae, S. pneumo-niae, Moraxella.*

B. **Treatment.** There is little evidence that antibiotics are useful in non-smokers. Cough suppression and inhaled beta-agonists are the mainstay of treatment. Albuterol and other beta-agonists are excellent for cough suppression in the patient with bronchitis and hasten symptomatic reso-lution. Erythromycin, doxycycline, and TMP/SMX are good antibiotic choices if antibiotics are indicated (only in acute exacerbations of chronic bronchitis in smokers). Benzonatate 100 mg PO Q6h will sup-press cough as will codeine (such as acetaminophen and codeine).

EVALUATION OF THE CHRONIC COUGH

I. **Most common causes in order of frequency.** Postnasal drip/chronic si-nusitis, asthma, including postviral reactive airways, GE reflux disease. Consider also medication (ACE inhibitors), CHF, pertussis, TB. Pertussis in adults may present only with chronic cough and may be present de-spite childhood immunization and represent 21% of those with chronic cough in one series (check acute and convalescent titers).

II. **One Approach.**

A. Treat with antihistamine or decongestant empirically. Consider course of antibiotics for sinusitis if appropriate.

B. If positive titer for pertussis, treat with erythromycin or other macrolide.
C. If this fails, do bronchoprovocation testing for asthma and treat patients with positive results with beta-agonists and prednisone (if fail, beta-agonists alone).
D. If cough continues or bronchoprovocation is negative, do CXR and sinus CT. Treat positives.
E. Evaluate negatives for GE reflux and give trial of H_2-blocker.
F. If patient still coughing, consider bronchoscopy.
G. This approach leads to successful treatment in 96% (though there are recurrences).

OBSTRUCTIVE SLEEP APNEA

Obstructive sleep apnea Affects 2% to 4% of the population

I. **Clinically complain of:**
A. Daytime sleepiness, snoring, headache, personality changes, intellectual deterioration, sexual dysfunction. Partners may note restless sleep, periods of apnea. Daytime sleepiness, depression, unrefreshing sleep, etc. are not specific and may occur with other sleep disorders, depression, etc.
B. 40% of women with sleep apnea have amenorrhea or dysmenorrhea that resolves with treatment.
C. May have secondary hypertension, right- and left-sided heart failure, dysrhythmias, MI, CVA, increased risk of MVA (sevenfold increase).
D. Only 50% are obese.

II. **Diagnosis By**
A. **Polysomnography (sleep study).** Expensive and time consuming but is the gold standard. Criteria include:
   1. Cessation of air flow for 10 seconds even with maintenance of respiratory effort.
   2. Five or more episodes of apnea per hour.
   3. Decrease in oxygen saturation of at least 4% during episodes.
B. **Continuous nocturnal oxygen saturation measurement at home.** Using 10 desaturations per hour as the cutoff, it has a 98% sensitivity but only a 48% specificity with a positive predictive value of 61% and a negative predictive value of 97% in those with a history suggestive of sleep apnea.
   1. Not valid in those receiving oxygen therapy.
   2. Can use to screen before ordering a sleep study, since it has a high negative predictive value and is inexpensive.

III. **Treatment.**
A. Relieve nasal obstruction including polyps, allergic causes, and structural abnormalities (such as septal deviation).
B. Avoid sedatives, androgens and alcohol.
C. Weight loss.
D. Treat hypothyroidism if present.
E. Mask or nasal CPAP (continuous positive airway pressure) is the treatment of choice. Need to customize positive pressure by observing result in a sleep study. Only 46% will have adequate compliance.

4

PULMONARY MEDICINE

F. Drugs including medroxyprogesterone, protriptyline (centrally stimulates respiration), and fluoxetine have some benefit but only in mild cases.

G. Oxygen alone can be used if mild desaturation or not able to tolerate other modalities.

H. Surgical therapy, including tonsillectomy, uvulopalatopharyngoplasty (efficacy only 30% to 50% but no good controlled studies), tracheostomy.

SARCOIDOSIS

I. **General.** A diffuse inflammatory process of unknown cause leading to the formation of noncaseating granulomas, which may form in any organ. The lungs are the primary site of involvement with chest radiograph findings in 95% of those with sarcoidosis.

II. **Clinically.**

A. Affects those 20 to 40 years of age but may occur at any age.

B. **Much more common** in African-Americans and tends to be more severe in this group.

C. **Must differentiate** from tuberculosis and fungal illnesses (histoplasmosis etc.), which may have a similar clinical appearance. Also must exclude carcinoma and lymphoma.

D. Symptoms and signs are related to organ involved.

   1. **Pulmonary manifestations** include bilateral hilar adenopathy, dyspnea, reduced vital capacity, cough, pleural effusion and reduced diffusion capacity.

   2. **Systemic manifestations** include fever, erythema nodosum, infiltrative skin lesions, ocular involvement with uveitis (causes about 4% of uveitis).

   3. **CNS** involvement may present as meningitis, seizure disorder, and cranial nerve abnormality.

   4. **Endocrine** including hypercalcemia and hypercalciuria, pituitary dysfunction secondary to mass lesions.

   5. **Cardiac involvement** with arrhythmias, heart block, sudden death.

   6. **Bone and joint** involvement with pain, arthritis, etc.

   7. **Liver and pancreas** involvement are common.

III. **Diagnosis.** Demonstration of noncaseating granulomas by biopsy.

A. Transbronchial biopsy or mediastinal biopsy generally diagnostic.

B. May biopsy granulomatous skin lesions (but not erythema nodosum) or peripheral adenopathy, if present.

C. Classically, elevated levels of angiotensin-converting enzyme (ACE) have been used to make the diagnosis of sarcoid. However, this is nonspecific, and ACE levels may be elevated in miliary TB, silicosis, asbestosis, and other conditions. However, once diagnosis is made, one can follow ACE levels as measure of disease activity though this is generally not needed.

IV. **Treatment of Sarcoidosis.**

A. Treatment is difficult, and efficacy is controversial. Generally reserve treatment for those with progressive disease, or those with airway or ocular involvement. Even in those with pulmonary impairment, delaying treatment for three months to monitor for progression is not dangerous.

B. Many patients go into remission spontaneously, negating the need for treatment. Spontaneous remissions tend to not relapse. However, in those who obtain remission through corticosteroids, there is a high rate of relapse upon discontinuing therapy. Again therapy should be reserved for progressive disease, and patients should be followed (radiographs and pulmonary function) for several years after withdrawing therapy.

C. Corticosteroids are the mainstay in those who require treatment. Generally will respond to low-dose steroids (5 to15 mg prednisone QOD).

D. Methotrexate and chlorambucil have been used as steroid-sparing agents, but have toxicities of their own.

WEGENER'S GRANULOMATOSIS

I. **General.** Systemic illness that primarily affects the nasal and sinus mucosa, the lung, and the kidney. Necrotizing granulomas are found in the perivascular areas. Generally occurs in middle-aged adults but may occur in younger patients (mean age 40 years).

II. Clinical symptoms.

A. **Pulmonary symptoms** such as cough, recurrent pneumonia, hemoptysis

B. **Renal symptoms** including hematuria, pyuria, renal failure from glomerulonephritis.

C. **Recurrent sinusitis.**

D. **Systemic symptoms** including fever, arthralgias, and polyarthritis, weight loss.

III. Diagnosis.

A. **Central antineutrophil cytoplasmic antibody (c-ANCA)** is 85% sensitive. However, it is not 100% specific since other vasculitides may also present with a positive c-ANCA.

B. **Multiple pulmonary nodules** (may be cavitary) or infiltrates on chest radiograph (90%).

C. **Biopsy specimen** that shows classic granulomas.

D. **Lab.** May have anemia, ESR, leukocytosis, pyuria, and hematuria. Complement levels are normal, and the ANA is negative.

IV. Treatment and Course.

A. **It is suggested that a consultation be obtained before initiating treatment of Wegener's granulomatosis.** Wegener's has a 90% mortality within 1 to 2 years if not treated.

HEMOPTYSIS/PULMONARY HEMORRHAGE

I. **Defined as** the expectoration of blood or bloody sputum.

II. **Divided into two categories** based on whether the problem is a primary pulmonary abnormality or of an extrapulmonary etiology.

A. **Intrapulmonary source.**

1. **Infectious,** including bronchitis, TB, pneumonia, abscesses, fungal infections.

2. **Structural,** including arteriovenous malformation, tumor, infarction (e.g., from pulmonary embolism), foreign body.
3. **Vascular,** including Goodpasture's syndrome, pulmonary vasculitis, traumatic vessel disruption, Henoch-Schonlein purpura.
4. **Cardiac,** including CHF, mitral stenosis.
5. **Wegner's granulomatosis.**
6. **Connective tissue** diseases such as RA, lupus, and other vasculitis.
7. **Pulmonary hemosiderosis.** The majority are children or young adults with episodic hemoptysis, occasionally massive.

B. **Extrapulmonary sources.**
1. **GI, including** hematemesis (aspirated blood).
2. **Extrapulmonary structural,** including epistaxis, oral, or nasopharyngeal lesions.
3. **Systemic coagulopathies,** including DIC.
4. **Cocaine and penicillamine.**

III. **Diagnosis.**
A. **History.** Concomitant illness, presence of shock, vomiting, other bleeding sites, etc.
B. **Lab.** CBC, platelet count, PT/PTT, fibrinogen, fibrin degradation products, sputum for culture, gram stain, and AFB. Sputum for cytology.
C. **Imaging.** A CXR should be done and a chest CT or angiogram may be indicated, depending on the clinical situation.
D. **Bronchoscopy** should be considered in those at risk for malignancy (smokers, older patients, prior malignancy of any source, family history of malignancy).

IV. **Management.**
A. **General.** Treat the underlying disease state.
B. **Massive hemoptysis** should be treated as per the *hypovolemic shock* section in Chapter 2. Obtain surgery and pulmonary consults if acute intervention is required to stop the bleeding.
C. **Admission.** Use clinical judgment about the need for admission and imminent work-up. If the bleeding is minor and from a self-limited cause (e.g., bronchitis), patients may be followed as outpatients. In those with greater than 200 cc of bleeding in 24 hours, admission is indicated.

PLEURAL EFFUSION

I. **Definition.** An abnormal collection of fluid within the pleural space.
II. **Clinical symptoms and signs** are nonspecific. Dyspnea, orthopnea, and pleuritic pain are common. On exam, will have decreased breath sounds and dullness to percussion over the effusion.
III. **Diagnosis.**
A. **Radiographic.** Lateral radiograph is more sensitive than PA film. Blunting of costophrenic angle on PA view suggests at least 500 cc of fluid. Larger effusions may show loss of diaphragm border. Decubitus x-rays will show layering of fluid if not loculated. Ultrasound or CT may help if x-rays are not clear.
B. **Thoracentesis.** Fluid analysis helps define etiology of the effusion. Most

fluid should be sent for protein, LDH, glucose, cell count and differential, gram stain and bacterial culture, and pH (must be sent in heparinized syringe on ice!). Additional studies as indicated, include AFB stain and culture, anaerobic culture, cytology, amylase, cholesterol.

IV **Etiologies.**

A. **Transudate.** Caused by fluid leaking from normal capillaries, ascites crossing the diaphragm, or failure of normal pleural drainage through lymphatic channels. Differential diagnosis includes elevated hydrostatic pressure (CHF, renal failure, portal hypertension), decreased oncotic pressure (liver failure, nephrotic syndrome), or thoracic duct obstruction. Transudates meet none of Light's Criteria (listed below).

B. **Exudate.** Caused by "active processes" within the pleural space. Defined by one or more of the following Light's criteria:

1. Pleural fluid to serum protein ratio greater than 0.5
2. Pleural fluid to serum LDH ratio greater than 0.6
3. Pleural fluid LDH greater than 150 mg/dl (two-thirds the upper limit of normal serum LDH)
4. **Differential diagnosis.** Parapneumonic effusion, malignancy (especially with bloody effusion), empyema (infection in the pleural space), collagen vascular disease, TB, other inflammatory diseases. Exudates are caused by abnormal pleural tissue; work-up for underlying etiologies may include chest CT, bronchoscopy, pleural biopsy, or thoracoscopy

V. **Management.** Treat the underlying problem. Draining large effusions by thoracentesis may relieve symptoms of dyspnea and improve cardiac function; however, on objective exercise testing, exercise tolerance is not altered. Empyemas and parapneumonic effusions with pH less than 7.1 require complete drainage with repeated thoracentesis, tube thoracostomy, or surgery; some have used thrombolytics (e.g., streptokinase or urokinase) to successfully clear loculated effusions. No controlled studies to date. Recurrent malignant effusions may be palliated with pleurodesis.

4

PULMONARY MEDICINE

BIBLIOGRAPHY

Bartlett JG et al: Community-acquired pneumonia in adults: guidelines for management (Guidelines from the Infectious Diseases Society of America), *Clin Infect Dis* 26: 811-38, 1998.

Breiman RF et al: Emergence of drug-resistant pneumococcal infections in the United States, *JAMA* 271(23):1831, 1994.

Brochard L et al: Comparison of three methods of gradual withdrawal from ventilatory support during weaning from mechanical ventilation [see comments], *Am J Respir Crit Care Med* 150(4): 896-903, 1994.

Campbell GD et al: Hospital-acquired pneumonia in adults: diagnosis, assessment of severity, initial antimicrobial therapy, and preventative strategies, *Am J Respir Crit Care Med* 153: 1711-25, 1996.

Craig WA: Pharmacokinetic/pharmacodynamic parameters: rationale for antibacterial dosing of mice and men, *Clin Infect Dis* 26(1): 1-10, 1998.

de Moerloose P, Michiels JJ, Bounameaux H: The place of D-dimer testing in an integrated approach of patients suspected of pulmonary embolism, *Semin Thromb Hemost* 24(4): 409-12, 1998.

Dalton AM: A review of radiological abnormalities in 135 patients presenting with acute asthma, *Arch Emerg Med* 8(1):36, 1991.

Den Jeijer M et al: Hyperhomocysteinemia as a risk factor for deep-vein thrombosis, *N Engl J Med* 334 (12):759, 1996.

Drummond N et al: Effectiveness of routine self monitoring of peak flow in patients with asthma, *Br Med J* 308(6928):564, 1994.

Esteban, A et al: A comparison of four methods of weaning patients from mechanical ventilation. Spanish Lung Failure Collaborative Group [see comments], *N Engl J Med* 332(6): 345-50, 1995.

Esteban A et al: Effect of spontaneous breathing trial duration on outcome of attempts to discontinue mechanical ventilation. Spanish Lung Failure Collaborative Group, *Am J Respir Crit Care Med* 159(2): 512-8, 1999.

Ewig S et al: Pneumonia acquired in the community through drug-resistant Streptococcus pneumoniae, *Am J Respir Crit Care Med* 159(6): 1835-42, 1999

Ewig, S, Torres A: Severe community-acquired pneumonia, *Clin Chest Med* 20(3): 575-87, 1999.

Ginsberg JS et al: Sensitivity and specificity of a rapid whole-blood assay for d-dimer in the diagnosis of pulmonary embolism, *Ann Intern Med* 129:1006-11, 1998.

Goldhaber SZ: Pulmonary embolism, *N Engl J Med* 339(2): 93-104, 1998.

Guilleminault C et al: Upper airway sleep-disordered breathing in women, *Ann Intern Med* 122(7):493-501, 1995.

Hunninghake GW et al: Statement on sarcoidosis, *Am J Respir Crit Care Med* 160 (2): 736-755, 1999.

Imperiale TF et al: A meta-analysis of methods to prevent venous thromboembolism following total hip replacement, *JAMA* 271(22):1780, 1994.

Janssen MC et al: Rapid D-dimer assays to exclude deep venous thrombosis and pulmonary embolism: current status and new developments, *Semin Thromb Hemost* 24(4): 393-400, 1998.

Koopman MMW et al: Treatment of venous thrombosis with intravenous unfractionated heparin administered in the hospital compared with subcutaneous low-molecular-weight heparin administered at home, *N Engl J Med* 334(11):682, 1996.

Lanter PL et al: Safety of thrombolytic therapy in normally menstruating women with acute myocardial infarction, *Am J Cardiol* 74(2):179, 1994.

Levine M et al: A comparison of low-molecular-weight heparin administered primarily at home with unfractionated heparin administered in the hospital for proximal deep-vein thrombosis, *N Engl J Med* 334(11):677, 1996.

National Heart, Lung, and Blood Institute, National Asthma Education and Prevention Program, Expert Panel Report 2: *Guidelines for the diagnosis and management of asthma,* National Institutes of Health publication no 97-4051, 1997.

Pratter MR et al: An algorithmic approach to chronic cough, *Ann Intern Med* 119(10):977, 1993.

Remy-Jardin M et al: Spiral CT of pulmonary embolism: diagnostic approach, interpretive pitfalls and current indications, *Eur Radiol* 8(8):1376-90, 1998.

Séries F, Marc I, Cormier Y, La Forge J: Utility of nocturnal home oximetry for case finding in patients with suspected sleep apnea hypopnea syndrome, *Ann Intern Med* 119:449-453, 1993.

Strollo PJ Jr, Rogers RM: Obstructive sleep apnea, *N Engl J Med* 334(2):99, 1996.

Taylor DR et al: Regular inhaled beta agonist in asthma: effects on exacerbations and lung function, *Thorax* 48(2):134, 1993.

Vallés J, Artigas A, Rello J et al: Continuous aspiration of subglottic secretions in preventing ventilator-associated pneumonia, *Ann Intern Med* 122:179-186, 1995.

Wells PS et al: Graduated compression stockings in the prevention of postoperative venous thromboembolism: a meta-analysis, *Arch Intern Med* 154:67, 1994.

Wright SW et al: Pertussis infection in adults with persistent cough, *JAMA,* 273(13):1044, 1995.

Yang KL, Tobin MJ: A prospective study of indexes predicting the outcome of trials of weaning from mechanical ventilation, *N Engl J Med* 324(21): 1445-50, 1991.

GASTROENTEROLOGY AND HEPATOLOGY

Jatinder P. S. Ahluwalia
Mark A. Graber
William B. Silverman

DYSPEPSIA (SEE ALSO GASTROESOPHAGEAL REFLUX DISEASE)

I. **General.** The symptoms of dyspepsia can include intermittent or persistent pain and discomfort in the upper abdomen or lower part of the chest, regurgitation, postprandial bloating or distension, heartburn, nausea, early satiety and a feeling of postprandial fullness. Any or all of these symptoms may also be present in patients with ulcer disease. **Unfortunately, it is not possible to differentiate non-ulcer dyspepsia from "functional" dyspepsia based on history and physical.**

II. **Etiology** is multifactorial and may include food intolerance, motility problems (30% to 80% have delayed gastric emptying), and psychologic overlay. Visceral hypersensitivity, in which patients are oversensitive the postprandial distension of the stomach, etc., is also hypothesized as a mechanism.

III. **Differential includes** ulcer disease, gastritis, reflux esophagitis and **aerophagia. Aerophagia,** which is caused by swallowing excess air during meals, presents as bloating (to the point that patients may need to loosen their clothing), and belching.

IV. **Evaluation** may include endoscopy, testing for food intolerance (e.g., elimination diet), upper abdominal ultrasound, abdominal CT scan, gastric emptying studies. However, for the younger patient, an empiric trial of treatment is reasonable.

V. **Treatment.** Treating *H. pylori* in patients with dyspepsia is controversial and does not seem to yield any benefit, although there are conflicting data. A trial of H-2 blockers, proton pump inhibitors, or a promotility agent (e.g., metoclopramide) is reasonable. Have patients slow their eating and chew well. However, treatment is often unsatisfactory.

PEPTIC ULCER DISEASE

I. **General.** Predisposing factors for both duodenal and gastric ulcers include alcohol, tobacco, aspirin and other NSAIDS, and physiologic stress such as multiple trauma, sepsis, neurosurgical problems, gastrinoma, other "ICU" stresses.

II. **There is no symptom complex that can adequately differentiate gastric from duodenal ulcers and nonulcer dyspepsia.** Classically, food is reported to alleviate the pain of duodenal ulcers and exacerbate the pain of gastric ulcers. However, food may exacerbate or relieve the pain of either type of ulcer; the pain of gastritis is reliably worsened by food. The

151

pain of either type of ulcer may be felt as a gnawing pain in the chest, back, mid-abdomen, or either upper quadrant. Additionally, many ulcers are asymptomatic (especially those related to NSAIDS) and first present with a perforated viscus or GI bleed.

III. **Physical exam and lab** should include a CBC to rule out anemia secondary to bleeding, as well testing stool for fecal occult blood.

IV. **Who needs a study to visualize the upper GI tract:** Those over 45 years of age with new onset of dyspeptic/ulcer symptoms or with other symptoms suggesting malignancy, such as fever, weight loss, early satiety, vomiting, and so on, should be referred for endoscopy. Others can be treated presumptively but should have a work-up if they have recurrent disease or disease that is difficult to control. Work-up can be either a barium upper GI study or endoscopy. Endoscopy is a superior test for diagnosis but is more costly and has less patient acceptance.

V. **The role of *H. pylori*.** Excluding patients with Zollinger-Ellison syndrome, NSAID-induced ulcer disease, and some other rare causes of ulcers, *H. pylori* (a urease-producing flagellated bacterium) infection is believed to play an etiologic role in up to 95% of those with duodenal ulcers and greater than 80% of those with gastric ulcer. There is also evidence that *H. pylori* infection is highly correlated with atrophic gastritis, intestinal metaplasia, gastric carcinoma, gastric non-Hodgkin's lymphoma, and mucosa-associated lymphoid tissue lymphomas of the stomach. **Treating for *H. pylori* increases healing and decreases relapse rate.**

A. **Testing for *H. pylori*:** If the patient is not on an NSAID, consider presumptive treatment for *H. pylori* without a work-up. Presumptive treatment has been shown be clinically and cost effective.

B. **Available tests include:**

1. **Invasive tests.** CLO test (pH change in medium secondary to the urease activity of the organism), direct culture or stain of the organism.

2. **Noninvasive tests.** The *H. pylori* antibody test is sensitive and specific for *H. pylori* infection. Alternatives include the breath urea test in which urea is ingested and radioactive CO_2 is exhaled if *H. pylori* is present. Another form of the urea test checks for radioactive CO_2 in the blood after the ingestion of urea. A stool test for *H. pylori* will soon be available.

3. **Caveats.**

a. You cannot follow antibody levels to determine effectiveness of treatment. Only 57% of patients become antibody negative at 1 year. Use the CLO test or breath urea test if documentation of *H. pylori* clearance is required.

b. Recent therapy with H-2 blocker or proton pump inhibitors can cause false negative CLO and urea tests by suppressing the organism. Stop therapy for 2 weeks in advance of testing.

C. **Treating *H. pylori* infection.** All of the options in Table 5-1 have a greater than >90% cure rate.

TABLE 5-1

TREATMENT FOR *H. PYLORI*

Regimen	Number of Days
Omeprazole 20 mg BID + Clarithromycin 500 mg BID + Amoxicillin 1 g BID (Prevpac)	14 days
Lansoprazole 30 mg BID + Clarithromycin 500 mg BID+ Metronidazole 500 mg BID	14 days
Bismuth Subsulfate-525 mg (2 tablets) BID + Metronidazole 500 mg PO TID + tetracycline 500 mg QID + Lansoprazole 30 mg PO QD	14 days
Omeprazole 20 mg BID + Clarithromycin 500 mg BID + Metronidazole 500 mg BID	10 days
Helidac (BSS, Metronidazole, tetracycline) QID + famotidine 40 mg QD	14 days

VI. **The role of acid control measures.** The H-2 blockers and proton pump inhibitors, cimetidine, ranitidine, famotidine, omeprazole, lansoprazole, and others, are all effective in treating duodenal ulcers when given for 6-8 weeks. Lansoprazole has fewer drug interactions than does omeprazole. **However, be sure to address *H. pylori* as noted above. Using acid control measures alone is not optimal treatment!** Sucralfate is indicated as therapy for duodenal disease but only works in the presence of acid (so cannot use H-2 blockers or proton pump inhibitors concurrently). Additionally, it is difficult to maintain a QID regimen.

VI. **The role of lifestyle factors.** To be successful at treating ulcer disease, it is important that the patient be advised to avoid factors that predispose to ulceration, including alcohol, NSAIDS and aspirin, and tobacco use.

VII. **Preventing recurrence.** Continue maintenance for 2 additional weeks after 6-8 weeks of treatment and consider long-term suppression in those at high risk of recurrence (smokers, alcohol abusers) and in those with a high risk of bleeding. Treating for *H. pylori* is effective at preventing recurrence.

VIII. **Special considerations in duodenal ulcers**

A. **Recurrent ulcers.** Patients with recurrent ulcers should have a full work-up, including endoscopy and serum gastrin levels (to rule out Zollinger-Ellison syndrome). However, remember that proton pump inhibitors and to a lesser degree H-2 blockers can increase serum gastrin levels. Consider also:

  1. Surgical consult for vagotomy/antrectomy.
  2. Consider causes such as carcinoma. In the immunosuppressed, cytomegalovirus should be considered a potential cause.

B. **Complications of duodenal ulcer disease:**

  1. **Gastric outlet obstruction** with early satiety and reflux symptoms.
  2. **Perforation.** Usually occurs posteriorly and presents as an acute abdomen with free air in the abdomen.
  3. **GI bleeding.** See section on GI bleeding.

IX. **Special considerations in gastric ulcers.**

A. **Endoscopy:** All lesions found on x-ray should be biopsied to rule out gastric carcinoma. Several samples should be taken of each ulcer, as well as brushings for cytology. **Resolution of symptoms and healing of ulcer with treatment does not ensure that it is not a carcinoma. All gastric ulcers require biopsy.**

X. **NSAID-Induced Gastroduodenal Ulcers**

A. **General.** NSAIDs are the most widely prescribed drugs in the world. They are potent cyclooxygenase inhibitors and prevent the gastric synthesis of prostaglandins, which are necessary for the production of gastric protective mucus and bicarbonate. There is contradictory evidence about whether or *H. pylori* plays a role in NSAID-induced ulcers, **although it seems reasonable to look for and treat *H. pylori* in patients with NSAID-induced ulcers.**

B. **Presentation.** Many NSAID-related ulcers are painless because NSAIDs are such potent pain relievers. Dyspeptic symptoms do not correlate well with NSAID-induced ulcers; those with symptoms frequently do not have ulcers and those without symptoms frequently do.

C. **Treatment.**

1. **Stop offending drug** and use acetaminophen for pain control if possible. If not, choose one of the NSAIDs with lower GI side effects such as ibuprofen or salsalate. COX-2 inhibitors may also be used but are expensive, and the efficacy is no better than that of traditional NSAIDS. Additionally, even one aspirin per day such as for stroke and MI prophylaxis may erase any GI advantage of the COX-2 inhibitors.

2. **Prevention.** The only drugs shown to prevent both NSAID-induced gastric and duodenal ulcers are the proton pump inhibitors. Generally, lansoprazole is preferred because of fewer drug interactions. Misoprostol plus an H_2-blocker is an alternative but is more expensive and has more side effects (e.g., diarrhea, abdominal pain, and abortion).

XI. **Zollinger-Ellison Syndrome (ZES).**

A. **ZES is caused by hypersecretion of gastrin,** from a gastrinoma. ZES is responsible for 0.1% to 1% of all cases of peptic ulcer disease.

B. **Serum gastrin levels can be elevated both in acid hypersecretory states (e.g., ZES), as well as in states of low acid secretion.** Gastrin levels can be elevated by gastric atrophy, stomach surgery, pernicious anemia with achlorhydria, ZES, and proton pump inhibitor use.

C. **A normal gastrin level reliably rules out ZES.** If the serum gastrin level is elevated, the test should be repeated simultaneously with a gastric pH. If the gastrin level remains high and the gastric pH is less than 2.5, there is a high likelihood that the patient may have ZES and needs to be referred to an appropriate specialist for definitive diagnosis and treatment.

D. ZES is often associated with hyperparathyroidism and pituitary dysfunction (Multiple Endocrine Neoplasia [MEN I]) at a rate of 20% to 25%.

Appropriate tests to evaluate for the presence of MEN I include serum calcium levels and serum PTH levels, as well as tests for pituitary function.

ESOPHAGEAL DISEASES

I. **Dysphagia** is the sensation of difficulty swallowing and feeling as though food is getting stuck in the esophagus. This is a common presenting complaint of many esophageal diseases. Esophageal disease may also present as "cardiac-like" chest pain

A. Consider infectious esophagitis (e.g., candida, Herpes simplex) in the appropriate setting.

B. Always consider esophageal malignancy when dysphagia is present.

C. See also specific disease entities below.

II. **Esophageal Foreign Bodies**

A. **Clinically presents as** inability to swallow, including the inability to swallow saliva; everything is regurgitated.

    1. Usually occurs after eating a large bolus of meat.

    2. May have a previous history of esophageal obstruction.

B. **Diagnosis can be made clinically.** Barium swallow can define area of obstruction, although is not indicated since endoscopy may be needed.

C. **Treatment.** Should not allow impaction to remain for >12 hours because of the risk of perforation.

    1. **Glucagon** 1mg IV followed in 20 minutes by another 2 mg. Carbonated beverages, such as Pepsi, have been used with success in some cases.

    2. **IV diazepam** may be helpful to relax the patient.

    3. **Nifedipine** or SL NTG have been used with some success.

    4. **Endoscopy** is the treatment of choice if the above are not successful.

    5. **Proteolytic enzymes** (e.g., Adolf's meat tenderizer) have been associated with esophageal perforation and are therefore not recommended.

D. **Evaluation.** All patients should be evaluated for esophageal rings and strictures after the foreign body is removed.

III. **Swallowed Foreign Bodies (excluding food)**

A. **Coin ingestion.**

    1. 35% or more of children are asymptomatic.

    2. Esophageal coins are generally visible as disk on AP, while those in trachea tend to be on edge.

    3. If within 24 hours, consider passing a Foley under fluoroscopy, inflate Foley, and pull out coin. Must protect airway.

    4. Endoscopy is the treatment of choice. If the coin passes into the stomach, there is no need to proceed to endoscopy. Simply observe the patient and assure passage by radiograph or observation of stool.

B. **Button Battery Ingestion**

    1. **A true emergency!! May have perforation in 4 hours!! Endoscopy is required if a button battery is lodged in esophagus.**

    2. If in stomach, may watch for 24 to 48 hours to see if passes. If not, endoscopy.

    3. Call the National Button Battery Ingestion Hotline (202)-625-3333 for questions.

C. **Ingestion of sharp objects**

    1. **If longer than 5 cm or wider than 2 cm,** may not pass through stomach and should be removed.

    2. Remove sharp objects, such as razor blades, safety pins, etc, if possible.

    3. If not, document passage with serial x-rays.

    4. If symptomatic, get surgical consult.

IV. **Achalasia.** Motility disorder of the esophagus secondary to the loss of neurons from the myenteric plexus in which there is aperistalsis of the esophageal body, failure of the lower esophageal sphincter (LES) to relax with swallowing, and elevated LES pressures. Absence of peristalsis is the cardinal finding and is sufficient to make a diagnosis of achalasia.

A. **Clinically.** Dysphagia, regurgitation, and chest pain eventually leading to weight loss.

    1. Presenting age is 20 to 40 years.

    2. Have about 5% chance of developing esophageal carcinoma.

B. **Diagnosis.** Barium swallow will demonstrate narrowing of the distal esophagus (bird beaking) and dilatation of the proximal esophagus.

C. **Treatment.**

    1. **Medication, including** isosorbide dinitrate 5-10 mg SL before meals (may be the most effective modality) or calcium channel blockers such as nifedipine 10 to 30 mg PO ½ hour before meals. An alternative is nitroglycerin 0.4 mg SL ½ hour before meals and QHS.

    2. **Physical modalities, including** esophageal dilatation with a bougie, surgical myomotomy, or endoscopic balloon dilatation.

    3. **Botulinum toxin injection.**

V. **Diffuse esophageal spasm:** A motor disorder with large amplitude, long duration, and repetitive contractions of esophageal smooth muscle with the absence of coordinated peristalsis.

A. **Clinically,** patient may have chest pain and dysphagia. Symptoms may be precipitated by stress or cold liquids.

B. **Diagnosis:**

    1. Barium swallow shows diffuse esophageal spasm.

    2. Manometry shows normal LES pressures and uncoordinated contraction but some normal peristaltic activity.

C. **Treatment:** With medications as noted under Achalasia.

VI. **Zenker's Diverticulum**

A. **Generally presents** after age 60 but may have years of symptoms.

B. **Clinically**

    1. Regurgitation of undigested food when patient bends over or lies down.

    2. May lead to aspiration pneumonia.

C. **Diagnosis** is by barium swallow or endoscopy.

D. **Treatment** is by surgical resection.

VII. Scleroderma

A. **Clinically.** Dysphagia and acid reflux secondary to lower esophageal sphincter incompetence. Have predisposition to Barrett's metaplasia and stricture of the esophagus. Also predisposed esophageal adenocarcinoma.

B. **Diagnosis:** Barium swallow shows dilatation of the lower esophagus with poor sphincter tone. Manometry shows low pressures especially at LES.

C. **Treatment** is symptomatic as for reflux esophagitis (below).

VIII. **Gastroesophageal reflux/reflux esophagitis.** Reflux of gastric contents (including acid, pepsin, and bile salts) into the esophagus resulting in mucosal damage. Caused by transient relaxation of the lower esophageal sphincter muscle. These episodes of relaxation are more common after meals and are stimulated by fat in the duodenum.

A. Clinically

   1. **Presents as** heartburn, dysphagia, frequently found in asthmatics.

   2. **Predisposing factors include:** Increased gastric volume (from meals, pyloric obstruction, diabetic gastroparesis), increased abdominal pressure such as with obesity, pregnancy, ascites, hiatal hernia. Other factors include smoking, caffeine, alcohol, chocolate, fats.

B. Diagnosis

   1. **By history.** Esophagoscopy will show esophagitis. Barium swallow may show reflux from stomach to esophagus.

   2. **Manometry** will show decreased LES pressure.

   3. **Bernstein test:** Solution of 0.1 M HCl is dripped into the distal esophagus at 8 cc/hr. A positive test reproduces the patient's symptoms. Saline should be used as a control.

   4. **24-hour esophageal pH monitoring.**

C. Treatment:

   1. **Eliminate precipitating factors** (see above).

   2. **Elevate head of bed** on blocks (adding pillows does not work).

   3. **Histamine receptor antagonists** (cimetidine, ranitidine, nizatidine, and Famotidine) **and proton pump inhibitors** (omeprazole, lansoprazole, etc.) are the only agents known to heal erosive esophagitis. The proton pump inhibitors are more expensive and should be reserved for those patients unresponsive to an H-2 blocker. For long-term control, omeprazole and lansoprazole have been shown to be superior to ranitidine at 1 year.

   4. **Agents that increase LES tone:**

      a. **Metoclopramide** (Reglan) 5 to 10 mg PO ½ hr AC and QHS. Generally needs to be used in conjunction with an H2 antagonist. Additionally, metoclopramide promotes stomach emptying.

      b. **Omeprazole** (Prilosec) 20 mg PO QD for 4 to 8 weeks, or lansoprazole. These agents act by suppressing acid formation and increasing LES tone.

     c. Cisapride may cause dangerous arrhythmias and is not recommended.

  5. **Surgical fundoplication** for incapacitating disease.

D. **Complications:** aspiration pneumonia, acid laryngitis, asthma, pulmonary fibrosis, Barrett's esophagus, stricture formation, and predisposition to carcinoma if chronic.

ACUTE DIARRHEA

I. **Definition and pathophysiology.** Abnormally increased frequency or decreased consistency of stools for less than 3 weeks.

II. **Pathophysiology.**

A. **Osmotic.** Caused by ingestion of a poorly absorbed solute (carbohydrate malabsorption: ingestion of mannitol, sorbitol, lactulose; disaccharidase deficiency: lactose intolerance; pancreatic insufficiency; small intestinal mucosal disease: celiac sprue (gluten sensitive enteropathy); ingestion of magnesium-containing antacids in excess).

B. **Secretory diarrhea.** Increased small intestinal secretion or reduced absorption. This may result from bacterial enterotoxins, infections in patients with AIDS (*Cryptosporidium* spp. and *M. avium* complex); hormonal secretagogues, e.g., vasoactive intestinal peptide (VIP), which is secreted by pancreatic tumors and causes "pancreatic cholera"); carcinoid (5-HIAA excess); gastrin hypersecretion (e.g., Zollinger-Ellison Syndrome); or laxatives. Usually large-volume, watery stools without blood or leukocytes.

C. **Exudative diarrhea.** Inflammatory states such as inflammatory bowel disease and eosinophilic gastroenteritis; radiation enterocolitis; infection with invasive organisms; cytotoxins, ischemia, or vasculitis. Intestinal mucosa is inflamed, causing mucus, blood, and pus to leak into lumen.

D. **Motility disturbance.** Normal output (<250 g/day) diarrhea characterized by small, frequent and formed stools associated with urgency. Causes include hyperthyroidism, anorectal disease, proctitis or fecal impaction, irritable bowel disease.

III. **Causes of Acute Diarrhea**

A. **Infectious.** Contaminated food is the most frequent source of organisms causing diarrhea (less commonly contaminated water). Table 5-2 contains details of common causes of food poisoning.

  1. **Bacteria.** *Campylobacter,* enterotoxigenic *Escherichia coli, Salmonella, Shigella, Clostridium difficile, Yersinia enterocolitica, Vibrio cholerae, Aeromonas, Plesiomonas shigelloides,* and noncholera vibrios.

  2. **Viruses.** Rotavirus, Norwalk agent, enterovirus, hepatitis-associated virus.

  3. **Fungi.** *Candida, Actinomyces, Histoplasma.*

  4. **Parasites.** *Giardia lamblia* (fairly ubiquitous), *Entamoeba histolytica, Cryptosporidium, Strongyloides.*

B. **Toxin.**

1. **Bacterial toxins.** *Staphylococcus* (food poisoning), *Clostridium perfringens, C. botulinum, C. difficile, Bacillus cereus, Shigella* spp, *E. coli.*
2. **Chemical poisons.** Heavy metals, mushroom poisoning.

C. **Dietary.** Nonabsorbable sugar substitutes (sorbitol), food intolerance or allergy, irritating foods, milk and excessive caffeine.

D. **Drugs.** Laxatives, magnesium-containing antacids, colchicine, antibiotics, cholinergic agents, lactulose, quinidine.

E. **Visceral causes.** Appendicitis, diverticulitis, GI hemorrhage, fecal impaction, ischemic colitis, pseudomembranous colitis.

IV. **Diagnosis**

A. Acute diarrhea is often self-limited, and the diagnosis can be made by history and physical examination.

B. If the patient develops systemic toxicity, severe pain, dehydration, or bloody stools, or if symptoms persist more than 24 hours without improvement, then consider:

1. **CBC** with differential.
2. **Stool studies,** including ova and parasites, occult blood, *Giardia,* and *Cryptosporidium* antigen.
   a. Stool for occult blood is only 36% sensitive and 86% specific in patients with culture proven *Salmonella, Shigella, Campylobacter.* Stool for leukocytes is only 57% sensitive and 86% specific for infectious diarrhea. Fecal testing for lactoferrin is more sensitive.
3. *Clostridium difficile* **toxin** particularly if recent antibiotic use, operation or other intervention.
4. **Serum electrolytes,** if needed to manage dehydration.
5. **Sigmoidoscopy.** Particularly indicated in patients with bloody diarrhea. It can also be useful in diagnosing inflammatory bowel disease, Shigellosis, and amebic dysentery.
6. **Abdominal radiographs, flat and upright.** Obtain if there is abdominal distension, severe pain, obstructive symptoms (e.g. vomiting), or a suspected perforation. In general, however, abdominal radiographs are not useful in the patient with diarrhea.

V. **Treatment**

A. **Volume repletion** (see also Chapter 12).
1. **Oral** (clear liquids, sodium- and glucose-containing oral rehydration solutions). See Chapter 12 for instructions on making a rehydration solution at home.
2. **Intravenous** (normal saline or lactated Ringer's solution, especially if severely dehydrated or if the patient has intractable vomiting).

B. **Absorbents** (Kaopectate, aluminum hydroxide). These do not alter the course of the disease or reduce fluid loss, but allow the patient more control over the timing of defecation. Medications should be taken **at least** ½ hour before or 2 hours after absorbents are used.

C. **Antisecretory agents** such as bismuth subsalicylate (Pepto-Bismol). Usual dose is 30 ml every 30 minutes for 8 doses.

TABLE 5-2

SOME COMMON CAUSES OF FOOD POISONING

Poisoning	Foods	Food Taste	Symptoms
Bacillus cereus	Fried rice, other cooled rice, or vegetables	Normal	1. Vomiting 2. Diarrheal form
Ciguatera	Red snapper, amber-jack, grouper, warm water fish	Normal	GI symptoms (75%) followed by perioral numbness, diffuse dysesthesias, hot-cold reversal on face (pathognomonic), cranial nerve palsies, hallucinations, unusual sensory symptoms (e.g., feel teeth are loose), cardiac abnormalities, hypotension
Clostridium perfringens	Meats ubiquitously infected	Normal	Watery diarrhea, nausea, cramps Vomiting rare
Salmonella	Eggs, poultry	Normal	Diarrhea with blood, cramps Occasional sepsis
Scombroid	Dark meat fish (tuna, mackerel, swordfish, mahi mahi), including canned	Peppery, metallic	Skin flushing, wheezing, diarrhea, headache, urticaria
Shigella organisms	Poor hygiene, person to person	NA	Nausea, vomiting, diarrhea with progression to invasive diarrhea (heme positive stool) Neurologic symptoms, including seizures in young patients
Staphylococcus organisms	Any protein rich food	Normal	Cramps, vomiting, diarrhea mild, occasional fever

Onset	Duration	Heat Stable/ Other Toxin Characteristics	Treatment
1. ½ to 3 hrs 2. 6 to 10 hrs	1. 10 hrs 2. 20 to 36 hrs	Vomiting: heat stable Diarrhea: heat labile	Supportive
Minutes to 30 hrs (most common 1-6 hrs)	Up to months or years	Yes, calcium channel blocker	Supportive: gastric decontamination, calcium gluconate, atropine as needed
6-12 hrs (but up to 24)	24 hours	Ingestive organisms Usually meats cooked and cooled	Supportive (IV fluids, etc)
8-48 hrs	2-5 days	Heat labile but organisms occasionally survive cooking	Supportive, if severe levofloxacin or IV ceftriaxone
20-30 min	3 hrs-days	Yes, histamine-like	Like anaphylaxis (see Chapter 2)
36-72 hrs	3 days to 2 weeks	Shiga toxin inhibits water resorption	Supportive, fluoroquinolones
1-2 hrs	5-8 hrs (occasionally days)	Heat stable, CNS toxin	Supportive

5

GASTROENTEROLOGY AND HEPATOLOGY

D. **Antiperistaltics,** such as anticholinergics and opiate derivatives. Do not use in patients with fever, systemic toxicity, or bloody diarrhea. Discontinue if no improvement or if patient deteriorates. However, antiperistaltics are otherwise safe in the adult patient with diarrhea. Antiperistaltics have been used in children safely but this **is not** the standard of care and they should be used only after careful consideration.

1. **Diphenoxylate with atropine (Lomotil).** Available in tablets (2.5 mg of diphenoxylate) and liquid (2.5 mg of diphenoxylate/5 ml). The initial dose for adults is two tablets QID (20 mg/day). For children the dose is 0.1 mg/kg/dose QID. The dose is tapered as diarrhea improves. It is not indicated for diarrhea caused by pseudomembranous colitis or enterotoxin-producing or invasive bacteria. Lomotil should not be used in ulcerative colitis or in children under 2 years of age. **Lomotil is quite toxic with a low therapeutic range in children.**

2. **Loperamide (Imodium).** Available over the counter in 2 mg capsules and liquid (1 mg/5 ml). It increases the intestinal absorption of electrolytes and water and decreases intestinal motility and secretion. The dose in adults is 4 mg initially, followed by 2 mg after each diarrhea stool, not to exceed 16 mg in one 24-hour period. In children the dose is based on age, with 2 to 5 year olds receiving 1 mg TID 6 to 8 year olds 2 mg BID, and 9 to 12 year olds 2 mg TID on the first day of treatment. Thereafter 0.1 mg/kg is administered after each diarrhea stool, not to exceed the total daily dose recommended for the first day of therapy. Loperamide is safe and decreases the number of unformed stools and the duration of diarrhea in patients with *Shigella*-induced dysentery who are treated with ciprofloxacin.

E. **Antibiotics.** Not necessary for most episodes of diarrhea. Once cultures are done, empiric treatment with an agent that covers *Shigella* and *Campylobacter* is reasonable in those with severe diarrhea, systemic signs or heme positive diarrhea. A 3-day course of a fluoroquinolone (ciprofloxacin 500 mg PO BID or norfloxacin 400 mg PO BID) is the first-line therapy. TMP/SMX (Bactrim DS 1 tab PO QD) is an alternative therapy, but resistant organisms are common. If the diarrhea is caused by seafood ingestion, infection with either *Vibrio cholerae* or *Vibrio parahaemolyticus* is possible and can be treated with either a fluoroquinolone or with doxycycline 100 mg PO BID. **Antibiotics may increase the risk of hemolytic-uremic syndrome in those infected with E. coli O157:H7.**

CHRONIC DIARRHEA

I. **Definition.** Loose stools with or without increased stool frequency persisting for more than 4 weeks.

II. **Etiology:** See acute diarrhea above for additional discussion.

A. **Infection.** Giardiasis, amebiasis, *Clostridium difficile, Cryptosporidium* (see Chapter 11).

1. **Whipple's disease,** caused by *Tropheryma whippleii,* is a unique cause of diarrhea. Begins as a nondeforming arthritis in middle age, which may be manifest for years before GI symptoms begin. The illness progresses to include abdominal pain, diarrhea, weight loss, fever, lymphadenopathy, and occasionally CNS symptoms. Diagnosis is by biopsy of the small intestine yielding the offending organism.

B. **Inflammation.** Ulcerative colitis, Crohn's disease, ischemic colitis, diverticulitis, AIDS-related chronic diarrhea, collagenous colitis (very common in middle-aged and elderly women), microscopic (lymphocytic) colitis.

C. **Drugs.** Laxatives, antibiotics, NSAIDs, magnesium-containing antacids, alcohol.

D. **Malabsorption.** Short bowel syndrome, celiac sprue (gluten sensitive enteropathy), carbohydrate malabsorption, pancreatic insufficiency, bacterial overgrowth.

E. **Endocrine.** Hypothyroidism or hyperthyroidism, diabetes, adrenal insufficiency, hypoparathyroidism, Zollinger-Ellison syndrome.

F. **Motility disorders.** Irritable bowel syndrome, dumping syndrome.

G. **Infiltrative disorders.** Amyloidosis, diffuse intestinal lymphoma, scleroderma.

H. **Hormone-producing tumors.** VIPoma, carcinoid tumor, pheochromocytoma, ganglioneuroma, villous adenoma, medullary thyroid carcinoma or systemic mastocytosis.

I. **Others.** Fecal incontinence, food allergy, radiation enteritis or colitis.

J. Most patients with chronic watery diarrhea and abdominal pain have no identifiable cause for diarrhea except for irritable bowel syndrome.

III. Evaluation

A. **History.** Inquire about diurnal variation, relationship to meals, weight loss, and character of stools (such as foul-smelling or greasy stools characteristic of malabsorption or chronic bloody stools and abdominal pain or tenesmus suggestive of inflammatory bowel disease or tumor). Absence of stools at night suggests (but does not prove) a non-organic etiology.

B. **Physical examination.** Look for abdominal tenderness, distension, organomegaly, anal fistulas, rectal mass, and hyperactive bowel sounds.

C. **Laboratory analyses.**

1. **CBC with differential.** Anemia is suggestive of chronic blood loss, infection, malabsorption, or neoplasm. Eosinophilia may be secondary to parasitic disease or allergic reaction. Megaloblastic anemia may result from vitamin B_{12} or folate malabsorption.

2. **ESR, C-reactive protein.** If elevated, may indicate chronic inflammation.

3. **Serum electrolytes, magnesium, iron, renal function, albumin, cholesterol.** Calcium, phosphate, and alkaline phosphatase levels to evaluate for parathyroid disease. A fasting or random glucose can be used to screen for diabetes. Carotene levels may be low because of fat malabsorption. PT/PTT may be abnormal because of decreased

vitamin K absorption. Thyroid function abnormalities should be ruled out. Hypocalcemia may be due to vitamin D malabsorption.

4. **Stool exam for occult blood, leukocytes, and ova and parasites.** A stool specimen should be sent for culture and sensitivity; one culture is sufficient. Stool antigen test (sensitivity 92%, specificity 98%) is available for *Giardia* organisms and is more sensitive than an "O & P." The same type of test is available for Cryptosporidium (see Chapter 10 for details of this and other causes of infectious diarrhea). Generally 3 stools are sent of ova and parasites.

5. Special tests.
   a. **A 72-hour fecal fat quantitation** or Sudan staining of stool if steatorrhea (fat malabsorption) is suspected.
   b. **d-Xylose absorption** (decreased in disorders of proximal small intestine).
   c. **A stool pH** <5.3 is diagnostic of a carbohydrate intolerance. Breath hydrogen test for lactase deficiency. Can also check for reducing substances in stool or therapeutic trial of lactose-free diet.
   d. **Small intestinal biopsy** (useful for Whipple's disease, celiac sprue, regional enteritis, some parasitic infestations).
   e. **Smooth muscle endomysial antibody** titers may be positive in celiac sprue/gluten insensitivity. Tissue transglutaminase is starting to be utilized as an alternative test (see Sprue below).
   f. **Small bowel culture** for bacterial overgrowth.
   g. **Stool test with phenolphthalein** (test for factitious laxative abuse). Bring stool pH to 8.0. If the specimen turns maroon in color, this indicates the presence of phenolphthalein, an ingredient in over-the-counter laxative products. Urine tests are available to detect aloes, senna alkaloids, and bisacodyl.
   h. **Sigmoidoscopy** should be done to detect inflammation of the colon or rectum, neoplasms, and parasites.
   i. **Radiographic studies.** Plain abdominal radiography and barium studies of the upper GI tract, small intestine, and colon.

IV. Treatment
A. **Should be directed toward underlying cause** of the chronic diarrhea.
B. **Occasionally, when a definitive diagnosis cannot be made, one might empirically try:**
   1. **Dietary restriction.** Restricting lactose, gluten, or long-chain fatty acids in the diet. Restrictions should be done systematically so that if symptoms improve, the restricted factor can be identified and removed permanently from the diet. Lactase replacements (such as Lactaid caplets) are available OTC for patients intolerant to lactose.
   2. **Pancreatic enzyme supplementation** (Creon [pancrelipase] capsules) for suspected pancreatic exocrine deficiency (such as cystic fibrosis, chronic pancreatitis).
   3. **Increase dietary or supplemental fiber.**
   4. **Cholestyramine,** which tends to have a constipating effect.

5. **Antimicrobials** (such as metronidazole).
6. **Judicious use of antidiarrheal medication** may be appropriate for symptomatic relief in some patients. Avoid opiates in the treatment of chronic diarrhea. See acute diarrhea section for dosages and cautions.

TRAVELER'S DIARRHEA

I. **Definition and clinical features.** Loose stools with or without increased frequency acquired when going from an industrialized country to a developing country or starting up to 7 to 10 days after return to a developed area. Most people have 3 to 5 loose stools per day, and the illness generally last for 3 to 5 days in untreated individuals. Fever, bloody stools, or both can be found in 2% to 10%.

II. **Etiology**

A. **Bacterial pathogens** are responsible for 80% of cases and include enterotoxigenic *E. coli*, *Campylobacter jejuni*, *Aeromonas*, *Shigella*, *Salmonella* and non-*Cholera vibrios*.

B. **Viral pathogens** account for ~10% of the cases.

C. **Others:** *Giardia, cryptosporidium, cyclospora* organisms.

III. **Prophylaxis**

A. **Not routinely recommended** because of the risk of adverse effects from the drugs (rash, anaphylaxis, and vaginal candidiasis) and the development of resistant gut flora.

B. **Possible regimens for prophylaxis** include bismuth subsalicylate (Pepto-Bismol) 524 mg PO QID with meals and QHS, doxycycline 100 mg PO QD (resistant strains common), TMP/SMX 160 mg/800 mg (1 double-strength tablet) PO QD (resistance strains common), or norfloxacin 400 mg PO QD (fluoroquinolones should not be prescribed to children or pregnant women). No significant resistance to the fluoroquinolones has yet been reported in high-risk areas, and they are the most effective antibiotics in regions where susceptibilities are not known.

IV. **Treatment. Although routine prophylaxis is discouraged, sending the traveler with a prescription to take at the onset of acute diarrhea is reasonable.** (For doses, see prophylaxis.) **Loperamide can be added to the fluoroquinolones or TMP/SMX** when treating traveler's diarrhea. These medications should be continued for 1 or 2 days after patient returns home. A course of metronidazole to cover for *Giardia* organisms may also be sent with the patient.

CELIAC SPRUE (GLUTEN-SENSITIVE ENTEROPATHY)

I. **Etiology.** Celiac sprue is caused by the interaction of gluten of particular grains (e.g. wheat) with the small intestinal mucosa. Gluten causes the intestinal mucosa to lose its villous structure and absorptive capacity.

II. **Clinical features.** The severity of symptoms will depend upon the amount and the specific location of small intestine involved but may include diarrhea, steatorrhea, foul-smelling flatulence, and weakness. Dehydration, electrolyte losses, neuropathy, and acidosis may ensue.

The incidence of dermatitis herpetiformis is increased among these patients. Anemia may result from alterations in iron, folate and vitamin B_{12} absorption. Impaired fat soluble vitamin absorption may also occur leading to osteopenia, increased clotting times, and night blindness.

III. **Diagnosis.**

A. Serum IgA antiendomysial and tissue transglutaminase are found in up to 95% of patients with gluten sensitivity. Anti-gliadin levels are less specific for sprue.

B. Intestinal biopsy is the most sensitive means of making the diagnosis.

C. To make the diagnosis unequivocally, the patient's symptoms must be relieved with an adequate trial (a few weeks) of a gluten-free diet. An objective means of demonstrating improvement may be to repeat the intestinal biopsy and evaluate for histologic improvement or repeat the serum titers for anti-endomysial antibodies which should decrease in the absence of gluten exposure.

IV. **Therapy.** Remove all foodstuffs containing rye, barley, oat, or wheat gluten. The patient must be encouraged to compulsively read food labels. Corn, rice, and soybean flours are safe. If there is an incomplete response, the diet must be reviewed and other potential sources of toxic gluten removed.

V. Patients with celiac sprue are at increased risk for both intestinal and extraintestinal lymphomas, esophageal squamous cell carcinomas, and small intestinal adenocarcinomas. If symptoms so indicate, a search for these malignancies should be performed.

LACTOSE INTOLERANCE

I. **Lactose intolerance** is an unpleasant reaction to lactose ingestion caused by a deficiency of lactase, a disaccharidase responsible for hydrolyzing lactose into glucose and galactose. Lactose intolerance is the most prevalent genetic deficiency worldwide, affecting Asians, persons from the Mediterranean, African-Americans, native Americans, and Mexicans.

II. **Types of Lactase Deficiency.**

A. **Late-onset or acquired.** Adult lactase deficiency is inherited as an autosomal recessive trait. Onset most common in adolescence and early adulthood. Symptom severity depends on intestinal lactase activity and the size of the lactose load.

B. **Secondary.** Temporary lactase deficiency produced by acute infectious gastroenteritis or mucosal damage from NSAIDs, chronic alcohol use or other medications. Chronic small intestinal disorders (celiac sprue, cystic fibrosis, Whipple's disease, regional enteritis, HIV-induced enteropathy) may also cause a lactase deficiency because of brush border mucosal damage.

C. **Congenital (alactasia).** This condition is extremely rare and is the result of complete absence of lactase expression because of a genetic defect.

II. **Symptoms**

A. Include abdominal distention and pain, gaseous bloating, borborygmi, flatulence and diarrhea resulting from increased distension and de-

creased transit time of lactulose in the small bowel, and production SCFAs and gases in the colon.

B. People who are "lactose intolerant" by their own report rarely have symptoms if they limit themselves to about 240 ml of milk per day.

III. **Evaluation**

A. **Trial of lactose-free diet.** Withdrawal of lactose from diet for 2 weeks. Improvement in symptoms strongly implicated lactose intolerance.

B. **Lactose tolerance test.** Measurement of blood glucose after ingestion of 50 g of lactose. Normal individuals show a rise of >20 mg/dl.

C. **Breath hydrogen test.** Most practical and non-invasive test. However, false positives may occur in patients with bacterial overgrowth.

D. **Small-bowel biopsy.**

E. **Stool pH of less than 5.3** is diagnostic of carbohydrate intolerance.

IV. **Management**

A. **Dietary measures.** Study ingredient labels on foods and decrease or avoid products that contain milk, lactose, and dry milk solids. Use lactose-reduced milks or milk supplemented with exogenous lactase.

B. **Lactase supplements** (Lactaid, Lactrase, Dairy Ease) may be taken 30 minutes before the consumption of a lactose-containing product. Two capsules provide enough lactase to hydrolyze the lactose in an 8 oz glass of whole milk.

C. The consumption of yogurt containing live bacterial cultures can result in the release of bioactive bacterial lactase into the gut.

IRRITABLE BOWEL SYNDROME

I. **General Features**

A. **History.** Patients often describe a long history of chronic or intermittent diarrhea, which usually starts before age 50 and is exacerbated by anxiety or stress. Diarrhea is often worse in the morning and after meals. These patients often complain of a sensation of incomplete evacuation, distention, passage of mucus, or associated abdominal, pelvic, and back pain. Pain is relieved by evacuation. Alternating constipation, diarrhea, and bloating is typical. Diarrhea is not bloody unless accompanied by an anorectal lesion such as hemorrhoids or a fissure. Systemic symptoms or weight loss are not present. Nutritional status is not compromised. Proposed criteria for diagnosis of IBS are found in Box 5-1.

B. **Etiology.** The following factors are believed to play a mechanistic role in IBS and more than one may operate in a given individual: (1) abnormal motility, (2) abnormal visceral perception, (3) psychologic factors, (4) luminal compounds (lactose, short chain fatty acids, food allergens, and bile acids), which may irritate the bowel.

C. **Physical examination** is usually normal.

D. **A work-up should be done** to exclude other causes. Stool will usually be negative for occult blood. Sigmoidoscopy and barium enema are also usually normal.

BOX 5-1

CRITERIA FOR IRRITABLE BOWEL SYNDROME

- At least 3 months of continuous or recurrent symptoms of abdominal pain within a 12-month period, which is:
- Relieved by defecation *or*
- Associated with a change in stool consistency *or*
- Associated with a change in stool frequency

Supporting (but not necessary) symptoms for the diagnosis of IBS include:

- Altered stool frequency (>3 times per day or <3 times per week)
- Altered stool form
- Altered stool passage (straining, urgency, incomplete evacuation)
- Passage of mucous
- Abdominal bloating

E. **Associated symptoms and signs** which increase the likelihood of organic disease include: blood in stools, nocturnal diarrhea, recent onset, weight loss, painless diarrhea, positive HIV status. The absence of the above supports the diagnosis of functional bowel disease.

F. **Treatment**
   1. **Supportive.** Stress reduction, reassurance.
   2. **Diet and fiber therapy.** Avoid foods that the patient notices increase symptoms. High fiber diet or fiber supplements help some patients.
   3. **Antispasmodics.** Dicyclomine 10-20 mg QID may be helpful, side-effects may limit use.
   4. **Eliminate laxatives.**
   5. Patients with diarrhea may have some relief with low doses of diphenoxylate or loperamide prn (see section on Acute Diarrhea).
   6. **Long-term follow-up studies suggest** that most symptoms may resolve with time and the survival of these patients is unaffected by IBS. Maintaining a positive, sympathetic physician-patient relationship, addressing patient concerns and expectations, setting limits, and involving the patient in treatment decisions contribute to better results and fewer follow-up visits.

CLOSTRIDIUM DIFFICILE INFECTION

I. **General.** *Clostridium difficile* is a gram-positive, anaerobic, spore-forming bacterium associated with antecedent antibiotic therapy and most often responsible for antibiotic-associated diarrhea and colitis. The infection clinically ranges from asymptomatic carrier states to severe pseudomembranous colitis.

II. **Although classically associated with clindamycin use, *C. difficile* colitis can be caused by almost any antibiotic including the cephalosporins and penicillins.** Symptoms may develop within a few days or even 6 to 10 weeks after antibiotic therapy is completed. Risk of acquisition depends on the number of antibiotics used concurrently and the number of days they are used.

III. **Clinical manifestations. Any of these manifestations may be absent, and pseudomembranous colitis should be considered in any patient with otherwise unexplainable diarrhea.**

A. Profuse watery diarrhea that may be foul smelling.

B. Abdominal pain, cramping, and tenderness.

C. Stools may be guaiac positive and occasionally grossly bloody.

D. Fever.

E. White blood cell count 12,000 to 20,000.

F. In severe cases, toxic megacolon, colonic perforation, and peritonitis may develop. Other complications: electrolyte abnormalities, hypovolemic shock, anasarca caused by hypoalbuminemia, sepsis, and hemorrhage.

IV. **Toxin detection by latex agglutination,** immunobinding assay, or ELISA make the diagnosis. Since *C. difficile* may be a normal bowel organism (especially in children), simply culturing the organism does not mean that diarrhea is caused by *C. difficile.*

V. **Treatment.** Those patients with mild symptoms will usually resolve infection spontaneously once the causative antibiotic is withdrawn. More severe cases warrant therapy with oral antibiotic therapy. Metronidazole (250 mg PO QID) for 10 days is an effective initial therapy. Oral vancomycin (500 mg PO QID) can be used in patients not responding to metronidazole. Patients with relapse may be treated with another course of the aforementioned antibiotics.

GIARDIASIS

I. **General.** Caused by the parasite, *Giardia intestinalis,* also known as *G. lamblia.* The disease varies from asymptomatic colonization (15%) to explosive diarrhea (25% to 50%) with weight loss and malabsorption. Approximately 50% of those ingesting *Giardia* organisms will not become colonized or develop diarrhea. Generally transmitted through water especially from wells on farms, streams, or lakes. Has also occurred from public water systems (especially Eastern Europe), but this is uncommon in the United States.

II. **Groups with Increased Risk.**

A. Travelers to developing countries (also see Traveler's diarrhea) with latency of onset of symptoms of approximately 7-10 days.

B. Children in day care centers where most infections are asymptomatic.

C. Homosexual men.

III. **Clinically.** Clinical presentation varies. Diarrhea, weight loss and abdominal cramping are the most common symptoms. However, fever (initially), nausea, increased flatus and chronic diarrhea with malabsorption may occur. Moreover, the infection may be asymptomatic, and any of the above may be absent.

IV. **Diagnosis.** The diagnosis is made by detecting Giardia antigen in the stool by immunofluorescence (most common) or ELISA. This is from

85% to 98% sensitive. *Giardia* can also be diagnosed by duodenal biopsy (90% sensitivity) or stool for O & P with a 50% sensitivity.

V. **Treatment.** Mainstay of treatment is metronidazole 250 mg PO TID for 5 days. Higher dose of 750 mg PO TID for 5 is indicated for treatment failures. The 250 mg dose has a cure rate of about 85%. Quinacrine 100 mg TID after meals for 5 days is an alternative.

DIVERTICULAR DISEASE

I. **Definitions and General Features**
A. **Diverticulum (plural, diverticula).** Outpouching of the bowel wall usually between 0.1 to 1 cm in diameter. Most occur in the sigmoid and descending colon. Common colonic diverticula are pseudodiverticula, which are herniations of mucosa and submucosa but not muscularis at sites of penetration of nutrient arteries.
B. **Diverticulosis.** Presence of multiple diverticula. Does not imply a pathologic condition. In industrialized countries, up to half of the population older than 50 years of age has colonic diverticulosis.
C. **Diverticulitis.** Inflammation and infection in one or more diverticula.

II. **Symptomatic Diverticulosis**
A. **Symptoms.** Most (80% to 85%) patients with colonic diverticula are asymptomatic. Some have mild intermittent left lower quadrant abdominal pain, bloating and constipation or diarrhea. The symptoms overlap with those of irritable bowel syndrome.
B. **Differential diagnosis.** IBS, diverticulitis, colon cancer, inflammatory bowel disease, or a urologic or gynecologic disorder.
C. **Physical exam.** Possible tenderness and firm feces-filled sigmoid colon in the left lower quadrant of the abdomen. Rectal exam may reveal firm, guaiac-negative stool.
D. **Studies are not indicated** if symptoms are mild and the patient is otherwise healthy.
E. **Studies are indicated** if symptoms are more severe or if the patient has occult blood in stool, weight loss, or other symptoms of concern. Obtain a CBC, UA, and perform a flexible sigmoidoscopy and barium enema or colonoscopy.
F. **Treatment.** Recommend high-fiber diet. Antispasmodics such as dicyclomine may help with cramping. Avoid cathartic laxatives.

III. **Diverticulitis.** See Chapter 15 for diagnosis of abdominal pain.
A. **General.** Microperforation of diverticulum leads to peridiverticulitis. Free perforation is rare, but localized abscess, sinus tracts or fistulas into the bladder, vagina, etc. may occur. Most cases occur in the sigmoid colon and the incidence increases with age.
B. **Symptoms.** When full blown, may have acute abdominal pain with chills, fever, and tachycardia but more often develops over hours to days with left lower quadrant pain, anorexia, fever, nausea, vomiting. May have pneumaturia (air passage per urethra) if there is erosion into the bladder.

C. **Differential diagnosis.** Appendicitis, inflammatory bowel disease, is-chemic colitis, colon cancer, other causes of bowel obstruction, urologic or gynecologic disorders. See Chapter 15 for a more complete discussion.

D. **Physical examination.** Abdominal tenderness to palpation with possible rebound tenderness. A palpable mass may be present, representing an abscess or inflammatory phlegmon. Bowel sounds may be active if there is partial obstruction; hypoactive or absent if peritonitis has developed.

E. **Diagnostic studies.** CBC with a differential and UA. Abdominal plain films (flat and upright) and chest x-ray to evaluate for ileus, obstruction, and free air (perforation). Ultrasound of abdomen and pelvis may be helpful in identifying an inflammatory mass or abscess, but a CT scan is the imaging procedure of choice especially if the diagnosis is uncertain. Sigmoidoscopy may be performed cautiously if there is no evidence of perforation and if necessary for diagnosis. However, sigmoidoscopy and barium enema are both best delayed until after acute symptoms resolve. Colonoscopy is contraindicated in the case of acute diverticulitis.

F. **Treatment.** Keep NPO, place nasogastric tube if vomiting, and maintain hydration with IV fluids. Broad-spectrum antibiotics such as ampicillin/gentamycin/(clindamycin or metronidazole) or cefoxitin alone should be used for inpatients. Oral antibiotics may be given to patients who have no peritoneal signs. Either [TMP/SMX (DS 1 tab PO BID) + metronidazole] or [fluoroquinolone + metronidazole 500 mg PO QID] are good regimens for outpatients **(although occasional seizures have been reported with the combination of a fluoroquinolone and metronidazole).** Antibiotics should be continued for 7 to 10 days. Abscess may require percutaneous drainage under ultrasound or CT guidance. Surgery may be required if there is peritonitis, with or without evidence of perforation, unresolved obstruction, inability to exclude neoplasia, development of a fistula, failure to improve after several days of medical treatment or recurrent diverticulitis.

CONSTIPATION, FECAL IMPACTION AND FECAL INCONTINENCE

See Chapter 12 for pediatric considerations.

I. Constipation

A. It is a symptom and not a disease.

B. Affects ~10% of the general and up to 25% of the elderly population.

C. Defined as two or more of the following for at least 12 weeks:
  1. <3 bowel movements/week
  2. Excessive straining during at least 25% of the bowel movements
  3. Feeling of incomplete evacuation during at least 25% of the bowel movements
  4. Passage of hard stools during at least 25% of the bowel movements

II. **Etiology and Differential Diagnosis**

A. **Drugs.** Aluminum-containing antacids, calcium supplements, iron supplements, opiates, antihypertensives (calcium-channel blockers, clonidine, methyldopa), anticholinergic agents (antidepressants, neuroleptics, antihistamines), some antiparkinsonian drugs, antispasmodics, estrogen and progestins, among many others.

B. **Dietary.** Inadequate fluid and fiber intake.

C. **Lack of exercise.**

D. **Metabolic and endocrine.** Hypercalcemia, hypokalemia, hypothyroidism diabetes mellitus, Addison's disease, Cushing's syndrome, and other electrolyte abnormalities.

E. **Neurogenic.** Multiple sclerosis, parkinsonism, spinal cord disease, autonomic neuropathy, Chagas' disease and Hirschsprung's disease.

F. **Colonic disease.** Tumors, diverticular disease, diverticulitis, irritable bowel syndrome, inflammatory strictures, abnormal colonic or anal musculature junction.

G. **Other.** Anal fissure (pain), hemorrhoids, ulcerative colitis (proctitis), rectal neoplasms, dementia, many others.

III. **Evaluation and Diagnosis**

A. **History.** A detailed history is key and should include stool frequency and consistency; extent of straining; sensation of incomplete evacuation; need for incomplete evacuation; repeatedly ignoring the urge to stool; need for digital disimpaction of stool; dietary history (amount of fiber and fluid intake, frequency and time of eating); drug history; other history including obstetrical surgery, back injury, neurological problems and sexual abuse.

B. **Physical Exam.** May note palpable colon in the left lower quadrant of the abdomen due to the presence of stool. Perianal inspection may reveal fissures or hemorrhoids. Rectal examination should include evaluation of the anal sphincter tone both at rest and with a squeeze. Bearing down should cause relaxation of the anal sphincter along with perineal descent—absence of either component suggests obstructive defecation.

C. **Diagnostic studies.** Consider CBC, serum electrolytes including calcium, glucose, thyroid function tests, stool examination for occult blood and ova and parasites, and flexible sigmoidoscopy.

D. **Infants and young adults usually need minimal work-up.** Exceptions would be suspected Hirschsprung's disease or chronic refractory constipation. See Chapter 12.

E. **In older adults** the extent of the evaluation depends on the nature and duration of symptoms. Presence of iron deficiency anemia, with or without blood in the stool (occult or frank) warrants a work-up for colon cancer in older adults with constipation. Colonoscopy is more cost effective than barium enema as it can be used both diagnostically and therapeutically at the same time (mucosal biopsy and polypectomy).

F. **Exclusion of secondary causes listed above suggests idiopathic constipation, a colorectal motility disorder.** Simplest method of evaluating colonic transit involves giving patients Sitzmark capsules (containing 24 radiopaque markers) and obtaining a abdominal flat plate 5 days later. The presence of 5 or more markers suggests slow colonic transit. In obstructive defecation, patients usually have more markers in the rectosigmoid colon.

IV. **Management**

A. **Patient education.** Avoid irritant and combination laxatives. Allow adequate time and a relaxed environment to have a bowel movement. Increase ambulation/exercise and advise patients to move their bowels at the same time daily.

B. **Fluid and fiber.** If no pathology is uncovered by diagnostic tests indicated above, a trial of high-fiber diet or psyllium supplementation can be instituted. Soluble fiber is more important than insoluble fiber in treating constipation. Soluble fiber is found in grains and legumes, as well as in commercial psyllium preparations (Metamucil). Increase fluid intake to several glasses per day.

C. **Stool softeners and lubricants.** Avoid products that combine stool softeners with irritant laxatives unless specifically indicated. An example of a stool softener is docusate (usual dose 100 mg BID). However, the efficacy of docusate is limited in chronic constipation. Mineral oil is an alternative that works as a lubricant. Usual starting dose is 1 tablespoon QHS and the dose can be increased as needed to a maximum of 4 tablespoons per day. Mineral oil may interfere with the absorption of fat-soluble vitamins. Be cautious in the elderly or those with swallowing problems because of the danger of aspiration.

D. **Hyperosmotic preparations.** Mainstay of therapy for slow-transit constipation. Examples include 1 to 2 tablespoons of magnesium hydroxide (MOM) QD BID. Half to 1 bottle of magnesium citrate (17.7 g/300 cc) can be used in patients not responding to MOM. Nonabsorbable sugars such as lactulose or sorbitol can also be used. The usual dose of lactulose is 1 or 2 tablespoons up to QID; start with a low dose and titrate to desired effect. Sorbitol (70%) is less expensive and also effective, but should be used cautiously in diabetic patients. Polyethylene glycol (e.g., Miralax) 17 g daily (1 tablespoon) titrated up to desired effect is well tolerated and effective.

E. **Local agents (enemas, suppositories).** Initiate reflex evacuation by distending or irritating colon and rectum. Common enema solutions include water, saline, soap suds and milk of molasses. However, soap suds and milk of molasses enemas should be used with caution as the former can cause injury to colonic mucosa and the latter can cause colonic distension. Bisacodyl and glycerin suppositories work as local irritants.

F. **Prokinetic agents,** such as metoclopramide and misoprostol, may be effective in treating slow-transit constipation but can be expensive.

G. Patients with obstructive defecation should be referred for further evaluation and bowel retraining.

H. **Surgical treatment** may be required in certain circumstances (Hirschsprung's disease, idiopathic megacolon, and pseudoobstruction). It is also an option of last resort in patients with slow-transit constipation refractory to all treatment methods described above.

I. **Psychosocial issues** concerning defecation (embarrassment, aversion, anxiety, and depression) may also have to be explored.

IV. **Fecal Impaction.** Firm, immobile mass of stool, most often in the rectum but may also occur in sigmoid or descending colon. Most common in elderly, inactive patients. Differential diagnosis is similar to that for constipation. Impaction may present with involuntary leakage of stool around the impaction, which may be mistaken for diarrhea (AKA overflow diarrhea). May have fever, symptoms of acute abdomen, or mental status changes. Treatment involves softening of stool with glycerin or bisacodyl suppositories and enemas (warm water, saline or phosphate). Manual disimpaction may be necessary.

FECAL INCONTINENCE

I. **General Information.** Occurs in between 0.5%-1.5% of the general population and 3.7% of the population over the age of 65 but is under diagnosed. Fecal incontinence is more prevalent in women and institutionalized patients.

II. **Etiology**

A. **Normal pelvic floor**
   1. Fecal impaction, especially in the elderly.
   2. Carcinoma of the anal canal or lower rectum.
   3. Spinal cord injuries and other neurological conditions including lesions of the cauda equina, diabetes, frontal lobe lesions and multiple sclerosis.
   4. Rectal prolapse.
   5. Aging with decreased anal canal pressures and rectal compliance.
   6. Other conditions that cause diarrhea may predispose to fecal incontinence.

B. **Abnormal pelvic floor**
   1. Damage to the anal sphincter related to operative or obstetric injury, especially forceps deliveries.
   2. Pudendal nerve injury associated with childbirth or stretch injury due to prolonged straining during defecation.
   3. Anorectal surgery including hemorrhoidectomy and fissure repair.

III. **Evaluation**

A. **History.** A good history including onset of incontinence, precipitating event(s), frequency and severity of incontinence. A detailed obstetric history including the use offorceps, perineal tears and weight of the baby. Review of past medical history should assess the presence of other conditions that may cause or be associated with fecal incontinence (e.g. diabetes mellitus, neurological symptoms, pelvic irradiation, urinary incontinence

B. **Physical examination**
   1. Perineal inspection for soiling, chemical dermatitis (suggestive of chronic problem), a gaping anus (indicative of loss of sphincter function), fistula or rectal prolapse.

2. Assess perianal sensation and check the anocutaneous reflex by stroking the skin in all 4 quadrants around the anus. Its absence indicates pudendal nerve damage.

3. Evaluate the length of anal sphincter and its tone at rest and with a squeeze.

4. Asking the patient to strain may reveal rectal prolapse or excessive perineal decent.

C. **Diagnostic procedures**

1. Work-up of diarrhea if it is reported.

2. Patients should be referred for anorectal manometry, anal endoscopy, electrophysiologic testing, etc., if they are unresponsive to therapy.

IV. **Treatment**

A. Treat the underlying cause if identified.

B. Mild incontinence may respond to bulk forming agents, high-fiber diet or adjusted doses of antidiarrheals such as loperamide and Lomotil.

C. Bowel retraining for elderly patients with fecal impaction and patients with mild pudendal neuropathy and a weak anal sphincter.

D. Weak or damaged anal sphincter in a patient with intact pudendal nerve may benefit from surgical repair of the sphincter

INFLAMMATORY BOWEL DISEASE

I. **Crohn's Disease (Regional Enteritis, Granulomatous Colitis)**

A. **Definition and General Information.** A focal, transmural inflammatory process potentially involving **any portion** of the GI tract. Most commonly it involves the ileum and colon but frequently also involves the anus (perianal fistulas and abscesses) and mouth (oral ulcerations). Incidence and prevalence in the US and other developed countries is estimated to be 5 and 10 per 100,000, respectively. It is more common in teenagers and young adults, although any age group may be affected. Crohn's disease is not "curable" and has systemic and extraintestinal manifestations. It is exacerbated by cigarette smoking.

B. **Clinical presentation.** Chronic or nocturnal diarrhea, abdominal pain especially in the right lower quadrant, anorexia, weight loss, fever, fatigue, recurrent oral apthous ulcers, and bowel obstruction. Recurrent perianal fissures, fistulous tracts and abscess formation are not uncommon. Extraintestinal manifestations involve the skin, eyes, or joints. Acute presentation of ileitis may be confused with appendicitis. Patients with disease limited to the colon present with rectal bleeding and perianal complications. Gastric and duodenal involvement presents with epigastric pain, nausea, vomiting or gastric outlet obstruction. Disease involving the small bowel may result in partial small bowel obstruction, bacterial overgrowth, or protein-losing enteropathy causing cachexia and growth retardation in the affected child. Associated complications of metabolic disorders may cause anemia, metabolic bone disease, cholelithiasis, or nephrolithiasis.

C. **Diagnosis.**
1. X-ray contrast studies (small bowel follow through, air contrast barium enema) showing typical areas of stricture with regions of normal bowel. **Contrast studies should not be done in patients who present with fulminant disease because of the possibility of inducing a toxic megacolon.**
2. Small bowel enteroclysis is more sensitive in evaluating the jejunal and ileal involvement.
3. Endoscopy is used to confirm the diagnosis of Crohn's disease and obtain tissue for histopathological evaluation.

D. **Laboratory finding and evaluation.**
1. Patients may have anemia or elevated erythrocyte sedimentation rate.
2. ANCA may be positive.
3. Other causes of chronic diarrhea should be ruled out. See chronic diarrhea section above.

E. **Complications.**
1. Toxic megacolon (more common with ulcerative colitis).
2. Dehydration and malnutrition from diarrhea and malabsorption. Fat-soluble vitamins and vitamin B_{12} tend to be particularly affected.
3. Bowel perforation and abscess formation.
4. Chronic fistula formation.
5. Bowel cancer (five times the rate of age-matched controls).
6. Renal disease including urolithiasis (due to steatorrhea promoting excess colonic absorption of oxalate causing hyperoxaluria).
7. Metabolic bone disease (due to chronic steroid use or calcium or vitamin D malabsorption).

F. **Extraintestinal manifestations** include joint disease, erythema nodosum, pyoderma gangrenosum, episcleritis or keratoconjunctivitis, and sclerosing cholangitis.

G. **Differential diagnosis.** See section on diarrhea.

H. **Treatment.**
1. **Acute treatment.**
   a. **Steroids.** Start prednisone 40 to 60 mg PO QD or its IV equivalent once an abscess has been excluded (see below). In severe or fulminant case, most patients will respond to 7 to 10 days of IV steroid therapy. When bowel function is restored and the patient is tolerating a diet, IV steroids may be discontinued and the patient switched to oral prednisone or prednisolone therapy with rapid tapering down and discontinuation. In an effort to decrease the severity of steroid side effects, new steroid preparations that minimize systemic effects have been developed. Budesonide (a steroid with high receptor affinity and high first-pass hepatic metabolism) is particularly promising and is available as both an enema and an oral controlled-release preparation that target the ileum and colon. Corticosteroid enemas can be used in patients with isolated rectal or left colic disease.

  b. **Metronidazole** has been shown to be useful acutely in doses of 10 to 30 mg/kg/day divided into 3 or 4 doses especially when perianal disease develops.
  c. **Intravenous cyclosporin A** (4 mg/kg/day IV for 6 days followed by 8 mg/kg/day orally for 3 to 6 months) or surgery should be considered for patients with severe disease who are refractory to steroid therapy.
  d. **A surgical consultation** should be obtained in patients with obstruction or tender abdominal mass which should be evaluated by ultrasound or CT scan.
  e. **Appropriate antibiotic therapy** and drainage is required for infection or abscesses.
  f. **Total parenteral nutrition** may be needed during the acute phase of disease.
  g. **Tincture of opium and other antidiarrheal agents** may be useful during therapy. These should be avoided, however, if the possibility of toxic megacolon is present.

2. **Long-term management.**
  a. **Steroids** should be tapered and discontinued as quickly as possible because of their significant side effects. Many patients do require chronic use of steroids, however.
  b. **Long-term metronidazole** use has been associated with a reversible peripheral neuropathy but can be used to keep steroid doses at the lowest possible levels.
  c. **Sucralfate** suspension has been used effectively for oral ulcers.
  d. **Azathioprine and 6-mercaptopurine** (6-MP) have been used as steroid-sparing agents and are safe for long-term use. Watch for significant side effects, including bone marrow suppression and pancreatitis (3% to 15%). Long-term follow-up suggests that 6-MP is effective and is associated with no higher rate of neoplasm than is placebo.
  e. **Aminosalicylates** such as sulfasalazine and mesalamine are frequently used to treat mild to moderate Crohn's disease and to maintain remission. Sulfasalazine 3 to 4 g PO QD divided Q8h may be used to help induce a remission but is seldom effective on its own. Sulfasalazine decreases folate absorption and patients receiving sulfasalazine should receive folate supplementation.
  f. **Mesalamine** (Asacol 200 to 400 mg PO TID; Pentasa 1 g PO QID) provide the active moiety (5-ASA) without the sulfapyridine, which causes most of the side effects
  g. **Antidiarrheal agents,** including loperamide or atropine sulfate-diphenoxylate HCl, can be helpful.
  h. **Infliximab** (a chimeric monoclonal antibody to tumor necrosis factor-alpha) has been shown to be effective in healing Crohn's patients with fistulous disease. Hyperbaric oxygen therapy may also be considered in patients with poorly healing fistulas.

5

GASTROENTEROLOGY AND HEPATOLOGY

    i. **Thalidomide,** which is thought to exert its antiinflammatory effect by inhibiting tumor necrosis factor, has been reported to be effective in refractory Crohn's disease. Caution should be used in women of reproductive age because of the risk of birth defects.

    j. **Treatment with recombinant human interleukin-10** is beneficial in Crohn's disease.

    k. **Low dose methotrexate** has recently been shown to maintain remission in patients with Crohn's disease who enter remission after treatment with a relatively higher dose methotrexate.

    l. Based on the geographic prevalence of Crohn's disease in "Western" countries, a role for recolonization of the GI tract with helminths (such as *Trichuris suis*) is being explored.

II. **Ulcerative Colitis**

A. **Defined as** inflammation limited to the mucosal surface and submucosa (as opposed to Crohn's disease, which is transmural).

B. **Involvement is limited to the colon** and rectosigmoid area in a continuous pattern without skip areas.

C. **Clinical presentation consists of** diarrhea (frequently bloody), passage of blood and mucus per rectum, abdominal pain, fever, tenesmus, and toxic megacolon.

D. **Diagnosis is by** endoscopy and biopsy or contrast studies showing superficial ulcerations. Carcinoembryonic antigen is elevated in chronic cases and does not suggest the development of a carcinoma. Bowel ANCA may be positive. Eosinophilia is also common (15% to 30%). As with Crohn's disease, contrast studies are contraindicated in those with acute disease since barium may induce a toxic megacolon.

E. **Complications include** those listed above for Crohn's disease. Additionally, the development of a toxic megacolon or anemia from hemorrhage is more common with ulcerative colitis as is the development of malignancy.

F. **Extra colonic manifestations** are the same as those found in Crohn's disease except for renal disease which is exclusively found in those with Crohn's disease.

G. **Treatment:**

  1. **Acute management:**

    a. **Symptomatic treatment** with antidiarrheal agents (see section on diarrhea). These should be avoided is there is any evidence of toxic megacolon.

    b. **If disease is moderate or mild,** hydrocortisone enemas (100 mg BID) may be helpful. Mesalamine enemas, 4 g in 100 cc QHS, have been shown to be efficacious. Mesalamine suppositories (1 g QHS) may be used for isolated rectal disease. Oral mesalamine, olsalazine, sulfasalazine and prednisone can be used in doses similar to those note above for Crohn's disease.

    c. **For more severe disease** (systemic signs or symptoms, severe abdominal pain) parenteral steroids should be administered as per Crohn's disease. Treatment for severe disease should be continued for 7 to 10 days and then tapered as disease allows.

    d. **Cyclosporine** 4 mg/kg/day IV added to steroids will frequently induce remission when steroids alone fail.

  2. **Long-term management includes the treatments noted for Crohn's disease (see above).** Oral forms of 5-ASA (olsalazine, mesalamine, and sulfasalazine) are effective for treating mild to moderate ulcerative colitis and in maintaining its remission. Budesonide enemas are helpful in distal colonic disease.

  3. **Surgical management** is indicated for uncontrolled hemorrhage, toxic colitis, and perforation. Total proctocolectomy is curative.

III. Toxic Megacolon

A. **A true emergency** defined as dilatation of the colon of >6 cm and accompanied by fever, abdominal pain, and shock.

B. **Treatment**

  1. Make patient NPO and pass long NG tube.

  2. **Treat shock aggressively** (see Chapter 2).

  3. **Hydrocortisone succinate** 300 mg/day continuous IV drip.

  4. **IV antibiotics** should be given (cefoxitin, ampicillin/sulbactam, or combination ciprofloxacin and metronidazole).

  5. **A surgical consult** should be obtained.

ANORECTAL DISEASES

I. Hemorrhoids

A. **Definition.** Dilated vein within the anal canal and distal rectum. Internal hemorrhoids are derived from the internal hemorrhoidal plexus above the dentate line and are covered by rectal mucosa. External hemorrhoids are derived from the external hemorrhoidal plexus below the dentate line and are covered by stratified squamous epithelium.

B. **Etiology.** Increased abdominal pressure secondary to straining during bowel movements, heavy lifting, childbirth, and benign prostatic hypertrophy.

C. **Classification.**

  1. First-degree: no prolapse.

  2. Second-degree: prolapses, but reduces spontaneously.

  3. Third-degree: reduces with manual reduction.

  4. Fourth-degree: permanently prolapsed, will not reduce.

D. **Symptoms** are bright red bleeding with defecation, external protrusion, tenderness (severe pain unusual unless thrombosed), itching.

E. **Treatment.**

  1. **General principles.** High fiber diet, stool softeners, avoid straining during bowel movements, avoid heavy lifting. Warm sitz baths BID and lubrication with glycerin suppositories may help to reduce symp-

toms. Medicated suppositories such as Anusol HC (contains hydrocortisone) may help to decrease inflammation. Limit steroid containing medications to less than 2 weeks of continuous use to avoid atrophy of anal tissues.

2. **Thrombosed external hemorrhoids.** Often can be treated nonsurgically. However, if a patient presents within 48 to 72 hours of onset, excision of thrombus often provides dramatic relief of pain. Incision and drainage is not adequate; the entire thrombus should be excised.

3. **Infrared photocoagulation** is the treatment of choice for first-degree hemorrhoids that cannot be managed with the conservative measures outlined above.

4. **Rubber band ligation** is useful for second-degree and small third-degree hemorrhoids. Limit treatment to two hemorrhoidal areas at one time. Subsequent treatments can be performed at 4 to 6 week intervals. Consider surgical referral if symptoms persist after 3 to 4 treatments.

5. **Work-up for bleeding presumed to be from hemorrhoids.** Digital rectal exam and anoscopy is the minimum work-up for the patient who presents with rectal bleeding. If the bleeding source is not apparent, or if the history is not consistent with hemorrhoids as the source, then do sigmoidoscopy. If the patient is >40 years of age, do sigmoidoscopy as part of the initial evaluation of rectal bleeding. A barium enema (in addition to sigmoidoscopy) or colonoscopy should be done in patients over 50 with rectal bleeding, or in patients whose stools remain guaiac positive after treatment of their hemorrhoids.

II. **Anal Fissures**

A. **Definition.** Superficial tear in the distal lining of the anal canal, usually posteriorly in the midline. Consider inflammatory bowel disease, leukemia, syphilis, and TB as possible secondary causes of lesions located outside the midline.

B. **History.** Usually acute onset of sharp anal pain, brought on by a bowel movement. The pain lasts several minutes to hours. A small amount of bleeding may be present.

C. **Treatment.** Bulk laxatives, stool softeners, sitz baths. Usually heal in 2 to 4 weeks. There is no proven benefit to topical ointments, suppositories, or injections of local anesthetic. **Local injections of botulinum toxin** to relax the sphincter muscle results in healing in up to 96% of patients. **Nitroglycerin ointment 0.2%** (1-inch 2% NTG paste mixed with 9 inches of petroleum jelly, etc.) applied BID results in a healing rate of 68%. Surgery may be required in refractory cases.

III. **Anorectal Abscess**

A. **Etiology.** Obstruction of the anal glands, leading to infection and abscess formation.

B. **Locations.** Perianal (40% to 50%), ischiorectal (20% to 30%), intersphincteric (20% to 25%), supralevator (5% to 7%).

C. **Signs and Symptoms.** Pain, swelling, and redness for superficial abscesses. Deeper abscesses may present only with systemic symptoms such as fever, malaise, and an elevated white blood cell count. Examination will reveal fullness or a tender mass. MRI may be indicated when the diagnosis is unclear.

D. **Treatment.** Incision and drainage. Antibiotic therapy is not needed if external drainage is adequate. However, antibiotics may be necessary for patients with surrounding cellulitis and in diabetic patients. Antibiotics must cover both aerobes and anaerobes (e.g., amoxicillin/clavulanate, TMP/SMX + metronidazole). If there is substantial soft tissue inflammation, hospitalization, IV antibiotics, drainage and debridement, and surgical referral may be warranted. Intersphincteric and supralevator abscesses are treated by internal drainage into the rectum, performed under anesthesia. Warn patient that fistulas develop in approximately 25% of cases, usually occurring several weeks after the abscess is drained.

GASTROINTESTINAL BLEEDING

I. **Types**
A. **Hematemesis.** Vomiting of blood.
   1. May be bright red blood or coffee grounds-like material. Usually from bleeding proximal to the ligament of Treitz.
   2. **Sources**
      a. Peptic ulcer disease: may be asymptomatic until first bleed especially in patients taking NSAIDS.
      b. Gastritis, especially from alcohol.
      c. Mallory-Weiss tear, a tear of the gastric mucosa, which occurs after prolonged vomiting/retching and is generally a self-limited bleed. Look for mediastinal air on CXR.
      d. Esophageal varices from portal hypertension especially secondary to chronic alcohol consumption.
      e. Swallowed blood from epistaxis or other source of bleeding.
B. **Melena.** Passage of black, tarry stools secondary to GI bleeding with intestinal transit time allowing for the digestion of hemoglobin.
   1. May be of upper or lower GI origin (Table 5-3).
   2. Black, tarry stools can be the result of ingested iron, licorice, or bismuth but the stool will be guaiac negative.
C. **Hematochezia.** Bright red blood per rectum.
   1. Can be secondary to anal disease (hemorrhoids, rectal fissure).
   2. May be secondary to a bleeding diverticulum, other colonic disease such as angiodysplasia, Crohn's disease, ulcerative colitis, carcinoma (very rarely causes gross bleeding), dysentery (especially amebiasis, campylobacter, shigella, or other invasive organisms).
   3. Ingestion of beets may simulate hematochezia.
II. **Evaluation of the GI Bleed**
A. **Laboratory studies** should include CBC and platelets, PT/PTT, electrolytes, BUN/creatinine (GI bleeders will frequently have elevated BUN secondary to the increased ingestion of nitrogen from digested blood). Type and crossmatch for at least 2 units of packed RBCs.

5

GASTROENTEROLOGY AND HEPATOLOGY

TABLE 5-3

ETIOLOGY OF GI BLEEDING

Category	Upper GI Bleed	Lower GI Bleed
Inflammatory	Peptic ulcer	Ulcerative colitis
	Esophagitis	Crohn's disease
	Gastritis	Diverticulitis
	Stress ulcer	Enterocolitis
Mechanical	Mallory-Weiss tear	Anal fissure
	Hiatal hernia	Diverticulosis
Vascular	Esophageal varices	Hemorrhoids
		Hemorrhoids/A-V malformations
		Angiodysplasia
Neoplastic	Carcinoma	Carcinoma/polyps
Systemic	Blood dyscrasias	Blood dyscrasias

B. **Physical examination** often reveals hyperactive bowel sounds secondary to intraluminal blood. If an acute abdomen is present, consider CXR and an upright abdominal film to look for free air.

C. **Endoscopy** may be done acutely for upper GI bleeding to help define the source and treat endoscopically if able.

D. **Angiography** or nuclear medicine studies can be useful to localize lower GI bleeding.

III. **Acute management of the GI Bleed**

A. **Upper GI bleeding.**

1. Start IV fluid resuscitation and manage shock as per Chapter 2. Transfuse as needed.

2. An NG tube should be placed to document the source and relative rate of bleeding (blood is usually (but not always) present in the NG aspirate during an upper GI bleed). The NG tube may be removed after the diagnosis is made unless it is needed to prevent nausea and vomiting. **Ice saline lavage does not serve a useful purpose and may prolong bleeding.** An NG tube will not induce variceal bleeding.

3. When examining the studies in aggregate, neither the H-2 blockers (e.g. cimetidine or ranitidine) nor the proton pump inhibitors (e.g. omeprazole) have been shown to decrease mortality, the need for blood transfusion or the length of hospital stay (although one study of high dose omeprazole 40mg PO BID for 5 days showed some benefit).

4. **Vasopressin has fallen out of favor** since treatment yields no benefit in the need for transfusion, surgery or mortality. Ischemic bowel, cardiac events, and arrhythmias are complications of vasopressin use. If used at all, it should be used in conjunction with IV NTG to prevent ischemic events.

5. **Endoscopy with thermocoagulation** is the treatment of choice.
6. **Esophageal varices.**
   a. Avoid volume over-expansion since this can precipitate CHF and worsen ascites. **However, do not withhold fluids from the unstable, hypotensive patient.** If bleeding has stopped, there is no need to completely normalize PT/PTT/INR.
   b. **The combination of sclerotherapy and octreotide** (a synthetic somatostatin analogue, 50 μg bolus followed by 50 μg/hr) is superior to sclerotherapy alone in controlling acute variceal bleeding in patients with cirrhosis. However, a recent metaanalysis suggests that octreotide alone does not have any advantage over placebo. Octreotide may be most useful as adjunct to banding and patients should be transferred for endoscopic intervention once octreotide is started and the patient is stabilized.
   c. **Transjugular intrahepatic portosystemic shunt (TIPS).** This is regarded as a safe and established means of treating variceal hemorrhage in patients with portal hypertension who fail sclerotherapy. The shunt decreases the portal venous pressure gradient by an average of 57% and helps to prevent variceal rebleeding in 92% and 82% of patients at 6 and 12 months after therapy, respectively. However, 10% to 35% of patients suffer from mental status changes and shunts may become occluded.
   d. **Endoscopic band ligation** of the varices is superior to sclerotherapy and propranolol with respect to the rebleeding rate and the mortality rate. Moreover, band ligation also reduces the frequency of significant esophageal strictures in comparison to sclerotherapy.
   e. Use of octreotide for a 5 day period in conjunction with band ligation reduces the relative risk of rebleeding in comparison to band ligation alone but does not change mortality.
   f. Before discontinuing octreotide, a nonspecific beta-blocker should be initiated. Propanolol to reduce portal pressure can be started initially at a dose of 10 mg BID and the dose titrated up to decrease the baseline heart rate by 25%. In patients intolerant of beta-blocker or those with bronchospasm, isosorbide mononitrate may be utilized.
   g. Balloon tamponade with a 4 lumen Sengstaken-Blakemore (Minnesota) tube can be used as a temporizing measure to control variceal bleeding. Its use is fraught with complications including esophageal perforation, aspiration pneumonia and asphyxia. The tube should be used for no more than 24 hours due to the risk of necrotic ulcers at compression sites.
   h. Actively bleeding patients with ascites should receive antibiotics due to an increased risk of spontaneous bacterial peritonitis (see section on ascites and peritonitis below).
   i. Up to 50% of the patients die with their first variceal bleed.

7. **Gastric varices.**
   a. While endoscopy is important to make the diagnosis, endoscopic therapeutics are not felt to be effective in the treatment of gastric varices.
   b. Nonspecific beta-blockers can reduce portal hypertension and the likelihood of recurrence of bleeding.
   c. Minnesota tube can be used as a temporizing measure as described above for esophageal varices.
   d. TIPS or a surgical shunt should be considered.
   e. The triad of isolated gastric varices, splenomegaly, and normal hepatic function should raise the suspicion for splenic vein thrombosis.

B. **Lower GI bleeding.**
   1. Start IV fluid resuscitation and manage shock as per Chapter 2.
   2. Work-up may include colonoscopy, barium enema, selective angiography, and radionuclide bleeding studies.
   3. A recent study shows a role for urgent therapeutic colonoscopy with epinephrine injection or bipolar coagulation in patients with **severe hematochezia and diverticulosis.** In this population, approximately 20% have diverticular hemorrhage and colonoscopic treatment may decrease the risk of recurrent bleeding or the need for surgery.
   4. A surgical consultation should be obtained in case operative intervention is needed.
   5. Most causes of lower GI bleeding are initially self limited.

DIFFERENTIAL DIAGNOSIS OF ELEVATED LIVER ENZYMES

I. See Boxes 5-2, 5-3, and 5-4 for the differential diagnosis and work-up of elevated liver enzymes.

II. **GGT is too nonspecific to be helpful** in the diagnosis of any specific liver disease. It is inducible by drugs, alcohol, renal failure, pancreatic disease, etc.

III. **If the alkaline phosphatase is noted to be elevated** a GGT and 5′-nucleotidase should be drawn or the alkaline phosphatase should be fractionated to determine if it is of bone or liver origin. However, fractionation is more expensive and not widely available. **A normal GGT and 5′-nucleotidase in the presence of an elevated alkaline phosphatase suggests a bone origin of the alkaline phosphatase.**

IV. General Principles.

A. **Even mild elevation** of liver enzymes may indicate the presence of potentially significant liver disease. **Levels do not always correlate with extent of hepatocellular damage.**

B. **Mild elevations of transaminases (less than 2 to 3 × normal)** are seen in patients with fatty liver, nonalcoholic steatohepatitis, and chronic viral hepatitis.

C. **Moderate elevations of transaminases (3 to 20 × normal)** typical of acute or chronic hepatitis including alcoholic hepatitis.

BOX 5-2

DIFFERENTIAL DIAGNOSIS OF ELEVATED TRANSAMINASES

ELEVATED ALT AND AST CAN BE CAUSED BY THE FOLLOWING:

Viral agents: Hepatitis (A, B, C, D, E), CMV, Epstein-Barr, and other viruses.

Drugs and chemicals: Acetaminophen overdose, the "glitizones," HMG-CoA reductase inhibitors, INH, griseofulvin, anti-convulsants, NSAIDs, chemicals (carbon tetrachloride, etc), alcohol, and many other agents.

Primary liver diseases: Primary sclerosing cholangitis, primary biliary cirrhosis (positive antimitochondrial antibody).

Metabolic diseases: Gilbert's disease (mild elevation in unconjugated bilirubin, especially with dehydration), Wilson's disease (decreased ceruloplasmin), hemochromatosis (see Chapter 6), alpha$_1$-antitrypsin deficiency, and cystic fibrosis.

Mechanical difficulties: Ductal obstruction secondary to common duct stone or carcinoma (especially pancreatic, hepatoma, metastatic), Budd-Chiari syndrome (thrombosis of the hepatic vein).

Cholestasis from central venous nutrition, pregnancy, or ceftriaxone therapy.

Infiltrative processes: Fatty liver (especially those with diabetes, hypothyroidism, obesity; determine by U/S), amyloid, granulomatous hepatitis, liver abscess (including amebic or echinococcal; diagnosis by U/S or CT; may have eosinophilia), AIDS-related lymphoma, or other neoplasm.

Other. CHF, celiac sprue, muscle diseases (e.g., polymyositis)

BOX 5-3

CAUSES OF ELEVATED ALKALINE PHOSPHATASE

CAUSES OF ELEVATED ALKALINE PHOSPHATASE

- Pregnancy, type O or B blood after a fatty meal.
- Liver: cholestasis, partial obstruction of the biliary ducts, primary sclerosing cholangitis, adult bile ductopenia, primary biliary cirrhosis, sarcoidosis, and other granulomatous diseases.
- Bone diseases such as Paget's disease, metastatic disease, etc.

Work-up:

Includes imaging study of the liver

5

GASTROENTEROLOGY AND HEPATOLOGY

D. **High elevations** occur in acute viral hepatitis, drug reaction, other toxins (e.g., acetaminophen toxicity) or ischemic injury related to shock.

E. **AST:ALT ratio of >2:1** is characteristic of alcoholic liver disease.

F. **ALT and AST may rise in common duct obstruction** (e.g., from cholelithiasis).

G. **Coagulation factors** reflect liver synthetic function. **Less than 20% factor V activity,** a non-vitamin K–dependent factor, is a poor prognostic factor in fulminant hepatic failure, indicating need for liver transplant.

H. **Prothrombin time may be prolonged in cholestatic liver disease** due to vitamin K deficiency; try to correct with vitamin K 10 mg SC/IV QD for 3 days.

BOX 5-4

EVALUATION OF ELEVATED LIVER ENZYMES

First step is to re-test. No further work-up if normal.

ELEVATED ALT/AST

Work-up proceeds in the following order:

- Rule out toxin exposure (alcohol, drugs)
- Hepatitis A, B, and C serology
- ANA and anti-smooth muscle antibody (autoimmune hepatitis but only 28% to 40% sensitive)
- Serum Fe, TIBC, transferrin saturation (hemochromatosis)
- Serum alpha$_1$-antitrypsinase
- Serum protein electrophoresis (elevated levels of autoimmune hepatitis, 80% sensitive)
- Anti-endomysial antibodies or tissue transglutaminase (gluten-sensitive sprue)
- Ultrasound or CT imaging (ultrasound first)
- Serum ceruloplasmin (Wilson's disease)

ELEVATED ALKALINE PHOSPHATASE

Ultrasound or CT imaging (ultrasound first)

VIRAL HEPATITIS

I. **General.** Classified into acute hepatitis (self-limited liver injury of <6 months) and chronic hepatitis (hepatic inflammation >6 months)

II. **Clinical Presentation.** Fever, nausea, vomiting, anorexia, vague RUQ abdominal pain, jaundice, headache, myalgia and/or arthralgia. Smokers may find tobacco tastes bad. Pronounced elevation of liver enzymes in acute hepatitis and low and variable increase with chronic disease.

III. **Etiologic Agents** (Table 5-4)

A. **Hepatitis A.** Causes ~200,000 cases of acute hepatitis annually (more than all of the other hepatatrophic viruses combined). No reinfection or chronicity. Of adults in the United States 50% to 75% are positive for antibodies to hepatitis A. Often produces subclinical disease especially in children. Transmission is primarily feco-oral (contaminated food and water) and rarely by parenteral exposure. Hepatitis A is generally self-limited **but may be serious with underlying liver disease.**

1. **Risk factors:** travel to developing countries, household contacts, consumption of raw mollusks, male homosexuality.

2. **Diagnosis:** based on elevated IgM (acute disease) or elevated IgG (prior disease) antibodies to hepatitis A.

3. **Prophylaxis:** IgG (gamma globulin) 0.02 ml/kg IM for close contacts or travelers to endemic areas. Immunization can be achieved with an inactivated hepatitis A vaccine (Havrix) if given IM at least 4 weeks before anticipated exposure, with a second dose 6 months to 1 year later. **Can administer both IgG prophylaxis and hepatitis A vaccination at the same time but at different sites.**

B. **Hepatitis B.** Serologic evidence precedes clinical symptoms by approxi-

TABLE 5-4

COMPARISONS OF TYPE A, TYPE B, AND TYPE C HEPATITIS

FEATURE	Hepatitis A	Hepatitis B	Hepatitis C
Incubation	15 to 45 days (mean 30)	30 to 180 days (mean 60 to 90)	15 to 160 days (mean 50)
Onset	Acute	Often insidious	Insidious
Age preference	Children, young adults	Any age	Any age but more common in adults
TRANSMISSION ROUTE			
Fecal-oral	+++	−	Unknown
Other nonpercutaneous routes	±	++	++
Percutaneous	±	+++	+++
OTHER CHARACTERISTICS			
Severity	Mild	Often severe	Variable
Prognosis	Generally good	Worse with age, debility	Moderate
Progression to chronicity	None	Occasional (5% to 10%)	Frequent (65% to 85%)
Prophylaxis	Immunoglobulin or hepatitis A vaccine	Standard IG (not documented) HBIG, HBV	?
Carrier	None	0.1% to 30%	Exists but prevalence unknown

mately 1 month. Hepatitis B is the leading cause of liver-related deaths from cirrhosis and hepatocellular carcinoma worldwide; is especially frequent in drug abusers, male homosexuals, and chronic dialysis patients; 5% to 10% of adults in the US have had the disease; and 10% develop a chronic carrier state and constitute an infectious pool.

1. Diagnosis.
   a. **Hepatitis B surface antigen (HBsAg) is found in acute illness** and becomes positive 1 to 7 weeks before clinical disease. It remains positive 1 to 6 weeks after clinical disease **and in chronic carrier states. Blood containing HBsAg is considered potentially infectious.**
   b. **Hepatitis B antibody (Anti-HBs)** is an antibody against the surface antigen of hepatitis B and appears weeks to months after clinical illness. The presence of this antibody confers immunity and indicates prior disease (if hepatitis B core antibody positive) or vaccination (if hepatitis B core antibody negative).
   c. **Anticore antibody (Anti HBc)** appears during the acute phase of

the illness and its presence can be used to diagnose acute HBV infection especially in the "window period" when both HBsAg and HbsAb may be undetectable. Presence of HBcIgM denotes acute infection and IgG appears chronically. The latter may be protective against reinfection.

   d. **Hepatitis B e antigen (HBeAg)** is a mark of infectivity both acutely and chronically.
   e. **Those who are hepatitis B carriers or have chronic active hepatitis will be HBsAg positive.**

2. **Prophylaxis.** Hepatitis B vaccine at time 0, 1 and 6 months given in the deltoid muscle. Hepatitis B immune globulin (0.05-0.07 ml/kg) should be given soon (preferably within 48 hours) after a sexual or needle Stick exposure along with concurrent vaccination. See Chapter 23 for pediatric immunization schedule.

3. **Treatment.** Lamivudine and famciclovir have been used to treat chronic hepatitis B; protocols are not well developed. Interferon alpha-2b is approved and is in more widespread usage.

C. **Hepatitis C.** Accounts for 20% to 40% of acute hepatitis in the United States. Hepatitis C also causes 90% of posttransfusion hepatitis. The virus has an extremely high mutation rate and is thus not easily neutralized by the body's antibody response. Acute infection is usually asymptomatic, 20% of patients develop jaundice, 75% of those infected develop chronic disease with chronically elevated ALT (2- to 8-fold normal), and 20% of patients eventually develop cirrhosis. This can take years to decades to occur. The degree of ALT elevation does not correlate with the severity of disease. The severity of disease can be evaluated only with a liver biopsy. Hepatitis C infection is a risk factor for the development of hepatocellular carcinoma.

1. **Risk factors.** Most patients with hepatitis C have a history of intravenous drug abuse. Other risk factors include history blood transfusion, tattoos, alcohol abuse and cocaine snorting. Epidemiological evidence suggests that it can be transmitted sexually with risk of transmission increasing with duration of a relationship but with a very low incidence (<5%).

2. **Diagnosis**
   a. **Serologic tests that probe for antibodies** produced in response to several viral antigens are now available for the diagnosis of hepatitis C. These tests are highly sensitive and specific. If testing low risk populations, RIBA (recombinant immunoblot assay) test should be obtained since the ELISA has a higher false-positive rate.
   b. **Polymerase chain reaction (PCR)** can detect minute quantities of HCV RNA present in blood as early as 1-2 weeks after infection. Qualitative PCR tests detect as few as 100 HCV RNA copies, and quantitative tests detect a lower limit of 500-2000 copies.
   c. **Genetic heterogeneity of HCV** identifies at least 6 distinct genotypes (with numerous subtypes). Different genotypes have geo-

graphic and epidemiological differences, and they are good predictors of response to interferon.

3. **Treatment:** Aim is to eradicate the virus and halt progression of the disease.

   a. Liver fibrosis can be reversed to some degree with treatment.

   b. **Who refer for treatment.** Anti-HCV- positive patients with persistently elevated ALT levels, detectable HCV RNA, and a liver biopsy that indicates either portal or bridging fibrosis or at least moderate degrees of inflammation and necrosis. **There is no benefit of treatment in patients with a normal ALT.**

   c. **Screening of those with normal initial liver biopsy but elevated ALT.** Patients with elevated ALT but a normal initial biopsy should have repeat biopsy every 3-5 years to determine progression and need for treatment. **There is no need for screening biopsies in those with normal transaminases.**

   d. **Therapy.** The goal of therapy is to eradicate HCV RNA. Alpha-interferons can be useful in treating chronic hepatitis C but should be administered under the care of a hepatologist. The usual dose is 3 million units 3 times per week for 6 months. There is a less than 40% response rate, and multiple courses may be necessary to achieve normalization of ALT. There may be multiple side effects of therapy, including flu-like symptoms, anorexia, malaise, fatigue, myalgias, fever, myelosuppression, hair loss, thyroid dysfunction and depression.

      (1) **Combination therapy with ribavirin and IFN alfa-2b** is superior to IFN monotherapy is becoming the treatment of choice. Ribavirin is teratogenic, an abortifacient and can cause hemolytic anemia. Therefore, hemoglobin needs to be checked frequently and patients should use birth control measures for up to 6 months after completing therapy.

      (2) **Future therapies include** the use of IFN attached to polyethylene glycol ("pegylated IFN") that prolongs the drug's $t_{1/2}$ and delivers a higher amount of the drug.

D. **Hepatitis D** is an RNA virus most often seen in intravenous drug users in North America.

   1. **Requires coinfection with hepatitis B.** It can occur as "superinfection" in the presence of chronic HBV infection or as a "coinfection" with HBV.

   2. Diagnosis made with antibody to hepatitis D antigen, but they are detectable in only ⅓ of the cases.

   3. Clinical course is identical to that of hepatitis B, since it requires coinfection to be active but with increased likelihood for worsening of manifestations of HBV infection including fulminant hepatitis.

E. **Hepatitis E.** Most cases occur in developing countries.

   1. Consider in travelers returning from abroad.

   2. Diagnosis made by hepatitis E antibodies.

F. **Chemical agents** that can cause acute hepatitis/injury include acetaminophen (overdose), carbon tetrachloride, alcohol, isoniazid, oral contraceptives, halothane and many, many others.

G. **General Management.** Management is supportive and includes nutritional support but limitation of protein intake. Discontinue hepatotoxic drugs and prescribe prophylaxis for contacts. Those with hepatitis A should have enteric precautions, whereas those with hepatitis B and C should have blood and body fluid precautions.

ASCITES AND SPONTANEOUS BACTERIAL PERITONITIS

I. **Ascites. General Information**

A. **Ascites is a pathologic accumulation of serous fluid** within the abdomen. It may be caused by decompensated liver disease (alcohol- and virus-related cirrhosis), heart failure, abdominal carcinomatosis, tuberculosis, fulminant liver failure, pancreatic disease, pelvic inflammatory disease, connective tissue diseases and hypoproteinemia.

B. **Cirrhosis is the underlying cause in ~80%** of the patients with ascites.
   1. Unlike nonalcohol-related causes of liver disease, ascites may be reversible in alcoholic liver disease with abstinence and salt restriction.
   2. An abrupt development of ascites after many years in a patient with stable cirrhosis should suggest the possibility of hepatocellular carcinoma.

II. **Physical Examination and Radiologic Assessment**

A. Percussion of the flanks helps differentiate ascites from other causes of increased abdominal distention. The dullness should shift upon rotating the patient in the right or left lateral positions. Shifting dullness indicates the presence of at least 1.5 liters of ascites.

B. Plain abdominal X-ray may show the ground glass appearance with centrally located bowel loops, but is not necessary or recommended in the assessment or treatment of ascites.

C. Ultrasonography may be necessary to determine the presence or absence of ascites. Doppler studies of the portal system are helpful in cases in which Budd-Chiari syndrome or a vena caval web are suspected.

D. A chest X-ray and an echocardiogram are helpful in assessing patients suspected to have ascites of cardiac origin.

III. **Paracentesis and Ascitic Fluid Analysis**

A. **Diagnostic paracentesis** should be performed routinely in all patients with new onset ascites and in all patients admitted to the hospital with ascites. A 22-gauge needle can be inserted in a Z-tract fashion, to minimize leakage of fluid after the paracentesis, in midline between the umbilicus and the pubis symphysis in order to avoid collateral vessels. In the presence of a midline scar, a position ~1.5 inches above and medial to the anterior superior iliac spine can be used safely.

B. **Ascitic fluid is mostly straw colored** or yellow tinged. Cloudiness or opacified appearance is due to the presence of neutrophils. Milky appearing ascites is due to the presence of triglycerides and is also known as chylous ascites. Non-traumatic bloody ascites should raise the suspicion for tuberculosis and malignancy. A tea-colored fluid is occasionally seen in pancreatic ascites.

C. **The initial ascitic fluid analysis should include the following studies:** cell count with WBC differential (mandatory test in all cases), albumin, total protein and culture (in blood culture bottles to increase the yield). Glucose, amylase, and Gram stain are of little or no value except in cases of suspected gut perforation.

1. **Patients with >250 polymorphonuclear leukocyte count** (PMN) per milliliter are assumed to be infected and need to be treated. In cases of bloody taps, only 1 PMN per 250 red cells can be attributed to contamination of the ascitic fluid with blood.

2. **In ascites due to tuberculous peritonitis** and peritoneal carcinomatosis, lymphocytes predominate.

3. **The serum-ascites albumin gradient (SAAG)** is equal to [albumin]$_{serum}$ − [albumin]$_{ascites}$. A gradient of ≥1.1 g/dl is indicative of portal hypertension with greater than 90% reliability.

IV. **Other causes of Ascites**

A. **High SAAG**

1. **Cardiac ascites** is due to congestion of hepatic sinusoids and has high total protein.

2. **Nephrogenous ascites** occurs in patients on hemodialysis with volume overload and tends to have high total protein as well.

3. **Massive liver metastases** can result in portal venous inflow obstruction and tumor emboli in portal vein radicals cause- portal hypertension. The ascites total protein is <2.5 mg/dl in two-thirds of the cases. Consider also Budd-Chiari syndrome, etc.

4. **In myxedema,** ascites forms due to congestive heart failure and also has high protein (>2.5 mg/dl).

B. **Low SAAG**

1. **Tuberculous peritonitis** is most often diagnosed in Asians and immigrants from Central America.

2. **Peritoneal carcinomatosis** accounts for ~50% of all cases of ascites due to a malignancy. Cytology is positive in 97% to 100% of the cases.

3. **Pancreatic ascites** accounts for <1% of ascites. Patients often have underlying liver disease due to alcohol abuse. The fluid has high amylase and the total protein of the ascites is usually high.

4. **Biliary ascites** is due to leakage of bile into the peritoneum, is dark brown, has bilirubin value ≥6 mg/dl and an ascitic fluid/serum bilirubin ratio of >1.

5. **Ascites with low SAAG may be seen in patients with connective tissue diseases** due to serositis in the absence of portal hypertension.

6. **Nephrotic syndrome** is a cause of ascites with low protein.

7. **Ascites in a febrile,** sexually active young woman should raise a suspicion for chlamydia peritonitis. This ascites has high protein and has elevated WBC.

V. **Treatment of Ascites.**

A. **Discontinue any prostaglandin inhibitors or other drugs which reduce GFR (e.g., NSAIDS).**

B. **Sodium restriction** is the key to successful treatment of ascites. Patient should be instructed to follow a 2 g/day sodium diet. **Fluid restriction is not necessary unless hyponatremia is present.**

C. **Avoidance of salt substitutes** that contain KCl and potassium-enriched foods should be emphasized especially if the patient is also on a potassium-sparing diuretic.

D. **If salt restriction alone is not effective,** oral diuretics can be initiated. A combination of spironolactone and furosemide is usually successful in causing natriuresis without precipitating hyper- or hypokalemia. The usual beginning doses are spironolactone 100 mg QD and furosemide 40 mg QD.

E. **Random urinary sodium and urinary potassium can be checked** and the diuretics' doses adjusted to effect Na/K ratio >1. (Increase in furosemide dose causes increased urinary sodium and potassium loss and increase in spironolactone dose causes increased potassium retention.)

F. **The doses of spironolactone and furosemide can be titrated** to a maximum of 400 mg qd and 160 mg QD, respectively, using the 100 mg:40 mg ratio to maintain normokalemia. The goal of diuretic therapy should be to effect a 1-2 lb weight loss daily.

G. Body weight, serum electrolytes, urea and creatinine are important parameters to follow.

H. **Diuretic therapy should be stopped** in the event that encephalopathy, hyponatremia (Na <120 mmol/L despite fluid restriction), or renal insufficiency (creatinine >2 mg/dl) develop. Overaggressive diuresis can also lead to hepatorenal syndrome, a non-reversible condition resulting in progressive renal failure due to renal hypoperfusion in patients with advanced liver disease. Avoid diuresis of greater than 1 liter per day.

I. **Large volume paracentesis** can be performed in patients with tense ascites affecting satiety and respiration. Approximately 4-6 L can be removed resulting in improvement of symptoms. No albumin replacement is recommended for removal of up to 5 liters of ascitic fluid. Intravenous albumin (8 g/liter of ascitic fluid removed) can be given for larger volume paracentesis.

J. **Refractory or diuretic-resistant ascites,** defined as minimal to no weight loss despite diuretics or development of complications of diuretic therapy, occurs in <10% of cirrhotic patients with ascites. It can be managed by repeated therapeutic paracenteses, peritoneovenous shunt or TIPS placement. TIPS is superior to repeated large volume paracentesis in resolving ascites and there is a trend towards better survival. However, patients with TIPS must be monitored for shunt malfunction and hepatic encephalopathy which may be more frequent than in those undergoing paracentesis (data is contradictory). While orthotopic liver transplantation should be considered initially after the onset of ascites, eligible patients who are diuretic-resistant need to be prioritized for transplantation as 50% die in 6 months.

K. **Spontaneous Bacterial Peritonitis.** Patients with ascitic fluid total protein concentration <1.0 g/dl and gastrointestinal hemorrhage are at high risk for spontaneous bacterial peritonitis. There is good evidence that Bactrim (1 DS tablet daily 5 days a week) is effective in preventing spontaneous bacterial peritonitis and decreasing mortality. Norfloxacin 400 mg qd has been used but there is rapid development of resistant organisms. Weekly use of ciprofloxacin 750 mg, as well as levofloxacin 250 mg qd are being used increasingly. Also see treatment for SBP below.

HEPATIC HYDROTHORAX

I. **Defined as** the presence of a large pleural effusion that is seen as a complication of ascites in 5% to 9% of the cirrhotic patients with ascites, is often right-sided and can occasionally be found in the **absence of ascites.** It is most likely due to defect(s) in the tendinous portion of the right hemi-diaphragm. The pleural fluid tends to recur and, like ascites, is usually transudative in nature.

II. **The diagnosis can be confirmed by** obtaining a nuclear study that establishes the presence of a peritoneo-pleural communication. The study involves the instillation of ^{99m}Tc-sulfur colloid into the peritoneum and documenting the presence of the radiotracer in the pleural space.

III. **Hepatic hydrothorax is a relative contraindication to chest tube placement** due to the potential for life-threatening fluid and electrolyte depletion. **Rather, it is treated like ascites.** In cases not responding to usual therapy, pleurodesis with tetracycline or thoracotomy to repair the diaphragmatic defect can be performed.

SPONTANEOUS BACTERIAL PERITONITIS (SBP)

I. General Information

A. **SBP is a common complication** in patients with cirrhosis and ascites, and occurs mostly in the setting of low ascitic fluid total protein level (<1 g/dl).

B. **Pathogenesis** involves bacterial translocation from the gut to the systemic circulation and then to ascitic fluid.

C. *E. coli, Klebseilla pneumoniae,* and *pneumococcus* are the three most common isolates.

D. **Renal failure occurs in approximately one-third of the patients despite treatment** of the infection.

II. Presentation and Diagnosis

A. **Abdominal pain and fever are the most characteristic symptoms,** but hepatic encephalopathy, gastrointestinal bleeding, vomiting, diarrhea, shock, or hypothermia may be the presenting symptom(s) in a large number of patients.

B. It can also be totally **asymptomatic.** Therefore one must have a low threshold for performing a paracentesis to obtain ascitic fluid for analysis.

C. **SBP is diagnosed when there is a positive ascitic fluid culture or when the ascitic fluid PMN count is ≥250 cells/mm³** in the absence of an identifiable intraabdominal source of infection.

D. **Ascitic fluid culture** must be placed directly into blood culture preferably at bedside to increase the sensitivity of culture.

E. **Secondary peritonitis** due to perforated viscus usually results in PMN count in the thousands, multiple organisms on gram stain and culture, and at least 2 of the following: total protein >1 g/dl, LDH > the upper limit of normal for serum, and glucose <50 mg/dl.

III. **Treatment.**

A. **Empiric antibiotic** treatment should be begun before the culture results become available to prevent demise of the patient.

B. **A broad-spectrum therapy is recommended in suspected ascitic fluid infection** until culture results and susceptibility are available. Cefotamine 2 g IV Q8h or a comparable third-generation cephalosporin is the treatment of choice. Five days of treatment is appropriate. **A repeat paracentesis** can be performed after completion of 5 days of therapy with IV antibiotics to ensure efficacy of the treatment especially in patients with atypical presentation or response.

C. **Intravenous albumin** at a dose of 1.5 g per kilogram body weight on day 1 and 1 g per kilogram on day 3 has been shown to reduce significantly the incidence of renal impairment and death in comparison with treatment with antibiotics alone.

D. Subsequently, these patients should be placed on SBP prophylaxis therapy (norfloxacin 400 mg QD or levofloxacin 250 mg QD) for the remaining part of their hospital stay.

ALCOHOLIC LIVER DISEASE, LIVER FAILURE, AND CHRONIC LIVER DISEASE

I. Alcoholic Liver Disease (ALD).

A. General Background.

1. It is caused by chronic alcohol ingestion-consumption exceeding 80 g/day (equivalent to six 12 oz cans of beer, 1 liter of wine, or 5-6 liquor drinks).

2. It is the most prevalent form of liver disease in the developed countries and affects women and those with hepatitis C infection at a lower consumption level than men.

3. Three histologic forms of ALD are recognized: hepatic steatosis (fatty liver), alcoholic hepatitis, and alcoholic cirrhosis.

4. An increased prevalence of hepatitis C in patients with ALD.

B. Clinical Presentation.

1. Presenting features range from non-specific signs and symptoms to frank liver failure. Also see **chronic liver disease** below for signs and symptoms.

2. Parotid gland hypertrophy may be present due to recurrent emesis.
3. Epigastric or right-sided abdominal pain, progressive jaundice, increasing abdominal girth or lower extremity swelling may be the reasons compelling the patient to seek medical attention.
4. Anorexia, nausea, and vomiting are also reported by these patients.
5. Fever and tachycardia may be noted in the absence of an infection.
6. Tender hepatomegaly may occur due to acute inflammation of the liver.
7. Progressive jaundice, palmar erythema, Dupuytren's contractures, cutaneous telangiectasias, feminization (gynecomastia and testicular atrophy) and complication of portal hypertension *(see below)* are some of the other findings.
8. Alteration in mental status may be noted due to **hepatic encephalopathy** (see below) and/or alcohol withdrawal.

C. **Diagnosis and laboratory evaluation.** A thorough history of alcohol use, complete liver panel, biochemical profile, CBC and PT with INR should be obtained on all patients. The *CAGE* questionnaire can be used to screen for alcohol abuse or dependency.
   1. **Elevated GGT in most.**
   2. **AST:ALT ratio is** typically between **2:1** to 8:1 with both usually being <300 IU/L. Unless associated with acetaminophen toxicity, transaminase values higher than seven times the upper limit of normal should make one question the diagnosis of ALD.
   3. **Leucocytosis** (with neutrophilia) in the absence of an infection may be present due to inflammation of the liver.
   4. **Coagulopathy** persisting despite replacement of vitamin K is indicative of decreased hepatic synthetic function.
   5. **Prognosis.** Patients with alcoholic hepatitis and discriminant function (DF) >32 have a poor prognosis with a predicted probability of mortality within 1 month of ~ 50%. *DF = 4.6 (PT − normal PT) + total bilirubin (mg/dl).*
   6. **A liver biopsy may be necessary** if the diagnosis is unclear or if there are atypical features. It aids in the selection of patients being considered for steroid therapy as up to 28% of patients with a clinical picture of alcoholic hepatitis do not have histological features consistent with alcoholic hepatitis on the biopsy.

D. **Treatment.**
   1. **Alcohol abstinence** and supportive care are key to the successful treatment of ALD. Liver enzyme abnormalities persisting for 6 months after the cessation of alcohol intake should prompt workup to rule out other causes of liver disease including a liver biopsy.
   2. **Symptomatic patients** should be hospitalized and given thiamine 100 mg via IV fluids initially to prevent Wernicke-Korsakoff's syndrome.
   3. **Treat alcohol withdrawal** (see Chapter 18 for details).

4. **Patients with ALD are usually malnourished** so protein intake should not be restricted severely. At least 60 g of protein should be given daily.

5. **Steroids.** If an infectious process has been ruled out, patients with severe alcoholic hepatitis (hepatic encephalopathy or DF > 32 may benefit from corticosteroids. Prednisolone 40 mg qd × 4 weeks followed by tapering over several days to weeks should be used.

6. Patients with end-stage alcoholic liver disease should be referred for liver transplantation especially if they have been abstinent of alcohol for 6 months.

II. **Liver Failure and Chronic Liver Disease**

A. **Fulminant hepatic failure (FHF).**

1. **FHF** develops within 2 weeks and subfulminant hepatic failure develops within 2-8 weeks of the onset of jaundice. It occurs due to acute onset of massive hepatocellular necrosis resulting in sudden and severe impairment of liver function. Encephalopathy is usually present.

2. **Causes include** acetaminophen toxicitiy, viral hepatitis, drug reaction, toxins *(mushroom poisoning),* ishemic hepatitis, Wilson's disease, autoimmune chronic active hepatitis, fatty liver of pregnancy and Reye's syndrome.

3. **FHF needs intensive monitoring** and emergent evaluation for orthotopic liver transplant.

B. **Cirrhosis.**

1. Cirrhosis of the liver is a diffuse process characterized by the formation of islands of regenerated liver surrounded by dense fibrosis (abnormal nodules) that occurs after a protracted insult (such as alcohol, chronic active hepatitis, etc.).

2. Most complications of cirrhosis occur as a result of development of portal hypertension or decreased synthetic function of the liver.

C. **Signs and symptoms of liver failure.**

1. **FHF.** One of the earliest signs of FHF is a change is personality. Uncooperative and violent behavior is not uncommon. Jaundice does not correlate with neuropsychiatric changes in the early stages and is deep in the late stage. Fetor hepaticus, flapping tremor and hyperreflexia may be present. Spontaneous bleeding from mucosal surfaces may occur due to coagulopathy. In later stages, decerebrate rigidity with spasticity can be noted. In contrast to chronic liver disease, the liver is non-nodular and splenomegaly and vascular telangiectasias are **not** present.

2. **Chronic liver disease (CLD).** Weight loss, malnutrition, fatigue, easy bruising (caused by reduced levels of factors II, VII, IX, and X), jaundice, pruritus, edema, ascites and encephalopathy with asterixis. The patient may also have GI bleeding from esophageal varices (caused by portal hypertension) or coma. **GI bleeding is a common precipitant of hepatic encephalopathy and coma in liver failure patients because of the large gastrointestinal protein load.**

D. **Laboratory Evaluation and Monitoring.**
 1. **FHF.** Obtain routine biochemical profile and complete liver panel. Serum albumin is usually normal initially. Hypoglycemia is found in a large percentage of patients with FHF. Lactic acidosis develops in approximately half the patients with grade 3 coma. Hyponatremia and hypokalemia are found especially in the later stages. **Coagulopathy** develops due to decreased hepatic synthesis of coagulation factors. The prothrombin (PT) time is also a good prognostic indicator. Cerebral edema can also lead to respiratory depression and respiratory acidosis. Hence, **neurologic status** and **PT/INR** should be followed closely in patients with FHF.
 2. **CLD.** Laboratory evaluation may show normal liver enzymes in end-stage disease because of the small amount of residual hepatic tissue. These patients will usually have low serum albumin. Anemia and **thrombocytopenia** may also be present. Blood ammonia levels may be elevated. Electrolyte abnormalities include **hyponatremia, hypokalemia,** and **free water overload.** There may also be concomitant acidosis or alkalosis.
E. **Management.**
 1. **Acute treatment.**
  a. For patients in FHF, a referral to a specialist should be obtained promptly.
  b. Since cerebral edema is an important cause of death in patients with fulminant hepatic failure, intracranial pressure (ICP) monitoring is used in specialized units.
  c. Hypoglycemia is corrected with 50% glucose. If patient is to be moved to an another medical center, patient is started on 20% glucose infusion during transport.
  d. Coagulopathy is managed by parenteral vitamin K 5-10 mg SQ QD × 2-3 days and by transfusion with blood, platelets, and fresh frozen plasma.
  e. Hepatic encephalopathy is treated as described below.
  f. Hypokalemia and other electrolyte abnormalities are corrected with appropriate replacement.
  g. Infections are sought after early and the patient should be pancultured.
  h. Charcoal hemoperfusion for removal of toxic metabolites is also being tried in some centers.
 2. **Chronic treatment.**
  a. A nonselective beta-blocker, such as propanolol or nadolol, reduces the risk of initial bleeding from esophageal varices. Propanolol can be started at a dose of 10 mg BID and titrated (to 60 mg QD) to effect a 25% reduction in the base-line heart rate. Nonselective beta-blockers are also the treatment of choice for bleeding from portal hypertensive gastropathy. Isosorbide may have an additive effect to the beta-blocker. New studies show that

endoscopic band ligation of esophageal varices is more effective than propanolol for the primary prevention of variceal bleeding. Endoscopic ligation can be repeated every 4-6 weeks until the esophageal varices have all been obliterated.

b. Management of other complication of chronic liver disease is as described below under individual sections.

HEPATIC ENCEPHALOPATHY

I. **General Information.** Hepatic encephalopathy (HE) is a reversible metabolic encephalopathy with global central nervous system depression that occurs as a result of hepatocellular failure. Associated with increased portosystemic shunting of nitrogenous compounds derived from the gut.

II. **Precipitated or exacerbated by** GI hemorrhage, excess dietary protein, constipation, infection (SBP), hypokalemia, and systemic alkalosis.

III. **Ammonia** is thought to play an important role in the pathogenesis of HE, but its plasma level correlates poorly with the severity of HE.

IV. **Manifestation and evaluation.**

A. Its clinical presentation ranges from subtle changes in behavior and sleep inversion to deep coma.

B. Subclinical HE can be detected by number connection tests *(trail test).*

C. Rule out other causes of encephalopathy and attempt to identify any precipitating factor(s). Absence of any precipitating factors of HE indicates worsening liver function.

D. Check ammonia level and electrolytes, BUN and creatinine.

V. **Treatment.**

A. Conventional therapy aims to lower the production and absorption of ammonia. Lactulose, a nonabsorbable dissacharide, is used usually in doses of 30-60 g daily. However, the dose can be titrated up to 20-40 g TID-QID to effect 2-3 semiformed bowel movements per day. If lactulose cannot be administered orally or per nasogastric tube, it may be given as a 300 cc (200 g) retention enema. Lacitol is as effective as lactulose but with fewer side effects.

B. In severely constipated patients, tap water enemas can be given to evacuate the bowels.

C. Hypokalemia should be corrected with potassium supplementation.

D. In patients with inadequate response to lactulose alone, sodium benzoate 2-8 g/day and/or neomycin 4-6 g/day PO can be added in divided doses.

E. Dietary protein may be restricted to 0.8-1 g/kg per day **initially** in comatose patients not responding to therapy outlined above.

F. Sedatives should be **avoided** if possible.

ACUTE PANCREATITIS

Should be in the differential of any acute abdomen.

I. **Etiology.**

A. **Cholelithiasis** is the most common cause in the United States, Western Europe, and in Asia (45% of cases). Biliary sludge has also been implicated in some cases.

B. **Chronic alcohol ingestion** is the second leading cause (35% of cases).

C. **"Traumatic" causes,** including **postoperative stress,** ERCP, direct trauma, manometry of the sphincter of Oddi, endoscopic sphincterotomy, and perforation of a duodenal ulcer.

D. **Metabolic insults** including hypertriglyceridemia (>1000 as in type V hyperlipoproteinemia), hypercalcemia (e.g., hyperparathyroidism), and renal failure.

E. **Drugs** including DDI, DDC, azathioprine, mercaptopurine, valproic acid, acetaminophen, and others.

F. **Infectious causes** including viruses (mumps, rubella, cytomegalovirus, adenovirus, HIV, coxsackievirus B), bacteria mycoplasma, Campylobacter, legionella, Mycobacterium tuberculosis, M. avium complex), and parasitic (ascariasis, clonorchiasis).

G. **Connective tissue disorders** (SLE, polyarteritis nodosa, Sarcoidosis) and idiopathic causes.

II. **Clinical presentation.**

A. Generally have abdominal pain in mid-epigastric region radiating to the left upper quadrant back, nausea, vomiting. Depending on severity may have low grade fever and signs of shock. **However, patients may be pain free and manifest only shock.** Patients may also have evidence of retroperitoneal bleeding (Cullen's, Grey Turner's sign). Complications include the following:

1. Multisystem organ failure (ARDS, renal failure from ATN), shock, DIC and hemorrhage
2. Pleural effusions, pneumonia, and atelectasis
3. Formation of pancreatic fluid collections (pseudocysts and abscesses (account for 70% to 80% of mortality)
4. Ileus, CNS hypoperfusion with confusion, and so on.

III. **Diagnosis.**

A. **Amylase and lipase** levels should be determined. Amylase is elevated in 80% of those with pancreatitis and is more sensitive early on. Lipase is more sensitive if symptoms have been present for more than 24 hours. Both the amylase and lipase may be normal in a patient with CT-proven pancreatitis. Urinary trypsin activation peptide (TAP) is a promising new test.

B. **Ultrasound or CT of the pancreas** may show pancreatic glandular edema, peripancreatic fat stranding, or pancreatic/peripancreatic fluid collections.

C. **Ultrasound of the gallbladder** may show a common bile duct (CBD) stone in gallstone pancreatitis.

D. **X-ray may reveal a "sentinel loop,"** a localized ileus in the midepigastric region. Pleural effusions may also be present.

IV. **Laboratory studies.**
A. CBC, electrolytes, liver enzymes, calcium, magnesium, PT/PTT.
   1. May have hemoconcentration secondary to third spacing of fluid.
   2. May have hypocalcemia due to "soap" formation (saponification of fat and calcium).
   3. Frequently have hypomagnesemia.
   4. White count usually elevated.
   5. Liver enzymes (ALT and AST) may be elevated from biliary obstruction in gallstone pancreatitis these are more sensitive (but less specific) of early CBD obstruction in acute biliary pancreatitis.

V. **Prognosis.**
A. **Based on Ranson's criteria.** The presence of three or four signs on admission is associated with a mortality of 15-20%. If 7 or more signs are present, mortality approaches 100%.
   1. On admission:
      a. Age >55 years.
      b. WBC count >16,000.
      c. Blood glucose >200 mg/dl.
      d. LDH >350 IU/L.
      e. AST >250 IU/l
   2. At 48 hours:
      a. Fall in Hct >10%.
      b. Rise in BUN >5mg per dl.
      c. Serum calcium <8mg per dl.
      d. Arterial pO2 <60mm Hg.
      e. Base deficit >4 meq/l.
      f. Estimated fluid third spacing of >6 liters.

VI. **Acute management:** Treat underlying cause!
A. **Treat shock** (see Chapter 2). Invasive hemodynamic monitoring may be required. May need up to 6-8 liters of fluid per day.
B. **An NG tube** useful for those with vomiting. However, NG tubes have not been shown to reduce the duration of hospitalization nor do they decrease pain intensity associated with pancreatitis.
C. **Keep the patient NPO** until pain resolves and analgesia is no longer required.
D. **Prevent hypocalcemia and hypomagnesemia.**
E. **Manage pain** with parenteral patient-controlled narcotics (see Chapter 15 for details of PCA). Meperidine is preferred in the case of a common duct stone. Morphine is otherwise a good choice.
F. Keep stomach pH close to neutral.
G. Octreotide **has not been shown** to be useful in treating pancreatitis.
H. **Urgent ERCP** to clear the biliary tract has been shown to reduce morbidity and mortality in severe acute biliary pancreatitis. Antibiotics (for the associated ascending cholangitis) are indicated. **However, routine antibiotics are not used.**

VII. **Long-term sequelae.**
A. **Chronic pancreatitis.** Characterized by chronic and progressive loss of pancreatic parenchyma. Both endocrine (diabetes mellitus) and exocrine (steatorrhea, azotorrhea) insufficiency develop when 80-90% of the gland is destroyed. Pancreatic calcification (resulting from intraductal calcium carbonate deposition) may be apparent on plain abdominal radiography. Patients may require therapy with insulin, pancreatic enzyme replacement (Creon), and medium chain triglycerides.

B. **Pseudocyst formation.** Result from the formation of granulation tissue within the pancreas. They may be asymptomatic and resolve spontaneously. Treatment (needle or endoscopic drainage or surgical resection) is indicated if they are enlarging, and are symptomatic. If asymptomatic, then they should generally be managed expectantly.

C. **Pleural fistulas and pancreatic ascites.** These entities result from pancreatic fluid entering the pleural space or abdomen, respectively. Treatment includes octreotide, ERCP (with pancreatic duct stenting), or surgical correction.

BIBLIOGRAPHY

Achkar J-P, Hanauer SB: Medical therapy to reduce postoperative Crohn's disease recurrence, *Am J Gastroenterol* 95:1139-1146, 2000.

Agarwal N et al: Evaluating tests for acute pancreatitis, *Am J Gastroenterol* 85:356- 366, 1990.

Angelico M et al: Isosorbide-5-mononitrate versus propanolol in the prevention of first bleeding in cirrhosis, *Gastroenterology* 104:1460-1465.

Anonymous: American gastroenterological association medical position statement: guidelines for the evaluation and management of chronic diarrhea, *Gastroenterology* 116:1461-1463, 1999.

Besson I et al: Sclerotherapy with or without octreotide for acute variceal bleeding, *N Engl J Med* 333:555-559, 1995.

Butterworth RF: Complications of cirrhosis III: hepatic encephalopathy, *J Hepatol* 32 (Supp 1):171-180, 2000.

Camilleri M et al: Efficacy and safety of alosetron in women with irritable bowel syndrome: a randomised, placebo controlled trial, *Lancet* 335:1035-1040, 1999.

Camilleri M: Therapeutic approach to the patient with irritable bowel syndrome, *Am J Med* 107:27S-32S, 1999.

Cleary RK: *Clostridium difficile*-associated diarrhea and colitis, *Dis Colon Rectum* 41:1435-1449, 1998.

Committee of the American College of Gastroenterology, *Am J Gastroenterol* 92:1962-1975, 1997.

Cordoba J, Blei AT: Treatment of hepatic encephalopathy, *Am J Gastroenterol* 92:1429-1439, 1997.

De las Casas C et al: Review article: Traveller's diarrhoea, *Aliment Pharmacol Ther* 13:1373-1378, 1999.

De Vault KR, Castell DO: Updated guidelines for the diagnosis and treatment of gastroesophageal reflux disease, *Am J Gastroenterol* 94:1434-1442, 1999.

DeBanto JR et al: What could be causing chronic abdominal pain? Anything from common peptic ulcers to uncommon pancreatic trauma, *Postgrad Med* 106:141-146, 1999.

Dupeyron C et al: Rapid emergence of quinolone resistance in cirrhotic patients treated with norfloxacin to prevent spontaneous bacterial peritonitis, *Antimicrob Agents Chemother* 38:340-344, 1994.

5

GASTROENTEROLOGY AND HEPATOLOGY

DuPont HL: Guidelines on acute infectious diarrhea in adults. The Practice Parameters.

Ehrenpreis ED, Kane SV, Cohen LB, et al: Thalidomide therapy for patients with refractory Crohn's disease: an open-label trial, *Gastroenterology* 117:1271-1277,1999.

Elliott DE et al: Does the failure to acquire helminthic parasites predispose to Crohn's disease? *Faseb J* 14:212, 2000.

Feagan BG et al: A comparison of methotrexate with placebo for the maintenance of remission in Crohn's disease. North American Crohn's Study Group Investigators, *N Engl J Med* 342:1627-1632, 2000.

Feldman M et al: *Sleisenger & Fordtran's Gastrointestinal and liver disease: pathophysiology/diagnosis/management,* ed 6, Philadelphia, 1998, WB Saunders.

Fine KD, Schiller LR: AGA technical review on the evaluation and management of chronic diarrhea, *Gastroenterology* 116:1464-1486, 1999.

Fisher BL et al: Obesity correlates with gastroesophageal reflux, *Dig Dis Sci* 44:2290-2294, 1999.

Graham DY et al: Duodenal and gastric ulcer prevention with misoprostol in arthritis patients taking NSAIDS, *Ann Intern Med* 119:257-262, 1993.

Graham DY et al: Effect of triple therapy (antibiotics plus bismuth) on duodenal ulcer healing: a randomized controlled trial, *Ann Intern Med* 115:266-269, 1991.

Guarner C, Soriano G: Spontaneous bacterial peritonitis, *Semin Liver Dis* 17:203-217, 1997.

Gumaste V et al: Serum lipase: a better test to diagnose acute alcoholic pancreatitis, *Am J Med* 92:239, 1992.

Hanauer SB: Management of Crohn's disease in adults, *Am J Gastroenterol* 92:559-566, 1997.

Hill DB, Kugelman M: Alcoholic liver disease: treatment strategies for the potentially reversible stages, *Postgrad Med* 103:261-264, 267-268, 273-275, 1998.

Imperiale TF et al: A meta-analysis of somatostatin versus vasopressin in the management of acute esophageal variceal hemorrhage, *Gastroenterology* 109:1289-1294, 1995.

Jaeckel E, Manns MP: Experience with lamivudine against hepatitis B virus, *Intervirology* 40:322-336, 1997.

Jensen DM et al: Urgent colonoscopy for the diagnosis and treatment of severe diverticular hemorrhage, *N Engl J Med* 342:78-82, 2000.

Karjoo M: Caustic ingestion and foreign bodies in the gastrointestinal system, *Curr Opin Pediatr* 10:516-522, 1998.

Kim PS et al: Optimum duration of treatment with 6-mercaptopurine for Crohn's disease, *Am J Gastroenterol* 94:3254-3257, 1999.

Koch KL: Diabetic gastropathy, *Dig Dis Sci* 44:1061-1075, 1999.

Korelitz BI et al: Malignant neoplasms subsequent to treatment of inflammatory bowel disease with 6-mercaptopurine, *Am J Gastroenterol* 94:3248-3253,1999.

Kornbluth A et al: Cyclosporin for severe ulcerative colitis: a user's guide, *Am J Gastroenterol* 92:1424-1428, 1997.

Kornbluth A, Sachar DB: Ulcerative colitis practice guidelines in adults, *Am J Gastroenterol* 92:204-211, 1997.

Kuipers EJ el al: Long-term sequelae of *Helicobacter pylori* gastritis, *Lancet* 345:1525-1528, 1995.

LaBrecque DR: A commonsense approach to variceal bleeding, *Clin Liver Dis* 1:121-127, 1997.

Lagergren J et al: Symptomatic gastroesophageal reflux as a risk factor for esophageal adenocarcinoma, *N Engl J Med* 340:825-831, 1999.

Lake JR: The role of transjugular portosystemic shunting in patients with ascites, *N Engl J Med* 342:1745-1747, 2000.

Lamah M, Kumar D: Fecal incontinence, *Dig Dis Sci* 44:2488-2499, 1999.

McCullough AJ, O'Connor JFB: Alcoholic liver disease: proposed recommendations of the American college of gastroenterology, *Am J Gastroenterol* 93:2022-2036, 1998.

McHutchison JG: Differential diagnosis of ascites, *Semin Liver Dis* 17:191-202, 1997.

Menon KVN, Kamath PS: Managing the complications of cirrhosis, *Mayo Clin Proc* 75:501-509, 2000.

Mentes BB et al: Hepatic hydrothorax in the absence of ascites: report of two cases and review of the mechanism, *Dig Dis Sci* 42:781-788, 1997.

Miller-Catchpole R: Transjugular intrahepatic portosystemic shunt (TIPS): diagnostic and therapeutic technology assessment (DATTA), *JAMA* 273:1824-1830, 1995.

O'Brien B et al: Cost-effectiveness of *Helicobacter pylori* eradication for the long-term management of duodenal ulcer in Canada, *Arch Intern Med* 155:1958-1964, 1995.

Peterson WL et al: COX-1–sparing NSAIDs—is the enthusiasm justified? *JAMA* 282(20):1961-1963, 1999.

Peterson WL et al: Helicobacter pylori-related disease: guidelines for testing and treatment, *Arch Intern Med* 160:1285-1291, 2000.

Pope CE Acid-reflux disorders, *N Engl J Med* 331:656-660, 1994.

Present DH et al: Infliximab for the treatment of fistulas in patients with Crohn's disease, *N Engl J Med* 340:1398-405, 1999.

Rao SSC: Chronic anal fissure, *Curr Treat Op Gastroenterol* 4:385-391, 1999.

Rao SSC: Functional colonic and anorectal disorders, *Postgrad Med* 98: 115-119, 124-126, 1995.

Raskin JB et al: Misoprostol dosage in the prevention of nonsteroidal anti-inflammatory drug-induced gastric and duodenal ulcers: a comparison of three regimens, *Ann Intern Med* 123:344-350, 1995.

Ricca P, Horowitz BR: Current approach to the management of irritable bowel syndrome, *Hosp Phys* 34:52-55, 1998.

Rocke DC: Occult gastrointestinal bleeding, *N Engl J Med* 341:38-46, 1999.

Rossle M et al: A comparison of paracentesis and transjugular intrahepatic portosystemic shunting in patients with ascites, *N Engl J Med* 342:1701-1707, 2000.

Rössle M et al: The transjugular intrahepatic portosystemic stent-shunt procedure for variceal bleeding, *N Engl J Med* 330:165-171, 1994.

Runyon BA: Management of adult patients with ascites caused by cirrhosis (AASLD Practice Guidelines), *Hepatology* 27:264-272, 1998.

Rutgeerts P et al: A comparison of budesonide with prednisolone for active Crohn's disease, *N Engl J Med* 331:842-846, 1994.

Saab S, Martin P: Tests for acute and chronic viral hepatitis, *Postgrad Med* 107:123-126, 129-130, 1999.

Sarin SK et al: Comparison of endoscopic ligation and propanolol for the primary prevention of variceal bleeding, *N Engl J Med* 340:988-993.

Schmulson MW, Chang L: Diagnostic approach to the patient with irritable bowel syndrome, *Am J Med* 107(5A):20S-26S, 1999.

Schoenfeld PS, Butler JA: An evidence-based approach to the treatment of esophageal variceal bleeding, *Crit Care Clin* 14:441-455, 1998.

Shaw AD, Davies GJ: Lactose Intolerance, *J Clin Gastroenterol* 28:208-216, 1999.

Singh N et al: Trimethoprim-sulfamethoxazole for the prevention of spontaneous bacterial peritonitis in cirrhosis: a randomized trial, *Ann Intern Med* 122:595-598, 1995.

Sort P et al: Effect of intravenous albumin on renal impairment and mortality in patients with cirrhosis and spontaneous bacterial peritonitis, *N Engl J Med* 341:403-409, 1999.

Stein RB, Hanauer SB: Medical therapy for inflammatory bowel disease, *Gastroenterol Clin North Am* 28:297-321, 1999.

Steinberg W, Tenner S: Acute pancreatitis, *N Engl J Med* 330:1198-1210, 1994.

Summers RA et al: TH2 conditioning by *Trichuris suis* appears safe and effective in modifying the mucosal immune response in inflammatory bowel disease, *Gastroenterology* 116:A828, 1999.

Sung JJ et al: Prospective randomized study of effect of octreotide on rebleeding from esophageal varices after endoscopic ligation, *Lancet* 346:1666-1669, 1995.

5

GASTROENTEROLOGY AND HEPATOLOGY

Taha AS et al: Famotidine for the prevention of gastric and duodenal ulcers caused by nonsteroidal antiinflammatory drugs, *N Engl J Med* 334(22):1435, 1996.

The Mesalamine Study Group: An oral preparation of mesalamine as long-term maintenance therapy for ulcerative colitis: a randomized, placebo-controlled trial, *Ann Intern Med* 124:204-211, 1996.

Thomas GA et al: Transdermal nicotine as maintenance therapy for ulcerative colitis, *N Engl J Med* 332(15):988-992, 1995.

Thompson WG et al: Functional bowel disorders and functional abdominal pain, *Gut* 45(suppl II):II43-II47, 2000.

Thompson WG et al: Irritable bowel syndrome in general practice: prevalence, characteristics, and referral, *Gut* 46(1):78-82, 2000.

Vaezi MF, Richter JE: Diagnosis and management of achalasia, *Am J Gastroenterol* 94:3406-3412, 1999.

Vasiliauskas EA et al: An open-label pilot study of low-dose thalidomide in chronically active, steroid-dependent Crohn's disease, *Gastroenterology* 117:1278-1287, 1999.

Vesy CJ, Peterson WL: Review article: the management of *Giardiasis, Aliment Pharmacol Ther* 13:843-850, 1999.

Walsh JH, Peterson WL: The treatment of *Helicobacter pylori* infection in the management of peptic ulcer disease, *N Engl J Med* 333:984-991, 1995.

Wolfe MM et al: Gastrointestinal toxicity of nonsteroidal antiinflammatory drugs, *N Engl J Med* 340:1888-1899, 1999.

Wolfe MM, Sachs G: Acid suppression: optimizing therapy for gastroduodenal ulcer healing, gastroesophageal reflux disease, and stress-related erosive syndrome, *Gastroenterology* 118(2 suppl 1):S9-S31, 2000.

Yamada T et al: *Handbook of gastroenterology,* Philadelphia, 1998, Lippincott-Raven.

Zimmerman HJ: Acetominophen hepatotoxicity, *Clin Liver Dis* 2:523-541, 1998.

HEMATOLOGIC, ELECTROLYTE, AND METABOLIC DISORDERS

Ke Chen
Mark A. Graber

BLEEDING DISORDERS

I. **Presentation.**

A. Can often determine type of bleeding disorder by history and physical. Is there a family history of bleeding after minor surgical procedures, dental procedures, childbirth, or other trauma? Is this an isolated event, or has the patient had other bleeding episodes?

B. Is the patient receiving medications that can cause a bleeding problem? Many drugs can contribute to bleeding, including semisynthetic penicillins, calcium channel blockers, cephalosporins, dipyridamole, thiazides, alcohol, quinidine, chlorpromazine, sulfonamides, INH, rifampin, methyldopa, phenytoin, barbiturates, warfarin, heparin, thrombolytic agents, NSAIDs and ASA, diuretics, allopurinol, TMP/SMX, and many others.

C. Look for physical signs and symptoms of diseases related to capillary fragility. Examples include Cushing's syndrome and Marfan syndrome. Consider also "senile purpura," petechiae secondary to coughing, sneezing, Valsalva maneuver, blood pressure measurement, vasculitis ("palpable purpura"), scurvy (vitamin C deficiency), or exogenous steroids. Telangiectasias are suggestive of Osler-Weber-Rendu syndrome.

II. **Differentiation of Platelet versus Coagulation Defect**

A. **Platelet defects.** Generally have immediate onset of bleeding after trauma. Bleeding is predominantly in skin, mucous membranes, nose, GI tract, and urinary tract. Bleeding may be observed as petechiae (<3 mm) or ecchymoses (>3 mm). Must differentiate from vasculitic "palpable purpura."

B. **Coagulation system defects.** "Deep" bleeding (in the joint spaces, muscles, and retroperitoneal spaces) is common. Observed on exam as hematomas and hemarthroses.

III. **Physical Exam**

A. Assess volume status and correct shock if present (see Chapter 2). Look for hepatosplenomegaly (evidence of platelet destruction, extramedullary hematopoiesis). Do a rectal exam for evidence of GI bleeding and examine oropharynx for evidence of bleeding.

IV. **Tests of Coagulation**

A. **PT** (INR) to assess extrinsic system. Elevated in DIC, warfarin use, liver failure, myelofibrosis, vitamin K deficiency, fat malabsorption, circulating anticoagulants, factor deficiencies (vitamin K dependent), etc.

B. **PTT** to assess intrinsic system. Elevated in factor deficiencies (such as hemophilia), circulating anticoagulants as in lupus (mix patient's serum with equal amount of normal serum; if PTT corrects, PTT elevation is not caused by circulating anticoagulant, which will prevent coagulation even with adequate clotting factors present), heparin use, other drugs such as antipsychotics. PTT is the best screening test for coagulation defects and is elevated in 90% of those with coagulopathy. Patients with an elevated PTT may paradoxically have increased thrombotic events depending on cause (e.g., antiphospholipid antibody syndrome).

C. **Platelet count and bleeding time.** If <100,000/mm³, expect a mild prolongation of bleeding time. <50,000 results in easy bruising, and <20,000 is associated with an increased incidence of spontaneous bleeding. If bleeding time is lengthened and there is a normal platelet count, consider qualitative platelet defect. Can also perform tests of platelet aggregation.

D. **Fibrin degradation products** (or fibrin split products). Provides a measure of fibrin activation. Elevated in DIC but may also be elevated in other states such as trauma and inflammatory diseases.

E. **D-dimer.** A byproduct of clot breakdown, D-dimer is a sensitive measure of intravascular fibrinolysis (and therefore coagulation). D-dimer will be present in most individuals (especially with cancer, trauma) so it is sensitive for active clotting but not specific for abnormal intervascular clotting (e.g., DVT, PE). See Chapter 4 for further details.

F. Can also assay for specific factors.

V. **Differential Diagnosis of Abnormal Bleeding**

A. **Bleeding caused by qualitative platelet disorders.**

1. **Von Willebrand disease.**

   a. Most common hereditary coagulation disorder. Autosomal dominant. Abnormal synthesis of von Willebrand factor (vWF) causing decreased platelet adhesion and decreased serum levels of factor VIII:C (vWF is carrier for factor VIII:C). Type I is absent vWF; type II is abnormal, nonfunctional vWF.

   b. **Testing.** May need to test a single patient at multiple times since the level of vWF is variable within a patient.

   c. **Treatment** involves administering factor VIII:C to achieve 30% to 50% activity (**Humate-P or Koate-HS contain some von Willebrand factor; other factor VIII:C concentrates do not.** See hemophilia below for calculations). Another alternative is cryoprecipitate (1000 to 1250 units of factor VIII:C, generally about 10 bags). However, this carries the risk of virus transmission. A single infusion is enough to control mild bleeding. If bleeding persists, repeat the infusion every 12 hours. Desmopressin is also useful for type I von Willebrand disease (see hemophilia below for dose). If neither of these modalities works, consider platelet transfusion.

2. **Defective aggregation.** Rare.

3. **Defective activation or secretion.**

   a. Ingestion of aspirin or NSAIDs.

   b. High-dose penicillin.

    c. Storage pool defects. Vary rare. The platelets are activated but secrete "inactive" granules, for example, gray platelet syndrome and dense granule deficiency syndrome.

    d. Can treat these with platelet transfusion.

B. **Bleeding caused by quantitative platelet disorders.**

  1. **Thrombocytosis.** Occurs in myeloproliferative disease (including polycythemia vera, myeloid metaplasia with myelofibrosis, essential thrombocytosis). In these states platelets are often poorly functioning leading to a bleeding disorder, although there may also be abnormal thrombosis. The platelets in those with a reactive thrombocytosis (such as cancer, inflammation, iron deficiency anemia, etc.) function well leading to thrombosis, if anything. Treatment of bleeding is by platelet transfusion to bring the pool of normal platelets to 50,000/ml (generally about six platelet packs). For those with thrombotic complications, aspirin 325 mg/day is indicated. Definitive treatment with chemotherapy will also help.

  2. **Thrombocytopenia.** Causes include decreased production, increased splenic sequestration, or increased platelet destruction. Consider also HELLP syndrome and preeclampsia in pregnant women.

    a. **Decreased production can be caused by:**

      (1) **Marrow aplasia.** Infiltration secondary to malignancy or fibrosis. Also from vitamin deficiency. Diagnose by bone marrow biopsy.

      (2) **Multiple drugs,** including ethanol, estrogens, thiazides, and cytotoxic drugs (cytosine arabinoside, daunorubicin, cyclophosphamide, busulfan, methotrexate, 6-mercaptopurine, etc.).

      (3) **Infectious causes,** including sepsis, AIDS, EBV, ehrlichiosis, Colorado tick fever, Rocky Mountain spotted fever, babesiosis, malaria, etc.

    b. **Increased sequestration** in spleen secondary to portal hypertension (for example from cirrhosis), myeloproliferative disease.

    c. **Increased platelet destruction caused by:**

      (1) **Immunologic destruction.** Bacterial or viral infections, drugs (sulfonamides, quinidine, INH, sedative or hypnotics, chlorpromazine, digoxin, methyldopa, heparin), idiopathic thrombocytopenic purpura (ITP).

      (2) **Nonimmunologic destruction.** Vasculitis, DIC, thrombotic thrombocytopenic purpura (TTP), hemolytic uremic syndrome (HUS), and prosthetic heart valves.

    d. **Idiopathic thrombocytopenic purpura (ITP).** Antibodies form against platelets.

      (1) **Frequently preceded by** URI or other viral infection. More frequent in women, those with HIV, mononucleosis (EBV), Graves' disease, and hyperthyroidism.

6

HEMATOLOGIC, ELECTROLYTE, AND METABOLIC DISORDERS

(2) **Presents as** petechiae and other bleeding such as CNS bleeding or bleeding gums. Women may have increased uterine bleeding.

(3) **Diagnosis.** By bone marrow showing increase in megakaryocytes. Also may have antiplatelet antibodies (90% sensitive but only 25% specific). Many clinicians will not order antiplatelet antibodies and make the diagnosis by clinical presentation and bone marrow.

(4) **Treatment.**
  - May choose to follow and not treat if no bleeding. In children 70% recover in 4 to 6 weeks.
  - Platelet transfusions are not helpful, and infused platelets will be destroyed along with the patient's platelets. May want to use to try to stop acute bleeding, though.
  - **Steroids.** If bleeding or platelet count <20,000, treat with prednisone 1 to 2 mg/kg/day or methylprednisolone 1 g/day for 3 days. May take 2 to 3 weeks to see response.
  - Intravenous IgG concentrates transiently increase platelet count (1 to 2 g/kg IV for 2 days). $Rh_0(D)$ immune globulin (WinRho-SD) is indicated as IV therapy for ITP in **non-splenectomized patients** who are **Rh positive.** The dose is 250 IU/kg given either at one time or as split doses and must be reduced for those with anemia. **See package information for details.**
  - **Splenectomy** for patients who are bleeding and are not responding to other measures and bleeding. Other options include danazol, vincristine/vinblastine, cyclophosphamide, and azathioprine.
  - Experimental monoclonal antibodies are also available.

e. Disseminated intravascular coagulation (DIC).

(1) Occurs as a result of:
  - **Complications of obstetrics,** including abruptio placentae, saline abortion, retained products of conception, amniotic fluid embolism, and eclampsia.
  - **Infection,** especially gram negative with endotoxin release.
  - **Malignancy,** especially adenocarcinoma of pancreas and prostate, acute leukemia.
  - **Other.** Head trauma, prostatic surgery, venomous snake bites, etc.

(2) **Clinically may mimic liver failure** with elevated PT/INR and decreased platelets.
  - **Subacute.** Thromboembolic events including DVT, heart valve thrombosis, stroke, extremity infarction, etc.
  - **Acute.** Serious bleeding complications with depletion of clotting factors.

(3) **Diagnosis.** Elevated PT/INR or elevated PTT, thrombocytopenia, reduced level of fibrinogen, elevated D-dimer, and ele-

vated fibrin degradation products (fibrin split products). Will also have evidence of microangiopathic hemolysis, including schistocytes, helmet cells, etc.

    (4) **Treatment.** Correct the problems that led to DIC in the first place.

- **If no complications** of DIC (no bleeding or thrombosis), no need to institute replacement therapy.
- **For bleeding complications,** can infuse platelets to replace platelets, cryoprecipitate or fresh frozen plasma to replace clotting factors. Maintain fibrinogen level at 100 to 150 mg/dl and other factors above 50% activity if possible.
- **If patient has thrombotic complications,** use heparin 500 U/hr (about 5 to 10 U/kg/hr) after a 500 to 1000 U bolus **(note these are lower doses than with usual heparin use)** *but only if able to correct underlying process.* This should be followed in 2 to 3 hours by fresh frozen plasma. Consider increasing heparin to 750 to 1000 U/hr after administering fresh frozen plasma.
- **Aminocaproic acid and tranexamic acid,** which prevent fibrinolysis, have fallen out of favor because they may increase thrombotic complications.

C. **Bleeding caused by defects of the intrinsic pathway.**

  1. Products available for factor replacement.

    a. **Fresh frozen plasma.** Contains all the coagulation factors in nearly normal concentrations. This is useful for patients with liver disease who have multiple factor deficiencies and require infrequent therapy. Contains about 200 to 250 U of each factor (about 1 U of factor VIII per milliliter).

    b. **Cryoprecipitate.** Contains factor VIII, vWF, and fibrinogen. This is treatment of choice for von Willebrand disease if virus-free factor VIII not available. Contains about 100 U of factor VIII per bag.

    c. **Factor VIII concentrate.** A lyophilized powder prepared from multiple donors that contains a high concentration of factor VIII and a variable amount of vWF **(Humate-P or Koate-HS have adequate amounts).** Most preparations have some risk of transmission of hepatitis and HIV. Virus-free preparations are available (Monoclate-P and Hemofil-M) although they are much more expensive.

    d. **Genetically engineered factor VIII** available. Carries no risk of disease transmission.

    e. **Prothrombin complex concentration.** Contains 500 to 1000 IU of prothrombin factor X and factor IX.

  2. **Hemophilia A.** Deficiency of factor VIII, X-linked recessive. Diagnose by factor VIII assay. PT and thrombin clot time are normal. PTT generally elevated but may be normal if >30% activity (mild disease).

a. **Treatment of factor VIII deficiency.**
  (1) **Minor cuts and abrasions,** superficial ecchymosis, and non-traumatic hematuria may require no therapy. CNS trauma requires prophylactic therapy.
  (2) **Uncomplicated hemarthrosis,** noncritical hematomas, and traumatic hematuria are treated with factor VIII to achieve a factor VIII level of 25% to 50% for at least 72 hours.
  (3) **Life-threatening hemorrhage** and hematomas in critical locations require factor VIII to achieve a factor VIII level of >50% for 2 weeks.
  (4) **If mild hemophilia** (baseline factor VIII activity of 5% to 10%), desmopressin 0.3 μg/kg in 50 ml NS IV over 15 to 30 minutes will transiently increase factor VIII and von Willebrand factor enough for minor surgery. Levels will return to baseline value with a half-life of 8 to 10 hours. Epsilon-aminocaproic acid 75 mg/kg PO 6 hours (4 g Q6h in adults) should be used to prevent fibrinolysis. An alternative is tranexamic acid 25 mg/kg TID (1.5 g PO TID in adults).
  (5) **To calculate factor VIII dose needed:** 1 U/ml = 100% activity; 0.5 U/ml = 50% activity; etc. Units of factor VIII needed = Wt in kg × 44 × (Required activity in U/ml − Patient's current activity in U/ml). For example, if a 25 kg patient has 10% activity and you want to raise it to 50% activity for an uncomplicated hemarthrosis: Units of factor VIII needed = 25 kg × 44 × (0.5 U/ml − 0.1 U/ml) = 440 U.
  (6) **Consider using e-aminocaproic acid or tranexamic** acid after factor infused (see above, minor hemophilia, for dose).
3. **Hemophilia B.** Deficiency of factor IX (Christmas disease), X-linked recessive. Diagnose by factor IX assay.
  a. **Treatment of factor IX deficiency.**
    (1) Minimal bleeding can be treated with FFP.
    (2) Major hemorrhage is treated with prothrombin complex concentrate or FFP.
4. **Factor XI deficiency.** Autosomal recessive disease occurring primarily in Ashkenazi Jews. Treatment is generally not required because bleeding tends to be minor.
D. **Bleeding caused by defects of the extrinsic and common pathway.**
  1. **Hepatocellular insufficiency.** Have decreased production of vitamin K–dependent factors II, VII, IX, X.
  2. **Vitamin K deficiency from:**
    a. **Cholestasis and other GI disease** causing impaired absorption of lipid-soluble vitamin K.
    b. **Poor dietary intake** of vitamin K.
    c. **Broad-spectrum antibiotics.** Gut bacteria produce vitamin K. Loss of these bacteria from antibiotics can lead to vitamin K deficiency.

3. Coumarin anticoagulants.
4. Treatment.
   a. **Vitamin K deficiency.**
      (1) **For serious hemorrhage,** infuse FFP 15 ml/kg IV and then 5 to 8 ml/kg IV Q8-12h.
      (2) **Mild vitamin K deficiencies** can be treated with 10 to 15 mg IM or IV QD for 1 to 3 days. The administration of vitamin K may make it difficult to achieve anticoagulation with warfarin for several days.
   b. **Liver disease.**
      (1) Fresh frozen plasma.
      (2) Vitamin K 10 to 15 mg IV or SQ for 1 to 3 days.
   c. **Warfarin overdose.**
      (1) Do not treat the INR. If INR < 9 and patient has a low risk of bleeding, observation and withholding of warfarin for one or two doses is adequate. Expect a response in 24 to 48 hours. Alternatively, for an INR < 9, give 1 to 2.5 mg PO vitamin K; if INR > 9, give 3 to 5 mg PO vitamin K. If INR > 20, give 10 mg IV vitamin K.
      (2) For bleeding, administer vitamin K and fresh frozen plasma.
E. **Bleeding caused by vascular defects.**
   1. **Paraproteinemias.** Cryoglobulinemia, macroglobulinemia, myeloma.
   2. **Thrombotic thrombocytopenic purpura.** Due to inhibitor of vWF-cleaving protease and unchecked platelet aggregation.
      a. **Criteria for diagnosis include** microangiopathic hemolytic anemia (schistocytes, helmet cells on smear) with elevated LDH, fever, renal failure, and mental status changes or fluctuating focal neurologic deficits.
      b. **Etiology.** See HUS. Also may be inherited and related to ticlopidine or clopidogrel.
      c. **Epidemiology.** Generally occurs in those 10 to 40 years of age with peak about 25 years. May occur in postpartum period.
      d. **Diagnose** by biopsy of vessels, clinical presentation.
      e. **Outcome.** Mortality is now 5%, much better than in the past. There is a 40% 10-year recurrence rate if survive initial insult.
      f. **Therapy.** The most effective therapy is plasma exchange 40 ml/kg/day (more effective than plasma infusion) until platelets are >100,000. Other modalities have been tried, including high-dose steroids (prednisone 200 mg/day). **Plasma exchange has largely replaced other modalities of treatment (including steroids) and is more effective.**
      g. Transfuse if Hb < 6 g or patient is symptomatic.
   3. **Hemolytic uremic syndrome.** Patient does not have inhibitor of vWF-cleaving protease.
      a. Usually in infants, children, or pregnant or postpartum women.

6

HEMATOLOGIC, ELECTROLYTE, AND METABOLIC DISORDERS

      b. Presents with thrombocytopenia, fever, microangiopathic hemolytic anemia, hypertension, acute renal failure with anuria.

      c. **Etiology.**

         (1) **Bacteria.** In some cases, induced by a diarrheal illness caused by *Escherichia coli* O157:H7, which produces Shiga toxin (also known as verocytotoxin) but also may be from *Shigella, Staphylococcus,* other *E. coli* subtypes. Has been found in pond water, apple cider, and uncooked or undercooked hamburger. Day care is also a risk. **May not have diarrheal prodrome. Recent data suggest that treatment of *E. coli* O157:H7 with amoxicillin increases the rate of HUS in children.**

         (2) **Drugs/other.** Some cases are related to use of drugs (especially chemotherapeutic agents, tacrolimus, ticlopidine, oral contraceptives), HIV, sepsis, glomerulonephritis, vasculitis, or cancer.

      d. 5% mortality in children and adults.

      e. Treatment: See TTP above.

  4. **Henoch-Schönlein purpura.** A generally self-limited IgA vasculitis.

      a. May follow URI or streptococcal infection. Peak incidence ages 4 through 11.

      b. Causes purpura, arthralgias, colicky abdominal pain, vomiting, diarrhea, and hematuria (from nephritis).

      c. Aspirin and corticosteroids have been used for joint pain and GI symptoms, respectively. Corticosteroids do not change the course of the associated renal disease but may be given (prednisone 1 mg/kg/day or 60 mg in adults).

  5. **Miscellaneous.** Causes of vascular defects include SLE, rheumatoid arthritis, Sjögren syndrome, amyloidosis.

F. **Bleeding caused by heparin.** Treatment is protamine sulfate, which forms an inactive complex with heparin. 1 mg of protamine zinc will neutralize about 90 to 115 U of heparin depending on derivation of heparin. Calculate dose and administer over 10 minutes. Do not exceed 50 mg. Heparin half-life is 30 to 180 minutes; therefore dose of protamine needed will decrease rapidly with time. **Administer slowly to prevent hypotension. Protamine is an anticoagulant when not complexed with heparin. Therefore follow dosing guidelines carefully.**

MANAGING ANTICOAGULATION (TABLES 6-1 TO 6-3)

A. **For problems with bleeding,** see above.

B. **Low-molecular-weight heparin:** enoxaparin—for anticoagulation use 1 mg/kg SQ BID. No need to follow PT/INR/PTT.

C. **To initiate warfarin (Coumadin and others)**

TABLE 6-1

RECOMMENDED THERAPEUTIC RANGE FOR ORAL ANTICOAGULANT THERAPY

Indication	INR
Prophylaxis of venous thrombosis (high-risk surgery)	Optimal INR 2.0-3.0
Treatment of venous thrombosis	
Treatment of pulmonary embolism	
Prevention of systemic embolism	
Tissue heart valves	
AMI (to prevent systemic embolism)*	
Valvular heart disease	
Atrial fibrillation	
DVT **while on warfarin** with INR 2.0-3.0	No good studies. Several strategies can be tried, including the following: increase INR to 3.5, add aspirin or change to SQ low-molecular-weight heparin. Vena caval filters can be used but are of questionable efficacy.
Symptomatic anticardiolipin antibody syndrome (if no history of DVT, no need to anticoagulate)	Only a few studies. Generally need higher doses than for other indications. Target is INR >2.5-3.5 but generally >3.0 is more effective.
Mechanical prosthetic valves (high risk)	2.5-3.5
Bileaflet mechanical valve in aortic position	2.0-3.0

Modified from Hirsh J et al: *Chest* 114(5):445, 1998.
*If oral anticoagulant therapy is elected to prevent recurrent myocardial infarction, an INR of 2.5 to 3.5 is recommended, consistent with FDA recommendations. However, this is of questionable efficacy.

6

1. Warfarin should be started the same time as heparin. Heparin should be continued for at least 4 days total and for at least 2 days after a therapeutic INR is obtained.

2. **Warfarin:** begin with 5 mg QHS. This has been shown to be as effective as 10 mg QHS and less frequently leads a supertherapeutic INR. The INR will change 24 to 48 hours after a dose of warfarin. Therefore wait at least 48 hours to see how a change affected the INR before making any additional changes to the warfarin dose.

3. **Hereditary resistance** to warfarin occurs, which may require doses that are 2 to 20 times the usual dose to achieve a therapeutic INR. However, noncompliance is the most common cause of a subtherapeutic INR. Other patients are highly sensitive to warfarin

---

TABLE 6-2

BODY WEIGHT–BASED DOSING OF IV HEPARIN*

APTT (sec)	Dose Change (U/kg/hr)	Additional Action	Next APTT (hr)
<35 (<1.2 × mean normal)	+4	Rebolus with 80	6
35-45 (1.2 -1.5 × mean normal)	+2	IU/kg	6
46-70 (1.5 -2.3 × mean normal)	0	Rebolus with 40 IU/kg	6
71-90 (2.3 -3.0 × mean normal))	−2	0	6†
>90 (>3 × mean normal)	−3	Stop infusion 1 hr	6

From Heyers T et al: *Chest* 114:561, 1998.

*Initial dosing; loading 80 IU/kg; maintenance infusion: 18 IU/kg/hr (APTT in 6 hr). The therapeutic range in seconds should correspond to a plasma heparin level of 0.2 to 0.4 IU/ml by protamine sulfate or 0.3 to 0.6 IU/ml by amidolytic assay. When APTT is checked at 6 hr or longer, steady-state kinetics can be assumed. Heparin, 25,000 IU in 250 ml D_5W. Infuse at rate dictated by body weight through an infusion apparatus calibrated for low flow rates.

†During the first 24 hr, repeat APTT every 6 hr. Thereafter, monitor APTT once every morning unless it is outside the therapeutic range.

---

and need only low doses of the drug to achieve a therapeutic INR.

4. **Monitor daily** until patient is therapeutic and has been therapeutic with a stable INR for 2 days, then **2 to 3 times weekly** for 1 to 2 weeks, and then **monthly.**

D. **To initiate heparin (IV, unfractionated):** Weight-based dosing (bolus with 80 U/kg and start a drip at 18 U/kg/hr) is preferred over the traditional regimen (bolus of 5000 U with a drip starting at 1000 U/hr) (see Table 6-2). Therapeutic levels are reached much more quickly with weight-based dosing.

1. **Caveats.** Remember that unfractionated and low molecular weight heparin can cause thrombocytopenia and that a hypercoagulable state will exist when heparin is stopped if the duration of heparin has been at least 72 hours.

2. **Check PT/INR/PTT in 6 hours.** Adjust dose as per protocol in Table 6-2. These are guidelines. **Use clinical judgment!**

E. Encrod (Viprinex), Argatroban (Acova), and Lepirudin (Rfludan) can be used as substitutes for heparin in patients who develop or have a history of heparin-induced thrombocytopenia. Ancrod is not FDA approved for this indication. Argatroban is hepatically eliminated and can be used in those with renal failure.

TABLE 6-3

PREOPERATIVE MANAGEMENT OF ANTICOAGULATION[a]

Indication for Anticoagulation	Type of Preoperative Anticoagulation	When to Stop Oral (e.g., Warfarin) Anticoagulation	Heparin Coverage Needed Preoperatively?	Restart Anticoagulation Postoperatively with (Note: Simultaneously Resume Prior Oral Anticoagulation If No Bleeding Noted)
After thromboembolism, month 1	Warfarin	If INR 2-3: 4 days before	Yes, IV heparin[b]	IV heparin[b]
After thromboembolism, month 2-3	Warfarin	If INR >3: 4-5 days before	No[c]	IV heparin
Recurrent thromboembolism[d]	Warfarin	Same as above	No[c]	SQ heparin
Arterial embolism, month 1	Warfarin	Same as above	Yes, IV heparin	IV heparin[e]
Mechanical heart valve	Warfarin	Same as above	No[c]	SQ heparin
Nonvalvular atrial fibrillation	Warfarin	Same as above	No[c]	SQ heparin
Asprin, all indications		48 hrs to 10 days before surgery (no significant prolongation of bleeding time after 48 hrs)	Generally no	Generally no

Modified from Kearon C, Hirsh J: *N Engl J Med* 336:1507, 1997; Sonksen JR et al: *Br J Anaesth* 82:360, 1999.

[a]These are guidelines based on risk of an adverse event with heparin versus risk of thromboembolic disease when off warfarin or aspirin. Use clinical judgment. Restart heparin 12 hours after surgery unless there is bleeding, in which case it should be delayed. IV heparin denotes intravenous heparin at therapeutic doses, and SQ heparin denotes subcutaneous unfractionated or low-molecular-weight heparin in doses recommended for prophylaxis against venous thromboembolism in high-risk patients.

[b]Vena caval filter should be considered if acute venous thromboembolism has occurred within 2 weeks or if the risk of bleeding during intravenous heparin therapy is high.

[c]If patients are hospitalized, subcutaneous heparin may be administered, but hospitalization is not recommended solely for this purpose.

[d]This term refers to patients whose last episode of venous thromboembolism occurred more than three months before evaluation but who require long-term anticoagulation because of a high risk of recurrence.

[e]IV heparin should be used after surgery only if the risk of bleeding is low.

HEMATOLOGIC, ELECTROLYTE, AND METABOLIC DISORDERS

6

ANEMIA

I. **Overview (Table 6-4).**

A. **Definition.**
1. Normal hematocrit (HCT) = 36% to 48%, hemoglobin (Hb) = 12 to 16 g/dl. *Anemia* is defined as a low HCT and Hb.
2. Changes in intravascular volume can be reflected in the hematocrit. Fluid overload leads to hemodilution and a lower HCT, whereas volume contraction can yield a spuriously elevated HCT even in the face of anemia. Fluids and blood products equilibrate in the circulation within 15 to 30 minutes.

B. **Signs and symptoms of anemia.**
1. **Symptoms.** Dyspnea on exertion, palpitations, angina pectoris, lightheadedness, syncope, anorexia, tinnitus.
2. **Signs.** Pallor of mucous membranes and skin, mild tachycardia, peripheral edema, systolic ejection murmurs from increased flow though not sensitive or specific.

TABLE 6-4

DIFFERENTIAL DIAGNOSIS OF ANEMIA BASED ON CELL SIZE AND MARROW RESPONSE (RETICULOCYTE COUNT)

Microcytosis and Unresponsive Marrow*	Normocytosis and Unresponsive Marrow*	Macrocytosis with Unresponsive Marrow*	Anemia with Responsive Marrow (reticulocytosis)
Iron deficiency anemia	Iron deficiency anemia (rarely)	Vit B-12 and Folate deficiency	Hemolytic anemia including
Anemia of chronic disease (microcytic 30% of cases)	Anemia of chronic disease	Some drugs	• Microangiopathic
Thalassemias	Primary marrow disorders	Arsenic	• HUS/TTP
Sideroblasti anemia	• Aplastic anemia	Alcohol (occasionally)	• Warm and cold antibody induced
	• Toxin-induced anemia (some)	Hypothyroidism	• Valve prosthesis
	• Infectious anemia (e.g., HIV)		• Eclampsia/HELLP
	• Graft versus host disease		• Malignant hypertension
			• Red blood cell defects (e.g., spherocytosis, paroxysmal nocturnal hemoglobinuria)

*Low or normal reticulocyte count.

3. **May be asymptomatic** if it is long-standing. Patients can adapt to a gradual change in Hb and HCT.

C. **History.** Obtain history, including presence of jaundice or gallstones (hemolysis), history of blood loss, alcohol abuse, diarrhea, other chronic disease, drugs.

D. **Laboratory evaluation.**

   1. All anemic patients should have the following labs:

      a. CBC with differential, platelet count.

      b. Mean corpuscular volume (MCV). In hemolysis, elevated MCV reflects reticulocytosis.

      c. Serum ferritin (estimate of Fe stores).

      d. TIBC (mmol/L) = transferrin (mg/L) $\times$ 0.025. Transferrin saturation = serum iron/TIBC (normal $>$ 16).

      e. Reticulocyte count.

         (1) The reticulocyte count is expressed as a percentage of total cells counted and must be corrected to a total number of reticulocytes per microliter. This is done by multiplying the red blood cell count by the percentage of reticulocytes. Normal is 50 to 100,000 reticulocytes per microliter.

         (2) Reticulocyte counts that are normal or low (in the face of anemia) are suggestive of the inability of the bone marrow to respond to anemia (marrow failure).

         (3) Reticulocyte counts that are increased are indicative of acute blood loss or hemolysis with a marrow that is able to respond.

         (4) If reticulocyte count is low or normal reflecting the inability of the marrow to respond to anemia ("marrow failure"), the MCV is helpful in diagnosing anemia. The MCV is either normocytic at 80 to 100 femtoliters (fl), microcytic $<$80 fl, or macrocytic $>$100 fl.

         (5) Consider serum haptoglobin, serum free hemoglobin to evaluate for hemolysis.

II. **Microcytosis and Unresponsive Marrow.** Low or normal reticulocyte count and anemia.

A. **Iron deficiency anemia** generally has microcytic MCV but may occasionally be normocytic.

   1. **Causes.** Increased iron requirements (during infancy, adolescence, pregnancy, etc.), inadequate iron intake, decreased iron absorption (gastrectomy, achlorhydria, chronic diarrhea), blood loss from menses or GI tract.

   2. **Exam.** Skin and conjunctivae may show pallor; nails may be dry and brittle with ridges; cardiovascular exam may reveal tachycardia and flow murmur. Stomatitis or glossitis may be present. However, physical signs and symptoms are not sensitive enough to rule in or out the diagnosis of anemia.

   3. **Lab tests.**

      a. **CBC** will show microcytic, hypochromic cells. May have elevated platelet count.

6

HEMATOLOGIC, ELECTROLYTE, AND METABOLIC DISORDERS

    b. **Low serum ferritin** (overall best test for outpatients). Serum ferritin elevated by fever, cancer, and other inflammatory processes and is therefore a poor predictor of iron deficiency anemia in hospitalized patients. Reticulocyte hemoglobin content may be a more accurate reflection of bone marrow iron stores and is a promising technology.

    c. **Increased TIBC** with transferrin saturation <15% and low serum iron. Bone marrow biopsy specimen will show decreased iron stores.

    d. Must differentiate from the thalassemias and anemia of chronic disease. Red cell distribution width (RDW) is increased in iron deficiency anemia, normal in thalassemias.

4. **Other work-up.** All adults with iron deficiency anemia should be evaluated for upper and lower GI bleeding (determining what to evaluate first by symptoms). If a source is found in the upper GI tract, there is little chance of there being a second lower GI source, and vice versa. However, use clinical judgment when deciding whether to work up both upper and lower GI.

5. **Treatment.** Ferrous sulfate 325 mg PO TID. Enteric-coated and timed-release products are poorly absorbed. Iron is better absorbed if administered between meals on an empty stomach, but less GI upset if taken with meals. Vitamin C will increase absorption. Calcium and magnesium may impair Fe absorption. Iron may impair absorption of thyroxin. Treat for 6 months to replace body stores. Iron is toxic and should be kept away from children.

6. **If marrow does not respond to iron,** consider another superimposed cause of anemia such as inflammation, vitamin B_{12} or folate deficiency, continued bleeding, etc.

B. **Anemia of chronic disease.** Microcytic in 30% of cases. See IIIB later in this section for details.

C. **Thalassemias.**

1. **Background.** Hemoglobin made up of paired alpha and beta chains. Thalassemia caused by a defect in the synthesis of either alpha or beta chains. Normally there are four genes to produce alpha chains but only two to produce beta chains.

2. **Alpha-thalassemia.** Caused by decreased synthesis of alpha subchain of Hb. Because there are normally four copies, it is generally a mild disease.

    a. **Silent carrier state.** One of the four genes is deleted. No hematologic abnormalities.

    b. **Alpha-thalassemia trait.** Two of four genes are deleted. RBCs are microcytic, hypochromic. No significant anemia. Hemoglobin shows a decrease in Hb A_2.

    c. **Beta-thalassemia minor.** Caused by decreased synthesis of beta chains. One of two genes not present (heterozygous).

        (1) **Presentation.** Symptoms of anemia, splenomegaly, icterus. Cells are microcytic. Examination of peripheral smear shows target cells, cigar-shaped cells, and basophilic stippling.

(2) **Diagnosis.** Hb electrophoresis shows increased Hb A$_2$, usually >4%, and possibly an increase of hemoglobin F. May occur with a normal Hb A, however.

(3) **Treatment.** None. Genetic counseling is necessary.

3. **Beta-thalassemia major (Cooley's anemia).**

a. Both genes for beta-chain synthesis defective or missing.

b. **Presentation.** Manifestations begin at approximately 4 to 6 months of life. Usually present with severe anemia (HCT less than 20%). There is pronounced wasting, jaundice, slow growth and development, and delayed onset of secondary sex features. The patient will have skeletal abnormalities secondary to bone marrow expansion.

c. **Diagnosis.** Hb electrophoresis shows large amounts of Hb F, variable amounts of Hb A, and increased Hb A$_2$. Nucleated RBCs.

d. **Treatment.** Transfusion, splenectomy, deferoxamine (to prevent iron overload from transfusions), folic acid supplementation. Watch for development of hemochromatosis. Cord blood stem cell transplantation and compatible relative bone marrow transplantation have been used with success.

e. **Prognosis.** Many die before puberty secondary to hemochromatosis.

D. **Sideroblastic anemia.** Amorphous iron is deposited in RBC mitochondria, which may form a ring around the RBC nucleus during development (therefore ringed sideroblasts).

1. **Causes.** Ineffective erythropoiesis.

a. **Hereditary.** Multiple forms, but most are X-linked recessive.

b. **Acquired.** Drugs and toxins (alcohol in the presence of malnutrition and folate deficiency, lead, INH, chloramphenicol), neoplasia and inflammation (rheumatoid arthritis, carcinoma, lymphoma, leukemia), malnutrition (folate deficiency), idiopathic. May also represent a myelodysplastic syndrome with deletion of either chromosome 5 or chromosome 7.

2. **Lab tests.** CBC may show normochromic or hypochromic cells; anisocytosis and poikilocytosis are pronounced. May have normocytic or microcytic cells. Sideroblasts may or may not be present. Iron studies show increased serum iron, increased ferritin, increased transferrin saturation, decreased TIBC. LDH may be elevated. If appropriate, determine if there is chromosomal abnormality.

3. **Clinically** may have anemia or hemochromatosis.

4. **Treatment.**

a. Withdraw offending agent, especially alcohol.

b. Pyridoxine 200 mg QD for 2 to 3 months with or without folate. One third of hereditary cases will respond.

c. Depending on anemia and iron stores, may require phlebotomy or deferoxamine, 40 mg/kg/day SQ by infusion pump over 12 hours 5 days per week.

d. Splenectomy is contraindicated.

6

HEMATOLOGIC, ELECTROLYTE, AND METABOLIC DISORDERS

III. **Normocytosis and Unresponsive Marrow.** Low or normal reticulocyte count and anemia.

A. **Iron deficiency.** Generally there is microcytosis but may be normal (see above).

B. **Anemia of chronic disease.** Probably the most common anemia except for blood loss–related iron deficiency anemia.

1. **Causes.** Chronic infections (subacute bacterial endocarditis, osteomyelitis, AIDS), chronic inflammatory disorders (RA, SLE, sarcoidosis, renal failure), neoplasms, hypothyroidism, liver disease, alcoholism, CHF, and diabetes. Some authors do not classify those anemias associated with kidney, liver, and endocrinologic diseases in this category.

2. **Multifactorial causes.** Decreased RBC life span, unresponsive bone marrow, inability to mobilize iron stores.

3. **Lab tests.** Hemoglobin generally between 9 and 11 mg/dl. Cells may be normocytic or microcytic. Serum ferritin usually increased but may be normal. Serum transferrin, TIBC, and serum iron will be decreased. Transferrin saturation is decreased. Erythropoietin levels will be low compared with similarly anemic patients with iron deficiency anemia (but higher than those in normal individuals). Bone marrow will show adequate iron stores.

4. **Treatment.** Treat underlying disease. Transfuse only as needed for symptoms. Erythropoietin may be used as well. Start with 100 to 150 U/kg SQ 3 times per week and increase to 300 U/kg SQ 3 times per week if no response in 3 weeks. If no response by 12 weeks, the patient is not going to respond, and erythropoietin should be discontinued. Reduce dose when HCT reaches 36% and hold dose if HCT = 40.

C. **Primary marrow disorders.**

1. **Include** congenital aplastic anemia, acquired aplastic anemia, and marrow depression from drugs and toxins (antineoplastic agents, immunosuppressive drugs, ionizing radiation, benzene, chloramphenicol, antithyroid agents, oral hypoglycemics, TMP/SMX, ticlopidine), infections (hepatitis, mononucleosis, graft-versus-host disease, lupus, HIV).

2. **Clinical manifestations.** Weakness and fatigue from anemia, bleeding from thrombocytopenia, infection from leukopenia.

3. **Aplastic anemia.**

a. In aplastic anemia, course may be mild or severe though predicting the course based on marrow cellularity is imprecise; 70% mortality by 1 year with "severe" disease.

b. **Diagnosis.** CBC may show pancytopenia with normochromic-normocytic anemia. Reticulocyte count will be very low. Serum iron will be elevated with normal TIBC. Bone marrow will be hypocellular.

c. **Therapy.** Requires hematology consultation.

IV. **Macrocytosis with Unresponsive Marrow.** Low or normal reticulocyte count and anemia.

A. **Causes.**

1. **Vitamin B_{12} deficiency** (malabsorption from pernicious anemia, gastrectomy, Crohn's disease, celiac sprue). Strict vegetarians are at high risk but not a problem in ovolactovegetarians. In the elderly, achlorhydria and lack of intrinsic factor may decrease vitamin B_{12} absorption.

2. **Folic acid deficiency** (usually caused by poor intake in alcoholics, indigent; or increased demand in pregnancy).

3. **Drugs** (including methotrexate, trimethoprim, pentamidine, AZT, hydroxyurea, alkylating agents, chloramphenicol).

4. **Alcohol** also causes macrocytosis independent of nutritional effects.

5. **Arsenic.**

6. **Endocrine, including hypothyroidism.**

B. **Clinical presentation.**

1. **Vitamin B_{12} deficiency.**

   a. **Symptoms include** gastrointestinal symptoms (glossitis, taste bud atrophy, anorexia, weight loss, diarrhea). Neurologic symptoms including numbness, paresthesias, weakness, ataxia, sphincter dysfunction, positive Babinski sign (toe upgoing).

   b. **Signs** include those of anemia (pallor, tachycardia, etc.) and neurologic signs of hyperreflexia or hyporeflexia, positive Romberg sign, impaired positional and vibratory sensation, depressed mentation, hallucinations, and personality changes. Neurologic disease may occur with normal hematocrit.

   c. Some suggest periodic screening of those >55 years of age, because symptoms of deficiency may exist before hematologic changes occur. If 258 pmol/L is used as cutoff, 40.5% of the elderly may be deficient.

2. **Folate deficiency.** Signs and symptoms are the same as in vitamin B_{12} deficiency, except that the patient is more likely to be malnourished. Neurologic abnormalities are generally absent, as is glossitis.

C. **Diagnosis.** Elevated MCV, low reticulocyte count. **However, many have normal indices because of coexistent thalassemia or iron deficiency, etc.** Low vitamin B_{12} or low RBC folate levels, respectively. RBC folate is preferred because serum folate level varies with meals and is an unreliable indicator of base state. Thrombocytopenia (50%) and leukopenia are late findings. Smear shows anisocytosis, poikilocytosis, basophilic stippling, and hypersegmentation of neutrophils. Once the diagnosis of vitamin B_{12} deficiency is made, a Schilling test can identify the etiology, although it is optional.

D. **Therapy.**

1. **Vitamin B_{12} deficiency.** IM cyanocobalamin 1000 μg per week for 6 weeks and then 1000 μg IM every month for life. Oral replacement works just as well even in the presence of pernicious anemia. Use 1000 μg PO per day.

2. **Folate deficiency.** One milligram of folic acid PO QD is sufficient.
3. Blood transfusions are usually not required. Empiric therapy before a diagnosis is established can be dangerous. A patient deficient in vitamin B_{12} may have a hematologic response to folic acid but an exacerbation of neurologic symptoms.
4. Esophageal, stomach, and colorectal tumors have a higher incidence in those with pernicious anemia. They also have a higher rate of hypothyroidism; therefore screen these patients.

V. **Anemia with Increased Red Blood Cell Production.**

A. Usually acute anemias primarily associated with blood loss or hemolysis. May be caused by prolonged running or marching, as well as microangiopathic changes as with HUS/TTP or artificial valves.

B. **Hemolytic anemia.**
1. **Presentation.** Patients usually have classic signs of anemia. See section IB for symptoms. Hemolytic crisis, which is rare, manifests with fever, chills, tachycardia, tachypnea, backache, and hemoglobinuria. This can progress to renal failure from hemoglobinuria. In addition to the causes below, consider malaria, ehrlichiosis, etc. May develop cholelithiasis secondary to pigment stones.
2. **Lab tests.**
   a. Often normochromic-normocytic but may be macrocytic.
   b. Generally elevated indirect bilirubin with normal direct bilirubin. Haptoglobin is decreased; serum LDH is increased; hemosiderinuria and hemoglobinuria may be present. Serum free hemoglobin may be increased.
   c. Coombs' tests. Direct Coombs' test measures antibody that is attached to RBCs (antibody directly on RBC). Indirect Coombs' tests for circulating anti-RBC antibodies in serum. Example: In Rh disease, mother has positive indirect Coombs' test (circulating anti-D antibody). Rh-positive child has positive direct Coombs' test because mother's antibodies are coating cells (tested after birth).
3. **Hemolytic anemia secondary to acquired hemolytic disorders.**
   a. **Warm-antibody induced hemolytic anemia.** Antibodies most active at temperature of 37° C. About 70% of those with antibody-related hemolytic disease have warm antibodies.
      (1) May be primary (60%) or secondary (40%) to underlying disease affecting the immune system (such as CLL, non-Hodgkin's lymphoma, SLE, myeloma, HIV, ulcerative colitis). Commonly occurs with drugs (penicillin, alpha-methyldopa, INH, sulfonamides).
      (2) Usually have positive direct Coombs' test, generally an IgG antibody.
      (3) Often severe with Hb of 7.0 or less; can be fatal.
      (4) May have enlarged spleen, liver, jaundice.
      (5) No therapy required if disease is mild. With significant hemolysis, prednisone at dose of 1 to 1.5 mg/kg/day, transfusions,

splenectomy (50% to 75% response; may relapse), and cyto-toxic agents (cyclophosphamide 50 to 150 mg/day or azathio-prine 50 to 200 mg/day) have been used with some success, as have androgens. Hematology consultation is recommended. Also need folic acid 1 mg/day.

b. **Cold-antibody induced hemolytic anemia.** Represents about 15% of those with antibody-related hemolysis. Generally there is agglutination of cells followed by hemolysis.

    (1) These IgM antibodies agglutinate RBCs, generally at temperature of 4° to 35° C but occasionally up to 37° C. Seen with *Mycoplasma pneumoniae,* infectious mononucleosis, lymphoid neoplasms (e.g., CLL, Waldenstrom's macroglobulinemia), etc.. Most patients are over 60.

    (2) Diagnose by red cell agglutination on smear, absurdly elevated MCV (secondary to clumping), blood bank will detect cold agglutinin.

    (3) May note cold-related symptoms such as acrocyanosis, which gets better on warming.

    (4) Maintain patient in warm environment. Chlorambucil, 4 to 6 mg/day, is the most common agent used. Splenectomy and steroids are generally not helpful, but an occasional patient will respond to prednisone 100 mg/day if low titers of cold agglutinins. If related to infectious process, generally resolves spontaneously in weeks.

c. **Trauma in the circulation.**

    (1) Abnormalities of the vessel wall: seen in malignant hypertension, eclampsia, TTP, valve prostheses, and microvascular thrombi.

    (2) Diagnosis. Fragmented and nucleated RBCs. See appropriate section on underlying disease.

    (3) **Therapy.** Directed toward underlying illness.

d. **Red blood cell defects.** Hereditary spherocytosis (220/million, inherited but one third of cases are de novo), hereditary elliptocytosis, hereditary stomatocytosis can cause a hemolytic anemia. May develop aplastic crisis secondary to parvovirus B19.

e. **Paroxysmal nocturnal hemoglobinuria.** Onset in adulthood, hemoglobinuria after sleep, venous thrombosis and embolism, evidence of chronic hemolysis, diagnose with Ham test (measures hemolysis in acidified serum at pH of 6.8). Average life span after diagnosis is 10 years.

SICKLE CELL ANEMIA

A. **Incidence.** 0.3% of African Americans are homozygotes (have sickle cell disease); 13% of African Americans are heterozygotes (carriers).

B. **Genetics.** Autosomal recessive. Abnormal hemoglobin S, leading to sickling of RBCs.

C. **Clinical.**
  1. **Anemia** (see IA and IB under anemia above for clinical symptoms).
  2. **Sickle crisis:** 60% incidence per year. Defined as sickling of cells causing vaso-occlusive disease with bone, lung, renal infarctions, often precipitated by exposure to cold and, **importantly, infection.** Most common sites of pain are lumbar spine, abdomen, femur, knees, sternum, ribs, shoulder, and elbows. Joint involvement may be symmetric. May be associated with abdominal distension or ileus. May have fever, pulmonary infarctions (see acute chest syndrome below). It may be difficult to differentiate abdominal pain from a sickle crisis from the pain of a surgical acute abdomen. May develop priapism.
  3. **Fever.** From infections, especially pneumonia and especially in children. If temperature >38° C (101° F), start broad-spectrum antibiotics while searching for a cause of infection; **de facto splenectomized** secondary to repeated infarction. Need to treat fever aggressively because encapsulated organisms such as pneumococci and *Haemophilus influenzae* cause high mortality.
  4. **Increased bilirubin** secondary to increased RBC destruction. Cholelithiasis is common (75%).
  5. **Acute chest syndrome.** Occurs in 40% of patients with sickle cell anemia.
     a. Characterized by "pleuritic" chest pain, fever, hypoxia, cough, dyspnea, rales, and rhonchi (any combination). Usually there is a rapid decrease in Hb with increased platelets and WBC.
     b. Major source of mortality in those with sickle cell disease (15% of deaths in adults). There may be a delayed development of infiltrates on CXR. Must differentiate from pneumonia.
  6. **Acute splenic sequestration syndrome,** which causes hemoglobin to drop from 3 to 6 g/dl. May also have aplastic crisis in response to parvovirus B19.
  7. **Sickle trait.** May have hematuria and sloughing of papilla, trouble concentrating urine, very rarely a sickle crisis.
D. **Microscopic examination of blood smear** shows typical sickle-shaped RBCs.
E. **Treatment.**
  1. **Acute treatment of sickle crisis and acute chest syndrome.**
     a. Pain control (such as IV morphine), hydration, transfusion for evidence of cardiopulmonary failure or a Hb <5 mg/dl. Admission as required to treat infection, to maintain hydration, or for parenteral analgesics.
     b. If fever >38° C (101° F), start antibiotics (e.g., ceftriaxone) while looking for source of infection.
  2. **Chronic/prophylactic treatment.**
     a. **Infection prophylaxis** including pneumococcal (age 2, booster age 5) and *H. influenzae* vaccines during childhood. Start prophylactic penicillin 125 mg PO BID at 2 months of age and increase to 250 mg PO BID starting at 3 years of age. Can stop this prophy-

laxis at age 5 **but only if the child has not had a severe pneumo-coccal infection.** However, any fever should be aggressively treated with antibiotics (e.g., ceftriaxone).

b. **Folic acid,** 1 mg/day.

c. **Hydroxyurea** has been shown to increase fetal hemoglobin and decrease frequency of sickle cell crises. Long-term effects (e.g., malignancy induction) unknown. Start at 500 mg in adults, 10 to 15 mg/kg/day in children (>2 years). Increase to 1000 to 2000 mg/day (20 to 30 mg/kg/day). Keep track of blood counts, etc.

d. **Transfusions. Any child with a stroke should have prophylactic transfusions.** Exchange transfusions to keep HbS at below 30% will prevent recurrent strokes. Allow HbS to increase to 50% at age 4 years. Even though it is not yet standard of care, **prophylactic transfusions for those with abnormal intracranial blood flow by Doppler will prevent strokes** and should be considered (see *N Engl J Med* 339:5–11, 1998, for protocol.). Patients age 2 through 16 should be screened twice yearly by Doppler.

e. **Surgery.** Transfuse to **hematocrit** of 30% before surgery (as effective as getting HbS to below 30% with fewer complications).

f. **Bone marrow transplantation** has been used with success in some cases.

GLUCOSE-6-PHOSPHATE DEHYDROGENASE (G6PD) DEFICIENCY

A. **Incidence.** X-linked disorder that is expressed in 10% of African-American men and fewer African-American women. Also occurs in people of Mediterranean ancestry. There are over 300 variants of G6PD deficiency.

B. **Clinically.** Get variable degree of hemolysis in RBCs after exposure to substances that cause oxidative stress, including:

1. **Drugs.** Sulfonamides, nitrofurantoin, salicylates, vitamin C, quinine, quinidine, dapsone.

2. **Foods.** Fava beans cause particularly severe hemolysis (generally only in those with the Mediterranean variant).

3. **Infections.** Fever, viral illnesses, bacterial infections.

4. **DKA and renal failure.**

C. **Diagnosis.** Check G6PD levels **when reticulocyte count is normal.** If checked after acute hemolysis, those cells surviving in the circulation and the young reticulocytes may have a normal G6PD level.

D. **Treatment.**

1. Since only old RBCs are vulnerable, generally <25% of the RBC mass is affected.

2. May develop renal failure secondary to hemolysis. Maintain hydration and withdraw offending agents.

IRON-STORAGE DISEASES

I. **Hereditary Hemochromatosis.**

A. **General.** Inherited disorder that results from excessive iron absorption from food. Fairly common:10% heterozygous and 0.5% homozygous.

Generally manifests in those 40 to 60 years of age. Men more commonly symptomatic than women (not because of menstrual loss of iron in women but probably secondary to X-linked gene that suppressed enhanced iron absorption).

B. **Clinically.** May have evidence of liver failure (cirrhosis), pancreatic failure (diabetes, specifically "bronze diabetes"), arthritis, congestive heart failure, hypothyroidism, impotence (secondary to hypogonadism), CNS symptoms, nonspecific right upper quadrant abdominal pain.

C. Alcohol intake may exacerbate the disease and hasten the onset of symptoms.

D. **Diagnosis.** Elevated serum iron, elevated transferrin saturation (>50%), elevated serum ferritin (>700 ng/dl). Follow-up with liver biopsy to evaluate iron deposition.

E. **Treatment.** Based on phlebotomy. Remove 500 ml of blood every week until HCT stabilized at 35 to 40, Hb about 12 g/dl. Avoid iron-fortified foods; consider drinking tea with meals because it reduces iron absorption.

II. **Transfusion-related Hemochromatosis.**

A. **General.** Related to iron overload from transfusions, especially in those with sickle cell disease, aplastic anemia, and thalassemia.

B. **Diagnosis.** Blood testing as in idiopathic hemochromatosis.

C. **Treatment.** Deferoxamine, 1 to 4 g/day IV or SQ. Hematology consultation is suggested.

TRANSFUSION MEDICINE: AVAILABLE PRODUCTS AND TRANSFUSION REACTIONS

I. **Blood Products and Indications.** Blood hemoglobin will stabilize 15 to 30 minutes after transfusion. It is not necessary to wait hours before checking Hb/HCT after transfusion.

II. **Indications for transfusion** (based on NIH, American College of Physicians guidelines). Following the guidelines in Table 6-5 will minimize transfusions and improve mortality rates when compared with a more liberal transfusion policy. **However, use clinical judgment!**

III. May need to use diuretics (such as furosemide, dose determined by underlying function) to maintain hemodynamic stability in those with CHF, etc.

A. **Packed red blood cells.** Used to reverse hemodynamically significant anemia in patients without compatibility problems. Expect the Hb to increase by 1 g/dl/U in the patient without active bleeding. Rate of transfusion dependent on clinical setting (faster with acute blood loss, over 3 to 4 hours with CHF).

B. **Leukocyte-poor RBCs.** Used in those with a history of two or more febrile reactions to packed RBCs and in those requiring a large number of transfusions to prevent immunization against donor WBCs. May also be useful in those with postoperative infections, graft-versus-host disease.

C. **Washed RBCs.** Used in those with a history of anaphylactic or allergic reactions to transfusions (such as those with IgA deficiency).

TABLE 6-5

INDICATIONS FOR TRANSFUSION

Indication	Transfuse to Maintain:
Transfuse any symptomatic patient (e.g., tachycardia, hypotension, CHF, angina)	Until no longer symptomatic
Asymptomatic, presurgical, stable patient	Hb 7-8 g/dl
Hemodynamically stable postsurgical stable patient	Hb 8 g/dl
Postsurgical patient at risk for ischemic disease (e.g., cardiac, bowel)	Hb 10 g/dl
Hemodynamically stable, nonpregnant, ICU patients >age 16 without ongoing blood loss	Transfuse at 7 g/dl to maintain Hb at 7-9 g/dl

6

HEMATOLOGIC, ELECTROLYTE, AND METABOLIC DISORDERS

D. **Irradiated RBCs.** Used in those with immunodeficiency to prevent transfusion-associated graft-versus-host disease (>90% mortality, rash, pancytopenia, diarrhea). Examples include those with bone marrow transplants, premature infants. No need to use this in patients with AIDS.

IV. **Transfusion Reactions.**

A. **Hemolytic reactions.**
   1. 1 in 1400 to 1 in 6200 transfusions. May be acute or delayed.
   2. **Symptoms** include fever with or without chills, back pain, pain in the extremity that is accepting the transfused blood, tachycardia, hypotension, DIC, renal failure, chest pain, wheezing, nausea, vomiting.
   3. **If suspected,** immediately discontinue transfusion and return transfused unit to blood bank along with specimen of patient's blood.
   4. **Treatment.** Fluids and mannitol (0.5 to 2.5 g/kg) to maintain urine output and prevent renal failure. Furosemide may also be useful. Dopamine may be needed for blood pressure support. Treat pain with narcotic analgesics, wheezing with albuterol, etc., as appropriate.

B. **Febrile reactions.**
   1. Complicate about 2% of transfusions.
   2. **Symptoms** include fever with or without shaking chills, headache, and malaise. Generally occur within 5 hours of transfusion. Must differentiate from sepsis.
   3. **Treatment.** Stop transfusion; use meperidine in 25 mg IV aliquots to control symptoms such as chills, acetaminophen for fever. Can try to pretreat with acetaminophen and ASA and meperidine to prevent febrile reactions. After two febrile transfusion reactions, consider use of leukocyte-poor cells in future transfusions.

C. **Allergic reactions.**
   1. Complicate about 2% of transfusions, especially in those who are IgA deficient. True anaphylaxis is 1 in 20,000.

    2. Symptoms include allergic manifestations such as pruritus, urticaria, bronchospasm with wheezing, possibly shock.

    3. See Chapter 2 for treatment of anaphylaxis.

    4. Use washed cells if reacting to plasma protein.

D. **Graft-versus-host disease.**

    1. **Rare.** Clinically have diarrhea, rash, pancytopenia, elevated liver enzymes.

    2. Most common in those with lymphoma, bone marrow transplants, hereditary immune deficiencies, premature infants, **but not AIDS.**

    3. **Treatment.** High mortality rate (>90%). Treatment not generally effective; requires consultation with hematology staff. Prevent by using irradiated cell products in those at risk.

E. **Transfusion-related pulmonary injury.**

    1. **Pulmonary infiltrates and noncardiogenic CHF** (ARDS) related to lung injury.

    2. Clinically note fever, chills, cough, and hypoxia.

    3. **Treatment.** Symptomatic and includes respiratory support, including mechanical ventilation if required.

F. **Infection.** Hepatitis B—1:200,000; hepatitis C—1:100,000; hepatitis A—too low to categorize; HIV—1:450,000 to 1:600,000.

POTASSIUM

I. **Overview.** Total body potassium is approximately 50 mEq/kg of body weight; 98% is intracellular; serum decrease of 1 mEq of K^+ corresponds to a 10% to 20% deficit in total body potassium. Serum K^+ concentration is not always a reliable indicator of total body K^+. Distribution is affected by multiple factors (see hyperkalemia and hypokalemia below). Total body K^+ is largely controlled by the kidney, with 90% of ingested K^+ excreted in the urine; 10% of the daily K^+ load is excreted in the GI tract (in uremic patients this may increase to 33%). Aldosterone promotes potassium excretion (and hypokalemia). Normally there is no significant K^+ loss through the skin. However, with profuse sweating the K^+ loss through the skin may approach 24% of the daily K^+ load. From 5 to 15 mEq of K^+ is lost daily in the urine even with no K^+ intake.

II. **Hypokalemia.** Serum K^+ level below 3.6 mmol/L.

A. **Etiology.**

    1. **GI losses** of K^+ seen in vomiting, NG suction, diarrhea, malabsorption syndrome, laxative or enema abuse. Villous adenomas may excrete K^+ and are associated with a large amount of mucus in the stools. GI losses distal to the stomach result in a low urine K^+ concentration and metabolic acidosis secondary to high bicarbonate losses. GI losses from the stomach result in a high urine K^+ concentration (usually >40 mEq/L) and metabolic alkalosis secondary to high hydrochloride loss. Hydrogen ions are retained by the kidney in an attempt to maintain acid/base balance in exchange for potassium.

2. **Drug-induced hypokalemia.** Can be due to abnormal losses (diuretics such as thiazides, furosemide, ethacrynic acid; mineralocorticoid or glucocorticoid; penicillin and aminoglycosides). May also be secondary to transcellular K^+ shift (epinephrine, decongestant, bronchodilators, tocolytics, theophylline, caffeine, insulin, and verapamil). There is more likely to be significant K^+ loss if patient has edema (edematous states are associated with elevated aldosterone level, which stimulates K^+ excretion). Serum K^+ concentration should be measured before initiation of a diuretic and 1 week after initiation of increase in dose of the diuretic.

3. **Other causes of hypokalemia.**
   a. **Insufficient dietary K^+** is an unusual cause, seen occasionally in alcoholics or cachectic patients.
   b. **Excessive renal losses.** Hypokalemia occurs with a urine K^+ concentration >20 mEq/L. **Causes:** hyperaldosteronism, Bartter's syndrome (hypokalemia, normotension, no edema, sodium wasting, metabolic alkalosis), glucocorticoid excess, magnesium deficiency, osmotic diuresis, renal tubular acidosis.
   c. **Extracellular to intracellular shift.** Metabolic alkalosis shifts potasium intracellularly, as do insulin and adrenergic excess (MI, inhaled beta-agonists).
   d. **Hyperaldosteronism.** May have hypertension and edema when severe. To evaluate, stop all antihypertensives if possible and liberalize diet (must have normal Na intake), get baseline serum aldosterone value, and then give fludrocortisone 0.2 mg PO TID for 3 days. Recheck serum aldosterone, which should be <3 ng/dl. Other protocols are used as well, such as spironolactone challenge.
   e. **Rarely hypokalemic familial periodic paralysis.**

B. **Presentation.** Mostly asymptomatic. However, can cause weakness (especially of proximal muscles), perhaps areflexia, decreased GI motility resulting in ileus. Hyperpolarization of the myocardium occurs with hypokalemia and may cause ventricular ectopy, reentry phenomena, and conduction abnormalities. The ECG frequently shows flattened T waves, U waves, and ST-segment depression. Hypokalemia also causes increased sensitivity of cardiac cells to digitalis preparations and may result in toxicity at therapeutic plasma levels of digitalis.

C. **Treatment.** Goal in all patients is 4.0 mmol/l.
   1. **Magnesium.** It is difficult or impossible to correct a potassium deficit in the face of hypomagnesemia, a frequent occurrence with potassium-wasting diuretics. A magnesium level should be checked if there is any difficulty increasing the serum potassium. Magnesium should be replaced if the serum level is low. Since serum magnesium levels do not reflect total body stores, empiric use of magnesium is indicated if despite a normal serum magnesium it is still difficult to increase the serum potassium (see section on hypomagnesemia).

6

HEMATOLOGIC, ELECTROLYTE, AND METABOLIC DISORDERS

2. **Oral therapy.** K$^+$ supplementation (20 mEq KCl) should be given at the start of non–potassium-sparing diuretic therapy if indicated. Recheck K$^+$ concentration 2 to 4 weeks after starting supplementation. Check periodically thereafter. In hypokalemic-hypochloremic metabolic alkalosis, a chloride supplement should be given as well (KCl). Consider potassium-sparing diuretics, which may not require potassium supplementation. Renal failure and ACE inhibitors are relative (but not absolute) contraindications to potassium-sparing diuretics.

3. **IV therapy** should be used for severe hypokalemia and in patients unable to tolerate oral supplementation. If serum K$^+$ concentrations >2.4 mEq/L and no ECG changes, K$^+$ can be given at a rate up to 10 to 20 mEq/hr with maximum daily administration of 200 mEq. Rapid treatment may be required if K$^+$ concentration <2 mEq/L with ECG changes (up to 40 mEq/hr on monitor, through peripheral line, diluted). Serum K$^+$ concentrations should be measured every 4 to 6 hours with the patient under continuous ECG monitoring. Use a nondextrose solution to prevent insulin release, which causes the shift of potassium intracellularly.

III. **Hyperkalemia.**

A. **Definition.** Serum K$^+$ above laboratory normal (generally 5.5 mEq/L).

B. **Causes.**

1. **Inadequate renal excretion.** Acute or chronic renal failure, potassium-sparing diuretics, ACE inhibitors.

2. **Potassium load** from massive cell death caused by crush injuries, major surgery, burns, acute arterial emboli, hemolysis, GI bleeding, or rhabdomyolysis. Exogenous sources such as ingestion of potassium supplements and salt substitutes, blood transfusions, IV potassium administration, and high-dose penicillin therapy must also be considered. Also consider water softeners as a potential source of exogenous potassium.

3. **Intracellular to extracellular shift.** Acidosis, digitalis toxicity, insulin deficiency, or rapid increase of blood osmolality.

4. **Adrenal insufficiency** (Addison's disease).

5. **Pseudohyperkalemia.** Secondary to hemolysis of blood sample or prolonged tourniquet time.

6. **Hypoaldosteronism.**

C. **Presentation.** Most important effect is a change in cardiac excitability. ECG shows sequential changes with a rising serum potassium level. Initially, tall peaked T waves are seen (K$^+$ >6.5 mEq/dl). This is followed by prolonged PR intervals, diminished P-wave amplitude, widened QRS complexes (K$^+$ = 7 to 8 mEq/L). Eventually the QT interval prolongs and leads to a sine-wave pattern. Ventricular fibrillation and asystole are likely with K$^+$ >10 mEq/L. Other findings include paresthesias, weakness, areflexia, and ascending paralysis.

D. **Treatment.** Continuous ECG monitoring is warranted if ECG changes are present or if serum potassium >7 mEq/L.

1. **Calcium gluconate** may be administered IV as 10 ml of a 10% solution over 10 minutes to stabilize myocardium and cardiac conduction system. This can be repeated twice at 5-minute intervals if no response. **Administration of calcium may cause digitalis toxicity in patients receiving digitalis therapy. Calcium gluconate should not be used in the face of digitalis toxicity.**

2. **Sodium bicarbonate** alkalinizes the blood, causing a shift of potassium from the extracellular fluid to the intracellular space. This is given as 40 to 150 mEq of $NaHCO_3$ IV over 30 minutes or as an IV bolus in an emergency; may worsen CHF because of sodium load. The effect is temporary but will work even when serum pH is normal.

3. **Insulin** causes a shift of potassium from the extracellular fluid into cells; 5 to 10 U of regular insulin should be administered with 1 ampule of 50% glucose IV over 5 minutes. A response may not be seen for 50 to 60 minutes, and the effect usually lasts for several hours.

4. **Cation-exchange resins** such as sodium polystyrene sulfonate (Kayexalate and others) remove potassium from the body by binding potassium in the GI tract in exchange for another cation (sodium in the case of sodium polystyrene sulfonate and most other drugs in this class). These drugs may be given orally or rectally. The initial oral dose is 15 to 30 g of sodium polystyrene sulfonate mixed with 50 to 100 ml of 70% sorbitol to counteract its constipating effect. The dose may be repeated every 3 to 4 hours if needed. A retention enema is given as 50 g of sodium polystyrene sulfonate mixed with 200 ml of 20% sorbitol or D20W and may be repeated every 1 to 2 hours initially and then every 6 hours or as necessary. These agents cause a significant sodium load and may precipitate CHF.

5. **Dialysis** may be required in severe, refractory cases of hyperkalemia.

6. **Aerosolized beta$_2$-agonists.** Will drive K^+ intracellularly and are particularly useful in renal failure. Can use constant nebulization of albuterol.

7. **Potassium restriction** is indicated in the late stages of renal failure (GFR <15 ml/min).

8. **Adrenal insufficiency** is treated acutely with hydrocortisone succinate. See discussion of adrenal insufficiency this chapter.

SODIUM

I. **Hyponatremia.** Defined as a serum sodium below normal (generally 135 mEq/L).

A. **Four possible states. Initial assessment is to measure urine osmolality** and urine sodium. **Then, assess the patient's volume status** based on clinical exam and lab data such as urine specific gravity and BUN/Cr. Hyponatremia is then classified as follows:

1. **Artifactual or spurious.**

2. **Dilutional.** Hypervolemic with expansion of total body water.

3. **Hypovolemic.** Sodium depletion in excess of water depletion.

6

HEMATOLOGIC, ELECTROLYTE, AND METABOLIC DISORDERS

TABLE 6-6

DIFFERENTIAL DIAGNOSIS OF HYPONATREMIA BASED ON VOLUME STATUS AND URINE SODIUM

Spurious (Sodium Decreased Because of Laboratory Interaction)	Hypovolemia (Dry)		Euvolemia (No Edema)	Hypervolemia (Edema)	
	Urine Sodium >20	Urine Sodium <10	Urine Sodium >20	Urine Sodium >20	Urine Sodium <10
Occurs only if using flame photometer and **not if measured by ion selective electrode**	Renal loss, including:	Extrarenal loss	Glucocorticoid deficiency	Renal failure	Other causes of fluid overload such as cirrhosis, CHF, nephrotic syndrome, etc.
Hyperglycemia	Diuretics	Vomiting, diarrhea, NG suction	Stress (physical, emotional)		SIADH (but may not appear edematous)
Hyperlipidemia	RTA, metabolic acidosis	Third-spacing such as with burns, pancreatitis, surgery, etc.	Drugs		
Hyperproteinemia (myeloma, macroglobulinemia, etc.)	Osmotic diuresis (e.g., mannitol, DM)	Sweating	SIADH		
Mannitol	Mineralocorticoid deficiency		Hypothyroidism		
Other osmotically active substances.	Hypoaldosteronism				
	Addison's disease				

4. **Euvolemic.** Sodium and water depletion in equal amounts.
5. See Table 6-6 for an overview.

B. **Artifactual or spurious.** Lab reporting error secondary to:
1. **Hyperglycemia.** Correct sodium for glucose. Each increase of blood glucose of 100 mg/dl decreases serum sodium by 1.7 to 2.4 mEq/L depending on how high the glucose is; 2.4 mEq/L is used as the correction factor when the glucose is >300mEq/L.
2. **Hyperlipidemia.** Measured serum osmolality will be normal and greater than the calculated osmolality (Osm = [2 × Na] + [Glucose/18] + [BUN/2.8]).

C. **Dilutional or hypervolemic.**
1. **Caused by defect in water excretion.**
   a. **Sodium-retaining (edematous) states.**
      (1) CHF, renal failure and nephrotic syndrome, cirrhosis and ascites.
      (2) **Diagnosis.**
      - Clinical situation and underlying disease are key to determining the cause.
      - Urine sodium concentration usually very low (<10 mEq/L). However, with acute and chronic renal failure, may have urine Na and Cl concentrations >20 mEq/L.
      - Urine osmolality is elevated (only valid in absence of diuretics).
   b. **Excessive water intake** without sodium retention in the presence of:
      (1) Renal failure, hypothyroidism, Addison's disease.
      - SIADH (see below).
2. **Diagnosis of dilutional or hypervolemic hyponatremia.**
   a. To diagnose most causes of hypervolemic or dilutional hyponatremia (renal failure, CHF, hypothyroidism, and Addison's disease), see the section appropriate to the individual illness.
   b. **SIADH:** nonosmotically driven ADH secretion (may also be euvolemic).
      (1) **Clinically.** May be caused by lung and other cancers, pulmonary processes (pneumonia, TB, contusion), CNS disorders including Guillain-Barré and subarachnoid hemorrhage, acute intermittent porphyria, multiple drugs including MAO inhibitors, desmopressin, paregoric, oral hypoglycemic agents, opioids, barbiturates, vincristine, clofibrate, carbamazepine, and NSAIDs. May also be seen with physical stress, including postoperatively. Postoperative hyponatremia is more common and more severe in menstruating females.
      (2) **Diagnosis.** Patients generally have a normal GFR and an inappropriately hypertonic urine with respect to serum sodium (urine osmolality should be <130 mOsm/kg if hyponatremic [kidneys should be conserving sodium and getting rid of free water]); in SIADH, urine osmoles are >130 mOsm/kg).

(3) **ADH can be measured** in the blood. However, ADH excretion can be erratic and may not be elevated at all times in SIADH.

(4) **Treatment for SIADH.** Fluid restriction to 1 liter per day. If this is unacceptable to patient, demeclocycline 3.25 to 3.75 mg/kg Q6h to antagonize the effect of ADH on the kidney may help. Doses up to 1200 mg/day (400 mg Q6h) have been used. Use with caution in those with liver disease, CHF, or renal failure.

D. **Hypovolemic hyponatremia.**

1. **Causes.** Combined water and sodium loss.
   a. **GI loss** such as vomiting, NG suction, diarrhea.
   b. **Third-space losses** as with burns, surgery.
   c. **Excessive sweating, diuretics.**
   d. **Renal and adrenal disease** including uncontrolled diabetes mellitus, hypoaldosteronism, Addison's disease, recovery phase of renal disease.

2. **Diagnosis.**
   a. If renal function is normal, the urine osmolality is high and the urine Na usually less than 10 to 15 mEq/L, thus the kidney is responding appropriately by conserving Na. The fractional excretion of sodium (FE_{Na}) is <1%. (See Chapter 23 for calculations.)
   b. In those with kidney or adrenal disease, the urine Na is usually >20 mEq/L and is not helpful. (See section on renal failure.)
   c. In the presence of metabolic alkalosis, urine Na may be high with a low urine chloride (<10 mEq/L).

E. **Euvolemic hyponatremia.**

1. **Causes.** SIADH; see above for diagnosis and treatment. May also be caused by water intoxication but usually requires intake of >10 L/day. Other causes include hypothyroidism, stress, and adrenal insufficiency. With these latter 3, the urine Na >20 mEq/L. Fluid restriction will be diagnostic (see diabetes insipidus below for protocol).

F. **Clinical presentation of hyponatremia.** Depends on severity and time course of onset.

1. Rapidly developing hyponatremia is more symptomatic.
2. If plasma Na drops 10 mEq/L over several hours, patients may have nausea, vomiting, headache, muscle cramps.
3. If plasma Na drops 10 mEq/L in an hour, may have severe headache, lethargy, seizures, disorientation, and coma.
   a. Mortality 50% if Na concentration falls to <113 mEq/L rapidly.
   b. Any geriatric patient with a change in mental status should have serum electrolytes to check for hyponatremia.
4. May have signs of the underlying illness (such as CHF, Addison's disease). If secondary to fluid loss, may have signs of shock including hypotension and tachycardia.

G. **Treatment of hyponatremia.**

1. Treat underlying condition (CHF, Addison's disease, hypothyroidism, SIADH). See specific section on treatment of underlying disease.
2. Stop any contributing drugs.
3. Correct a long-standing hyponatremia slowly and a rapidly developing hyponatremia more aggressively. **Do not overcorrect hyponatremia.** May precipitate central pontine myelinolysis. Consider early therapy with IV NaCl. This is associated with better outcomes than fluid restriction.
   a. Do not raise serum Na more than 12 mEq/L in 24 hours in asymptomatic patients. If the patient is symptomatic, can increase serum sodium by 1 to 1.5 mEq/L/hr until symptoms resolve.
   b. To calculate the amount of Na needed to raise the serum Na to 125 mEq/L: Amount of Na (mEq) = 125 mEq/L − Actual serum Na (mEq/L) × TBW (in liters); TBW = 0.6 × Body weight in kg.
   c. May replace Na with 3% or 5% NaCl solution (provide 0.51 mEq/ml and 0.86 mEq/ml, respectively).
   d. In those with ECF volume expansion, the use of diuretics may be necessary.

II. **Hypernatremia.** Defined as a serum sodium above normal (generally 135 to 140 mEq/L).

A. **Causes.**
   1. Hypernatremia will result if hypotonic fluid losses are not adequately replaced.
      a. If fluid losses are extrarenal (GI losses, perspiration, or hyperventilation), the urine osmolality will be greater than that of the serum, and urinary Na^+ will be <20 mEq/L.
      b. A urine osmolality less than or equal to that of the serum implies renal fluid losses (diuretic therapy, osmotic diuresis, diabetes insipidus, acute tubular necrosis, postobstructive uropathy, hypokalemic nephropathy, or hypercalcemic nephropathy).
   2. Hypernatremia may occur with hyperalimentation or other hypertonic fluid administration.

B. **Signs and symptoms.** Muscle irritability, confusion, ataxia, tremulousness, seizures, and finally coma. Additional manifestations usually occur secondary to the underlying abnormality and volume status (tachycardia and orthostatic hypotension with volume depletion; edema with fluid excess).

C. **Treatment.**
   1. **Hypernatremia with volume depletion** should be treated by administration of **isotonic saline** until hemodynamic stability is achieved. Can then correct the remaining water deficit with D_5W or hypotonic saline.
   2. **Hypernatremia with volume excess** is treated with diuresis or, if necessary, with dialysis. D_5W is then administered to replace the water deficit.
   3. Body water deficit is estimated by:
      a. Deficit = Desired TBW (liters) − Current TBW.

    b. Desired TBW = (Measured serum Na) × (Current TBW/Normal serum Na).

    c. Current TBW = 0.6 × Current body weight (kg).

4. One half the calculated water deficit should be given in the first 24 hours, and the remaining deficit is corrected over 1 or 2 days to avoid cerebral edema secondary to abrupt change in serum sodium concentration.

5. **Diabetes insipidus** (may also have normal sodium if no access to free water): Caused by either renal resistance to ADH or decreased secretion of ADH (including granulomatous disease, CNS trauma or hypoxia, tumor, drugs (especially lithium carbonate), etc. May have polyuria and polydipsia.

    a. **Diagnosis.** An initial urine osmolality of <300 mOsm/kg indicates possibility of diabetes insipidus (though occasionally will have urine osmolality of 300 to 500 mOsm/kg). Patients with hypernatremia should have a maximally concentrated urine (800 to 1200 mOsm/kg). Next step is water deprivation **under direct observation because of risk of hypovolemia** for 6 to 12 hours. Check urine and serum osmolality. If concentrate urine to normal with fluid deprivation (>800 mOsm/kg), problem not diabetes insipidus (consider water intoxication, etc.). If not able to concentrate urine, probably diabetes insipidus. Confirm by administration of 10 to 20 μU of DDAVP by nasal spray **or** 5 U SQ. If urine concentrates by 50%, the diagnosis is diabetes insipidus. If urine does not concentrate, consider nephrogenic diabetes insipidus (e.g., kidney unresponsive to ADH) or other diagnosis causing hypernatremia.

    b. **Treatment.** DDAVP 10 to 25 μg intranasally BID to reduce polydipsia or polyuria.

CALCIUM

I. **Hypercalcemia.** An elevated serum calcium of over 10.5 mg/dl after correction for serum albumin. Corrected calcium = Serum calcium + (0.8 × [Normal serum albumin − Patient's albumin]).

A. **History.** "Bones, stones, abdominal groans."

1. **If mild, may be asymptomatic.** Frequently found on routine screening labs. Asymptomatic, incidental hypercalcemia secondary to hyperparathyroidism need not be treated.

2. **Moderate elevations.** Constipation, anorexia, nausea, vomiting, abdominal pain, ileus.

3. **More severe elevations** (>12 mg/dl). Emotional lability, confusion, delirium, psychosis, stupor, coma. Weaknesses and seizures. Nephrolithiasis or urolithiasis common. May have associated renal failure, QT shortening.

4. No symptom complex is sensitive enough to be diagnostic.

B. **Etiology and pathophysiology.** Either overabsorption of calcium as with milk-alkali syndrome; too little calcium excretion as with thiazide use; excess mobilization of bone as with hyperparathyroidism, metastatic cancer.

C. **Differential diagnosis.** See specific topic for additional information.

    1. **Spurious.** High-calcium meal before blood draw, long tourniquet application time; 53% will be found to be normocalcemic when calcium level is repeated.

    2. **Hyperparathyroidism.** Generally have high calcium, low phosphate, elevated serum parathyroid hormone.

    3. **Malignancy.** Breast cancer (50% of cases from malignancy), lung cancer, multiple myeloma, renal cancer, colon cancer, prostate cancer, ovarian cancer, others.

    4. Together, hyperparathyroidism and malignancy account for 80% to 90% of cases of hypercalcemia in adults.

    5. **Drugs.** Lithium carbonate, vitamin D, vitamin A, thiazide diuretics; milk-alkali syndrome.

    6. **Hyperthyroidism or hypothyroidism.** Will have low TSH, elevated free T_4 (hyperthyroidism), high TSH (hypothyroidism).

    7. **Immobilization and bed rest.**

    8. **Addison's disease.** Should have weakness, fatigue, weight loss, hypotension; may have hyperpigmentation, low sodium level, high potassium level.

    9. **Cushing's disease.** Should have physical stigmas such as truncal obesity, striae, moon facies.

   10. **Multiple endocrine neoplasia. MEN type I:** tumors of parathyroid, pituitary, pancreas, and possibly Zollinger-Ellison syndrome; **MEN type II:** medullary thyroid carcinoma, hyperparathyroidism, pheochromocytoma.

   11. **Paget's disease of the bone.** See Chapter 7.

D. **Work-up.**

    1. **History and physical exam,** including drug and vitamin history.

    2. **Repeat calcium to rule out artifact.** Get fasting A.M. calcium, electrolytes, BUN, creatinine, and alkaline phosphatase; look for evidence of renal failure, adrenal failure, bone disease. TSH to rule out hyperthyroidism or hypothyroidism. If repeat calcium is elevated and no other abnormality noted, continue workup.

    3. **Check parathyroid hormone level,** preferably using a two-site, double-antibody, immunoradiometric assay (immunoassay for intact parathyroid hormone). Obtain a simultaneous calcium. If parathyroid hormone is high, the diagnosis is hyperparathyroidism. Consider surgical referral for parathyroidectomy. Normal or low parathyroid hormone is suggestive of malignancy; continue work-up.

    4. **Search for malignancy,** including breast exam, mammogram, chest radiograph, stool guaiac, PSA value, abdominal CT, bone scan, bone radiographs, etc. as dictated by patient history and physical.

6

HEMATOLOGIC, ELECTROLYTE, AND METABOLIC DISORDERS

Serum and urine protein electrophoresis looking for myeloma if indicated (urine dipstick will not pick up Bence Jones proteins).

5. **If this work-up is negative** and patient has uveitis or erythema nodosum and has bilateral hilar adenopathy on CXR, can assume sarcoid. Serum ACE levels unreliable (see sarcoid section, Chapter 4).

6. If work-up is negative and patient asymptomatic, repeat calcium value, work-up in 6 months.

7. If work-up remains negative and high calcium maintained, consider neck exploration for parathyroid adenoma.

E. **Laboratory results.**

1. High chloride and low phosphate levels are suggestive of hyperparathyroidism.

2. Anemia, high sedimentation rate, abnormal serum globulins, low albumin level, proteinuria are suggestive of malignancy.

3. Elevated parathyroid hormone defines hyperparathyroidism.

4. Elevated BUN and creatinine levels are suggestive of renal failure.

5. Elevated alkaline phosphatase levels are suggestive of a bone process such as Paget's disease of the bone or metastatic breast or prostate cancer.

F. **Treatment for hypercalcemia.** Address underlying disorder (see under specific diagnosis).

1. **Acute treatment.**

a. If patient severely symptomatic or if serum Ca >15 mg/dl, need to reduce serum Ca rapidly.

b. **Promote diuresis** and replace intravascular volume with normal saline. If renal function intact, give 1 to 2 L of normal saline and furosemide 80 to 100 mg IV Q2-12h for the first 24 hours. Adjust furosemide and saline rates to prevent fluid overload **and** intravascular depletion. Replace urine losses with normal saline and KCl to prevent hypokalemia. Avoid thiazide diuretics, which can cause calcium retention.

c. If renal function is compromised and the patient is symptomatic, consider acute hemodialysis.

d. **Calcitonin** 4 to 8 U SQ Q6-12h. Not very potent but rapid acting; will lower serum calcium by 1 to 3 mg/dl. Use one or two doses as emergency therapy while waiting for other modalities to work. Short acting. Side effects include abdominal cramping, nausea, flushing, allergic reaction (to salmon calcitonin). Calcitonin nasal spray is now available for maintenance.

e. **Bisphosphonates** (inhibit osteoclastic activity), helpful in hyperparathyroidism, malignancy.

(1) Pamidronate 60 to 90 mg IV over 4 to 24 hours. More potent than etidronate; achieves control in 70% to 100% of cases. Effective within 2 days and reaches nadir at 7 days. Side effects are mild and include a transient increase in temperature ($<2°$ C), transient leukopenia, and a small de-

      crease in serum phosphate. Generally preferred over etidronate and plicamycin.

      (2) Disodium etidronate 7.5 mg/kg IV daily over 4 hours for 3 to 7 days. May cause increase in serum creatinine and phosphate. Long-term administration may lead to osteomalacia. Calcium will drop within 2 days and reach nadir at 7 days. Achieves control in 60% to 100%.

  f. **Plicamycin (mithramycin)** 25 µg/kg IV in 500 ml of D_5W over 3 to 6 hours is useful. May repeat several times at 24- to 48-hour intervals. Especially useful in hypercalcemia from malignancy. Side effects include nausea, local irritation, and cellulitis if extravasation occurs, hepatic toxicity, nephrotoxicity, and thrombocytopenia. Contraindicated in hepatic or renal dysfunction, thrombocytopenia, other coagulopathy. Works in 12 hours with peak at 72 hours. **Use becoming less common as bisphosphonates become more common. Is less well tolerated and less effective than pamidronate.**

  g. **Steroids.** Prednisone 60 mg/day PO, or hydrocortisone succinate 200 to 300 mg IV. Helpful for hypercalcemia from vitamin-D intoxication, myeloma, and breast carcinoma.

  h. *A very risky approach* is to administer 1 L of disodium phosphate and monopotassium phosphate (0.5 to 1 g can be given over 24 hours). This can cause soft-tissue calcification, renal failure, and death. This approach should be tried only if all other measures fail, hypercalcemia is life threatening, and you are unable to arrange for hemodialysis. A nephrology or endocrinology consultation is suggested before use of this modality.

2. **Chronic treatment.**

  a. Oral calcium binders including phosphates (1 to 3 g of elemental phosphorus per day). Do not use in those with renal failure.

  b. Oral etidronate 1200 to 1600 mg/day. May cause osteomalacia. Alendronate and risedronate may also be used but are not FDA approved for this indication.

  c. Pamidronate. May be repeated in initial dose (see above) weekly if needed. Does not cause osteomalacia.

II. **Hypocalcemia.** Defined as serum Ca <8.8 mg/dl (usually <7 mg/dl when symptoms present). Must correct for serum albumin. Corrected calcium = Measured serum calcium + (0.8 × [Normal serum albumin − Patient's albumin]).

A. **Causes.**

  1. Hypoparathyroidism.

  2. Spurious.

  3. Vitamin D deficiency or resistance.

  4. Renal tubular acidosis, renal failure.

  5. Magnesium depletion.

  6. Acute pancreatitis.

    7. Septic shock.

    8. Drugs: cisplatin, pentamidine, foscarnet, and ketoconazole.

B. **Clinical symptoms.**

    1. Primarily neurologic.

    2. If develops slowly, confusion, encephalopathy, depression, psychosis. May also note tetany, convulsions, laryngospasm, carpopedal spasm, muscle aches.

    3. Look for Chvostek's sign. Contraction of facial muscles elicited by light tapping of facial nerve.

    4. Trousseau's sign. Carpopedal spasms elicited by application of tourniquet for 3 minutes to extremity. Avoid in those with vascular disease or coagulopathy.

C. **Treatment.**

    1. **If tetany present,** can administer 10 ml of 10% calcium gluconate over 15 to 30 minutes. Lasts only a few hours and may require repeat infusions (60 ml of Ca gluconate in 500 ml of D_5W at 0.5 to 2 mg/kg/hr). Measure calcium every 2 hours.

    2. Calcium can cause digoxin toxicity and may cause arrhythmias in those taking digitalis.

    3. Must correct hypomagnesemia if present (see hypomagnesemia and hypokalemia, for discussion).

    4. Administer oral calcium 1 to 7 g/day divided with meals.

    5. **If secondary to renal failure:**

        a. Need to add phosphate binders (aluminum hydroxide gel).

        b. Dietary restriction of phosphate.

        c. Vitamin D may be hazardous in renal failure.

    7. **If secondary to vitamin D deficiency,** give vitamin D replacement, such as calcitriol (Rocaltrol), calcifediol (Calderol), etc.

    8. **If vitamin D resistant,** treat with inorganic phosphate 1 to 3.5 g/day and calcitriol 0.25 to 1 μg/day.

MAGNESIUM

I. **Hypermagnesemia.** Serum magnesium >2.5 mg/dl. Fifty percent of body stores is in bone; the remainder is mostly in the muscle. Less than 1% in ECF with 20% to 30% protein bound, and the remainder as free cation. Most is absorbed in small bowel, excreted by kidneys.

A. **Causes.**

    1. Renal failure in patients administered magnesium-containing products (laxatives and antacids).

    2. Administration IV (as in preeclampsia).

B. **Clinically.** Get impairment of neuromuscular transmission. Manifests as muscle weakness, respiratory depression, absence of deep tendon reflexes, widened QRS and prolonged PR interval, hypotension, heart block, asystole.

C. **Treatment.**

1. IV administration of 10 to 20 ml of 10% calcium gluconate IV over 10 minutes or 10% $CaCl_2$ 5 to 10 mg/kg IV to temporize. Without severe renal dysfunction 20 ml of 10% calcium gluconate in a liter of 0.9 NS can be given at 100 to 200 ml/hr.
2. Administration of furosemide or ethacrynic acid may enhance excretion.
3. Hemodialysis is effective.

II. **Hypomagnesemia.** Serum magnesium <1.9 mg/dl. However, serum levels do not reflect total body stores, and a patient (especially in CHF, using a diuretic, etc.) may be total body depleted with normal serum levels of magnesium.

A. **Causes.**
1. Relatively common in stress situations as in myocardial infarction, shock.
2. Alcoholism and nutritional deficiency (chronic TPN).
3. Loss from diarrhea, diuretics **(diuretics major cause of hypomagnesemia in those with CHF),** osmotic diuresis (diabetes).
4. **Renal.** Hyperaldosteronism and hypoparathyroidism. Hypercalcemia causes increased renal Mg^{++} excretion.
5. Amphotericin B and cyclosporin A.

B. **Clinically.** Anorexia, lethargy, vomiting, tetany, arrhythmias, seizures, prolonged PR and QT intervals.

C. **Treatment.**
1. In an emergency, can give 2 to 4 g of magnesium sulfate in 50 ml of D_5W over 5 to 15 minutes. Can repeat to a total of 10 g over the next 6 hours. Continue replacement for 3 to 7 days with 48 mEq/L/24 hr.
2. If it is a less severe situation, replace 0.03 to 0.06 g/kg/day in four to six doses until serum magnesium is normal.
3. Continue oral replacement therapy as long as precipitating factor is present (such as oral Mag-Ox one PO QD BID).

GLUCOSE

I. **Hypoglycemia.**

A. **Definition.** Plasma glucose <50 mg/dl. May be asymptomatic.

B. **Categories.**
1. **Postprandial hypoglycemia.**
   a. **Clinically.**
      (1) Generally have symptoms of adrenergic stimulation, including diaphoresis, anxiety, irritability, palpitations, tremor, and hunger.
      (2) Occurs 2 to 4 hours postprandially, sudden onset, and generally subsides in 15 to 20 minutes.
      (3) Caused by stimulation of epinephrine release.
   b. **Etiology.** Often idiopathic but may be caused by early diabetes, alcohol intake, status postgastrectomy, renal failure, drugs such as salicylates, beta-blockers, pentamidine, ACE inhibitors.
2. **Fasting hypoglycemia.**

6

HEMATOLOGIC, ELECTROLYTE, AND METABOLIC DISORDERS

    a. **Clinically.**

       (1) Generally have symptoms of neuroglycopenia, including headache, mental dullness, and fatigue. If hypoglycemia is more severe, it may progress to confusion, visual blurring, loss of consciousness, and seizures.

       (2) Occurs with fasting greater than 4 hours.

    b. **Etiology.**

       (1) Excess insulin including insulinoma, self-administered insulin or oral hypoglycemic agents.

       (2) Alcohol abuse and liver disease (decreased gluconeogenesis).

       (3) Pituitary or adrenal insufficiency.

  3. **Iatrogenic or exogenous.** May occur in diabetic patients with changes in dosage of medications or level of physical activity.

C. **Evaluation of hypoglycemia.**

  1. **Postprandial hypoglycemia.**

    a. 5-hour glucose tolerance test (GTT). Give 75 g glucose load and measure serum glucose every 30 minutes for 5 hours. 25% of asymptomatic individuals will have hypoglycemic symptoms and a blood glucose <50 mg/dl when challenged this way. Many have blood glucose <50 mg/dl but remain asymptomatic.

    b. **If cause of postprandial hypoglycemia is:**

       (1) Early diabetes. Normal or elevated fasting glucose; glucose is greatest during first 2 hours, an indication of diabetes, but may have low plasma level at glucose hours 3 to 4.

       (2) Status postgastrectomy. Rapid elevation of glucose by 1 hour; rapid decline with trough at 2 to 3 hours.

       (3) Idiopathic hypoglycemia. Normal plasma glucose hours 1 to 2, low glucose hour 3, return to baseline value by hour 5.

       (4) Idiopathic postprandial syndrome. Have postprandial adrenergic symptoms with normal GTT.

  2. **Fasting hypoglycemia.**

    a. For screening, measure plasma glucose after overnight fast.

       (1) If overnight value normal (>50 mg/dl), can try 72-hour fast (observed).

       (2) Some premenopausal women will normally have serum glucose <50 mg/dl after a 72-hour fast.

    b. **If cause for fasting hypoglycemia is:**

       (1) Insulinoma. Will have hunger, weight gain, hypoglycemic symptoms. Consultation with an endocrinologist important.

       (2) Surreptitious insulin or oral hypoglycemic administration.

         • Usually a diabetic or person with medical background.

         • Needle marks usually evident (with insulin).

         • Can measure for oral hypoglycemic agents in the blood.

         • Measure insulin C-peptide; will be low if exogenous insulin being administered to patient.

- The presence of anti-insulin antibodies supports the diagnosis of exogenous insulin being given.
      (3) Alcohol abuse. Should have other stigmas of alcohol abuse.
      (4) Liver disease.
         - Have elevated liver enzymes; other signs of liver failure.
         - Any patient with cirrhosis and hypoglycemia should be evaluated for a hepatoma.
      (5) Pituitary or adrenal insufficiency. See below for evaluation.
  D. **Treatment of hypoglycemia.**
    1. **Acute management.**
       a. Oral carbohydrates if possible.
       b. IV D_{50} at 1 ampule or more. There is no predictable response of blood glucose to D_{50}.
       c. If no IV access, glucagon 1 mg IM (may cause nausea, vomiting, and aspiration).
       d. Monitor blood glucose Q15-30 min.
       e. Those with hypoglycemia secondary to oral agents should be admitted for observation.
    2. **Long-term management.**
       a. Adjust drug dosages; give diabetic training where applicable.
       b. Institute an ADA diet with high proportion of complex carbohydrates.
       c. Propantheline 7.5 to 15 mg PO 1/2 hour before meals may delay gastric emptying in postgastrectomy patient, avoiding rapid peaks in serum glucose. This is not an approved use.

II. **Diabetes Mellitus.**
  A. **Overview.**
    1. **Definition.** Diabetes mellitus (DM) is hyperglycemia secondary to decreased insulin production or peripheral tissue resistance to insulin.
    2. **Classification and etiology** (1997 Report of the Expert Committee on the Diagnosis and Classification of Diabetes Mellitus).
       a. **Type 1 DM** (formerly type I or insulin-dependent DM) usually occurs in childhood or early adulthood and results in ketoacidosis when patients are without insulin therapy. This accounts for 10% of cases of DM. Type 1 DM is caused by beta islet cell failure, which is of multifactorial causes such as genetic predisposition, viral and autoimmune attacks on the beta islet cells.
       b. **Type 2 DM** (formerly type II or non–insulin-dependent DM) usually occurs in people >40 years of age, and 60% of the patients are obese. However, type 2 DM is being increasingly seen in the teenage years. Type 2 DM occurs with intact beta islet cell function but peripheral tissue resistance to insulin. There may be some decrease in insulin production or a hyperinsulin state. These patients are not ketosis prone but may develop it under conditions of stress.

6

HEMATOLOGIC, ELECTROLYTE, AND METABOLIC DISORDERS

    c. **Gestational onset DM** (GODM) occurs when diabetes onset is during pregnancy and resolves with delivery. These patients are at a higher risk for developing DM at a later date. See Chapter 14 for details on GODM diagnosis and management.

    d. Other specific types include diseases of the exocrine pancreas, various endocrinopathies (Cushing's syndrome, pheochromocytoma), drug- or chemical-induced DM (beta-blockers, oral contraceptives), or genetic syndromes (lipodystrophies) associated with diabetes.

  3. Evidence is accumulating showing the benefit of tight glycemic control in patients with DM. Tight glycemic control can delay the onset and slow the progression of diabetic retinopathy, nephropathy, and neuropathy in patients with type 1 DM. Improved blood glucose control in type 2 DM decreases the progression of microvascular complications by about 25%.

B. **Evaluation.**

  1. **Symptoms.** Presentations may include polyuria, polydipsia, polyphagia associated with weight loss, blurred vision, recurrent candidal vaginitis, soft-tissue infections, or dehydration. Many cases will be asymptomatic and picked up on routine screening.

  2. **Screening.** Test at age 45, repeat every 3 years. Test before age 45 and repeat more frequently if patient has the following risk factors: obesity (BMI >27 kg/m^2), first-degree relative with DM, member of high-risk group (African-American, Hispanic, Native-American, Asian), history of gestational DM or delivered a baby weighing more than 4032 g (9 lb), hypertensive, HDL <35 mg/dl or triglyceride level >250 mg/dl, history of impaired fasting glucose or impaired glucose tolerance glucose on prior testing.

  3. **Diagnosis** of diabetes mellitus is made if patient has:

    a. Random plasma glucose of >200 mg/dl and symptoms of diabetes.

    b. Two fasting plasma glucose of >126 mg/dl.

    c. 2-hour postprandial plasma glucose >200 mg/dl after a glucose load of 75 g (see caveats below).

    d. Elevated HbA_{1c}. However, the HbA_{1c} is not an adequate screening tool for DM because it may be normal in those with impaired glucose tolerance.

    e. The patient is said to have impaired glucose tolerance if the fasting plasma glucose is >110 mg/dl and <126 mg/dl.

  4. **The oral glucose tolerance test is being deemphasized. However, if you are going to use it,** the patient must fast for 10 to 16 hours before the ingestion of a 75 g glucose load and should not be under significant metabolic stress (e.g., no systemic infection). Plasma glucose is measured initially and at 2 hours after glucose administration.

    a. The test is normal if the fasting plasma glucose is <110 mg/dl and the 2-hour plasma glucose is <140 mg/dl.

b. **Impaired fasting glucose:** fasting plasma glucose level between 110 and 126 mg/dl.

c. **Impaired glucose tolerance:** 2-hour plasma glucose values between 140 and 200 mg/dl. Of these patients, 1% to 5% per year will develop DM.

d. **Diabetes diagnosed if any value >200 mg/dl.**

5. **Caveats.** Of those with a fasting plasma glucose between 110 and 126, only 0.02% will have an elevated HbA_{1c} and 80% will have a normal HbA_{1c} with the rest only slightly elevated. Of those with a fasting glucose between 126 and 140 mg/dl, 61% will have a normal HbA_{1c}, 35% will have a slightly elevated HbA_{1c}, and only 3% will have a "high" HbA_{1c}. If the HbA_{1c}, which is a reflection of blood glucose over the past several months, is 1% above the reference laboratory's upper range of normal, it has a specificity of 98% for diagnosis of DM.

6. **Differentiating type 1 and type 2.** It is usually possible to differentiate between type 1 and type 2 DM based on the clinical situation. On occasion, however, this may be difficult. The diagnosis can be clarified by the use of the C-peptide, a product of the cleavage of proinsulin to insulin. This will be present in those with type 2 DM and low or absent in those with type 1 DM. If the C-peptide is borderline, checking it after a glucose load may help. In those with type 2 DM, it will increase significantly after glucose load; this response will be absent in those with type 1 DM.

7. **Honeymoon period.** After the initial diagnosis of DM, there is often a "honeymoon" period during which small amounts of a hypoglycemic agent or insulin is needed. Frequently, diabetes first manifests during a situation of metabolic stress (such as infection or pregnancy). With the return to baseline metabolic demands, the pancreatic reserve may be adequate to maintain a normal or near-normal blood glucose.

8. **Somogyi phenomenon** refers to hyperglycemia secondary to a period of drug-induced hypoglycemia with metabolic compensation (increased gluconeogenesis and sympathetic outflow). If controlling high glucose becomes a problem (especially A.M. glucose), consider checking for hypoglycemia in the time leading up to high readings.

C. **Treatment.**

1. **Goal of therapy.** Eliminate symptoms and prevent the complications of diabetes.

2. **Patient education.** Crucial to proper management of DM. Patients must understand diet planning, home glucose-monitoring techniques, proper foot care, and symptoms and treatment of hypoglycemia.

3. **Diet therapy.** Patients should receive instruction from a registered dietitian. Alcohol ingestion should be limited. Diet should include 60% to 65% carbohydrates, 25% to 35% fat, and 10% to 20% protein.

a. **Type 1 DM.** Rigid dietary pattern must be followed to avoid wide fluctuations in plasma glucose. Some flexibility if intensive therapy is used. If a meal is delayed, patient should ingest 10 g of carbohydrate per half hour. Caloric needs may be estimated at 40 kcal/kg/day for an adult with average activity. Modest exercise requires 10 g of extra carbohydrate per hour, vigorous exercise requires an additional 20 to 30 g/hr.

b. **Type 2 DM.** In the obese patient, diabetes is usually reversible with weight loss. The patient who is not obese should follow the same diet as a type 1 DM patient. If patients are receiving oral drug or insulin therapy, their appetite may be stimulated, causing weight gain. This is not the case with the use of metformin.

4. **Pharmacologic therapy.** Type 1 DM patients must be started on insulin at the time of diagnosis. However, type 2 DM patients may need insulin, oral hypoglycemics, metformin, or other medication (see below) if control of hyperglycemia is not achieved by diet alone. The HbA_{1c} level may be helpful in deciding the need for drug therapy in relatively mild hyperglycemia. **Patients with diabetes and one other risk factor for cardiac disease should be started on an ACE inhibitor. This has been shown to decrease the risk of stroke and MI.**

   a. **Insulin.** Beef, pork, and recombinant human insulin (Humulin) are available. Humulin is generally preferable and tends to be less immunogenic than beef or pork insulin and therefore there is less insulin resistance secondary to anti-insulin antibodies. Although there was some thought that those using Humulin are less likely to manifest and therefore recognize symptoms of hypoglycemia, this has proved not to be the case.

      (1) Preparations.
         • Insulin lispro: Short-acting insulin with rapid onset (onset <1 hour, duration <4 hours). The main benefit is for those who cannot plan meals and need to cover erratic intake of calories because it can be used immediately before or after eating. Especially useful in children and toddlers. However, insulin lispro should always be used with a longer-acting, basal insulin. **No advantage of lispro over conventional insulin when it comes to control of HbA_{1c} or preventing hypoglycemia.** It is also more expensive than other insulins.
         • Short-acting insulin (regular or Semilente): onset (SQ) 15 to 30 minutes; peaks 2 to 4 hours; duration 6 to 8 hours.
         • Intermediate-acting insulin (NPH or Lente): onset 1 to 3 hours; peak action 6 to 12 hours; duration 18 to 26 hours.
         • Long-acting insulin (Ultralente PZI): onset 4 to 8 hours; peak action 14 to 24 hours; duration 28 to 36 hours.
         • Lantus is the first long-acting, basal insulin that reliably allows once-a-day administration. Patients can use this in conjunction with regular or lispro insulin before meals.

(2) **In type 1 DM, glucose control is initially obtained with a sliding scale** of regular insulin. Measure serum glucose every 6 hours and give SQ regular insulin to cover sugars. Once the glucose is stabilized with Q6h injections, a split-dosing regimen is introduced with two thirds of the total insulin requirement given as an A.M. dose and one third given as a P.M. dose. This should be given as NPH insulin. If the intermediate-acting agent does not give adequate control of daytime blood glucose, a short-acting agent should be added. The two types of insulin can be given in the same syringe unless they are regular and protamine zinc insulin (PZI).

- Intensive insulin therapy involves either an insulin pump, which administers continuous SQ insulin infusion with mealtime boluses, or multiple daily insulin injections with frequent blood glucose determinations. Another option is the use of a long-acting insulin (such as Ultralente) to provide a base of insulin delivery augmented by regular insulin at mealtimes.
- While adjusting insulin regimen, measure preprandial blood glucose four times daily (including bedtime).
- Only regular insulin can be given IV.

(3) **In type 2 DM,** insulin is usually added to an oral agent when glycemic control is suboptimal at maximal doses of oral medications. An intermediate-acting agent is used starting with a low dose and increasing as needed for glycemic control (such as 5 to 10 U of NPH increasing as needed). Adding NPH at bedtime is generally more efficacious than using it during the day. If using only insulin, start with an A.M. injection. The dose can be increased by 5 U every 3 to 7 days until adequate control is achieved. If fasting hyperglycemia is a problem, intermediate-acting insulin can be given twice daily as a split dose.

b. **Oral hypoglycemic agents are indicated in the management of type 2 DM only.**

(1) **Sulfonylureas** stimulate pancreatic beta cells to secrete insulin. Glyburide 2.5 to 20 mg and glipizide 5 to 20 mg are good choices for an oral hypoglycemic. There is little evidence that glipizide doses of greater than 20 mg/day are helpful and may actually result in decreased beta-cell function. Glyburide is more likely to result in glycemic control when used once a day than is glipizide. Glyburide should be used in a twice-daily dosing if 20 mg/day total is required. Newer agents, such as glipizide GITS and glimepiride, have persistent hypoglycemic effect with once-daily dosing.

- The effectiveness of sulfonylureas declines up to 10% annually as the failure of beta-cell function progresses.

- Contraindications include IDDM, severe renal or hepatic disease, pregnancy, and lactation. Glyburide does not cross the placenta and has been used successfully in the second and third trimesters of pregnancy but is not yet standard of care. Sulfonylureas should not be used in children.
- Complications of sulfonylureas include: *hypoglycemia,* which may be severe and prolonged; a *disulfiram-like effect,* which may be seen when taken with alcohol, with flushing, headache, tachycardia, nausea, and vomiting; and *severe hyponatremia* and *fluid retention,* which may result from the use of chlorpropamide in the elderly (drug-induced SIADH).
- Drug interactions include: propranolol and clonidine may mask the signs and symptoms of hypoglycemia; thiazide diuretics, chlorthalidone, furosemide, ethacrynic acid, and phenytoin may have antagonistic effects on sulfonylureas; and hypoglycemic effects of the sulfonylureas may be potentiated by beta-blockers, ACE inhibitors, salicylates, sulfonamides, phenylbutazone, methyldopa, clofibrate, warfarin, monoamine oxidase inhibitors, and chloramphenicol.

(2) **Metformin** reduces blood glucose levels by improving hepatic and peripheral tissue sensitivity to insulin without affecting the secretion of insulin. Metformin is used as monotherapy or in combination with sulfonylureas or insulin for type 2 DM. **It is especially useful in overweight patients because it does not cause weight gain.** Hypoglycemia is not a problem with metformin. Metformin also appears to improve plasma lipid and fibrinolytic profiles associated with type 2 DM. Initial dosage is 500 mg PO QD until initial nausea and anorexia are tolerated and then advanced to 500 mg BID and then increased 500 mg/day weekly to maximum dose of 2500 mg if needed to control sugars. Use with or after food may lessen the GI side effects. Main risk of metformin is the rare induction of lactic acidosis. Risk is minimized if metformin is avoided in patients with renal disease (creatinine 1.5 mg/dl or higher) and CHF or pulmonary disease. **Discontinue metformin for 48 hours before using IV contrast material because contrast material can contribute to the development of lactic acidosis. Cases of lactic acidosis occur after the initiation of NSAIDS.**

(3) **Alpha-glucosidase inhibitors,** such as acarbose and miglitol, are oral agents that reduce the absorption of carbohydrates. Alpha-glucosidase inhibitors can be used as monotherapy or in combination with insulin or sulfonylureas. Start with 50 mg PO TID with meals and increase weekly to 300 mg PO TID. Main side effects include asymptomatic elevation of liver en-

zymes, flatulence, and diarrhea. In general, this group of drugs is less effective than other classes.

(4) Thiazolidinediones (rosiglitazone [Avenida], pioglitazone [Actos]) increase the body's sensitivity to endogenous insulin by stimulating the peroxisome proliferator-activated receptor (PPAR-gamma). Can be used as monotherapy or in combination with metformin or insulin for type 2 DM; combination therapy led to 0.6% to 1.3% decrease in HbA_{1c}. Side effects include anemia, edema, and elevated LFT. Pioglitazone has the benefit of lowering triglycerides and increasing HDL. Troglitazone is no longer on the market in the United States because of significant liver toxicity.

(5) Repaglinide is very short acting and is the first benzoic acid derivative used to treat type 2 DM. It has a mechanism of action similar to sulfonylureas and promotes insulin release. It has been approved by FDA for monotherapy and in combination with metformin. Dosing is 0.5 to 4 mg TID before each meal. Side effects include hypoglycemia, and repaglinide should be used with caution in patients with diminished liver function. **It is expensive and requires frequent dosing** but may be useful in patients who do not eat regularly.

C. **Symptoms of hypoglycemia** may develop with the use of insulin or oral hypoglycemics. Symptoms include shakiness, tachycardia, weakness, sweating, and nightmares. If not treated with glucose, manifestations may progress to stupor and coma.

D. **Complications of DM.** Intensive glycemic control delays the onset and progression of diabetic retinopathy, nephropathy, and neuropathy in type 1 DM. There is a dose-response relationship between the level of hyperglycemia and both CVD deaths and all cause mortality. Current recommendations are to treat DM patients with closely monitored regimens to maintain blood glucose levels as close to their normal state as possible, with recognition that the number of hypoglycemic episodes may increase. Patient education and compliance are crucial.

1. **Control of blood pressure** is critical to the prevention of diabetes-related consequences and, at least in the case of DM 2, plays more of a role in preventing complications than does tight glycemic control. Target blood pressure should be less than 135/85.

2. **Diabetic nephropathy.** Diabetic nephropathy is the most common cause of end-stage renal disease in the United States. There is clear evidence to indicate that the use of ACE inhibitors in those diabetics with microalbuminuria can delay the development of renal failure; this is true even in the absence of hypertension. Accordingly, all diabetics over 12 years of age should be screened for microalbuminuria at least yearly. **There are three ways to reliably measure microalbumin:** measurement of the albumin-to-creatinine ratio in a random, spot collection; a 24-hour urine collection (can also measure creati-

nine clearance); or a timed collection (e.g., 4-hour collection). Dipsticks are also available to check for microalbumin. However, routine UA dipsticks are not sensitive enough and should not be used. Test is considered positive if >30 mg/24 hr of albumin or >20 µg/min of albumin.

3. **Macrovascular disease.** Atherosclerosis of the coronary and peripheral arteries is three times more common in diabetics and increases with time. Patients with type 2 DM may have higher plasma triglyceride and lower HDL cholesterol level, and many experts recommend lowering LDL level to less than 100 mg/dl in patients with CV disease and to less than 130 mg/dl in those without. Periodic BP checks and annual lipid profile is also recommended.

   a. **Coronary artery disease.** The leading cause of death in DM patients is myocardial infarction. 30% of myocardial infarctions in diabetic patients are "silent" (that is, painless). Therefore the possibility of an MI must be considered whenever a diabetic patient has CHF, dyspnea, diabetic ketoacidosis, or other secondary event. **Syndrome X** occurs in diabetics with microvascular disease but no overt CAD on cardiac catheterization. It manifests with typical angina-type symptoms but has an overall good outcome.

   b. **Peripheral vascular disease.** The most important risk is smoking. Other risk factors (in addition to DM) include HTN, elevated LDL, and elevated triglyceride level. This disease results in ischemia with ulceration, polymicrobial infection, and gangrene of the lower extremities.

4. **Diabetic neuropathy** (see chapter 9).

   a. **Diabetic polyneuropathy** is the most common type of neuropathy and results in distal pain, numbness, hyperesthesias, and variable weakness and muscle wasting. Other conditions, such as vitamin B_{12} deficiency, uremia, and alcohol abuse, must be excluded before diagnosis can be made. Polyneuropathy is closely associated with poor glycemic control and often improves with tight control of serum glucose. For pain management, low-dose tricyclic antidepressants (e.g., amitriptyline, nortriptyline), topical capsaicin, carbamazepine, and gabapentin (Neurontin) are options. Screening can be done using a 10 g monofilament nylon, which is sensitive for early peripheral neuropathy.

   b. **Mononeuropathies** manifest as sudden onset of a deficit (motor, sensory, or pain) in the distribution of single or multiple large nerves, most commonly in the femoral, sciatic, and peroneal nerves, usually with complete recovery within a few months. The cranial nerves may be involved; pupillary function is usually spared with third nerve palsy.

   c. **Autonomic neuropathy** may affect the cardiovascular reflexes, gastrointestinal function (diabetic gastroparesis, gastric atony), or genitourinary function. Symptoms may include syncope, resting tachycardia, nausea, vomiting, impotence, neurogenic bladder, diarrhea, and urinary or fecal incontinence. Orthostatic hypotension may be treated with fludrocortisone, 0.1 to 0.3 mg/day, or with NaCl 1 to 4 g PO QID (may cause fluid overload). Midodrine has also been approved for orthostatic hypotension, and fluoxetine (Prozac) and venlafaxine (Effexor) may also be used; care must be taken to avoid recumbent hypertension. Gastroparesis may be treated with metoclopramide 10 mg 1/2 hour AC and HS. Erythromycin has also been used to promote gastric emptying but has more drug interactions.

   d. **Diabetic amyotrophy** is a rare complication of DM with proximal muscle weakness and pain, most commonly involving the pelvic girdle. Onset may be rapid, and the patient may have a low-grade fever and an elevated ESR. Prognosis for improvement is good over months. Diabetic patients may also suffer spontaneous muscle infarctions that can be seen on MRI.

5. **Neuropathic arthropathy** (Charcot's joint). Degenerative changes of the joints of the feet and ankles that occasionally progresses to complete joint destruction. This is frequently a painless process secondary to recurrent trauma, which may have gone unnoticed by the patient.

6. **Diabetic foot problems.** Diabetic foot problems caused by sensory neuropathies, arthropathies, and peripheral vascular disease make care of diabetic foot important. **Compulsive attention to the feet does more to prevent amputations than any other factor.** Feet should be inspected daily for ulceration, and shoes must be properly fitted. Foot ulcers commonly become infected, and osteomyelitis may also develop. Staphylococci and streptococci are the most common pathogens, but gram-negative and anaerobic bacteria may also be involved. For early infection, can use cefotaxime. If patient is septic, consider imipenem, ticarcillin-clavulanate, or clindamycin and fluoroquinolones. Aggressive therapy with dressing changes and debridement is essential. Surgical revascularization should be considered if indicated. Amputation of the foot is occasionally necessary. See 4a above.

7. **Diabetic retinopathy** is the leading cause of blindness in the United States. In nonproliferative retinopathy, the findings include microaneurysms, punctate retinal hemorrhages, hard exudates, soft exudates ("cotton wool" spots), microvascular anomalies, and macular edema. With proliferative retinopathy, new vessels and fibrous tissue grow along the posterior surface of the vitreous; this may lead to contraction of the vitreous, causing traction on the vessels and on the retina, resulting in vitreous hemorrhages and retinal detachment. Diabetics should be evaluated annually by an ophthalmologist.

8. **Summary of diabetic follow-up** (Table 6-7).

TABLE 6-7

SUMMARY OF DIABETIC FOLLOW-UP

Follow-up	IDDM	NIDDM
Eye exam by ophthalmologist	5 years after diagnosis and then every year	At time of diagnosis and every year thereafter
HbA$_{1c}$	Every 3 months	Every 3 months
Blood pressure	Every visit	Every visit
Foot check	Every visit (use 10 g monofilament nylon)	Every visit (use 10 g monofilament nylon)
Urine microalbumin	Every 6 months to 1 year after 12 years of age	Every 6 months to 1 year

III. **Diabetic Ketoacidosis.**
A. **Overview.** When severe insulin deficiency occurs, a starvation-like state develops with breakdown of free fatty acids and increasing blood levels of acetoacetic acid, beta-hydroxybutyric acid, and acetone, resulting in acidosis. This occurs predominantly in type I DM but can occur in anyone who requires insulin to control glucose.
B. **Causes.** DKA frequently results from intercurrent infection, poor compliance with insulin, or dehydration.
C. **Evaluation.**
   1. **Symptoms.** Mental status changes, rapid respirations (to compensate for acidosis), acetone ("fruity") odor of breath, nausea and vomiting, dehydration, and a history of diabetes (unless first presentation). Frequently complain of abdominal pain.
   2. **Hyperglycemia** can be diagnosed with rapid blood glucose determination, and ketosis can be determined with bedside reagents. Urine ketone dipstick is 97% sensitive for serum ketones. These and the symptoms are adequate for initiation of treatment.
   3. **Additional laboratory evaluation** should include true glucose, serum ketones, electrolytes, BUN, creatinine, serum osmolarity, and arterial blood gases. CXR, urine and C&S, blood cultures should also be done. Be aware of hypokalemia and hypomagnesemia; acidosis will give a spuriously elevated potassium.
D. **Treatment.**
   1. **Acute management (adults).**
      a. **Supportive therapy.** Airway maintenance, supplemental oxygen as needed, and treatment of shock.
      b. **Fluid.** Initially 1 L of normal saline should be given over a half hour if no cardiac compromise is present. The rate should then be decreased to 1 L/hr if patient is clinically stable. This will result in a decrease of the blood glucose and restoration of adequate renal perfusion. If cardiac compromise is present, central venous pressure monitoring is indicated to guide fluid resuscitation.

TABLE 6-8

POTASSIUM REPLACEMENT IN ACIDOTIC ADULTS*

If Serum K+ (mEq/dl)	mEq/hr KCl in NS
<3	40
3-4	30
4-5	20
5-6	10
>6	0

*Rough guideline only. Use clinical judgment!

c. **Potassium replacement** in acidotic adults (Table 6-8). Monitor potassium; use judgment. This is only a guide.

d. **Insulin** (0.1 U/kg IV): 5 to 10 U of regular insulin IV bolus in adults can be given with the initial fluid resuscitation. However, a bolus is not necessary and one can start with an insulin infusion of 3 to 10 U/hr (or more if needed), adjusted according to subsequent glucose and electrolyte determinations. The ideal rate of fall in serum glucose is not greater than 100 mg/dl/hr. If the glucose fails to fall by at least 10%, insulin infusion should be increased each hour until response occurs. When blood glucose reaches a range of 250 to 300 mg/dl, glucose should be added to IV fluids so that infusing solution includes 10% glucose ($D_{10}W$). Insulin infusion should be adjusted if needed to maintain glucose level but should not be stopped. **It is preferable to give $D_{10}W$ with the infusion rather than stop the insulin because insulin is still required to clear the acidosis and ketotic state.**

e. **Bicarbonate** is controversial but may be indicated for coma, arterial pH of less than 7.0, or severe hyperkalemia. May be administered with one of the initial liters of fluid by mixing of two ampules of bicarbonate (88 mEq) in a liter of 0.45% saline, which is substituted for one of the liters of normal saline. Bicarbonate may induce hypokalemia and does not change outcomes.

f. **Monitor serum glucose and potassium** as well as urine output hourly. If bicarbonate therapy was administered, arterial blood gases should also be followed. Otherwise monitor acidosis by following plasma bicarbonate levels.

g. **Phosphate supplementation** may be required if patient is not able to initiate oral intake within first few hours. Potassium phosphate (4 mEq of K+ per 93 mg of phosphorus) may be added to maintenance fluids if necessary. Should not exceed total dose of 20 mEq K+, and great caution is required with renal insufficiency.

h. **Magnesium.** Should replace. Can give magnesium sulfate 2.5 g in 50 ml of NS over first hour.

i. **Maintenance fluids** should consist of 0.45% saline with additives as indicated; 150 to 200 ml/hr adjusted according to urine output.

    j. **Evaluate for potential precipitating factors,** including infection, pregnancy, MI, inappropriate use of insulin.

    k. **Diet.** Oral intake may resume when mental status and nausea and vomiting allow. Initial diet should consist of fluids, and full diet is not resumed until ketoacidosis is corrected.

2. **For children.** Avoid too rapid glucose lowering or overcorrection to prevent CNS injury. Be judicious with fluids as well.

    a. Assume 10% to 15% deficit (100 to 150 ml/kg). Goal is to replace 50% in first 8 hours.

      (1) For first hour give 20 ml/kg boluses of normal saline until patient out of shock.

      (2) Hours 2 to 8. Give enough normal saline to replace 50% total deficit taking into account percentage already replaced in first hour. Change to D_5W 0.5 NS when serum glucose <250 mg/dl.

      (3) Hours 9 to 24. Use 0.3 to 0.5 NS to replace remaining deficit (50% of baseline deficit) plus maintenance fluids (see Chapter 12 for additional information on pediatric fluid management).

    b. In most children, a bolus of regular insulin 0.1 U/kg followed by 0.1 U/kg/hr is a good starting point. Again, a bolus is optional.

IV. **Hyperglycemic-Hyperosmolar Nonketotic Syndrome.**

A. **Overview.** Severe hyperglycemia leads to mental status changes and dehydration with absence of serum ketones; occurs primarily in type 2 diabetics.

B. **Causes.** Hyperglycemic-hyperosmolar nonketonic syndrome occurs because of osmotic diuresis from severe hyperglycemia with elevation of plasma osmolarity, dehydration, and hypernatremia.

C. **Evaluation.**

    1. **Symptoms.** Mental status changes, obtundation or coma, dehydration or shock.

    2. **Laboratory studies.** Serum glucose, ketones, osmolarity, electrolytes, BUN, creatinine, and arterial blood gases. ECG should also be obtained. Treatment should not be delayed pending the results of these studies.

D. **Treatment.**

    1. **Acute management.**

      a. **Supportive measures** to provide adequate airway and ventilation and treatment of shock.

      b. **Fluid.** Initial therapy should be with normal saline at 1 L/hr until intravascular volume is restored. If hypernatremia is present, this may be switched to 0.45% saline. Caution must be exercised in the setting of renal impairment, CHF, possible MI.

      c. **Insulin.** Treatment is initiated with 5 to 10 U of regular IV bolus for serum glucose greater than 600 mg/dl and begin insulin drip as above under DKA.

2. **Long-term management.**
    a. **Monitor** glucose and electrolytes initially every hour. Urine output should be monitored continuously (via Foley catheter). ABGs should be followed if bicarbonate is given. Serum osmolarity should be checked every 2 to 3 hours initially to aid in fluid therapy.
    b. **Fluid.** After intravascular volume is restored, therapy should be guided by electrolyte determinations. Generally 0.45% saline will be appropriate. If significant hypernatremia is present, the initial resuscitation with 0.45% saline should be followed by 0.2% saline or D5W. Fluid should be administered at 150 ml/hr, adjusted according to vitals and urine output.
    c. **Electrolytes.** Potassium depletion may occur, and supplementation should be provided if levels approach low normal; 10 mEq/hr of KCl initially, adjusted accordingly.
    d. **Insulin.** After initial bolus, constant infusion should be started at 5 to 10 U of regular insulin per hour. Gradual decline in blood glucose (around 75 mg/dl/hr) is the desired goal. Glucose should be added to the maintenance fluids when blood glucose drops to the 200 to 300 mg/dl range.
    e. Patient should be evaluated for possible precipitating causes, including infection, MI, stroke.

HYPERTHYROIDISM

I. **Definition.** Hyperthyroidism is a disease caused by high levels of circulating thyroid hormone.
II. **Etiology.** Common causes of hyperthyroidism include:
A. **Graves' disease.** Most common cause of hyperthyroidism in the third and fourth decades. Causes a diffuse, symmetrically enlarged thyroid gland with normal to slightly soft consistency and possibly pretibial myxedema. The classic infiltrative ophthalmopathy may occur with or without overt hyperthyroidism.
B. **Toxic multinodular goiter.** Results in an irregular, asymmetric, nodular thyroid gland. It usually develops insidiously in the sixth or seventh decade in a patient who has had a nontoxic nodular goiter for years. A thyroid scan may be useful in establishing the diagnosis.
C. **Solitary hyperfunctioning adenomas.** Usually occur during the fourth and fifth decades. The thyroid gland contains a smooth, well-defined, soft to firm nodule that shows intense radioactive uptake on scan with absence of uptake in the rest of the gland. Most patients with solitary adenomas do not become thyrotoxic. When they do, they are usually less toxic than those with Graves' disease, and they do not develop ophthalmopathy or pretibial myxedema.
D. **Autoimmune thyroiditis.** Normal-sized or enlarged nontender thyroid gland. Thyroid antibodies, when present, are high in titer. ^{131}I uptake is suppressed or zero. This disorder improves spontaneously but frequently

6

HEMATOLOGIC, ELECTROLYTE, AND METABOLIC DISORDERS

recurs. Autoimmune thyroiditis, painless thyroiditis, lymphocytic thyroiditis, and Hashimoto's thyroiditis are probably all the same disorder.

E. **Excess exogenous thyroid.** May occur because of dosage errors or occasionally in individuals taking large doses of thyroid hormones to lose weight or increase their energy. The thyroid gland is normal or small in size, and ^{131}I uptake is suppressed.

F. **Subacute thyroiditis and viral thyroiditis.** Tender, diffusely enlarged thyroid gland with a normal or elevated T_4, a depressed ^{131}I uptake, and an elevated ESR. Probably of viral origin and may manifest as a sore throat.

G. **Rare causes.** Radiation thyroiditis, thyroid carcinoma, excessive TSH stimulation, excessive iodine intake, struma ovarii, and trophoblastic disease.

III. **Evaluation.**

A. **Symptoms.** Patients may have nervousness, heat intolerance, palpitations, tachycardia, weight loss, weakness, dyspnea on exertion (also CHF), emotional lability, poor concentration, itching and burning of eyes, fullness in the throat, diarrhea, and dysmenorrhea or amenorrhea. Diarrhea is a bad sign and can herald the onset of thyroid storm. Frequently geriatric patients may show withdrawal or depression (apathetic hyperthyroidism).

B. **Laboratory evaluation of hyperthyroidism.**

1. **Ultrasensitive TSH.** Best method for diagnosing hyperthyroidism. Will be decreased in response to increased circulating thyroid hormone in 98%.

2. **Free T_4.** A measure of the active thyroid hormone, unaffected by changes in the thyroxine-binding globulin (TBG), free T_4 will be elevated in most cases of hyperthyroidism.

3. **Total T_4.** Measurement affected by increases in TBG. Therefore elevated total T_4 is not sensitive or specific. Total T_4 will be elevated in states that increase the TBG, including pregnancy, estrogen therapy and oral contraceptives, infectious hepatitis, cirrhosis, breast carcinoma, hypothyroidism, acute intermittent porphyria.

4. **Free T_4 index.** Corrects the total T_4 for the serum TBG to allow one to estimate the free T_4.

5. **Free T_3/T_3 RIA.** About 5% of hyperthyroid individuals will have a normal T_4 level but an elevated T_3 level, indicating an isolated T_3 hyperthyroidism. If the patient is clinically hyperthyroid but the free T_4 is normal, checking a T_3 RIA is prudent.

6. **Antithyroid antibodies** (antimicrosomal antibody and antifollicular cell antibody, antithyroglobulin antibody, thyroid-stimulating antibody). Elevated especially in autoimmune thyroiditis (such as Hashimoto's thyroiditis). May be slightly elevated in other thyroid diseases.

IV. **Treatment.**

A. **Graves' disease.**

1. **Propylthiouracil** 100 to 150 mg every 8 hours, **or methimazole** 15 to 60 mg divided BID or TID every 12 hours depending on severity

of illness. Clinical improvement may be seen in 1 to 2 weeks, and the patient becomes euthyroid 2 to 3 months after beginning therapy. Propylthiouracil may achieve results faster because it prevents the peripheral conversion of T_4 to active T_3. After the euthyroid state is reached, the medication dose should be decreased by a third every few months if the patient remains euthyroid. A free T_4 level should be checked after 1 month of therapy and then every 2 to 3 months. These drugs are usually continued for 6 months to 1 year. Low-dose thyroxine may be needed during therapy. A significant number of patients will experience permanent remission of hyperthyroidism after discontinuing these medications. Side effects (which are more common with PTU) include rashes, agranulocytosis, thrombocytopenia, anemia, hepatitis, arthritis, fever. WBC count and liver enzymes should be obtained before drug therapy is started and rechecked after 1 month and 3 months of treatment; after that recheck labs only if new symptoms arise. These drugs cause no permanent thyroid damage.

2. **Inorganic iodine** rapidly controls hyperthyroidism by inhibiting hormone synthesis and release from the gland. One drop of saturated potassium iodide solution in juice is taken daily. This should not be used as the sole form of therapy. It may be used alone for 7 to 10 days before surgery to decrease the vascularity of the thyroid gland. It should not be used for at least 3 days after ^{131}I therapy but thereafter may be used alone until the ^{131}I becomes effective.

3. **Levothyroxine.** Despite initially positive data, it is unlikely that routine use of levothyroxine during treatment reduces the recurrence of Graves' disease.

4. **Propranolol,** 80 to 200 mg/day in divided doses Q6h, will reduce symptoms of tachycardia, palpitations, heat intolerance, and nervousness but will not normalize the metabolic rate. It should not be used alone except in the case of transient hyperthyroidism secondary to autoimmune (viral) thyroiditis.

5. **Iodine 131,** 5 to 15 mCi, renders most patients euthyroid within 3 to 6 months. Therefore treatment should be preceded and followed by antithyroid therapy. Most will eventually become hypothyroid. Pregnancy is an absolute contraindication to ^{131}I therapy.

6. **Surgery.** Usually reserved for those who are unable to take antithyroid drugs.

7. **Ophthalmopathy.** Smoking can worsen opthalmopathy. Ophthalmopathy may also worsen (usually transiently) with radioactive iodine. This can be prevented by treatment with prednisone (0.5 mg/kg PO for 3 months starting 2 to 3 days after radioactive iodine). However, this carries the risk of prednisone exposure. Symptomatic treatment for ophthalmopathy includes artificial tears or methylcellulose drops for the discomfort, patching or prisms for diplopia, diuretics and raising the head of the bed for circumorbital edema.

6

HEMATOLOGIC, ELECTROLYTE, AND METABOLIC DISORDERS

B. **Toxic multinodular** goiter is treated with ^{131}I or surgery. Antithyroid drugs will not induce permanent remission and should be used only as interim therapy. Large multinodular goiters do not respond well to [131]I. Hypothyroidism is rare after ^{131}I therapy for toxic multinodular goiter because normal thyroid tissue is suppressed as a result of the disease and does not take up [131]I.

C. **Solitary hyperfunctioning adenomas** are treated with ^{131}I or surgery with antithyroid drugs used only as interim therapy when needed. Hypothyroidism is rare after therapy.

D. **Autoimmune thyroiditis** is transient and does not require definitive treatment except in those patients with recurrent hyperthyroidism. Propranolol may be used alone if symptoms are mild. Antithyroid drugs may be needed for a short time in some patients.

E. **Subacute thyroiditis** and viral thyroiditis generally self-limited but should be treated with aspirin 650 mg QID. In more severe cases, prednisone may be used at 40 mg PO QD, tapering to 10 mg each day over 2 weeks, and then continued for 1 month after patient becomes asymptomatic. Resolution of symptoms usually occurs in 1 to 6 months, and relapse is common. Hypothyroidism may occur but is rare.

THYROID STORM

I. **Overview.** A severe life-threatening form of hyperthyroidism.

II. **Cause.** Increasing stress such as trauma or illness may cause this in a previously mildly hyperthyroid patient.

III. **Clinically.** Have signs and symptoms consistent with thyrotoxicosis (tachycardia, heat intolerance, weight loss), as well as fever, confusion, agitation, weakness, dyspnea, diarrhea, and shock.

IV. **Treatment.**

A. **When suspected, treatment should be instituted immediately.** If defervescence of fever does not occur within several hours, concurrent infection should be suspected. Other signs of hyperthyroidism may require several days of therapy before improvement is seen.

B. **Treatment is propranolol** 20 to 40 mg Q4h to control tachycardia, tremor, etc. (can give 0.5 to 1.0 mg IV Q5min to keep pulse about 100; may need greater than 15 mg IV). Give propylthiouracil 250 mg PO or per NG Q6h (alternative is methimazole 20 to 40 mg PO or per NG Q6-8h) and SSKI 30 gtt PO 1 hour after giving PTU to avoid iodine being used for additional thyroid hormone synthesis. Continue with 5 to 10 gtt QID. Alternative is 0.5 g of sodium iodide in 1 L of NS over 12 hours. Fluid and electrolytes should be replaced and fever controlled with acetaminophen and a cooling blanket.

C. **Avoid aspirin** because it may increase circulating active T_3 and T_4 by reducing protein binding.

D. **Give steroids** equivalent to about 300 mg of hydrocortisone per day (100 mg IV Q8h). Dexamethasone has some theoretical advantage because it prevents conversion of T_4 to T_3 peripherally. (This would be about 11.25 mg of dexamethasone divided TID.)

HYPOTHYROIDISM

I. **Overview.**
A. **Definition.** *Primary hypothyroidism* refers to a thyroid hormone deficiency as a result of thyroid gland disease. *Secondary hypothyroidism* results from TSH deficiency. *Tertiary hypothyroidism* results from thyrotropin-releasing hormone (TRH) deficiency.
B. **Prevalence.** Present in 1% to 6% of population.
II. **Etiology.**
A. **Without thyroid enlargement.** Commonly caused by ^{131}I therapy, thyroidectomy for hyperthyroidism. The second most common cause is idiopathic hypothyroidism. Developmental defects and TSH or TRH deficiency are less common causes.
B. **With thyroid enlargement.** Most commonly caused by Hashimoto's thyroiditis. Drugs, iodine deficiency, and inherited defects in thyroid hormone synthesis are rare causes.
III. **Evaluation.**
A. **Signs and symptoms.** Fatigue, weakness, slow movement, cold intolerance, constipation, hair loss, menorrhagia, carpal tunnel syndrome, dry skin, edema of the face and extremities, memory impairment, hearing loss, hoarseness, and occasionally bradycardia and hypothermia. Sparse eyebrows with loss of the lateral half is a nonspecific sign. Pericardial effusion and ascites occasionally occur. A delay in the relaxation phase of the deep tendon reflexes, especially at the ankles, is a specific finding. May have myalgias and arthralgias. Psychosis may develop with long-standing hypothyroidism and may be precipitated by thyroid hormone replacement. Infants may have hypotonia, umbilical hernia, delayed mental and physical development, and other signs and symptoms typical of adult patients. Mental retardation may result if hypothyroidism goes untreated in the first few years of life.
B. **Laboratory findings.** Low free T_4 (see hyperthyroidism for a discussion of thyroid tests). A low TSH value indicates secondary (pituitary) or tertiary (hypothalamic) hypothyroidism, whereas a high TSH value is diagnostic of primary thyroid failure. The ^{131}I uptake is not helpful. Other laboratory abnormalities may include high AST, low sodium, low blood glucose, elevated CPK, elevated cholesterol and triglycerides, mild anemia, elevated prolactin levels secondary to high TRH levels, and flat or inverted T waves with minor ST-segment depression and low amplitude on ECG.
IV. **Treatment.** Treatment is by levothyroxine with the average daily dose being 0.1 to 0.15 mg every day. Patients over 40 years of age or those with heart disease should be started on one fourth to one third (0.025 mg) of this dose with increases every 2 to 4 weeks until a

6

HEMATOLOGIC, ELECTROLYTE, AND METABOLIC DISORDERS

maintenance dose is reached. The goal is to normalize the TSH. Check the TSH 2 to 3 months after changing the levothyroxine dose. Elective surgery should be avoided in hypothyroid patients because respiratory depression commonly occurs. Increased sensitivity to narcotics and hypnotics is also common in the hypothyroid patient. Small doses of T_3 may be helpful for patients with a normal TSH who are still symptomatic.

MYXEDEMA COMA

I. **Overview.** Myxedema coma occurs with severe chronic hypothyroidism and is life threatening.
II. **Etiology.** The coma is precipitated in chronically hypothyroid patients by exposure to cold, infection, hypoglycemia, respiratory depressants, allergic reactions, or other metabolic stress.
III. **Treatment.**
A. 500 μg of thyroxine (T_4) IV followed by oral thyroxine 0.1 mg QD. May substitute 40 μg of T_3 IV for the IV T_4 if available.
B. Hyponatremia and hypoglycemia frequently occur and should be treated appropriately.
C. Hypothermia and heat loss should be avoided.

THYROID ENLARGEMENT

I. **Goiter.** A goiter is a simple enlargement of the thyroid gland. It is more common in females with the highest incidence in the second through sixth decades of life.
A. Diffuse goiters are caused by iodine deficiency or excess, congenital defects in thyroid hormone synthesis, and drugs (e.g., lithium carbonate).
B. Most are asymptomatic. It is unusual to have pain and rare to have hoarseness and tracheal obstruction. Thyroid function tests should be performed on all patients with goiter because it can be associated with hypothyroidism, euthyroidism, or hyperthyroidism.
II. **Multinodular Goiter.** Multinodular enlargement of the thyroid gland.
A. **Cause:** most often caused by iodine deficiency.
B. **Clinical presentation.**
   1. **Symptoms.** Thyromegaly, occasionally with rapid enlargement and tenderness secondary to hemorrhage into a cyst. Rarely, tracheal compression may occur, causing coughing or choking. Some patients may complain of a lump in the throat.
   2. **Physical exam.** Many nodules of varying sizes are usually palpable. Occasionally it may be difficult to distinguish from the typically lobulated, irregular Hashimoto's gland.
   3. **Thyroid function tests.** Performed to rule out toxicity. A thyroid scan is useful only if the diagnosis of multinodular goiter is in doubt based on physical exam. A scan will show a patchy radioisotope distribution. Malignancy is rare but should be considered if the gland is enlarging rapidly or hoarseness develops.

C. **Treatment.** The main indications for treatment are compression of the trachea or esophagus and venous-outflow obstruction. For nontoxic multinodular goiter, the treatments include surgery, radioiodine, or thyroxine therapy. Oversuppression of the TSH can cause bone demineralization. For toxic multinodular goiter, options are antithyroid agent, surgery, radioiodine, and more recently percutaneous injection of ethanol. Levothyroxine suppression should not be given to patients with angina or other known heart disease unless the patient is hypothyroid. If thyroid enlargement persists despite adequate TSH suppression, a needle biopsy or subtotal thyroidectomy should be considered.

III. **Solitary Nodules.**

A. **Usually benign.** Suspect malignancy in a patient with a history of radiation exposure, rapid enlargement, hoarseness or obstruction, and a solid nodule that is cold on scan.

B. **Diagnosis.** History and a thyroid scan should be done on every patient with a solitary nodule. Hot nodules that take up the radioisotope are generally benign but fine-needle aspiration of a solitary nodule is prudent.

C. **Treatment** is indicated if signs of compression of trachea, esophagus, significant growth, and recurrence of a cystic nodule after aspiration. Similar to multinodular goiter: surgery, thyroxine, or radioiodine for nontoxic nodule; antithyroid agent, surgery, radioiodine for toxic nodule. Suppressive therapy with levothyroxine is usually not effective, however.

IV. **Subacute Thyroiditis.** Causes diffuse enlargement of the thyroid gland and may be associated with hyperthyroidism, hypothyroidism, or euthyroidism. See section on hyperthyroidism for the discussion of this entity.

V. **Euthyroid Sick Syndrome.** There is decreased peripheral conversion of T_4 to active T_3. Labs show a decreased serum T_3, an increased reverse T_3, a decreased T_4, and a normal TSH. Patients are euthyroid but suffering from chronic disease.

ADRENAL DISEASE

I. **Hypoadrenalism (Addison's Disease).**

A. **Etiology.** Most idiopathic (autoimmune), others from adrenal destruction (neoplasm, TB, amyloidosis, inflammatory necrosis), iatrogenic (discontinuation of steroids, ketoconazole, other drugs). Primary Addison's: from adrenal destruction. Secondary Addison's: from pituitary destruction. Those with pituitary Addison's are more tolerant to metabolic stress because mineralocorticoids are intact.

B. **Clinically.**
   1. Weakness, fatigue, orthostatic hypotension.
   2. Hyperpigmentation, freckling (**not with central hypoadrenalism;** requires elevated ACTH to stimulate melanocytes).
   3. Nausea, weight loss, dehydration, hypotension, small heart size.
   4. Decreased cold tolerance, hypometabolism.

C. **Diagnosis.**

1. **Serum Na** <130 mEq/L, K >5 mEq/L, elevated BUN and creatinine. May be hypoglycemic. **Electrolytes may be normal, especially in central hypoadrenalism.** Electrolyte abnormalities are secondary to loss of aldosterone, which occurs only with adrenal destruction.
2. **Low fasting A.M. cortisol.**
3. **Cosyntropin stimulation test.** Get baseline cortisol level.
   a. Give cosyntropin 0.25 mg IV before 9:00 A.M.
   b. Cortisol should increase from baseline value of 5 to 25 μg/dl and be doubled by 60 to 90 minutes. Any level of >20 μg/dl is considered normal responsiveness. If still suspect hypoadrenalism, do metyrapone test.
4. **Metyrapone test.** Get baseline serum cortisol value.
   a. Administer 3 g of metyrapone orally at midnight.
   b. Measure cortisol and deoxycortisol at 8:00 A.M. the next day. If the pituitary-adrenal axis is intact, the plasma cortisol level should be less than 5 mg/dl and the 11-deoxycortisol level greater than 10 mg/dl.
   c. Measure serum ACTH. Will be elevated if primary adrenal failure; will be normal or low if primary pituitary failure.

D. **Treatment.**
1. **Emergency.** *Institute therapy immediately.*
   a. Administer hydrocortisone succinate 100 mg IV push and another 100 mg in NS over the next 2 hours and a total of 300 mg hydrocortisone succinate IV over the first 24 hours.
   b. Administer NS IV to correct hypotension and shock.
2. **Long-term therapy.**
   a. Hydrocortisone succinate 150 mg IV over the second 24 hours.
   b. Hydrocortisone succinate 75 mg IV over the third 24 hours.
   c. Maintenance doses are hydrocortisone 30 mg PO QD plus fludrocortisone acetate 0.1 mg PO QD.

II. **Hyperadrenalism (Cushing's Disease).**
A. **Cause.** Administration of exogenous steroids, ACTH secretion by pituitary or extrapituitary source (such as small cell carcinoma of lung).
B. **Clinically.** Moon facies, plethora, truncal obesity with wasted extremities, atrophic skin with senile purpura, abdominal striae, poor wound healing, hypertension, glucose intolerance, psychiatric symptoms.
C. **Diagnosis.**
1. **Elevated A.M. fasting cortisol and lack of diurnal variation.**
2. **Check 24-hour free cortisol in urine** (usually >150 μg/24 hr in Cushing's). 17-OHS not helpful because of false positive in obesity.
3. **Dexamethasone test.**
   a. Administer dexamethasone 1 mg PO at midnight. Measure serum cortisol at 7:00 A.M. the next day. Should be <5 μg/dl.
   b. If this is equivocal, can give dexamethasone 0.5 mg PO Q6h for 2 days. If the patient has Cushing's disease, there will not be a decrease of urinary free cortisol.

c. Can also administer dexamethasone IV 1 mg/hr for 7 hours by constant infusion. At the end of this time, a normal person should have reduced plasma cortisol by at least 7 mg/dl over baseline value.

2. Further diagnosis and therapy should be done under the guidance of an endocrinologist.

ACID-BASE DISORDERS

I. **Metabolic Acidosis.**

A. **Definition.** pH <7.4 and implies a loss of bicarbonate or accumulation of fixed acids. Divided into two groups based on the calculated anion gap (Na − [Cl + Bicarb]) normal up to 12. Compensatory response is hyperventilation with drop in P_{CO_2}.

B. **Normal anion-gap acidosis.**

1. **GI bicarbonate (HCO_3^-) losses**, including causes relating to diarrhea, ileostomy, and colostomy.

2. **Renal tubular acidosis (RTA).**

a. **Distal (type I) RTA.** Will be hypokalemic with urine pH >5.3. Caused by distal nephron acidification defect. Causes include familial and idiopathic hypercalciuria, Sjögren's syndrome, rheumatoid arthritis, primary hyperparathyroidism, multiple myeloma, and severe dehydration. Also lithium, amphotericin B, and toluene. Occasionally seen is a hyperkalemic form with SLE, obstructive uropathy, or sickle cell uropathy. Treat with bicarbonate repletion at 1 to 2 mEq/kg/day with any acute K^+ deficit corrected and maintenance oral K^+ if needed.

b. **Proximal (type II) RTA.** Caused by a defect in the ability of proximal tubules to recover bicarbonate. Acutely the urine pH is usually >5.5, but it decreases with falling serum bicarbonate levels, resulting in increased proximal reabsorption of bicarbonate; final result is pH 5.5. Causes include autoimmune diseases (as in type I RTA), multiple myeloma, heavy metals, acetazolamide, and outdated tetracycline. Treatment is to identify the primary cause and treat it. Bicarbonate at 5 to 15 mEq/kg/day may be required and can result in severe hypokalemia. Consider use of thiazide diuretics to cause ECF volume contraction to promote HCO_3^- reabsorption proximally.

c. **Type IV RTA.** Generally caused by moderate renal insufficiency with renal resistance to aldosterone (as in diabetes). Similar presentation to hyporeninemic hypoaldosteronism. K^+ may be normal but generally is increased. Bicarbonate will typically be >15 mEq/L. Urine pH, done under mineral oil at time of collection, is usually <5.5. Treat with K^+ restriction and consider use of loop diuretics such as furosemide (Lasix and others). Bicarbonate may be needed (see above for dosing). Fludrocortisone (Florinef) at 0.1 to 0.2 mg PO QD may be useful if primary adrenal insufficiency is the cause.

6

HEMATOLOGIC, ELECTROLYTE, AND METABOLIC DISORDERS

3. **Interstitial renal disease.** Same as type IV RTA; serum K^+ is increased.
4. **Ureterosigmoid loop.**
5. **Ingestion of acetazolamide,** ammonium chloride, cholestyramine, calcium chloride, or magnesium chloride.
6. **Small bowel drainage** or fistula, biliary drainage or fistula, or pancreatic drainage or fistulas.
7. **Calculating the urine ion gap** (urine Na + urine K − urine Cl) may help determine if acidosis is renal related. A **normal gap** implies normal renal NH_4^+ excretion and a nonrenal cause for the acidosis. An **abnormal (e.g., elevated) positive gap** denotes the opposite. Caveat: Only valid in absence of diuretics. Also, if volume depleted secondary to GI losses, may be a false-positive urine ion gap.

C. **Increased anion-gap acidosis.**
   1. **Methanol.**
   2. **Uremia** or renal failure.
   3. **Lactic acidosis.**
   4. **Ethanol** or ethylene glycol (antifreeze).
   5. **Paraldehyde.**
   6. **Alcoholic ketoacidosis** or diabetic ketoacidosis.
   7. **Others.** Salicylates, cyanide (may be caused by nitroprusside). Can measure for these substances directly, but the first step is to determine the osmolal gap as noted previously. Treatment depends on the underlying condition.

D. **Treatment.** Acidosis will usually resolve with aggressive IV hydration and correction the underlying disease (e.g., DKA). May consider sodium bicarbonate therapy if severe acidemia (blood PH <7.1, bicarbonate <8 mmol/L) However, there is little evidence that bicarbonate changes outcomes.

II. **Metabolic Alkalosis.**

A. **Definition.** Serum pH >7.40. Implies a loss of acid or gain of bicarbonate. ECF volume contraction, hypokalemia, and increased mineralocorticoids or glucocorticoids all impair the normal kidney's ability to excrete excess HCO_3^- and may result in a metabolic alkalosis. Additionally, excess exogenous bicarbonate should be in the differential. Metabolic alkalosis is separated into the two categories of chloride responsive and non–chloride responsive. The urinary Cl^- level is measured to help differentiate the causes of metabolic alkalosis. ECF contraction is usually rapid and because of overzealous diuretic use is commonly termed *contraction alkalosis*.

B. **Clinical findings.** Carpal-pedal spasms, tetany, neuromuscular irritability, hypotension, hypoventilation, impaired cognition, cardiac arrhythmias, and decreased levels of ionized Ca^{++}.

C. **Diagnosis.** Elevated serum HCO_3^- levels and alkalotic serum pH. There may be a compensatory respiratory acidosis with a decrease in the respiratory rate. The urine may be alkaline or paradoxically acidic, especially in the presence of K^+ wasting (hyperaldosteronism and diuretic use).

D. **Treatment.**

1. **Chloride-responsive alkalosis.** This alkalosis is the more commonly seen form with **urine Cl^- <10 mEq/L.** Usually secondary to contraction alkalosis caused by GI HCl losses (emesis, NG suctioning), or diuretic use. Occasionally seen with villous adenomas or cystic fibrosis. Treat underlying cause and correct concurrent hypokalemia (for IV KCl see section on hypokalemia). Chloride may be administered as NaCl tablets or as 0.9 NS if volume depleted. Use caution in those with CHF and those who are fluid overloaded. Consider acetazolamide if renal function is intact. Some physicians also recommend use of H_2-blockers to decrease gastric HCl losses.

2. **Non–chloride-responsive alkalosis.** Seen in primary hyperaldosteronism, Cushing's syndrome, and renal artery stenosis. Occasionally seen in patients who consume excessive amounts of licorice, or secondary to severe hypokalemia (<2.0 mEq/L) or Bartter's syndrome (see hypokalemia above). The primary treatment is to determine the underlying cause and to correct it. See hypokalemia for treatment of low levels of potassium.

3. **Other rare causes** include massive citrated blood transfusions, hypercalcemia of malignancy, sarcoidosis, vitamin D toxicity, and high-dose penicillin-carbenicillin. Also consider milk-alkali syndrome.

4. If the metabolic alkalosis is severe (pH >7.55 or bicarbonate >45 mmol/L) with systemic effects, consider HCl acid therapy, which is typically done in an ICU setting.

BIBLIOGRAPHY

Adrogue HJ et al: Management of life-threatening acid-base disorders. Part I, *N Engl J Med* 338(2):107, 1998.

Adrogue HJ et al: Management of life-threatening acid-base disorders. Part II, *N Engl J Med* 338(3):108, 1998.

Ayus JC et al: Chronic hyponatremic encephalopathy in postmenopausal women, association of therapies with morbidity and mortality, *JAMA* 281:2299, 1999.

Bailey CJ et al: Metformin, *N Engl J Med* 334(9):547, 1996.

Berkow R et al, editors: *The Merck manual of diagnosis and therapy,* ed 16, Rahway, NJ, 1999, Merck.

Brugnara C et al: Reticulocyte hemoglobin content to diagnose iron deficiency in children, *JAMA* 281:2225, 1999.

Buse JB et al: Troglitazone use in insulin-treated type 2 diabetic patients, *Diabetes Care* 21(9):1455, 1998.

Carey CF, editor: *Manual of medical therapeutics,* ed 29, Boston, 1999, Little, Brown.

Carson JL et al: Perioperative blood transfusion and postoperative mortality, *JAMA* 279:199, 1998.

Chan NN et al: Non-steroidal anti-inflammatory drugs and metformin: a cause for concern? *Lancet* 352:201, 1998.

6

HEMATOLOGIC, ELECTROLYTE, AND METABOLIC DISORDERS

Clinical association recommendations, American Diabetes Association: screening for type 2 diabetes, *Diabetes Care* 21(suppl):s11, 1998.

Coniff RF et al: Reduction of glycosylated hemoglobin and postprandial hyperglycemia by acarbose in patients with NIDDM: a placebo-controlled dose-comparison study, *Diabetes Care* 18(6):817, 1995.

Dale DC, Federman DD, editors: *Scientific American medicine,* New York, 1999, Scientific American.

Davey P et al: Clinical outcomes with insulin lispro compared with human regular insulin: a meta-analysis, *Clin Ther* 19(4):656, 1997.

Davidson MB et al: Relationship between fasting plasma glucose and glycosylated hemoglobin: potential for false-positive diagnoses of type 2 diabetes using new diagnostic criteria, *JAMA* 281(13):1203, 1999.

Diabetes Control and Complications Trial Research Group: The effect of intensive treatment of diabetes on the development and progression of long-term complications of diabetes mellitus, *N Engl J Med* 329(14):977, 1993.

Elizalde JI et al: Early changes in hemoglobin and hematocrit levels after packed red cell transfusion in patients with acute anemia, *Transfusion* 37(6):573, 1997.

Fauci AS et al, editors: *Harrison's principles of internal medicine,* ed 14, New York, 1999, McGraw-Hill.

Gennari FJ: Hypokalemia, *N Engl J Med* 339(7):451, 1998.

Goodman LS, Gilman AG, et al, editors: *The pharmacological basis of therapeutics,* ed 8, New York, 1990, Pergamon Press.

Hebert PC et al: A multicenter, randomized, controlled clinical trial of transfusion requirements in critical care, *N Engl J Med* 340:409, 1999.

Holleman F et al: Reduced frequency of severe hypoglycemia and coma in well-controlled IDDM patients treated with insulin lispro, *Diabetes Care* 1997 20:1827, 1997.

Hord JD et al: Long-term granulocyte-macrophage colony-stimulating factor and immunosuppression in the treatment of acquired severe aplastic anemia, *Pediatr Hematol Oncol* 17(2):140, 1995.

Huysmans DA et al: Treatment of benign nodular thyroid disease, *N Engl J Med* 338(20):1438, 1998.

Kitabchi AE et al: Management of diabetic ketoacidosis, *Am Fam Physician* 60:455, 1999.

Lam KSL et al: Acarbose in NIDDM patients with poor control on conventional oral agents, *Diabetes Care* 21(7):1154, 1998.

Lee G et al: *Wintrobe's clinical hematology,* ed 10, Baltimore, 1999, Lippincott, Williams & Wilkins.

McCartney MM et al: Metformin and contrast media: a dangerous combination? *Clin Radiol* 54:29, 1999.

Moses R et al: Additional treatment with repaglinide provides significant improvement in glycemic control in NIDDM patient poorly controlled on metformin, *Diabetes* 46(suppl):93A, 1997 (abstract).

Panzer RJ et al, editors: *Diagnostic strategies for common medical problems,* Philadelphia, 1991, American College of Physicians.

Rakel RE, Conn HF, editors: *Textbook of family practice,* ed 3, Philadelphia, 1995, Saunders.

Rutledge KS et al: Effectiveness of postprandial Humalog in toddlers with diabetes, *Pediatrics* 100:968, 1997.

Salreil AR: Thiazolidinediones in the treatment of insulin resistance and type II diabetes, *Diabetes* 45(12):1661, 1996.

Sanford JP: *Guide to antimicrobial therapy,* Dallas, 1999, Anti-Microbial Therapy.

Schrier RW: *Renal and electrolyte disorders,* ed 4, Boston, 1992, Little, Brown.

Shumak KH, Rock GA, Nair RC: Late relapses in patients successfully treated for thrombotic thrombocytopenic purpura. Canadian Apheresis Group, *Ann Intern Med* 122(8):569, 1995.

Silverberg SJ et al: A 10-year prospective study of primary hyperparathyroidism with or without parathyroid surgery, *N Engl J Med* 341:1249, 1999.

Steinberg MH: Drug therapy: management of sickle cell disease, *N Engl J Med* 13:340, 1999.

Tierney LM et al, editors: *Current medical diagnosis and treatment,* Stamford, CT, 1999, Appleton & Lange.

Tintinalli JE et al: *Emergency medicine: a comprehensive study guide,* New York, 2000, McGraw-Hill.

United Kingdom prospective diabetes study group: UKPDS 28: a randomized trial of efficacy of early addition of metformin in sulfonylurea-treated type 2 diabetes, *Diabetes Care* 21:87, 1998.

Wallach J: *Interpretation of diagnostic tests: a synopsis of laboratory medicine,* ed 5, Boston, 1992, Little, Brown.

Wei M et al: Effects of diabetes and level of glycemia on all-cause and cardiovascular mortality, the San Antonio Heart Study, *Diabetes Care* 21:1167, 1998.

Wilimas JA et al: A randomized study of outpatient treatment with ceftriaxone for selected febrile children with sickle cell disease, *N Engl J Med* 329(7):472, 1993.

Wyngaarden JB et al, editors: *Cecil textbook of medicine,* ed 19, Philadelphia, 1996, Saunders.

Zoorob RJ et al: Guidelines on the care of diabetes nephropathy, retinopathy and foot disease, *Am Fam Physician* 56:2023, 1997.

6

HEMATOLOGIC, ELECTROLYTE, AND METABOLIC DISORDERS

RHEUMATOLOGY

David C. Krupp
Mark A. Graber

RHEUMATOLOGY: GENERAL

I. Laboratory data can be used to support the diagnosis of a rheumatologic syndrome (Table 7-1). **However, rheumatologic diagnosis is primarily clinical, based on specific criteria outlined in the following sections. The ordering of "arthritis panels" is discouraged because the presence of an antibody in the absence of physical criteria is meaningless.**

RHEUMATOID ARTHRITIS

I. **Overview.** Chronic systemic inflammatory disease principally involving joints but also with extraarticular manifestations. Rheumatoid arthritis (RA) affects 0.03% to 1.5% of the population, with females affected 2 to 3 times more often than males. Life span is decreased on average by 7.5 years for men and 3.5 years for women.

II. **Diagnosis.**

A. To make a diagnosis of RA, at least four of the seven criteria of the American Rheumatology Association (ARA) must be present, and at least one of the first four must be present for at least 6 weeks. Be aware that a positive rheumatoid factor is only one criterion, and a positive rheumatoid factor need not be present for a diagnosis of RA to be made. Additionally, there should not be evidence of other disease that may account for the symptoms, such as polyarteritis nodosa or lupus.

   1. Morning stiffness in and around joints, lasting more than 1 hour.
   2. Arthritis of three or more joint areas involved simultaneously.
   3. Arthritis of at least one area in a wrist, metacarpophalangeal (MCP), or proximal interphalangeal (PIP) joint.
   4. Symmetric arthritis involving the same joint areas.
   5. Rheumatoid nodules.
   6. Positive serum rheumatoid factor.
   7. Radiographic changes typical of RA on hand and wrist radiographs, including erosions, or unequivocal bony decalcification in or adjacent to the involved joints.

B. Most patients have an insidious onset; however, a third of patients experience rapid onset in days or weeks. The disease may be rapidly progressive, causing joint destruction and other sequelae, or may progress slowly; many have a fluctuating course of exacerbations and remissions. Symptoms remit in 70% of women during pregnancy.

III. **Clinical Features.**

A. **Articular movement.**

   1. Synovium (synovial membrane) is the site of onset of inflammation, with proliferation of synovia ("pannus") and inflammatory destruction of soft tissue resulting in laxity of ligaments and tendons. Joint destruction occurs with erosion of juxtaarticular bone around the mar-

TABLE 7-1

LABORATORY PROFILES OF RHEUMATOLOGIC DISEASES

	Rheuma-toid Factor	ANA	Single-Stranded (Denatured) DNA	Anti-native DNA (anti DS-DNA)	Anti Smith	Anti Ro (SSA)
PATTERN OF FLUORESCENCE WITH POSITIVE RESULT						
	N/A	Variable	Negative	DIF ± Rim	SP	SP
DISEASE						
RA	+(90%)	+(40%)	−(20%)	−(<5%)	−	−(<5%)
SLE	−(20%)	+(95%)	+(75%)	+(60%)	−(15%)	−(15%)
Drug-induced SLE	−	+	+(80%)	−	−	−
SS	−(25%)	+(90%)	−	−	−	−
SS-L	−(25%)	+(90%)	−	−	−	−
PM/DM	−(30%)	+(90%)	−	−	−	−
Wegener's granuloma-tosis	+(50%)	−(15%)	−	−	−	−
MCTD	−	−	−	−	−	−
SJOG	+(75%)	+(95%)	−	−	−	+(65%)

+, Positive in most cases; −, negative in most cases (percentages included in parenthesis are an approximation of the percent that are positive); *SP,* Speckled; *DIF,* diffuse; *CENT,* centromeric; *CYTO,* cytoplasmic; *NUC,* nucleolar; *SS,* scleroderma; *SS-L,* scleroderma-limited (CREST syndrome); *SLE,* systemic lupus erythematosus; *RA,* rheumatoid arthritis; *PM/DM,* polymyositis/dermatomyositis; *MCTD,* mixed connective tissue disorder; *SJOG,* Sjogren's syndrome.
*Although 85+ for SLE with cerebritis/psychosis.

gins of pannus and invasion of subchondral tissue by pannus. Can see cysts, loss of cartilage, and bony erosion. Thickened pannus may be palpated around joints, and a joint effusion may be present.

2. The most common sites of joint lesions are MCP and PIP joints and wrists. Distribution is symmetric, and small joints are predominantly involved.

3. **Manifestations in specific joints.**
   a. **Cervical spine.** Frequently affected (40%). This may lead to atlantoaxial subluxation or, less commonly, subluxation at lower levels. Symptoms are those of a radiculopathy, including pain radiating up into the occiput, paresthesia, sudden deterioration in hand function, sensory loss, abnormal gait, and urinary retention or incontinence.
   b. **Joint involvement.**
      (1) Hand involved >85% of patients. May notice fusiform swelling of fingers and MCP joints, ulnar deviation of fingers, palmar subluxation of proximal area of phalanges. Distal inter-

Anti LA (SSB)	Anti-SCL70	Anti-centromere	Anti-Jo	ANCA	Ribosomal RNP	U1nRNP	Histone
SP	DIF + NUC	CENT	CYTO	PANCA CANCA	NUC + CYTO	SP	DIF
−	−	−	−	−	−	−	−(15%)
−(15%)	−	−	−	−	−(10%)*	−(40%)	+(70%)
−	−	−	−	−	−	−	+(90%)
−	−(45%)	−(<1%)	−	−	−	−	−
−	−(10%)	+(50-80%)	−	−	−	−	−
−	−(10%)	−	−(30%)	−	−	−(25%)	−
−	−	−	−	+(>90%)	−	−	−
−	−	−	−	−	−	+(100%)	−
+(65%)	−	−	−	−	−	−	−

PANCA, Perinuclear; *CANCA*, cytoplasmic.

phalangeal (DIP) joints are most often spared. Ulnar deviation at MCP joints often is associated with radial deviation at wrist. Swan-neck and boutonnière deformities are also common.
  (2) Hip involved in 50% of cases.
  (3) Knee involved in 80% of patients.
  (4) Foot and ankle involved in 80% of cases.
  (5) Metatarsophalangeal (MTP), talonavicular, and ankle joints are affected in descending order of frequency.
  c. **Constitutional features.** Fatigue, weight loss, muscle pain, excessive sweating, and low-grade fever are common. Most patients with active disease complain of morning stiffness for more than 1 hour.
B. **Extraarticular complications.**
  1. **Rheumatoid nodules.** Characteristic of RA and seen in up to 25% to 50% of patients, especially those with more severe disease. They occur in the lungs, heart, kidney, and dura mater, in addition to the ex-

tensor surface of the forearm, olecranon, Achilles tendons, and is-chial area. Usually asymptomatic.

2. **Rheumatoid vasculitis.** Usually occurs in patients with severe de-forming arthritis and a high titer of rheumatoid factor. Vasculitic le-sions include rheumatoid nodules, small nail fold infarcts, and palpa-ble purpura. May also manifest by mononeuritis multiplex, organ ischemia, CNS infarctions, MI.

3. **Sjögren's syndrome.** Keratoconjunctivitis sicca is the most common eye complication and results in dry eyes with slight redness and nor-mal vision.

4. **Episcleritis and scleritis.** Eye irritation and pain. May cause vision loss.

5. **Pleuropericarditis or obstructive pulmonary disease including pul-monary nodules.** Diffuse interstitial fibrosis with pneumonitis is com-mon. COPD is more common than in the general public. However, pleural disease is usually asymptomatic; can see subpleural nodules and exudative pleural effusions.

6. **Cardiac.** Symptomatic cardiac disease is not common. Most com-mon type is acute pericarditis, usually in seropositive individuals (unrelated to duration of arthritis). Rheumatoid nodules can in-volve valves and myocardium and may have MI secondary to vasculitis.

7. **Neurologic.** May have entrapment neuropathy secondary to tissue swelling (as in carpal tunnel). Mononeuritis multiplex may occur and is related to ischemic neuropathy from vasculitis.

8. **Miscellaneous.** RA is a common cause of carpal tunnel syndrome.

C. **Laboratory findings.**

1. May have anemia of chronic disease (normochromic or hypochromic, normocytic), thrombocytosis reflecting inflammation, elevated ESR, elevated C-reactive protein, elevated ferritin as acute-phase reactant, low serum iron, low total iron binding capacity, elevated serum globulin.

2. **Presence of rheumatoid factor.** Occurs in 90% of patients but is not specific for the diagnosis of RA. Rheumatoid factor is an immuno-globulin directed against IgG. Generally higher titers are found in those with more generalized disease and destructive arthritis. Extremely high titers are associated with the presence of rheumatoid nodules. False positives occur with infection and lung and liver disease.

3. **Synovial fluid white blood cell count.** 5000 to 20,000/mm³ with 50% to 70% neutrophils; cultures should be negative.

4. **Felty's syndrome.** Combination of (generally severe) seropositive RA, splenomegaly, and leukopenia (WBC <3500/μl). It is associated with serious infections, vasculitis (leg ulcers, mononeuritis), anemia, thrombocytopenia, and lymphadenopathy.

D. **Radiographic findings.** Characteristic changes in RA include periarticular osteoporosis, symmetric narrowing of the joint space, and marginal bone erosions.

IV. **Treatment. It is now clear that early use of disease-modifying drugs, including the judicious use of steroids, decreases joint destruction.**

A. **Education.** The basic treatment program consists of patient education, balancing rest, exercise (often with physical and occupational therapy), and medication. More than 95% of seropositive patients respond to therapy, and 70% of patients have partial or complete remissions.

B. **Aspirin, NSAIDs, and COX-2 inhibitors.** Provide symptomatic relief but do nothing to suppress the rate of cartilage erosion or to alter the course of the disease. Doses should be increased to the recommended maximum over 1 to 2 weeks; a medication should not be abandoned until the patient has been on a maximal dose for at least 2 weeks, because medications may take this much time to reach maximal efficacy. If after 2 weeks of receiving a maximal dose the results are disappointing, an alternative NSAID should be tried. Zero-order release aspirin products such as Zorprin and Easprin may make aspirin products easier to take. Naproxen 500 mg PO BID and ibuprofen 600 mg PO TID are some of the least expensive NSAIDs. The use of proton pump inhibitors with NSAIDs (and COX-2 inhibitors) reduces incidence gastric and duodenal ulcers.

C. **The COX-2 inhibitors,** rofecoxib (Vioxx) and celecoxib (Celebrex), have the same efficacy as other NSAIDs but fewer GI side effects. However, up to 12% of patients on a COX-2 inhibitor develop ulcers, and these drugs are expensive. Rofecoxib also interacts with warfarin, and both have renal side effects. They have no direct effects on platelets. **NOTE: Initial studies suggest that even one aspirin a day (e.g., for cardiac or stroke prophylaxis) may negate any GI advantage of the COX-2 inhibitors.**

D. **Disease-modifying antirheumatic drugs (DMARDs):** These drugs modify the fundamental pathologic process. No consensus exists as to which DMARD should be used in what order, but aggressive treatment with more than one drug is becoming the standard of care. Treatment must be individualized. Methotrexate is now the most prescribed DMARD. The use of methotrexate in combination with other drugs is increasing, and combination therapy of methotrexate, sulfasalazine, and hydroxychloroquine works better than either drug alone or sulfasalazine plus hydroxychloroquine. Another combination is methotrexate plus cyclosporine and methotrexate. Oral gold, sodium thiosulfate, tends to be less toxic than other medications but is less effective. Injectable gold, sodium thiomalate, is more toxic and no more effective than hydroxychloroquine and sulfasalazine. Because of the spontaneous waxing and waning of RA, these drugs should be used for approximately 6 months before one decides on efficacy. Disease-modifying drugs should be considered for use early in the course of RA.

1. **Steroids.** Glucocorticoids have anti-inflammatory and immunosuppressive effects and **reduce joint erosion when used long-term** (e.g., prednisolone 7.5 mg QD for 2 years). Low-dose corticosteroids (<10 mg of prednisone QD or its equivalent) can be used in combination with other DMARDs. They can also be useful for treating acute flares with systemic symptoms. Keep steroid doses at the minimum effective dose because of osteopenia and other side effects, such as skin thinning, increased susceptibility to infection, ecchymoses, and cushingoid appearance. Patients on chronic steroids should also be on vitamin D, calcium, and possibly alendronate or risedronate (depending on degree of bone mineral loss).

2. **Tumor necrosis factor inhibitors. Infliximab** (not FDA approved for this indication) **and etanercept (Enbrel) are suspected disease modifiers slowing progression,** and etanercept is approved for use in patients who have failed other DMARDs. The long-term efficacy of these agents is unclear. Combining them with another agent such as methotrexate seems to allow a sustained response. They have also been used alone. They are contraindicated in patients with ongoing infections and **cannot be used with live virus vaccines.** See package insert for prescribing information.

3. **Leflunomide.** A recently FDA-approved DMARD with efficacy similar to methotrexate and sulfasalazine. Leflunomide has been shown to reduce bone erosions. It has a long half-life of 14 to 16 days. A loading dose of 100 mg QD for 3 days is suggested followed by 20 mg/day. Leflunomide requires 4 to 6 weeks to reach a steady state. Long-term safety and efficacy are not yet established.

4. **Antibiotics.** Minocycline 100 mg PO BID has been shown to be effective for mild to moderate RA in a double-blind placebo-controlled trial. This is probably secondary to its anti-inflammatory effects.

5. **Antimalarials.** Hydroxychloroquine 400 to 600 mg PO daily for 4 to 6 weeks and then 200 to 400 mg daily. Baseline ophthalmologic examination with subsequent examinations every 6 months can allow one to detect early eye changes. May have ciliary muscle dysfunction or corneal opacities. Having the patient view an Ansler grid daily will give an early warning of visual changes. As safe as NSAIDs.

6. **Sulfasalazine** (not FDA approved for RA) 500 mg PO QD and then increasing doses to a maximum of 3000 mg daily. Reduce to 500 mg qid for maintenance. Contraindications include sulfonamide allergy. Side effects include bone marrow toxicity, hepatitis, reversible oligospermia, yellow discoloration of urine and of soft contact lenses, nausea, headache, and abdominal discomfort. Monitoring CBCs and liver enzymes is recommended.

7. **Penicillamine.** Start with 125 to 250 mg PO QD 1 hour before or 2 hours after eating, and then increase the dose by 125 to 250 mg/day every 1 to 2 months to a maximum of 750 to 1000 mg daily. Metallic taste and nausea are common early problems but re-

solve with continued use. Skin rashes, bone marrow toxicity, and proteinuria may occur. Autoimmune syndromes, including myasthenia gravis, polymyositis, pemphigus, and Goodpasture's syndrome have been reported as a result of penicillamine. A monthly urinalysis and CBC count are recommended, and penicillamine should not be used in those with renal disease.

8. **Methotrexate** 7.5 to 15 mg PO weekly. **Contraindications:** concomitant therapy with sulfonamide-containing antibiotics or HIV seropositivity. Alcohol consumption, gross obesity, and diabetes are aggravating factors to hepatic toxicity. May have nausea, vomiting, abdominal cramps. Serious side effects are bone marrow toxicity, alveolitis, and hepatic fibrosis. Monthly CBCs and liver enzyme studies every 2 to 3 months are recommended. Persistent elevation of liver enzymes or significant hypoalbuminemia may indicate the need for a liver biopsy. Should be administered with folic acid, at least 5 mg/wk, which decreases side effects but not efficacy.

9. **Azathioprine** 50 to 100 mg PO QD (1.0 to 1.5 mg/kg/day, which may be increased by 0.5 mg/kg/day weekly to 2.0 to 2.5 mg/kg/day after 3 months). Nausea is the main limiting factor. Azathioprine is more toxic than other disease-modifying drugs. Monthly CBC and quarterly liver function tests are recommended. The concomitant use of allopurinol increases toxicity and should be avoided. Dosage should be reduced if renal impairment is present.

10. **Cyclophosphamide. Tends to be toxic, with many patients having one or more side effects.** These include nausea or vomiting (58%), alopecia (26%), dysuria (26%), hemorrhagic cystitis (14%), herpes zoster (5%). Other adverse reactions included leukopenia, thrombocytopenia, and amenorrhea in premenopausal women.

11. **Cyclosporine** can be used for patients with severe, refractory disease. However, the potential for irreversible toxicity would suggest limiting the drug to those patients unresponsive to other therapy.

12. **Gold salts.**
    a. **Parenteral gold salts.** Gold sodium thiomalate and aurothioglucose. **Intramuscular:** single dose of 10 mg, followed by 25 mg 1 week later to test for sensitivity. Maintenance therapy is 25 to 50 mg weekly. If there is no improvement with a cumulative dose of 1 or 2 g or if toxicity develops, therapy should be discontinued.
    b. **Auranofin** 3 to 6 mg PO QD. Diarrhea is a common side effect. Monthly urinalysis and CBC counts should be performed.
    c. **Side effects.**
       (1) **Common.** Pruritic skin rash, mouth ulcers, transient leukopenia, eosinophilia, diarrhea (oral). Treatment can sometimes be temporarily halted and then restarted at lower doses, and side effects may not recur, but rash must be allowed to clear because it can lead to an exfoliative dermatitis.

7

RHEUMATOLOGY

(2) **Transient proteinuria** in 3% to 10% of patients. Usually requires only cessation of treatment until the urine clears.

(3) **Less common.** Thrombocytopenia, pancytopenia, agranulocytosis, and aplastic anemia. Usually responds to stopping drug. Gold-chelating agent (dimercaprol) can be used if response is not fast enough.

OSTEOARTHRITIS

I. **Overview.** Osteoarthritis (OA) is the most common joint disease. OA is a condition of synovial joints characterized by focal cartilage loss and an accompanying reparative bone response. Typical radiographic features are joint space narrowing and the presence of osteophytes and sclerosis. OA is strongly related to age. It is rare under 45 years of age without trauma, but at least half of those over age 65 years have radiographic evidence of OA.

II. **Types.**

A. **Primary OA.** Primary OA is a wear-and-tear phenomenon. OA generally spares the shoulders and MCP joints.

B. **Secondary OA.** May involve joints that are generally not involved with primary OA, including MCP joints, shoulder, or isolated large joints. It may be related to chondrocalcinosis or another secondary cause (below).

1. **Traumatic arthritis** secondary to slipped capital femoral epiphysis, congenital hip dislocation, destruction secondary to septic joint, hemophilia, or other injury.

2. **Paget's disease.** A defect in older individuals of bone resorption and redeposition. Radiograph shows typical scalloped pattern of bone deposition, and 85% have an elevated alkaline phosphatase with a normal γ-glutamyltransferase (GGT). A normal serum 5'-nucleotidase (a liver enzyme) has fewer false positives than GGT and thus is a better test. Patients may have associated deafness, cardiac abnormalities, etc. Urine hydroxyproline does not accurately reflect disease activity. However, N-telopeptides and pyridinoline crosslink assays can be used to follow disease course. Risedronate or alendronate can be used for treatment.

3. **Alkaptonuria with ochronosis.** Rare disorder of tyrosine metabolism.

4. **Hemochromatosis.** 50% of cases show chronic progressive arthritis, affecting predominantly MCP and wrist joints, as well as large joints, including shoulders, hips, and knees. Treatment for arthritis is symptomatic; see Chapter 6 for treatment of the underlying disease.

5. **Wilson's disease.** 50% of adults with Wilson's disease have arthropathy, characterized by mild OA of the wrists, MCP joints, knees, and spine.

6. **Neuroarthropathy (Charcot's joint).** Severe destructive arthropathy caused by impaired joint sensation. Diabetes mellitus, tabes dorsalis, and syringomyelia are common causes. The foot is involved most commonly.

III. **Clinical Features.**
A. Pain after joint use progressing to pain with minimal movement and at rest and at night. As opposed to RA, there is generally no early morning stiffness or gelling.
B. Patients often have pain on passive movement with crepitus and joint enlargement.
C. May develop genu valgus or varus deformity at knee if there is a dispro-portionate loss of cartilage on one side.
D. Pseudolaxity of collateral ligaments develops with degeneration of cartilage.
IV. **Radiographic Features.** Characteristic progressive changes include joint-space narrowing, subchondral osteosclerosis, marginal osteophyte for-mation, and subchondral cysts. Spondylolisthesis (subluxation of one vertebra on another with lateral spondylosis) may occur.
V. **Laboratory.** None.
VI. **Treatment.**
A. **Goal of treatment.** Relieve pain, preserve joint motion and function, and prevent further injury and wear of cartilage.
B. **Biomechanical factors.** Weight loss, use of canes or crutches, correction of postural abnormalities, and proper shoe support are helpful corrective measures.
C. **Pain control.**
1. **Analgesics,** such as acetaminophen 1 g PO QID in scheduled doses, are important. OA is not an inflammatory disorder, and acetami-nophen is equal or superior to NSAIDs in efficacy without NSAID side effects.
2. **NSAIDs** are helpful in those who have failed acetaminophen. However, they have many side effects and may hasten joint de-struction. When an NSAID is being chosen, patient side effects and cost should be a consideration. Two weeks at maximal dose is needed before one decides that a particular drug is a therapeutic failure. Naprosyn 500 mg PO BID or ibuprofen 600 mg PO QID are relatively inexpensive and well tolerated. COX-2 inhibitors may also be helpful but are expensive (see under RA earlier in this chapter).
3. **Corticosteroids.** Oral or parenteral corticosteroid therapy is not indi-cated. Intra-articular injection of steroid may be helpful in acute flares.
4. **Surgery.** Joint arthroplasty may relieve pain, stabilize joints, and im-prove function. Total joint arthroplasty is successful for the knee and hip.
5. **Sodium hyaluronate (Synvisc)/Hylan G-F 20** can be injected directly into the joint and may provide up to 6 months of pain relief.
6. **Alternative therapies.** Chondroitin sulfate and glucosamine have been shown to have some benefit in open label trials. Double-blind ongoing trials are underway.

7

RHEUMATOLOGY

CRYSTAL-INDUCED SYNOVITIS

I. **Primary Gouty Arthritis.**
A. **Overview.** An illness secondary to a chronic increase in the serum uric acid. Deposition of uric acid crystals occurs throughout the body and results in:
1. Multiple acute episodes of inflammatory arthritis.
2. Chronic, low-grade inflammation of joints.
3. Accumulation of articular, osseous, soft tissue, and cartilaginous crystalline deposits (tophi).
4. Renal injury (gouty nephropathy).
5. Uric acid kidney stones.
B. **Acute gouty arthritis.**
1. **Clinical features.** Onset is usually acute with (generally) nocturnal onset of monoarticular pain; rarely more than one joint can be involved acutely. Involved joints are red, swollen, warm, and exquisitely tender. Fever and leukocytosis may occur. The big toe (first MTP joint) is the classic site of gout (also called podagra). Other sites, such as foot, knee, hand, or shoulder, may also be involved. Acute attack lasts 3 to 10 days without treatment. It may be difficult to differentiate from a septic joint, so joint aspiration for synovial fluid examination is critical, especially with the first attack.
2. **Precipitating events.** Trauma, surgery, major medical illness (myocardial infarction, cerebrovascular accident, pulmonary embolus), fasting, alcohol use, and infection. Overeating and emotional stress may also trigger attacks.
3. **Differential diagnosis.** Septic arthritis, other arthritis including pseudogout, RA.
4. **Diagnosis.** Definite diagnosis can be made by demonstration of the presence of monosodium urate (MSU) crystals within synovial leukocytes or in material derived from tophi under polarizing microscopy.
   a. Recommendation is to demonstrate crystals in joint aspirate.
      (1) Synovial fluid typically reveals 2000 to 100,000 cells/mm^3, predominantly PMNs.
      (2) Urate crystals are rod or needle shaped and negatively birefringent **but can also be easily seen on a regular light microscope.**
      (3) **Crystals may be recovered from joints during asymptomatic periods.**
      (4) Fluid should be sent for Gram stain and culture to rule out infection.
   b. **Serum uric acid levels are generally not helpful in acute attacks and may be normal.** However, when levels are chronically greater than 10 mg/dl, the chance of an acute attack is >90%.
5. **Treatment.** Do not administer allopurinol or probenecid until acute attack completely subsides; these may prolong the attack. Although colchicine has classically been used for acute attacks of gout,

NSAIDs have replaced it as initial therapy. Steroids are another option for acute treatment.

   a. **Pain management.** Oral narcotics (e.g., hydrocodone [Lortab]) can be used for pain management, in addition to other medications.
   b. **NSAIDs. There is no advantage to using ketorolac** in an acute flare of gout. It is equal to indomethacin in time of onset and control of symptoms.
      (1) **Indomethacin (Indocin)** 50 to 75 mg PO and then 50 mg Q6h, tapering to 50 mg Q8h and to 25 mg Q6h and maintained until symptoms have completely resolved.
      (2) **Ketorolac (Toradol)** has no advantage, is expensive, and has a greater number of side effects than other NSAIDS.
      (3) **Ibuprofen** 800 mg PO Q8h.
   c. **Corticosteroids.** Methylprednisolone 125 mg IV or IM followed by prednisone 40 to 60 mg/day PO with or without colchicine 0.5 mg PO once or twice per day until symptoms resolve. Taper rapidly.
   d. **Colchicine.**
      (1) Colchicine should be reserved for cases in which the diagnosis of gout is not confirmed and a response may have diagnostic value and for cases in which NSAIDs and steroids are contraindicated or have failed.
      (2) Administer 1 mg PO initially, followed by 0.5 mg Q2h up to 6 times on first day. On second day, give 0.5 mg Q6h and then twice per day until side effects occur. Side effects include abdominal cramps, diarrhea, nausea, and vomiting. If diarrhea develops, the drug is discontinued.
      (3) The dose should be reduced in older patients and in patients with renal or hepatic disease.
6. **Intercritical period.** See section on treatment of hyperuricemia (below). The goal is to prevent recurrent attack of acute gout. Oral colchicine 0.5 to 1.5 mg QD is the most effective dosing. Side effects are uncommon at this dose, and it may be discontinued after the serum urate level becomes normal and stable for 2 to 3 months. A low dose of NSAIDs (indomethacin 25 mg PO BID) is effective, but the incidence of side effects is higher than that of colchicine.

C. **Chronic gout.**
   1. **Clinical features.** Chronic changes are the result of persistent hyperuricemia and recurrent acute attacks of gout. Tophi develop mainly in the helix of the ear. Other locations include the ulnar aspects of the forearm, olecranon, and prepatellar bursae, Achilles tendons, and hands. Extraarticular locations for tophus formation included myocardium, pericardium, aortic valves, and extradural spinal regions.
   2. **Clinical picture.** May mimic rheumatoid arthritis though generally less symmetric.

3. **Characteristic radiographic appearance.** Bony erosion with an overhanging margin of the involved joint.

4. **Treatment of hyperuricemia.** Treatment depends on cause: increased uric acid (about 10%) production versus decreased excretion (about 90%). Asymptomatic hyperuricemia should not be treated. Treatment should be undertaken only after the second attack of gout or in the presence of a history of uric acid stones. The goal is to reduce serum uric acid level below its saturation point in extracellular fluid (6.4 mg/dl).

a. There are two classes of drugs to reduce uric acid: **uricosurics,** such as probenecid, which increases excretion, and **xanthine oxidase inhibitors,** such as allopurinol, which reduce production. Before deciding on therapy, obtain a 24-hour urine specimen for uric acid. This will help determine if the patient is an over-producer of uric acid or an under-excreter. If excretion is >800 mg/day, patient is an over-producer of uric acid and will require allopurinol to prevent production. Those with decreased excretion can be treated with either class of drug.

b. Drugs that increase excretion.

(1) **Probenecid.** Blocks tubular reabsorption of filtered uric acid. Initial dose is 250 mg PO BID and gradually increased by 500 mg every 4 weeks, until daily maximum dose of 2000 mg is achieved. The goal is to decrease serum uric acid levels to between 5 and 6 mg/dl. It is recommended for patients under 60 years of age and those with normal renal function, uric acid excretion of less than 800 to 1000 mg/day, and no history of kidney stones. Advise the patient to increase fluid intake and consider alkalinization of the urine to a pH of 6.5 or more with sodium bicarbonate, 2 to 6 g/day, or acetazolamide (Diamox) 250 mg/day PO. Aspirin blocks probenecid's effect. Continue colchicine for prophylaxis as above.

(2) **Sulfinpyrazone (Anturane)** 50 to 100 mg PO BID may be given. Its dose may be gradually increased by 100 mg every week until the maximum dose of 800 mg/day is attained. This is especially useful for those patients who must take aspirin.

c. Drug that decreases production. **Allopurinol (Zyloprim):** starting dose is 100 mg PO QD. Usual dose is 200 to 300 mg/day, and maximum is 800 mg/day. Indications include a history of kidney stones, presence of tophi, renal insufficiency (GFR <60 ml/min), inability to lower the serum urate level below 7 mg/dl with other agents, urinary urate excretion >800 to 1000 mg/day, allergy to uricosurics, and hyperuricemia caused by hypoxanthine-guanine phosphoribosyltransferase deficiency. Side effects are rare but can be serious. These include drug fever, rash (including Stevens-Johnson syndrome), bone marrow depression, vasculitis, and hepatitis.

II. **Calcium Pyrophosphate Deposition Disease.**

A. **Overview.** A degenerative joint disease characterized by the accumulation of calcium pyrophosphate crystals in articular cartilage and periarticular tissues. May be idiopathic or associated with a variety of metabolic diseases.

1. **Pseudogout.** An acute inflammatory attack that involves one or more joints and that can last for several days. Attacks can be very similar to gout, though usually not so severe. The knees are involved in about half of patients, but any joint can be affected. Patients may have less severe attacks between acute flares. Crystal deposition can occur in tendons, ligaments, and synovia, as well as in cartilage. Surgery or illness can predispose to attacks.

2. **Pseudo-osteoarthritis.** Chronic calcium pyrophosphate disease may appear similar to osteoarthritis (termed *pseudo-osteoarthritis*) with progressive degeneration of multiple joints. Knees are most commonly affected, followed by wrists, MCP joints, hips, shoulders, and elbows. May have symmetric involvement.

3. **Pseudorheumatoid arthritis.** In 5%, calcium pyrophosphate disease causes symptoms similar to rheumatoid arthritis, including morning stiffness, fatigue, synovial membrane thickening, and elevated ESR. About 10% of patients with calcium pyrophosphate dihydrate (CPPD) have a positive rheumatoid factor.

4. **Diagnosis.**

   a. **Laboratory.** Joint should be tapped and will note crystals composed of calcium pyrophosphate dihydrate (CPPD). Crystals are rod shaped, often intracellular, and positively birefringent, or blue when parallel to the axis of a polarizing microscope compensator. However, crystals can also easily be seen under a light microscope. Evaluation should include serum calcium, magnesium, phosphorus, alkaline phosphatase, ferritin, serum iron and iron-binding capacity, glucose, T4, TSH, and uric acid.

   b. **Radiographic findings.** Typical findings are punctate and linear densities in articular hyaline or fibrocartilaginous tissues. Characteristic sites include articular cartilage of knee, acetabular labrum, symphysis pubis, articular disk of wrist, and anulus fibrosus of intervertebral disks. Radiologic screen for CPPD disease should include AP view of both knees, AP view of pelvis including hips and symphysis pubis, and PA view of both hands.

B. **Treatment of pseudogout.**

1. **NSAIDS are effective.** No one drug is superior. May be used in manner similar to that in acute episodes of gouty arthritis.

2. **Colchicine.** See section on gout for dosing. Oral form is less predictable than when used with gout but has been proved to reduce the number and duration of attacks (with 1.2 mg daily).

3. **Corticosteroid injections** are often combined with aspiration for large joints.

7

RHEUMATOLOGY

SPONDYLOARTHROPATHIES

Characterized by involvement of spine and entheses (insertions of tendons and ligaments). Associated with HLA-B27. The target organs are not only the joint, but also the axial skeleton, the enthesis, the eye, the gut, the urogenital tract, the skin, and sometimes the heart. The prevalence of this entity in the general population is estimated at 1%, equal to the prevalence of rheumatoid arthritis. Diseases included within this concept are ankylosing spondylitis, reactive arthritis/Reiter's disease, undifferentiated spondyloarthropathies, some forms of psoriatic arthritis, juvenile chronic arthritis, acute anterior uveitis, and arthritis associated with inflammatory bowel diseases such as Crohn's disease and ulcerative colitis, as well as infectious diarrhea such as *Yersinia*.

I. **Ankylosing Spondylitis** (Marie-Strumpell disease).

A. **Clinical features.** A disease primarily affecting the sacroiliac joints with varying involvement of the spine and less so the appendicular skeleton.

1. **Clinically.** Onset is usually insidious, generally between 10 and 40 years of age. Patients generally have back pain that is worse after rest and improves with exercise. Patients may notice morning back stiffness that improves during the day; the pain may be so severe at night that it keeps the patient awake or prompts the patient to get up and become mobile to reduce the symptoms. By definition, the back is always involved. However, peripheral joints are involved in up to 25% of cases. Proximal, large joints, such as hips, knees, shoulders, and ankles, are preferentially affected. TMJ involvement is common. Involvement is usually asymmetric but not always. May have mild systemic manifestations such as fever, malaise, or anorexia.

2. **Associated with HLA-B27** in >90% of cases. The diagnosis is made according to clinical and radiologic criteria. Offspring of those with the disease have a 10% to 20% risk of having disease.

3. **Enthesopathy.** Involvement of the sites of insertion of ligaments and tendons (entheses) is manifested clinically as Achilles tendinitis, plantar fasciitis, and costochondritis.

4. **Extraarticular manifestations.** May include uveitis (25%), cardiac involvement in 10%, especially aortic insufficiency, cardiomegaly, conduction defects, heart block, and renal and neurologic complications. Pulmonary involvement consists principally of upper lobe fibrocystic changes and chest wall restriction but may include *Aspergillus* infection in the pulmonary cavities.

5. **Late complications** secondary to bone involvement can include cord compression caused by spinal fractures; cauda equina syndrome (neurogenic bladder, fecal incontinence, leg pain); and severe chest wall restriction.

B. **Diagnosis.**

1. **Physical examination.**

a. **Flexion test.** Mark two points on the back, at the lumbosacral junction and 10 cm above, with patient standing erect. Have the patient bend forward and measure the distance between the two points. The normal spine should have an increase of greater than 5 cm. Less than 5 cm is suggestive of decreased spinal mobility.

    b. **Chest expansion.** Normally, chest circumference increases by 5 cm with full inspiration. This will be decreased in those with ankylosing spondylitis.

2. **Radiographic findings.** Sacroiliitis with sclerosis and fusion of the sacroiliac joints. May have an asymmetric erosive arthropathy. Spine involvement may be manifested by squaring of superior and inferior margins of vertebral body, syndesmophytes, and "bamboo spine."

3. **Lab tests.** The sedimentation rate is elevated in 75% of patients, as is the CRP. However, they do not always correlate with the activity of the disease. Immunofluorescence will show IgM deposition in the superficial vessels of the skin. HLA-B27 is present not only in 95% of whites with ankylosing spondylitis but also 6% to 8% of normal population. HLA-B27 should not be obtained as a screening test; the diagnosis is made on clinical and radiographic findings.

C. **Treatment.**

1. **NSAIDs.** Indomethacin is the drug of choice, with a starting dose of 25 mg PO TID. This may be increased to 50 mg TID. Side effects include nausea, gastric discomfort and diarrhea, headache, vertigo, and depression common in elderly. Other NSAIDs, such as naproxen and sulindac, are also effective.

2. **Aspirin.** For unknown reasons generally not effective.

3. **Sulfasalazine** 2 to 3 g PO QD. May be helpful, especially for peripheral joint disease. The effect starts within the first 2 to 3 months, and the drug continues to be effective acutely. The effect seems to be best in patients with high peak of disease activity and early disease. In very chronic cases, the response has not been different from the placebo. Monitoring includes CBC and liver enzymes every 2 weeks during the first 3 months.

4. **Methotrexate and cyclophosphamide** have also been used in recalcitrant cases.

5. **Education** about good posture. Exercise to promote extension of the back. Stop smoking. Avoiding pillows at night and encouraging sleep in the prone position are important.

6. **Physical therapy exercises** (especially swimming) and attention to posture are critical. Range-of-motion exercises, especially of the back, are important to maintain flexibility.

7. **Genetic counseling should be recommended.**

II. **Reiter's Syndrome.**

A. **Clinical features.**

1. **Reiter's syndrome.** A seronegative arthropathy (reactive arthritis) that preferentially involves the lower extremities. Reiter's syndrome is the most common type of polyarthritis in young men. It may manifest as insidious joint pain or acutely with fever (as high as 39° C), swollen, hot joints, severe weight loss, and diffuse poly-

7

RHEUMATOLOGY

articular involvement. When synovitis is limited to a few joints, low-grade fever or no fever at all is the rule. The onset may temporally be related to urethritis, diarrhea, or other infection with organisms such as *Yersinia, Salmonella, Shigella, Campylobacter,* or *Chlamydia.* The triad of arthritis, conjunctivitis, and urethritis should be suggestive of a diagnosis of Reiter's syndrome. However, the manifestation of these symptoms may be separated by months. Relapses begin 3 to 4 years after the first episode and can consist of recurrence of peripheral arthritis or enthesopathic pain of pelvi-axial symptoms, or of iritis or other extraarticular symptoms. These symptoms can be isolated or associated. Radiographic changes may now be observed.

2. **Other associated findings.** Skin disorders (balanitis, oral ulcerations, or keratoderma blennorrhagicum), conjunctivitis, and urethritis. In chronic disease, heart block or aortic regurgitation may occur. Diarrhea may precede the development of Reiter's syndrome. There is an association of Reiter's disease with HIV infection, and arthritis may be present before symptoms or signs related to the HIV infection appear.

3. **Lab tests.** Findings may include an elevated ESR/CRP and anemia of chronic disease; 80% of patients are HLA-B27 positive. Stool cultures and urethral cultures should be done. Offer HIV testing in the appropriate population.

B. **Treatment.**
1. **NSAIDs.** Indomethacin 25 mg PO QID (can be increased to 50 mg PO QID).
2. **Antibiotics.** Treatment of the underlying bacterial infection may hasten resolution. A 3-month course of tetracycline has been shown to hasten resolution of symptoms in those with disease related to *Chlamydia* organisms.
3. **Immunosuppressive drugs,** such as methotrexate or azathioprine, may be effective.
4. **Steroids.** Patients with large-joint involvement may benefit from intra-articular corticosteroid injection.

III. **Arthritis Associated with Inflammatory Bowel Disease (Enteropathic Arthritis).** There are two types of arthritis associated with ulcerative colitis and Crohn's disease: a nondestructive oligoarthritis of peripheral joints and ankylosing spondylitis.

IV. **Psoriatic Arthritis.**
A. **Clinical features.** Occurs in up to 7% of patients with psoriasis and is strongly associated with the presence of nail pitting. Most patients (95%) have involvement of multiple small joints of the hands and feet. Others have solely spine involvement or, more commonly (35% to 50%), a combination of spine involvement and peripheral joint involvement. There is a high prevalence (10% to 30%) of atlantoaxial subluxation in severe, chronic disease. The inflamed joints in patients with pso-

riatic arthritis often have a purplish discoloration, which is not commonly seen in other forms of arthritis.

B. **Treatment.** Basic management uses NSAIDs, exercise, physical therapy, and education; control of psoriasis is important. Other possible therapies include methotrexate, antimalarials, sulfasalazine, and other DMARDs.

SEPTIC ARTHRITIS

I. **Overview.**

A. Any infectious agent can cause arthritis, but bacterial arthritis is the most rapidly destructive form. The major responsible organisms are *Neisseria gonorrhoeae* and *Staphylococcus aureus. Streptococcus* species (including pneumococcal infections), *Enterobacter, H. influenzae,* and other gram-negative species are much less common. Brucellosis is rarely found as joint pathogen in those who work with cattle.

B. **Source of infection.**

1. **Hematogenous spread.** Secondary to a puncture wound, a skin infection, or an adjacent osteomyelitis. Rarely, septic arthritis may be secondary to intra-articular injection or joint aspiration (incidence ranges from 1 in 500 to 1 in 5000).

2. **IV drug use.** May cause infections in unusual joints such as the sternoclavicular or sacroiliac joints. Infections in IV drug users are frequently secondary to unusual organisms such as *Pseudomonas, Serratia,* and methicillin-resistant staphylococci.

3. **Underlying illness.** Steroid use, RA, and the presence of joint prosthesis also predispose to the development of septic arthritis. Those with underlying illness such as lupus, RA, renal failure, and diabetes may have gram-negative organisms.

II. **Gonococcal Arthritis.**

A. **Clinical features.** May have an acute arthritis involving one or more joints, usually the knees, ankles, or wrists, with the knee being the most commonly involved. Two thirds of patients have a dermatitis with one or multiple, usually asymptomatic lesions that progress from macular to papular and finally vesicular, or pustular. Any new acute inflammatory monarthritis in a sexually active person should be considered related to gonococcal infection until proved otherwise. Fever may be present, and genitourinary symptoms occur in 25%. Physical exam reveals an acute arthritis, synovitis, or tenosynovitis, or all three. In gonococcal infection the arthritis should subside dramatically within 3 days and completely within 10 days after the start of antibiotics.

B. **Laboratory features** (Table 7-2).

1. **The synovial fluid white blood cell count averages over 60,000/ml,** but low WBC counts have been reported. Gram stain may be positive, but only 25% of synovial fluid cultures are positive in gonococcal arthritis.

2. Obtain blood cultures and cultures of the throat, joint, anorectum, blood, and genitourinary tract.

TABLE 7-2

SYNOVIAL FLUID ANALYSIS

Classification	Condition	Color	Clarity	Viscosity	WBC/l	NTP (%)	Crystals	Glucose (% serum)	Complement	Culture/ smear
Normal	Normal	Yellow	Translucent	High	<200	<25	0	Same	Normal	0
Group 1 (noninflammatory)	Osteoarthritis	Yellow	Transparent	High	<2000	<25	0	Same	Normal	0
	Trauma	Pink or red	Transparent	High	<2000	<25	0	Same	Normal	0
	SLE	Yellow	Translucent	Slightly decreased	0-9000	<25	0	Same	Normal	0
Group 2 (inflammatory)	Acute rheumatic fever	Yellow	Translucent	Slightly decreased	0-60,000	25-50	0	Same	Normal	0
	Pseudogout	Yellow or white	Translucent or opaque	Low	50-75,000	90	+	Same	Normal	0
	Gout	Yellow or white	Translucent or opaque	Low	100-160,000	90	+	Same	Normal	0
	Rheumatoid arthritis	Yellow or purulent	Translucent or opaque	Low	3000-50,000	50-75	0	75-100	Normal	0
Group 3 (purulent)	Tuberculosis	Purulent	Opaque	Low	2500-100,000	50	0	50-75	Normal or low	+
	Bacterial arthritis	Purulent	Opaque	Low	50,000-300,000	>90	0	<50	Normal or low	+*

From Paget S et al: *Rheumatology and outpatient orthopedics*, 1993, Philadelphia, Lippincott-Raven.
WBC, White blood cells; *NTP,* neutrophils; *SLE,* systemic lupus erythematosus.
*Often negative in gonococcal arthritis.

III. **Nongonococcal Bacterial Arthritis.**

A. **Clinical features.** The acute onset of arthritis with a hot, swollen joint or joints. Generally one or two joints are involved. The knee is most commonly affected in adults, whereas the hip and knee are the most commonly involved joints in children. Fever is common but may be of low grade; chills are less common.

B. **Diagnosis.**
   1. **Obtaining synovial fluid sample is critical.** The definitive test is joint aspiration with fluid sent for Gram staining (positive in 75% for gram-positive cocci), culture, synovial fluid leukocyte count, and differential (greater than 50,000 cells/ml in 70% of patients, with over 80% neutrophils), and decreased synovial fluid glucose.
   2. **Blood cultures should be done.** Positive in 50% of patients with nongonococcal bacterial arthritis.
   3. **An elevated white blood cell count** with a left shift and an elevated ESR often occur but are nonspecific.
   4. **Radiographic examination.** Plain films obtained for baseline view and to look for osteomyelitis. Usually no initial changes are visible except effusions and perhaps juxta-articular osteopenia. The changes of osteomyelitis take 10 to 20 days to appear on plain films. Radionuclide imaging, gallium scanning, and CT or MRI can be helpful, particularly with suspected hip or axial joint infections. Ultrasonography may be used to establish the presence of effusion in the hip joint and aid with aspiration.
   5. **Surgical exploration.** May be necessary to obtain fluid from joints such as the sternoclavicular or sacroiliac.
   6. **Diagnostic considerations.** Occult celiac disease, sarcoid arthritis, Lyme disease, parvovirus arthropathies, Behçet's syndrome (recurrent oral or genital ulcers [>97%]), uveitis (50%), meningoencephalitis, arthritis (40% to 50%), and HIV-associated arthritis.

IV. **Treatment.**

A. **Antibiotic therapy.**
   1. **Gonococcal arthritis.** Ceftriaxone 1 g IV QD for at least 3 days, followed by cefuroxime axetil 500 mg PO BID. For penicillin-allergic patients, an alternative is spectinomycin 2 g IM Q12h.
   2. **Nongonococcal arthritis.**
      a. **In adults.** Make the initial choice based on Gram-stain results and clinical likelihood. Essentially all antibiotics reach high levels of activity within an inflamed joint after oral or parenteral administration. Consider a penicillinase-resistant penicillin (such as methicillin or nafcillin) or vancomycin plus an aminoglycoside or aztreonam. Imipenem has been proposed for single-agent therapy.
      b. **Neonates.** Methicillin, nafcillin, or vancomycin plus a third-generation cephalosporin.

   c. **Infants and young children.** Methicillin, nafcillin, or vancomycin plus cefuroxime.

   d. **Prosthetic joint infections.** Vancomycin plus aztreonam.

B. **Drainage.**

   1. **Needle drainage.** As good as open drainage in most situations but is not adequate for hip infections, especially in children. Aspirate with a large-bore needle daily while effusions accumulate rapidly. Can irrigate with sterile saline.

   2. **Open drainage.** Method of choice for hip infections.

   3. **Arthroscopy.** Early arthroscopy has been reported to be helpful.

C. **Immobilize the joint** in the functional position during the acute phase of infection, with early mobilization and muscle-strengthening exercises.

D. **Reassess therapy if:**

   1. Synovial fluid cultures are not negative within 72 hours (reculture with tap), or

   2. Synovial fluid leukocyte count is not greatly lower after 7 days.

E. **Prognosis.**

   1. Up to 10% mortality rate.

   2. Only 60% recover completely; many are left with a joint problem, especially if symptomatic for more than 7 days before therapy. *Staphylococcus aureus* and gram-negative bacilli tend to be more destructive. *Neisseria gonorrhoeae* and pneumococcus are rarely destructive.

   3. Sterile synovitis may develop after treatment but is usually self-limited and responds to NSAIDs.

RHEUMATIC FEVER AND RHEUMATIC CARDITIS

A. **Etiology and present significance.** Acute rheumatic fever (ARF) and rheumatic carditis represent the clinical sequelae of infection with group A streptococci. Peak age of incidence is 5 to 15 years. Primary and recurrent illness occurs in adulthood as well. The incidence has decreased markedly, but it is still a common problem in developing countries. Among patients with rheumatic heart disease the incidence of valvular disease is as follows: mitral valve 85%, aortic valve 44%, tricuspid valve 10% to 16%. In developed countries, patients with rheumatic fever may not meet the Jones criteria (Box 7-1).

B. **Cardiac manifestations.** From 40% to 60% of patients develop carditis during the initial episode of ARF. Manifestations include cardiomegaly, heart murmur (mitral regurgitation, aortic regurgitation), friction rub secondary to pericarditis, and congestive heart failure.

C. **Treatment and prophylaxis.** Antibiotics (such as benzathine penicillin G) are given to eradicate tonsillar and pharyngeal group A streptococci. Aspirin is used to treat the acute polyarthritis. Corticosteroids (such as prednisone) are used to treat carditis and are administered for 3 to 6 weeks. Secondary prevention consists of chronic administration of antibiotics to patients who have already sustained significant damage from rheumatic carditis. Monthly IM injection of 1.2 million units of penicillin

BOX 7-1

JONES CRITERIA FOR RHEUMATIC FEVER

The revised Jones criteria recognize both major and minor manifestations of the disease. The development of two major criteria or one major and two minor criteria suggests a high probability of rheumatic fever.

MAJOR CRITERIA	MINOR CRITERIA
Polyarthritis: May have any degree of arthritis; generally migratory and in large joints. Resolves in about 1 month.	Prevouis episodes of ARF or rheumatic heart disease
Carditis: See text.	Arthralgia
Sydenham's chorea (St Vitus' Dance)	Fever
Erythema marginatum	Elevations in acute phase reactants (ESR, CRP)
Subcutaneous (Aschoff) nodules (painless subcutaneous nodules over bony surfaces	Leukocytosis
	Prolonged PR interval on EKG

G benzathine appears to provide optimal prophylaxis. Prophylaxis in these patients should be lifelong. Alternative protocols are beyond the scope of this manual.

FIBROMYALGIA SYNDROME

I. Clinical Features.

A. **Characterized by diffuse aches, stiffness, and fatigue,** coupled with multiple, symmetric tender spots in specific areas (Fig. 7-1). Over 75% of patients are women, and the peak incidence is between 20 and 60 years of age. There is often discordance between symptoms and objective findings. The cause may actually be related to a sleep disturbance.

B. **Pain** is often aggravated by stress, cold, and activity. Patients often complain of subjective swelling of hands and feet, as well as paresthesia and dysesthesia of hands and feet.

C. **Fatigability** is often extreme, occurring after minimal exertion.

D. **Sleep disturbance.** Patients complain of nonrestorative sleep, waking unrefreshed. Research has shown alpha wave intrusion into non-REM delta wave sleep 70% greater than controls. May have depression and irritability and be weepy.

E. **Headache** is common as are diffuse abdominal pain and alternating diarrhea or constipation.

F. **Miscellaneous.** Paresthesias, numbness, decreased mentation, feeling of swollen hands and feet.

G. **Associated syndromes.** Irritable bowel syndrome (35% to 65%), reflex sympathetic syndrome (1% to 10%), female urethral syndrome (urethral spasm with dysuria and urgency, 12%).

II. **Diagnosis.** Fibromyalgia is a diagnosis of exclusion (nomal CBC, ESR, thyroid functions, rheumatoid factor, electrolytes, creatinine, calcium,

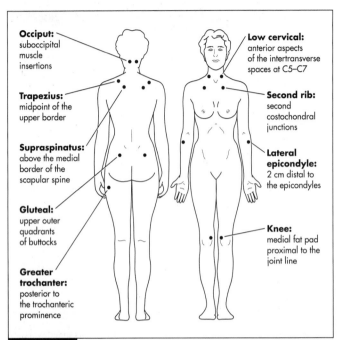

Occiput: suboccipital muscle insertions

Trapezius: midpoint of the upper border

Supraspinatus: above the medial border of the scapular spine

Gluteal: upper outer quadrants of buttocks

Greater trochanter: posterior to the trochanteric prominence

Low cervical: anterior aspects of the intertransverse spaces at C5–C7

Second rib: second costochondral junctions

Lateral epicondyle: 2 cm distal to the epicondyles

Knee: medial fat pad proximal to the joint line

FIGURE 7-1

Location of specific tender points in fibromyalgia. *(From Schumacher HR Jr, Klippel JH, Koopman WJ, editors: Primer on the rheumatic diseases, ed 11, Atlanta, 1997, Arthritis Foundation.)*

phosphorus, UA). Patients must meet the American College of Rheumatology (ACR) criteria: widespread pain of at 3 months' duration in combination with at least 11 of 18 specified tender points.

III. The World Health Organization views the ACR criteria as primarily for research purposes and determines that a patient has FMS based on the history and the finding of a nonspecific number of tender points.

IV. **Treatment.**

A. Treatment is aimed at controlling symptoms and restoring adequate sleep. Exercise programs and self-help strategies are the mainstay of treatment.

B. Treatment includes reassurance, education, graded aerobic exercise, massage, cognitive therapy, and increased flexibility. Patients may be assured that FMS is generally a self-limited illness that typically resolves within 2 to 3 years. Low-dose amitriptyline (Elavil), 10 to 75 mg PO QHS, or other tricyclic such as doxepin or nortriptyline taken before

---

BOX 7-2

CRITERIA FOR CHRONIC FATIGUE SYNDROME

Chronic fatigue defined as self-reported persistent or relapsing fatigue lasting 6 or more consecutive months with four or more of the following symptoms concurrently present.

Impaired memory or consciousness	Multi-joint pain
Sore throat	New headaches
Tender cervical or axillary adenopathy	Un-refreshing sleep
Muscle pain	Post-exertion malaise

Exclusion Criteria

Active medical conditions that may explain fatigue (e.g., hypothyroidism)

Previously diagnosed condition whose resolutions is not documented (e.g., hepatitis C)

Numerous psychiatric conditions (e.g., major depressive disorder, schizophrenia, dementia, anorexia, etc.)

Current alcohol or substance abuse or within the last 2 years

Unexplained physical, laboratory, or radiographic finding suggestive cause of fatigue

---

bedtime, as well as an SSRI in the morning if needed for depression/anxiety. Benzodiazepines should be avoided. NSAIDs are useful for achiness.

CHRONIC FATIGUE SYNDROME

I. A condition clinically characterized by severe disabling fatigue and a combination of symptoms described in Box 7-2. The patient is classified as having idiopathic chronic fatigue if diagnosis is suggested but inclusion criteria are not meet.

II. **Laboratory evaluation.** CBC with differential, ESR/CRP, ALT, protein, albumin, globulin, alkaline phosphatase, calcium, phosphorus, glucose, BUN, electrolytes, creatinine, TSH, urinalysis, and laboratory tests based on specific findings to exclude other diagnoses.

III. **Treatment** is beyond the scope of this manual.

POLYMYALGIA RHEUMATICA AND GIANT CELL ARTERITIS

Polymyalgia rheumatica (PMR) and giant cell arteritis form a spectrum of disease and affect patients of >50 years of age; up to 15% of patients with PMR have giant cell arteritis and 40% of patients with active giant cell arteritis have symptoms of PMR.

I. **Polymyalgia Rheumatica.**

A. **Clinical features.**

1. Pain and stiffness in the neck, shoulder, and pelvic girdle. Symptoms are bilateral and symmetric and more prolonged in the morning. May have diffuse aching.

    2. Systemic features may be present such as low-grade fever, fatigue, and weight loss.

    3. ESR and C-reactive protein are elevated with ESR elevation of 50 to 100 mm common. However, 15% of those with PMR may have a normal sedimentation rate and C-reactive protein.

B. **Diagnosis.**

    1. Rule out other causes such as claudication, disk disease, hypothyroidism, and myositis. In PMR thyroid functions are normal, CPK and aldolase are not elevated, ANA should be "normal" for age, and rheumatoid factor usually will be negative. Patients may have normocytic, normochromic anemia.

    2. Giant cell arteritis should be excluded.

C. **Treatment.** Prednisone: initial dose of 10 to 20 mg PO QD for 1 month and then reduce by 2.5 mg every 2 to 4 weeks until the lowest dose is reached that controls symptoms. Most patients require treatment for 3 to 4 years, but withdrawal after 2 years is worth attempting. Low-dose treatment should not be used in patients with symptoms suggestive of temporal arteritis.

II. **Giant Cell Arteritis (Temporal Arteritis).**

A. **Clinical features.** Predominantly affects persons >50 years of age with early symptoms of headache, fever, fatigue, and perhaps upper-limb girdle pain. May have associated ocular symptoms including partial visual loss and field cuts, diplopia, ptosis, and blindness. Tongue or jaw claudication may occur.

B. **Laboratory abnormalities.** Greatly elevated ESR, but 10% may have normal ESR and CRP, moderate normochromic anemia, and thrombocytosis.

C. **Diagnosis.** Temporal artery biopsy is most useful within 24 hours of starting treatment; however, steroids have little effect on the sensitivity of the biopsy, and treatment should not be delayed. A positive result helps to prevent later doubt about the diagnosis. Sensitivity of a biopsy is determined by length of artery taken and thinness of sections on microscopy.

D. **Treatment.** Prednisone: initial dose of 20 to 40 mg PO QD for 8 weeks. Patients with ocular symptoms may need up to 80 mg PO QD. Reduce the dose by 5 mg every 3 to 4 weeks until it is 10 mg QD and then taper slowly, based on symptoms and ESR. Treatment should last 24 to 30 months, at which time a trial off of steroids may be tried.

RAYNAUD'S PHENOMENON

I. **Overview.**

A. Episodic, biphasic or triphasic color change: white (ischemia), then often blue (stasis), then red (reactive hyperemia), of fingers or toes in response to cold or emotion.

B. More than 90% of patients with Raynaud's phenomenon are female.

II. **Types.**

A. **Raynaud's disease (primary Raynaud's phenomenon).** The cause is unknown, and the symptoms are usually stable.

B. **Secondary Raynaud's phenomenon.** Predisposing factors include atherosclerosis, arteritis, cancer, collagen vascular disease, thoracic outlet syndrome, embolic occlusions, occupational disease (working outdoors, using vibrating tools), and certain drugs (beta-adrenergic blockers, nicotine, ergotamine).

III. **Diagnosis.** Diagnosis is made on clinical grounds. The UK Scleroderma Study Group diagnostic terms for the diagnosis of Raynaud's phenomenon: (1) definite Raynaud's phenomenon consists of repeated episodes of biphasic color changes; (2) possible Raynaud's phenomenon consists of uniphasic color changes, plus numbness or paresthesia; and (3) no Raynaud's phenomenon is marked by no color changes on cold exposure.

IV. **Treatment.**

A. Treat the underlying condition. The mainstay of treatment relies on hygienic and dietetic measures (warm gloves, avoiding alcohol, smoking, etc).

B. Simple conservative measures include dressing warmly, relaxation and behavior modification (e.g., cold avoidance and stress management), and cessation of cigarette smoking.

C. Medications may be helpful.
1. Nifedipine extended release (such as Adalat CC) 30 mg PO daily.
2. Captopril 6.25 mg PO daily; may increase to 25 mg daily.
3. Transdermal nitroglycerin.

SYSTEMIC LUPUS ERYTHEMATOSUS

I. **Overview.** Systemic lupus erythematosus (SLE) is a systemic illness characterized by chronic inflammation; clinical manifestations are protean. It most commonly has its onset between 15 and 40 years of age and has an 8:1 female-to-male ratio. Genetic, environmental, and hormonal factors play a role in its etiology. The prevalence is 2.9 to 4 per 100,000; SLE is more common in blacks and some Asian populations.

II. **Diagnosis** of SLE requires the presence of 4 of 11 criteria (see A through K below). Keep in mind that a positive ANA is neither required for a diagnosis of lupus nor sufficient in itself to make a diagnosis of lupus. Initial workup for suspected lupus should include CBC, chemistry panel, ANA, ESR or CRP, CK, UA, ECG, and CXR.

A. Malar rash (fixed, raised, or flat).

B. Discoid rash.

C. Photosensitivity (by history or observation).

D. Oral ulcers (oral or nasopharyngeal, usually painless).

E. Arthritis (in two or more peripheral joints with tenderness, swelling, or effusion).

F. Serositis (pleuritis or pericarditis).

G. Renal disorder (proteinuria >0.5 g/day, >3+ proteinuria) or cellular casts.

H. Neurologic disorder (seizures or psychosis in the absence of other causes).

I. Hematologic disorder (hemolytic anemia, leukopenia <4000/mm, lymphopenia <1500/mm, or thrombocytopenia all in the absence of offending drugs and on two occasions).

J. Immunologic disorder (positive LE cell, anti–double-stranded DNA antigen, anti-Smith antigen, or false results of VDRL test with positive TPI or FTA, abnormal IgG or IgM anticardiolipin antibodies, or positive lupus anticoagulant using standard methods).

K. Positive results of fluorescent antinuclear antibody.

III. **Clinical Features.**

A. **Symmetric arthritis and arthralgias that are nondeforming and nonerosive.** Can be confused with RA early in course. May have deformity secondary to contractures. Tenosynovitis occurs in up to 10%, sometimes in absence of arthropathy. Ulnar deviation at MCP joints may be confused for RA.

B. **Mucocutaneous manifestations.**

1. **Acute cutaneous lupus.** Characteristic butterfly malar rash, often accompanied by a more widespread morbilliform eruption. Will flare with exacerbation of systemic disease or from sun exposure.

2. **Discoid lupus.** Erythematous raised patches with keratotic scaling, mostly on scalp, face, or neck. Alopecia and scarring are common (especially older lesions). Many with discoid lupus have no other systemic involvement.

3. **Subacute cutaneous lupus.** Skin lesions are symmetric, superficial, nonscarring, often annular, occurring on shoulders, upper arms, chest, back, and neck. Over half have diffuse nonscarring alopecia, and 20% have discoid lesions. Photosensitivity is prominent, but the incidence of nephritis is low.

4. **Mucosal manifestations.** Include recurrent oral and vaginal ulcers.

C. **Cardiac involvement.**

1. **Pericarditis.** May occur in up to 30% and may be asymptomatic. Often accompanied by pleural effusions. Rarely complicated by tamponade or restrictive pericarditis.

2. **Myocarditis.** May occur in up to 25%, often associated with pericarditis. Suggested by tachycardia, ST-T wave changes, and cardiomegaly. CK-MB elevation may occur and can result in CHF or arrhythmias.

3. **Endocarditis.** Typically asymptomatic without murmur or hemodynamic dysfunction. Mitral and aortic are the most commonly involved valves, and damage can be severe. Emboli are relatively rare.

4. **Myocardial infarction.** Usually considered secondary to accelerated atherosclerosis from long-term steroid use.

D. **Renal involvement.** Affects 50% of patients, with any pathologic form of glomerulonephritis. Clinical presentations include hematuria, proteinuria, hypertension, and uremia. Only 0.5% go on to end-stage renal disease. However, lupus nephritis is a poor prognostic marker, with a survival rate of 85% at 5 years and 65% at 10 years.

E. **Pulmonary.** Lung or pleura involved in 40% to 50%, with pleuritis or pleural effusion most common. Myopathy may affect the diaphragm.

F. **Central nervous system.** Frequently involved with highly varied presentation; depression is common. Headaches, strokes, TIAs, and memory loss or encephalopathy may occur. Seizures, chorea, and frank psychosis also occur.

G. **Gastrointestinal.** Less commonly involved. Serositis, oral ulcerations, and esophageal dysmotility may occur. Liver involvement not uncommon, but jaundice is rare.

H. **Raynaud's phenomenon.** Present in about half of patients at presentation.

I. **Vascular.** Terminal arterioles may be involved in vasculitis.

J. **Reticuloendothelial.** Lymphadenopathy is common.

IV. **Laboratory Findings.**

A. **Presence of ANA.** This result is found in 95% of those with SLE. Most common pattern is homogeneous and diffuse (pattern resulting in "LE cell"). Anti–double-stranded DNA and anti-Smith antigens are found only in SLE, whereas other antibodies such as anti–single-stranded DNA may also be present in other illnesses. Other antibodies such as anti-Ro and anti-La may also be present, suggesting Sjögren's syndrome. Those who are positive with inflammatory arthritis or Raynaud's but do not meet criteria for SLE are classified as having undifferentiated connective tissue disorder (UCTD). Of these, one third progress to SLE, one third maintain UCTD, and one third remit.

B. **Hematologic abnormalities.** A normochromic, normocytic anemia is seen in up to 40% of patients. Evidence of hemolytic anemia may be present, including decreased haptoglobin (see Chapter 6). Thrombocytopenia is found in up to 25% of patients. The ESR may be elevated but does not correlate with disease activity.

C. **Lupus anticoagulant.** Characterized by circulating anticoagulant with an elevated PTT or with circulating antiphospholipid (50% of those with lupus) or anticardiolipin antibodies (see below). Associated with venous or arterial thrombosis (see below).

D. Patients with SLE may have a false-positive VDRL test. However, FTA will be negative.

E. Hypocomplementemia (CH50, C3, C4) may be present and correlates with disease activity.

V. **Treatment.** Generally a rheumatologist should participate, although these patients can be followed by a primary care physician. Treatment should be individualized according to the activity of the disease and organs involved. Avoid sulfa antibiotics and be aware of oral contraceptives, both of which may induce flares.

A. **Preventive care.**

1. **Regular monitoring.** Patients should be seen every 3 to 6 months even if they are doing well.

2. **Energy conservation.** Fatigue is a common complaint.

3. **Photoprotection.** Sunscreen and avoidance of excess sun.

7

RHEUMATOLOGY

4. **Infection control.** Pneumococcal vaccine and yearly influenza vaccine. Consider antibiotic prophylaxis for procedures.

5. **Contraception.** Avoid pregnancy at time of increased disease activity or while using immunosuppressive therapy. Woman with anti-Ro (SSA) particularly run a risk of antibodies crossing the placenta and inducing neonatal lupus, congenital heart block, and miscarriage.

6. **Symptomatic.** Heat to affected joints, conditioning exercises, weight loss if necessary, and relaxation techniques.

B. **Medication.**

1. **NSAIDs/COX-2 inhibitors.** Useful for symptomatic relief of joint pain and the pain associated with pleurisy and pericarditis. Also useful for treatment of systemic symptoms such as fever and fatigue. May combine with a low-dose steroid to minimize side effects of both. Watch for adverse renal effects, especially in those who already have lupus nephritis. See section on RA for details.

2. **Antimalarial drugs (chloroquine, hydroxychloroquine).** Hydroxychloroquine is the most commonly used. Effective for cutaneous, musculoskeletal, and mild systemic symptoms. Mechanism of action is unknown. Begin 400 mg PO daily for 4 weeks and then taper to maintenance dose. Relapse is frequent with discontinuation of drug. See section on RA for side effects and monitoring.

3. **Steroids.** Topical preparations are effective for cutaneous manifestations. If fluorinated limit exposure to 2 weeks. Low-dose oral prednisone (10 mg/day) can be used for minor disease activity. Dose should be once daily in morning to reduce effect on pituitary-adrenal axis and high dose limited to 4 to 6 weeks if possible. Maintenance should be the lowest possible dose, using alternate-day therapy if possible. NSAIDs are used to try to lower steroid dose or for symptomatic treatment on the off day of alternate-day therapy. Prednisone at 1 mg/kg/day may be used for severe flares of joint symptoms, CNS symptoms, and nephritis. IV therapy with methylprednisolone may be needed in particularly severe disease. Consider alendronate, vitamin D, calcium, and low-cholesterol diet as prophylactic measures if oral steroids are required.

4. **Immunosuppressive drugs (azathioprine, cyclophosphamide).** For severe flare and renal or CNS involvement. These are generally reserved for patients who failed conventional therapy.

5. **Anticoagulation.** Persons with antiphospholipid syndrome should be treated with warfarin and low-dose aspirin but only if they have had symptomatic disease (e.g., thrombosis).

DRUG-INDUCED LUPUS

I. **Clinical Features.** A drug-induced lupus-like syndrome characterized by arthralgias, myalgias, fever, and serositis (pleurisy and pericarditis). CNS and renal disease are rare.

II. **Laboratory Tests.** Lab tests reveal cytopenias, ANA, LE. Anti-dsDNA is typically not present. Antihistone antibodies are present in >90% of cases but not specific for drug-induced lupus.

III. **Causative Agents.** Hydralazine and procainamide have been strongly implicated in drug-induced lupus. Other drugs include phenytoin, primidone, isoniazid, chlorpromazine, penicillamine, practolol, propylthiouracil, methylthiouracil, and methyldopa.

IV. **Treatment.** Symptoms usually resolve when the offending drug is withdrawn. Antinuclear antibodies may persist for months.

ANTIPHOSPHOLIPID SYNDROME

I. **General.** Antiphospholipid syndrome (APS) is a disorder characterized by recurrent venous or arterial thrombosis, recurrent fetal loss, and thrombocytopenia associated with the presence of lupus anticoagulant or anticardiolipin antibody, or both. The female-to-male ratio is 2:1. May occur as a manifestation of lupus or may occur as an isolated, discrete syndrome. *Anticardiolipin* and *antiphospholipid* are essentially interchangeable terms. Depending on the assay used to detect them, they cross-react. Several subtypes that do not cross-react have been identified but are currently of little clinical significance.

II. **Clinical Features.**

A. **Pregnancy loss.** Obstetric complications include recurrent fetal loss, often but not always in the late second or third trimester, severe preeclampsia, premature delivery, chorea gravidarum, and intrauterine growth retardation. Patients may also have "postpartum syndrome," which is manifested by pleuropericarditis and fever.

B. **Thrombosis.** All venous and arterial systems can be involved. The most common site for venous thrombosis is in the lower extremities. Patients may have recurrent DVT or PE. The most common arterial complications are embolic cerebrovascular accidents and transient ischemic attacks.

C. **Other features described.** Endocardial valvular vegetations, livedo reticularis, migraine headache, thrombocytopenia, and Coombs'-positive hemolytic anemia.

III. **Diagnosis.**

A. **Criteria for the presence of lupus anticoagulant (LA).** Prolonged partial thromboplastin time (PTT) not corrected by addition of normal plasma but corrected by freeze-thawed platelets or phospholipids.

B. **Anticardiolipin antibody (aCL)** as measured by ELISA.

C. Clinical diagnosis of APS can be made if the patient has experienced unexplained thromboembolism, thrombocytopenia, or recurrent fetal loss in conjunction with persistently elevated titers of aCL or LA.

IV. **Management.**

A. **There is no evidence that prophylactic therapy is helpful in patients who have been and are asymptomatic**

B. **For thrombotic events** chronic anticoagulation with warfarin and antiplatelet drugs (such as ASA) may be used. Heparin may need to be

7

RHEUMATOLOGY

substituted for warfarin during pregnancy. Intravenous immunoglobulin during pregnancy in women with APLS who have failed aspirin and subcutaneous heparin appear to be promising, and controlled trials are currently underway. Because patients may have an elevated PTT and occasionally PT, follow anticoagulation by measuring percent factor 2 activity.

C. Steroids and immunosuppressive drugs have been used for acute flares.

SYSTEMIC SCLEROSIS AND SCLERODERMA

I. **General.** Scleroderma is a diverse group of conditions that have in common fibrosis of skin and other tissues, including the microvascular system, visceral organs, and immunologic system. A subset is classified as having environmentally induced forms of scleroderma.

II. **Clinical Features.**

A. **Skin.** Bilateral symmetric swelling of the fingers and hands is often an early manifestation. Edema is replaced by induration in a few weeks to several months, resulting in thick, hard skin. Skin thickness spreads rapidly and within months may affect the forearms, upper arms, face, and finally the trunk.

B. **Raynaud's phenomenon.** Occurs in almost all patients.

C. **Joints.** Nondeforming symmetric polyarthritis similar to rheumatoid arthritis.

D. **Lungs.** Diffuse interstitial fibrosis occurs in 70% of patients.

E. **Heart.** Cardiac abnormalities, such as conduction defects and supraventricular arrhythmias, are seen in up to 70%.

F. **Gastrointestinal.** Esophageal dysfunction is the most frequent gastrointestinal abnormality but may have malabsorption, etc.

G. **Kidney.** Renal involvement frequently results in fulminant hypertension, renal failure, and death.

III. **Treatment.** No curative therapy available. Penicillamine 125 mg PO QOD may decrease skin thickness, delay internal organ involvement, and prolong life expectancy. A small, open-label trial suggests that minocycline 50 mg PO BID may be effective for early scleroderma. Other treatments are directed against symptoms including Raynaud's phenomenon, hypertension, gastroesophageal reflux, and digital sympathectomy for a critically ischemic finger.

BIBLIOGRAPHY

Amor B: Spondyloarthropathies, Reiter's syndrome, *Rheum Dis Clin North Am* 24(4):677, 1998.

Brennan P, Silman A, Black C, et al: Validity and reliability of three methods used in the diagnosis of Raynaud's phenomenon. The UK Scleroderma Study Group, *Br J Rheumatol* 32:357, 1993.

Bruce I, Gladman DD: Psoriatic arthritis. Recognition and management, *BioDrugs* 9:27, 1998.

Cohen S: Risedronate therapy prevents corticosteroid-induced bone loss, *Arthritis Rheum* 42(11):2309, 1999.

Deal CL, Moskowitz RW: Nutraceuticals as therapeutical agents in osteoarthritis. The role of glucosamin, chondroitin sulfate, and collagen hydrolysate, *Rheum Dis Clin North Am* 25(2):379, 1999.

Dougados M, van den Linden S, Leirisalo-Repo M, et al: Sulfasalazine in the treatment of spondylarthropathy: a randomized, multicenter, double-blind, placebo-controlled study, *Arthritis Rheum* 38:618, 1995.

Duhaut P, Berruyer M, Pinede L, et al: Anticardiolipin antibodies and giant cell arteritis: a prospective, multicenter case-control study, *Arthritis Rheum* 41:701, 1998.

Ellis CN, Fradin MS, Messana JM, et al: Cyclosporin for plaque-type psoriasis. Results of a multidose, double-blind trial, *N Engl J Med* 324:277, 1991.

Emery H: Pediatric scleroderma, *Semin Cutan Med Surg* 17(1):41, 1998.

Fraenkel L: Different factors influencing the expression of Raynaud's phenomenon in men and women, *Arthritis Rheum* 42(2):306, 1999.

Fraenkel L, Zhang Y, Chaisson CE, et al: The association of estrogen replacement therapy and Raynaud's phenomenon in post-menopausal women, *Ann Intern Med* 129:208, 1998.

Fukuda K et al: The chronic fatigue syndrome: a comprehensive approach to its definition and study, *Ann Intern Med* 121(12):953, 1995.

Gladman DD: Psoriatic arthritis, *Rheum Dis Clin North Am* 24(4):829, 1998.

Gladman DD: Psoriatic arthritis. In Maddison PJ et al, editors: *Oxford textbook of rheumatology*, Oxford, 1998, Oxford University Press.

Gladman DD, Brubacher B, Buskila D, et al: Psoriatic spondyloarthropathy in men and women: a clinical, radiographic, and HLA study, *Clin Invest Med* 15:371, 1992.

Gladman DD, Shuckett R, Russell ML, et al: Psoriatic arthritis—clinical and laboratory analysis of 220 patients, *Q J Med* 62:127, 1987.

Hunt JE, McNeil HP, Morgan GJ, et al: A phospholipid B_2-glycoprotein I complex is an antigen for anticardiolipin antibodies occurring in autoimmune disease but not with infection, *Lupus* 1:75, 1992.

Kirwan J, Edwards A, Huitfeldt B, et al: The course of established ankylosing spondylitis and the effects of sulphasalazine over 3 years, *Br J Rheumatol* 32:729, 1993.

Leirisalo-Repo M: Prognosis, course of disease, and treatment of the spondyloarthropathies, *Rheum Dis Clin North Am* 24(4):737, 1998.

LeRoy EC, Medsger TA Jr: Raynaud's phenomenon: a proposal for classification, *Clin Exp Rheumatol* 10:485, 1992.

McGonagle D: Enthesitis in spondyloarthropathy, *Curr Opin Rheumatol* 11(4):244, 1999.

Wallace DJ, Shapiro S, Panush R: Update on fibromyalgia syndrome, *Bull Rheum Dis* 48(5): 1-4, 1999.

Welsch S, Branch DW: Antiphospholipid syndrome in pregnancy: obstetric concerns and treatment, *Rheum Dis Clin North Am* 23:71, 1997.

7

RHEUMATOLOGY

NEPHROLOGY AND UROLOGY

Sudha Rajavel
Rosanna Yuk-Kuen Kao

URINARY TRACT INFECTIONS: FEMALES

I. **Acute Cystitis.**

A. **Signs and symptoms.** Dysuria, frequency, urgency, nocturia, enuresis, incontinence, urethral pain, suprapubic pain, low back pain, hematuria. Fever is unusual. The onset frequently follows intercourse ("honeymoon cystitis"). **Up to 30% of patients with symptoms of cystitis may have a smoldering pyelonephritis (especially if symptoms have been present for more than 1 week).**

B. **Differential diagnosis of urinary symptoms.** Urinary frequency and urgency can be caused by UTI, diuretic use, caffeine, tea, drugs (such as theophylline), interstitial cystitis, vaginitis, pregnancy, pelvic mass, PID, BPH (in the male), as well as other causes.

C. **Cause.** Colonization by fecal flora, usually *Escherichia coli* (75% to 95%). Other organisms include *Klebsiella* (5%), *Enterobacter, Proteus,* and *Pseudomonas.*

D. **Laboratory findings.**

1. **Urinalysis findings** (from clean catch midstream).

   a. **Positive leukocyte esterase, or pyuria.** Usually >5 WBCs per high-power field (HPF). However, 30% of urinalysis results are false negative, so patients may have bacterial cystitis and a negative urinalysis.

   b. **Bacteriuria.** Two organisms per HPF by microscopy; 10^5 organisms per milliliter on culture has classically been considered as a UTI. However, 10^2 organisms/ml is more predictive of symptoms of a UTI.

   c. **Positive dipstick** result for nitrates.

   d. **Hematuria,** gross or microscopic.

2. **C&S.** Not needed in simple UTI. Cultures should be done for recurrent UTIs, pyelonephritis, and in pregnant patients.

E. **Treatment.**

1. **Deciding who to treat.** Presence of classic symptoms in a patient who has had a previous documented UTI is about 70% predictive of a UTI, so one can consider treatment even in the absence of positive urine findings. However, also consider other causes as listed previously under signs and symptoms, especially vaginitis.

2. **Antibiotics.** Can be used in a 3-day regimen for young, sexually active women (preferred over single dose; decreases relapse without increase in side effects), or a standard oral regimen lasting 7 to 10 days. A 7- to 10-day course of antibiotics should be used in pregnant patients, those who have "complicated" UTIs such as the elderly, men, children, those with recurrent UTI, diabetic patients, and

patients with symptoms for more than 1 week who have a higher risk for pyelonephritis.

3. All of the following drugs can be used in a 3-day or 7- to 10-day course. **Failure of a short course of antibiotics generally indicates an upper tract infection and requires 10 to 14 days of antibiotics. Failure of a 14-day course suggests a deep-seated kidney infection and may require 4-6 weeks of antibiotics.**

   a. **TMP/SMX DS.** 1 PO BID. This is generally the preferred treatment, because it is inexpensive and has a cure rate superior to cephalosporins and amoxicillin.

   b. **Fluoroquinolone.** Ciprofloxacin 250 to 500 mg PO BID; levofloxacin 250 to 500 mg PO QD.

   c. **Oral cephalosporin.** Cephalexin 250 to 500 mg QID. Not as efficacious as TMP/SMX.

   d. **Nitrofurantoin.** 50 to 100 mg PO QID with meals and at bedtime. Absorption increased when taken with food.

   e. **Other antibiotics used.** Doxycycline 100 mg PO BID for 7 days; amoxicillin-clavulanic acid; amoxicillin alone has a lower cure rate than other drugs.

4. **Changing antibiotics.** If a culture is done and the organism is resistant to the drug prescribed, a change in antibiotics is indicated only if the patient is still symptomatic. Many drugs reach such high levels in the urine that standard sensitivity testing may not reflect in vivo activity.

5. **Other measures.**

   a. Consider a bladder anesthetic, such as phenazopyridine hydrochloride (Pyridium) 200 mg TID for 2 days to promptly relieve symptoms. Inform the patient that this will produce an orange tinge in tears and urine. Warn the patient not to wear contact lenses because they may become discolored.

   b. Instruct patient to increase fluid intake. See below for other measures.

II. **Chronic Cystitis.** Up to 20% of young females with acute cystitis develop recurrent UTIs. During these recurrences, the causative organism should be identified by urine cultures to differentiate between relapse and recurrence. Multiple infections caused by the same organism are by definition complicated UTIs.

A. **Symptoms.** Similar to simple cystitis but variable in severity.

B. **Laboratory findings.** UA shows a significant bacteriuria and may have any degree of pyuria. Urine culture will be positive, with *Escherichia coli* most common. Pyuria without bacteriuria should be suggestive of *Mycobacterium tuberculosis* or *Chlamydia* infection.

C. **Radiographs.** Excretory and retrograde urograms and voiding cystograms may demonstrate associated conditions: obstructive uropathy, vesicoureteral reflux, atrophic pyelonephritis, and vesicoenteric or vesicovaginal fistulas.

D. **Treatment.** Treat based on susceptibility testing but empirically as per cystitis (above) until sensitivities known.

E. **Prevention.** Women who have more than three UTI recurrences documented by urine cultures within 1 year can be managed using the following:

1. **Acute self-treatment** with a 3-day course of standard therapy.
2. **Postcoital prophylaxis** with TMP/SMX DS, 1 tab after coitus; single-dose fluoroquinolone may be used as second-line treatment. Patients should void immediately after intercourse, although the benefit is questionable.
3. **Continuous daily prophylaxis** with either TMP/SMX 1 single-strength tab daily, nitrofurantoin 50 to 100 mg/day, or a fluoroquinolone (e.g., levofloxacin 250 mg qd).

F. **Other preventive measures.**

1. Cranberry juice has been proven to reduce pyuria and bacteruria by preventing *E. coli* adherence to cells. Increasing fluids in general may be helpful as well.
2. The use of a diaphragm for birth control may exacerbate recurrent UTIs secondary to incomplete voiding. The use of nonoxynol-9 is associated with an increased incidence of bacteriuria.
3. Vaginal estrogen cream (0.5 to 2 g intravaginally daily) diminishes the incidence of UTIs for postmenopausal women.
4. Women should be instructed to wipe from front to back after a bowel movement to avoid bringing infective organisms toward the urethra.
5. There is no evidence that avoiding baths reduces the incidence of cystitis. However, irritating soaps should be eliminated.

III. **Interstitial Cystitis.**

A. **Signs and symptoms.** Frequency, urgency, and rarely urge incontinence with periurethral and suprapubic pain on bladder filling that is improved by voiding. May have terminal hematuria.

B. **Cause.** Unclear; possible autoimmune or allergic process.

C. **Treatment.** Refer to a urologist for cystoscopy and possible biopsy. Unable to diagnose without cystoscopy under anesthesia.

D. **May respond symptomatically** to phenazopyridine (Pyridium). Bladder washes with DMSO have been helpful, as has pentosan, although it is expensive and of limited efficacy (38% but may take up to 9 months for any changes). Hyaluronic acid (Cystistat) is available in Canada and has better efficacy in open trials. Heparin installations in the bladder, hydroxyzine (in standard doses up to 75 mg at bedtime), and tricyclics have also been helpful.

IV. **Radiation Cystitis.** Symptoms may develop months after cessation of treatment with history based on exposure to radiation. Urine may or may not be sterile.

V. **Noninfectious Hemorrhagic Cystitis.** Noninfectious hemorrhagic cystitis can occur after radiation therapy or treatment with cyclophosphamide.

There is often serious vesical hemorrhage. Urgent consultation with a urologist should be sought.

VI. **Urethritis.**

A. Patient may have UTI symptoms, pyuria, but negative cultures.

B. **Causes.** Infections with a low colony count, *Chlamydia, Neisseria gonorrhoeae, Trichomonas,* or vaginitis.

C. **Treatment.** Treat as *Chlamydia* and gonorrhea (see Table 8-1).

VII. **Asymptomatic Bacteriuria.**

A. **Diagnosis requires** >100,000 CFU/ml of urine of **same** organism in two clean-catch specimens **or** >100 organisms on a single catheterized specimen.

B. **Must be distinguished from** contamination from vaginal or urethral organisms attributable to poor technique in specimen collection. Treat based on C&S, not empirically.

C. **The only patients who should be treated for asymptomatic bacteriuria include** those who (1) are pregnant, (2) have had a past urologic procedure, (3) have recently had the removal of an indwelling catheter, (4) have diabetes mellitus, or (5) are children. Asymptomatic bacteriuria is not an indication for treatment with antibiotics in the elderly, because treatment does not affect the outcome in these patients.

URINARY TRACT INFECTION: CHILDREN

I. **Clinical Presentation.** Differs from adults in that symptoms may include only fever, new incontinence in a previously toilet-trained youngster, abdominal pain, diarrhea, vomiting, or lethargy. UTI is a common cause of fever in the neonatal period. Uncircumcised males <8 weeks of age are more prone to UTIs than are females or circumcised males.

II. **Diagnostic Criteria.** Same as for cystitis in females above. However, fever may cause pyuria; therefore culture is always indicated. Quick catheterization should be considered; "bag" urines generally yield poor specimens for culture because of contamination.

III. **Management.** All children with UTIs need a repeat culture 1 to 2 weeks after completing treatment. All children <3 months of age should be admitted for IV antibiotics, as should children who look ill. An older child with simple, uncomplicated UTI can be treated as an outpatient. A 10- to 14-day course of antibiotics is generally prescribed for UTI in children.

A. **IV regimens include** ceftriaxone 75 mg/kg Q24h, gentamicin 7.5 mg/kg/day divided Q8h, or ticarcillin 300 mg/kg/day divided Q6h. Ampicillin 100 mg/kg/day divided Q6h can be added to gentamicin but is often inadequate on its own because of resistance.

B. **PO regimens include** TMP/SMX, 6 to 12 mg TMP, 30 to 60 mg SMX per kilogram per day in two doses; cefixime, 8 mg/kg/day in two doses; or cephalexin, 50 to 100 mg/kg/day in four doses. Amoxicillin/clavulanate can also be used.

IV. **Evaluation.** Radiologic evaluation for anatomic abnormality (IVP, U/S, voiding cystourethrogram) should be obtained on all girls less than

5 years of age, all boys regardless of age, children with evidence of pyelonephritis, and any female >5 years of age with recurrent UTIs, as well as in those that are not responding as expected to antibiotics. The evidence for these recommendations is only fair. Some authors would not work up first cystitis in a girl but would defer work-up until there is a second infection.

LOWER UROGENITAL INFECTIONS: MALES

I. **Overview.**
A. **Cause.** Ascending infection from the urethra most common; reflux of infected urine into prostatic ducts and then into the posterior urethra likely an important cause of prostatitis. Hematogenous, lymphatic spread or extension from adjacent organs also possible.
B. **Pathogens:** *Escherichia coli* (80% to 91%), *Proteus, Enterobacter, Pseudomonas, Serratia, Streptococcus faecalis,* and *Staphylococcus* species are the most common.
C. **Localization of infection.** Divided urine collection may help localize the infection: urethra represented by first voided 10 ml, bladder represented by midstream collection, and prostate represented by the last 10 ml of voided urine. Prostatic massage before the last voided 10 ml will increase the yield.

II. **Urethritis.**
A. **Presentation.** Generally complain of a urethral discharge (watery to purulent), with or without urethral burning or itching, and burning on urination. May not note discharge but may have spotting in underwear.
B. **Cause.** *Neisseria gonorrhoeae* and *Chlamydia trachomatis* (causes 80% of non-GC) most common, followed by *Ureaplasma urealyticum, Mycoplasma hominis, Trichomonas vaginalis, Candida,* and herpesviruses.
C. **History.** Ask about first onset of symptoms, recent sexual contacts, prior history of STDs.
D. **Work-up.** Examination should be performed at least 1 hour after the last void. **Notice character of discharge:** watery and thin are suggestive of *Chlamydia,* whereas a purulent-looking discharge is suggestive of gonorrhea. Obtain a specimen by inserting a calcium alginate (Kalginate) swab 2 to 3 cm within the urethra (a drop of the discharge is not acceptable because *Chlamydia* organisms are intracellular and urethral cellular material is required for culture).
E. **Laboratory findings.** Gram stain of urethral discharge should show >4 WBCs per HPF. Demonstration of intracellular gram-negative diplococci within PMNs is strong evidence of gonorrhea. Absence of gram-negative cocci is strong evidence of nongonococcal urethritis (such as *Chlamydia*). However, Gram stain is only 95% sensitive for GC. Culture on modified Thayer-Martin medium for gonorrhea (<100% sensitive) and send for immunofluorescent testing and PCR, or culture for *Chlamydia.*

8

NEPHROLOGY AND UROLOGY

F. **Treatment** (see Table 8-1). Be sure to treat for both *Chlamydia* and *N. gonorrhoeae* and to treat partner.

III. **Bacterial Cystitis.**

A. **Signs and symptoms.** Similar to those in females. Also examine urethra for discharge (urethritis), prostate, and epididymis for tenderness to rule out other disorders.

B. **Laboratory findings.** UA shows pyuria, bacteriuria, no casts, occasionally gross or microscopic hematuria. **C&S should be done in males with history consistent with UTI.**

C. **Treatment.** Treat 10 to 14 days and then obtain follow-up culture. Antibiotic choices are similar to those for female UTI. After successful treatment (urine is sterile), consider intravenous pyelography (IVP) or cystoscopy to rule out structural obstruction to outflow.

IV. **Infections of the Prostate Gland.** Up to 95% of prostate complaints in men are related to nonbacterial prostatitis or prostatodynia. If symptoms are not relieved after a course of antibiotics, consider some of the following diagnoses.

A. **Acute bacterial prostatitis.**

1. **Signs and symptoms.** Acute febrile illness, chills, malaise, lower back pain, perineal pain, urinary urgency or frequency, nocturia, or dysuria. Varying degrees of urinary retention, tenesmus, or pain with bowel movement. The prostate is very tender, boggy, and warm to touch. (Do not massage because of risk of bacteremia.)

2. **Laboratory findings.** Leukocytosis with left shift, bacteriuria, hematuria, and pyuria. C&S required.

3. **Therapy.**

   a. Hospitalization for IV antibiotics if sepsis suspected. Start gentamicin or tobramycin and ampicillin pending culture results. An alternative is ofloxacin 400 mg PO then 300 mg PO BID.

   b. If hospitalization is not necessary (no fever; patient not toxic), prescribe TMP/SMX DS twice daily for 10 to 14 days, ciprofloxacin 500 BID, or ofloxacin 300 mg BID for 10 to 14 days. In young, sexually active men, treat for gonorrhea and *Chlamydia* infections for 14 days as well. In general, the fluoroquinoiones penetrate the prostate better and are preferred for this indication.

   c. Continuing oral antibiotics for l month after an episode of acute prostatitis may reduce recurrence and reduce transformation into chronic prostatitis.

   d. Avoid urethral catheterization if possible.

   e. After completion of successful therapy, the patient should be followed for at least 4 months with periodic examinations and cultures of prostatic fluids to ensure cure.

B. **Chronic bacterial prostatitis.**

1. **Signs and symptoms.** Low back and perineal discomfort; voiding symptoms similar to those of acute bacterial prostatitis but with a more insidious onset. No systemic signs; rarely painful ejaculation.

Prostate may feel normal, boggy, or focally indurated. Chronic prostatitis is the most common cause of recurrent UTIs in men.

2. **Laboratory tests.** UA and cultures should be done. Prostatic secretions reveal inflammatory cells, with macrophages containing oval fat bodies. UA will show WBCs and bacteriuria if secondary cystitis is present. Causative agents are usually *E. coli* or *Pseudomonas*. **But many cases of chronic prostatitis are not bacterial (see below).**

3. **Treatment.** Ciprofloxacin 500 mg PO or norfloxacin 400 mg PO BID for 4 to 6 weeks. Levofloxacin 500 mg PO QD is another option. This yields about an 80% cure rate. TMP/SMX DS twice daily for 3 months cures about one third of cases and improves symptoms in about three fourths. Failure of therapy may indicate the need for IV antibiotics or the presence of infected prostatic calculi. Chronic suppression with TMP/SMX or a quinolone at nighttime may be helpful.

C. **Nonbacterial prostatitis.**

1. **Cause.** Unknown. It is a diagnosis of exclusion. *Chlamydia, Ureaplasma,* and *Mycoplasma* infection and autoimmune processes are suspected but not proved. Consider also tuberculosis, mycotic infections, viral infections, or *Cryptococcus* infection in AIDS patients.

2. **Signs and symptoms.** Same as for chronic bacterial prostatitis.

3. **Laboratory findings.** Prostatic secretions reveal inflammatory cells but no bacteria. Never able to document UTI by culture.

4. **Therapy**

   a. A clinical trial of antibiotic therapy directed to aforementioned organisms is recommended: doxycycline 100 mg twice daily, erythromycin 500 mg 4 times daily, or ofloxacin 300 mg twice daily should be tried for at least 4 weeks. Because nonbacterial prostatitis usually does not respond to antibiotics, their continued empirical use is not justified beyond an initial 4-week course.

   b. Symptomatic flare-ups often respond to anti-inflammatory agents, such as ibuprofen 400 to 600 mg PO Q4-6h.

   c. Alpha-adrenergic receptor blocking agent may help: prazosin 2 to 4 mg orally twice daily, or terazosin 5 to 10 mg orally twice daily.

   d. Other measures: hot sitz baths, reassurance. The recurrent symptoms can often cause significant emotional stress, anxiety, and depression resulting in significant morbidity.

D. **Prostatodynia.**

1. Symptoms suggestive of prostatitis (prostatic or pelvic pain) but without infection or inflammation and negative labs and cultures. It is a syndrome of variable cause.

   a. In some men urodynamic testing discloses voiding dysfunction associated with apparent functional obstruction of the bladder neck and urethra. This "spasm" may result in intraprostatic reflux and chemical irritation of the prostate by urine. In such cases there is a favorable response to an alpha-adrenergic blocker such as pra-

8

NEPHROLOGY AND UROLOGY

zosin 2 to 4 mg orally twice daily or terazosin 5 to 10 mg orally once daily.

b. In other cases there is tension myalgia of the pelvic floor, which may respond to diathermy, muscle relaxants, and physiotherapy with or without the use of diazepam 5 mg orally TID. Tricyclics may also be helpful. Allopurinol hs been useful in some cases but is not considered standard of care.

E. **Epididymitis.**

1. **Causes.**

   a. Sexually transmitted form associated with urethritis and commonly caused by *Chlamydia* or *N. gonorrhoeae* or both.

   b. Nonsexually transmitted form associated with UTI or prostatitis, commonly caused by *Enterobacter* or *Pseudomonas* organisms.

   c. Causes such as trauma, tuberculosis, urine reflux, or as a complication of TURP or systemic infection are less common.

2. **Signs and symptoms.** Epididymis is painful, and swelling and tenderness may extend to groin, lower abdomen, or flank. Fever, urethral discharge, and reactive hydrocele may occur but are not common.

3. **Laboratory findings.** White count may be normal or elevated with left shift. UA may show pyuria or bacteriuria. C&S is indicated.

4. **Differential diagnosis.** Mumps orchitis, tumor, testicular abscess, torsion, and trauma must be considered.

5. **Therapy.**

   a. **General measures.** Bed rest, scrotal elevation and support, analgesics, ice (early), heat (late), and spermatic cord block with lidocaine may be used.

   b. **Antibiotics** (see Table 8-1).

   c. **NSAIDs.** Effective for inflammatory component.

UPPER URINARY TRACT INFECTION: MALES AND FEMALES

I. **Acute Pyelonephritis.**

A. **Definition.** Infection of the parenchyma and pelvis of the kidney, which may affect one or occasionally both kidneys.

B. **Causes.** Aerobic gram-negative bacterium, most commonly *E. coli*. All organisms causing acute cystitis can cause acute pyelonephritis. *Proteus* species are especially important because they produce urease, which causes alkaline urine and favors formation of struvite and apatite stones. Staphylococci may infect by hematogenous route and cause renal abscesses.

C. **Clinical findings.** Abrupt onset of shaking chills and fever >38.5° C, flank pain, malaise, and urinary frequency and burning. Often nausea, vomiting, and diarrhea as well. Generally have CVA tenderness. May be in septic shock. Children may complain of abdominal pain.

D. **Laboratory findings.** Leukocytosis with left shift. UA will show pyuria, white blood cell casts, hematuria, and mild proteinuria. C&S of urine is mandatory; some also obtain blood cultures, but the efficacy is questionable because the organism will be recovered in the urine. With the exception of WBC casts, bacteremia, and flank pain, none of the physical or lab findings is specific for pyelonephritis, so be sure to rule out other causes of fever, back pain, and so on. BUN and creatinine usually remain normal in uncomplicated pyelonephritis.

E. **Treatment.**

1. **Hospitalize.** If the patient is a child, is an infant, is pregnant, has a high fever, is dehydrated, appears "acutely ill," or is septic, hospitalization is indicated. Recent data indicate that "healthy-looking" pregnant patients can be treated as outpatients, but this is not yet the standard of care. Treat empirically with IV third-generation cephalosporin with or without gentamicin, IV or oral fluoroquinolone (oral fluoroquinolones attain the same serum levels as IV), gentamicin and ampicillin, ampicillin-sulbactam, or ticarcillin/clavulanic acid pending culture and sensitivity results. Avoid gentamicin and fluoroquinolones in pregnant patients. Treat IV for about 48 to 72 hours or more according to clinical response. Continue oral antibiotics and then complete with oral antibiotics for 2 to 6 more weeks. Medication should be given for pain, fever, and nausea. Ensure adequate hydration and maintenance of good urine output with either IV or oral fluids. See also septic shock in Chapter 10.

2. **If the patient is not acutely ill,** treat as outpatient for 10 days to 6 weeks with TMP/SMX, fluoroquinolone (e.g., ciprofloxacin 500 mg PO BID, levofloxacin 500 mg PO QD), amoxicillin/clavulanic acid, or a cephalosporin. Fluoroquinolones achieve the same levels in the blood orally and IV, making these a good choice. A good option is to give 1 g of ceftriaxone IV or IM at the time of diagnosis and then follow up the patient the next day. If required, an additional dose of ceftriaxone can be given at the follow-up exam if the patient warrants more than oral antibiotics but does not require hospitalization. Ensure good communication in case of worsening condition and establish follow-up care.

3. **If the patient is not improving** after 72 hours of appropriate antimicrobial therapy, consider infected stones or obstruction and treat early to avoid complications. If the patient is not responding to antibiotics and the organism is known to be sensitive to the current antibiotics, consider emphysematous pyelonephritis or abscess formation. CT scan will identify these patients. In the small percentage of patients who relapse after a 2-week course, a 6-week course is usually curative.

4. **Follow-up study.** Consider IVP or voiding cystourethrogram (VCUG) after resolution of UTI in all children and males or in females with frequent recurrences or unusual symptoms. Urine culture should be done 1 to 2 weeks after therapy in pregnant patients, children, patients who remain symptomatic, and those for whom suppression therapy is being considered. Follow-up cultures are optional for others.

SEXUALLY TRANSMITTED DISEASES

General note on testing: Because *Chlamydia* can be asymptomatic, it is important to screen high-risk populations such as those younger than 20 years of age, those with more than one sexual partner, and so on. There are now screening tests (PCR) that can be performed on the urine for *Chlamydia*, making a pelvic exam unnecessary. The sensitivity of gonorrhea (GC) culture is highly dependent on technique. At best, sensitivity is 85%. Gram stain is 95% sensitive in men and 48% in women. DNA testing and fluorescent antibody testing are also available for GC.

I. **Syphilis.** Caused by the spirochete *Treponema pallidum*.

A. **Primary syphilis.**

1. **Clinical presentation.** Characteristic sign is the chancre, a painless sore that usually develops 2 to 4 weeks after exposure. These are 1 to 2 cm in diameter, may be multiple, appear as shallow ulcerations with noninflamed margins, and occur most commonly on mucous membranes abraded during sexual contact. Chancres heal spontaneously and slowly without scarring in 2 to 12 weeks. Unilateral or bilateral inguinal lymphadenopathy may be present.

2. **Laboratory findings.** Dark-field exam of suspicious lesions will reveal spirochetes. VDRL test or RPR test is initially positive in 50% of patients but may remain negative for up to 3 weeks after the appearance of the chancre. The VDRL is nonspecific and may be positive in other disease states (e.g., connective tissue disorders). FTA-ABS is the quickest, least expensive, and most specific and sensitive examination. Following therapy, the VDRL and RPR should revert to negative. However, the FTA will remain positive in the great majority (80%+).

3. **Therapy** (Table 8-1). Patients may experience fever, chills, arthralgias, myalgias, and nausea several hours after treatment (the Jarisch-Herxheimer reaction), usually subsiding within 24 hours. VDRL titers usually return to nonreactive within 1 year of treatment.

B. **Secondary syphilis.**

1. **Clinical presentation.** Widespread, symmetric rash, often involving palms or soles (80%). Rash is usually erythematous but is otherwise variable in appearance (such as morbilliform, similar to pityriasis rosea, etc.) and normally occurs 4 to 8 weeks after chancre. Condylomata lata, oral or genital mucous patches (superficial mucosal erosions), systemic symptoms (50%), and symmetric adenopathy also occur. The lesions of secondary syphilis resolve with or without treatment in 2 to 10 weeks.

2. **Laboratory findings.** Dark-field exam of condylomata lata is often positive. VDRL test is highly reactive in 90% but should be confirmed with FTA-ABS.

3. **Therapy.** See Table 8-1.

C. **Tertiary syphilis.** May have gumma formation, tabes dorsalis (sensory loss in legs secondary to dorsal column changes), lymphocytic meningitis, aortic insufficiency, and dementia.

TABLE 8-1

TREATMENT OF SEXUALLY TRANSMITTED DISEASES

Type and Location	Drug of Choice	Alternatives
CHLAMYDIA TRACHOMATIS DISEASES		
Urethritis, proctitis, nongonococcal urethritis (treat also for gonorrhea)	Doxycycline 100 mg PO BID for 7 days* Azithromycin 1 g as single dose*	Erythromycin base 500 mg PO QID for 7 days (preferred in pregnancy) OR Ofloxacin 300 mg BID for 7 days
Persistent urethritis	Metronidazole 2 g orally in a single dose PLUS Erythromycin base 500 mg orally four times a day for 7 days OR Erythromycin ethylsuccinate 800 mg orally four times a day for 7 days	
Lymphogranuloma venereum	Doxycycline 100 mg PO BID for 21 days	Erythromycin 500 mg PO QID for 21 days
NEISSERIA GONORRHOEAE GONORRHEA		
Urethritis, proctitis, pharyngitis (treat also for Chlamydia)	Cefixime 400 mg orally in a single dose OR Ceftriaxone 125 mg IM in a single dose OR Ciprofloxacin 500 mg orally in a single dose OR Ofloxacin 400 mg orally in a single dose PLUS Azithromycin 1 g orally in a single dose OR Doxycycline 100 mg orally twice a day for 7 days	

From *MMWR* 47(RR-1), 1998.

Note: If treating for either *Neisseria gonorrhoeae* or *Chlamydia trachomatis*, treat for both organisms, because patients frequently have concurrent infections. **Always treat a sexual partner or partners as well.**

*Doxycycline is as efficacious as azithromycin for chlamydia even if the patient does not take all of the doses. Bacteriologic cure rates are 95% for both drugs (and doxycycline is less expensive).

Continued

8

NEPHROLOGY AND UROLOGY

TABLE 8-1

TREATMENT OF SEXUALLY TRANSMITTED DISEASES—cont'd

Type and Location	Drug of Choice	Alternatives
NEISSERIA GONORRHOEAE GONORRHEA—cont'd		
Disseminated	*Initial:* Ceftriaxone 1 g IV or IM Q24h until asymptomatic; follow with: Cefixime 400 mg orally twice a day OR Ciprofloxacin 500 mg orally twice a day OR Ofloxacin 400 mg orally twice a day for a total of 7-10 days	*Initial, alternative:* Cefotaxime 1 g IV Q8h OR Ceftizoxime 1 g IV Q8h OR For persons allergic to beta-lactam drugs: Ciprofloxacin 500 mg IV every 12 hours OR Ofloxacin 400 mg IV Q12h OR Spectinomycin 2 g IM Q12h; follow with regimen to left
PELVIC INFLAMMATORY DISEASE		
Initial treatment	Cefotetan 2 g IV Q12h OR Cefoxitin 2 g IV Q6h PLUS Doxycycline 100 mg IV or orally Q12h	Ofloxacin 400 mg IV Q12h PLUS Metronidazole 500 mg IV Q8h OR Ampicillin/sulbactam 3 g IV Q6h PLUS Doxycycline 100 mg IV or orally Q12h OR Ciprofloxacin 200 mg IV Q12h PLUS Doxycycline 100 mg IV or orally Q12h PLUS Metronidazole 500 mg IV Q8h
Follow-up treatment	Ofloxacin 400 mg orally twice a day for 14 days PLUS Metronidazole 500 mg orally twice a day for 14 days	Ceftriaxone 250 mg IM once OR Cefoxitin 2 g IM plus probenecid 1 g orally in a single dose concurrently once OR Other parenteral third-generation cephalosporin (e.g., ceftizoxime or cefotaxime) PLUS Doxycycline 100 mg orally twice a day for 14 days (include this regimen with one of the above regimens)

EPIDIDYMO-ORCHITIS

If likely an STD	Ceftriaxone 250 mg IM in a single dose PLUS Doxycycline 100 mg orally twice a day for 10 days
If likely enteric organism	Ofloxacin 300 mg PO BID for 10 days

TRICHOMONAS

Trichomonas urethritis or vaginitis	Metronidazole 2 g PO in single dose (recommended in pregnancy by the CDC) OR Metronidazole 500 mg BID for 7 days

GRANULOMA INGUINALE

Granuloma inguinale, Calymmatobacterium granulomatis	Trimethoprim-sulfamethoxazole one double-strength tablet orally twice a day for a minimum of 3 weeks OR Doxycycline 100 mg orally twice a day for a minimum of 3 weeks Therapy continues until all lesions have healed completely

CHANCROID

Chancroid (H. ducreyi)	Ceftriaxone 250 mg IM once OR Azithromycin 1 g PO in single dose OR Erythromycin base 500 mg PO QID for 7 days

SYPHILIS

Primary and secondary	Benzathine penicillin G 2.4 million units IM in a single dose

From *MMWR 47*(RR-1), 1998.

Note: If treating for either *Neisseria gonorrhoeae* or *Chlamydia trachomatis*, treat for both organisms, because patients frequently have concurrent infections. **Always treat a sexual partner or partners as well.**

(Right column continuation)

	Ampicillin/sulbactam or third-generation cephalosporin
	No effective alternatives
	Ciprofloxacin 750 mg orally twice a day for a minimum of 3 weeks OR Erythromycin base 500 mg orally four times a day for a minimum of 3 weeks
	Ciprofloxacin 500 mg PO BID for 3 days OR TMP/SMX DS 1 PO BID for 7 days
	Doxycycline 100 mg orally twice a day for 2 weeks OR Tetracycline 500 mg orally four times a day for 2 weeks

NEPHROLOGY AND UROLOGY

8

Continued

TABLE 8-1

TREATMENT OF SEXUALLY TRANSMITTED DISEASES—cont'd

Type and Location	Drug of Choice	Alternatives
SYPHILIS —cont'd		
Latent	*Early latent syphilis:* Benzathine penicillin G 2.4 million units IM in a single dose	§Doxycycline 100 mg orally twice a day OR Tetracycline 500 mg orally four times a day
	Late latent syphilis or latent syphilis of unknown duration: Benzathine penicillin G 7.2 million units total, administered as three doses of 2.4 million units IM each at 1-week intervals	
Teritiary	Benzathine penicillin G 7.2 million units total, administered as three doses of 2.4 million units IM at 1-week intervals	As above
HERPES SIMPLEX		
Initial episode†	Acyclovir 400 mg PO TID for 7-10 days OR Famciclovir 250 mg PO TID for 7-10 days	Valacyclovir 1000 mg PO BID for 7-10 days
Chronic suppression	Acyclovir 400 mg orally twice a day OR Famciclovir 250 mg orally twice a day OR ‡Valacyclovir 500 mg orally once a day OR Valacyclovir 1000 mg orally once a day	

| Recurrent | Acyclovir 400 mg orally three times a day for 5 days OR
Acyclovir 200 mg orally five times a day for 5 days OR
Acyclovir 800 mg orally twice a day for 5 days OR
Famciclovir 125 mg orally twice a day for 5 days OR
Valacyclovir 500 mg orally twice a day for 5 days | Valacyclovir 500 mg PO BID for 5 days |
| Disseminated herpes | Acyclovir 5-10 mg/kg body weight IV every 8 hours for 5-7 days or until clinical resolution is attained | |

From *MMWR* 47(RR-1), 1998.

NOTE: If treating for either *Neisseria gonorrhoeae* or *Chlamydia trachomatis*, treat for both organisms, because patients frequently have concurrent infections. **Always treat a sexual partner or partners as well.**

†May continue for longer than 10 days if lesions have not resolved.
‡Less efficacious than other regimens.
§For pregnancy, desensitize to penicillin and treat with penicillin.

NEPHROLOGY AND UROLOGY

8

D. **Therapy.** Treat based on duration of infection. Follow the VDRL test at 3, 6, and 12 months in all patients with syphilis. If the treatment is adequate, the VDRL test results should become negative.

II. **Gonorrhea.** Caused by gram-negative diplococcus *Neisseria gonorrhoeae.* (For discussion of gonococcal disease in the male, see previous section on urethritis.)

A. **Signs and symptoms.** The primary site of infection is the endocervix with secondary infection of the rectum or urethra. Yellow-white discharge may be present, but the infection is frequently asymptomatic. Findings may include friable cervix, yellow-green cervical discharge, sterile pyuria, positive cultures, or other evidence of gonorrhea. Other infections include proctitis, pharyngitis, salpingitis, and disseminated disease (pustulovesicular lesions with arthralgias and arthritis).

B. **Laboratory findings.** Gram stain of a vaginal smear reveals gram-negative intracellular diplococci (only 30% to 70%). Culture on Thayer-Martin (chocolate agar) medium to grow *Neisseria* organisms.

C. **Therapy.** See Table 8-1. Repeat cultures should be obtained 3 to 7 days after treatment to ensure adequate treatment. Sexual partner or partners should also be treated.

III. **Chancroid.** Caused by a gram-negative rod, *Haemophilus ducreyi.*

A. **Signs and symptoms.** A papule that becomes a pustule that subsequently ulcerates. In distinction to syphilis, the ulcers of chancroid are painful. Lesions are deep with flat, ragged erythematous borders that may extend into subcutaneous tissue. Adenopathy is common; systemic signs of fever, headache, and malaise occur in 50%.

B. **Laboratory findings.** Smear reveals gram-negative rods in chains ("school of fish"). Culture on enriched chocolate agar with vancomycin may be positive; biopsy specimen is diagnostic.

C. **Therapy.** See Table 8-1.

IV. **Lymphogranuloma Venereum.** Caused by a highly virulent strain of *Chlamydia trachomatis.*

A. **Signs and symptoms.** A papule or pustule that appears 5 to 21 days after exposure and ulcerates. This lesion often goes unnoticed. Painful adenopathy (usually unilateral) occurs 1 to 2 weeks later. May form buboes, become fluctuant, or form chronic draining sinuses. Generally have fever, chills, or rash. Rectal strictures from anorectal node involvement can be seen.

B. **Laboratory findings.** Complement fixation titers should show a fourfold increase after 4 weeks. Culture of aspirate for *C. trachomatis* is diagnostic but is positive in only 20% to 30%.

C. **Therapy.** See Table 8-1. I&D of nodes is rarely indicated.

V. **Herpes Simplex Genitalis.** Caused by herpes simplex virus type II (occasionally type I).

A. **Signs and symptoms.** Often asymptomatic. Incubation is 2 to 10 days. Primary lesion is manifest by grouped painful vesicles on an erythematous base that ulcerate and heal without scarring. Fever and adenopathy are common. Secondary lesions are similar to primary lesions except that the duration and severity are less and accompanying fever and adenopathy are rare.

B. **Laboratory findings.** Tzanck smear of a base of a fresh vesicle (Giemsa stain) reveals multinucleated giant cells. Culture requires 48 to 72 hours; rapid antigen test is available. Serologic tests are available for herpesvirus but are generally negative during a primary disease and do not reliably differentiate type I from type II herpesvirus.

C. **Therapy.** See Table 8-1.

VI. **Condyloma Acuminatum.** Caused by human papillomavirus.

A. **Signs and symptoms.** Soft, flesh-colored, verrucous lesions in genital area. Is associated with an increased risk of cervical dysplasia and cancer.

B. **Laboratory findings.** Serologic studies may be necessary to rule out condyloma latum of secondary syphilis. Biopsy specimen (rarely necessary) is diagnostic.

C. **Therapy.**

1. **Podophyllin (10% to 25% in tincture of benzoin).** Applied and then thoroughly washed off in 1 to 4 hours. Alternatively, home therapy with the preparation Podofilox 0.5% can be tried. Warts are treated twice daily for 3 days; an area of no more than 10 cm^2 should be treated. No further applications should be made for 4 days. This cycle can be repeated three times (a total of four cycles of 3 days of treatment over a 4-week period). If a poor or no response is noted, another therapeutic modality should be tried.

2. **Trichloroacetic acid.** Can be applied cautiously to lesions. It is highly caustic and will injure normal skin.

3. **Intravaginal 5-FU.** Use 5% 5-fluorouracil cream and apply one fourth of applicator QHS for 1 week and then once a week for 10 weeks. Alternatively, the cream can be used twice per week for 10 weeks. Many women will not tolerate these regimens because of erosion of vaginal mucosa.

4. **Alternative therapies.** Cryotherapy, electrosurgery, excision, laser vaporization, or intralesional interferon. Imiquimod is an immune modulator that is used three times per week and is 73% successful in women after 16 weeks of treatment. Its efficacy is only 30% to 40% in men.

5. **Condylomas.** Tend to recur in 7.5% to 80%.

VII. **Molluscum Contagiosum.** Caused by a poxvirus.

A. **Signs and symptoms.** Dome-shaped papules, 2 to 6 mm with central umbilication.

B. **Laboratory findings.** Incision of a papule reveals white waxy core. Smear of contents reveals swollen epithelial cells. Biopsy specimen is diagnostic.

C. **Therapy.** Curettage, cryosurgery, or electrodesiccation.

VIII. **Candidiasis.** Yeast infection caused by *Candida albicans* (see Chapter 13).

IX. **Trichomoniasis.** Caused by protozoon *Trichomonas vaginalis*. See Table 8-1 and Chapter 13.

X. **Chlamydia.** Caused by *Chlamydia trachomatis*. See Table 8-1 and Chapter 13.

XI. **Bacterial Vaginosis.** May present as malodorous vaginal discharge. See Chapter 13 for details.

BENIGN PROSTATIC HYPERTROPHY

I. **Cause.** Benign prostatic hypertrophy (BPH) rarely affects men <40 years of age, with symptoms generally beginning between 60 to 65 years of age.

II. **Clinical Presentation.**

A. **Signs and symptoms** include decreased force and caliber of urinary stream, hesitancy, retention, postmicturition dribbling, double voiding (patient voids and is able to void again in 5 to 10 minutes), and overflow urinary incontinence (on straining or coughing). Irritative symptoms such as dysuria, frequency, nocturia, urgency, hematuria, and incontinence occur frequently. Flank pain during micturition, suprapubic pain, and azotemic symptoms occur less commonly.

B. **Exam.** The bladder may be distended, and the prostate is enlarged, smooth, and symmetric. The prostate gland may be soft or firm and possibly nodular. However, the nodules lack the stony-hard consistency associated with carcinoma.

C. **Laboratory findings.** UA may reveal signs of infection. If the obstruction has been severe enough to impair renal function, BUN and creatinine may be elevated. PSA may be elevated.

D. **Radiographic findings.** IVP may show upper tract or bladder changes secondary to obstruction (hydroureteronephrosis, bladder trabeculation and thickening, bladder diverticula or calculi). VCUG may be indicated. Postvoid catheterization will reveal residual urine. Order an ultrasonogram with rectal probe and biopsies if indicated, to rule out carcinoma. Cystoscopy if indicated.

E. **Uroflowmetry.** It is the most frequently used and most informative though nonspecific method of diagnosing bladder neck obstruction. Maximum flow rate should be >15 ml/sec. Flow rate of <10 ml/sec usually indicates infravesical obstruction.

F. **Postvoid residual urine.** It is a useful tool for follow-up and evaluation of response to therapy.

G. **Pressure flow studies.** These are indicated in patients with normal peak flow rates but with symptoms suggestive of infravesical obstruction and patients with symptoms suggestive of bladder voiding dysfunction.

H. **Treatment.** Men with mild symptoms may be managed by watchful waiting. Those with moderate symptoms may be managed by medical treatment. Those with severe symptoms are candidates for surgical treatment. An indwelling Foley catheter may help acute episodes but is only a temporary measure.

1. **Medical measures.** Terazosin 1 to 2 mg/day is often helpful in relieving symptoms. Tamsulosin 0.4 to 0.8 mg/day may be helpful, but it is more expensive. Finasteride (Proscar) 5 mg PO QD blocks transformation of testosterone to 5a-dihydrotestosterone. Shrinks prostate tissue but may take 6 to 12 months to have a clinical effect. Hypertrophy recurs on stopping drug. Recent data indicate that finasteride may be no better than placebo at relieving symptoms of benign prostatic hypertrophy.

2. **Surgical measures.** Transurethral prostatectomy (TURP) is the gold standard surgical treatment, but it should not be performed in patients who want to remain fertile. There is a significant incidence of incontinence and impotence following TURP.

3. **Antibiotics** should be used to control infection when indicated.

4. If exam reveals nodularity of the gland, referral to a urologist is indicated.

5. **Phytotherapy.** See Chapter 22 for herbal formulary.

HEMATURIA

I. **Definition.** *Hematuria* is defined as >3 to 5 RBC/HPF. Incidence is 13% to 40% depending on the population studied. Hematuria in the anticoagulated patient has the same significance as that in the "normal" patient and should not be ignored.

II. **Cause.** Possible causes include trauma, tumor, kidney stones, cystitis, prostatitis, pyelonephritis, glomerulonephritis, urethral stricture, and foreign body. Consider systemic disorders that produce vasculitis (Wegener's granulomatosis, SLE, etc.), "malignant" hypertension, or bacterial endocarditis. Also crystalluria, familial thin basement membrane disease, and traumatic exercise such as running may cause hematuria. Schistosomiasis and sickle cell disease should be considered in the proper population. **If dipstick is positive for blood but microscopic exam is negative for cells, consider hemoglobinuria or myoglobinuria.**

III. **Evaluation** (for trauma-related hematuria, see Chapter 2).

A. **History and physical exam.** May provide evidence to indicate cause.

B. **Laboratory and radiologic investigation.**

   1. **Urinalysis and renal function tests.**

   2. **Different strategies.**

      a. The following strategy has been suggested by Black and colleagues (Black ER et al, editors: *Diagnostic strategies for common medical problems,* Philadelphia, 1999, American College of Physicians):

         (1) All patients over 50 years of age **or** with risk factors for urologic malignancy (smoking; dye exposure; chemical, textile, leather, or rubber industry work; cyclophosphamide history; use of phenacetin-containing products) or individuals with history consistent with a significant underlying cause (weight

loss, fevers, etc.) should be evaluated with urine cytologic analysis, IVP, and cystoscopy.

(2) Those <50 years of age without any risk factors require only a KUB (or preferably a renal ultrasound) and a serum creatinine to assess renal function (the incidence of a serious underlying cause in these asymptomatic individuals is <1%). If these are normal, a follow-up exam with recheck of the urine can be done. If hematuria is persistent and no other cause is evident (such as running), it seems prudent to work up the patient.

b. **Other authors argue for a full work-up of all patients with hematuria.** If one chooses watchful waiting, discussion with the patient of pros and cons of work-up versus waiting must be documented.

c. **All children with unexplained hematuria need a complete work-up including radiologic examination.**

IV. **Treatment.** Address underlying cause.

UROLITHIASIS

I. **Overview.** Urolithiasis is a common cause of both hematuria and abdominal, flank, or groin pain affecting about 4% to 5% of the population. Of these, 50% will have a second stone within 5 years and 60% within 9 years. Stones can be composed of calcium, oxalate, urate, cystine, xanthine, phosphate, or all of these.

II. **Clinical Presentation and Evaluation.**

A. **History.** Pain is usually of sudden onset, severe and colicky, not improved by position, radiating from the back, down flank, and into groin. Hematuria may be noted. Nausea and vomiting are common. Predisposing factors may be present: recent reduction in fluid intake, medications that predispose to hyperuricemia, history of gout, increased exercise with dehydration. Children <16 years of age make up 7% of those with stones and may present with only painless hematuria.

B. **Physical examination.** May reveal costovertebral-angle tenderness. Tachycardia may be present, or the patient may have bradycardia from a vasovagal reaction. Vitals are usually stable, and there should be no abdominal peritoneal signs.

C. **Laboratory findings.** Urinalysis will demonstrate gross or microscopic hematuria in 75% to 90% of patients with stones. In the other 10% to 25% the urine may be normal. **A normal urinalysis does not rule out urolithiasis.** Urine culture should be obtained, and a fresh urine sample should be examined for crystals. WBC may be increased on CBC secondary to pain and demargination. BUN and creatinine should be obtained.

D. **Differential diagnosis.** Abdominal aortic aneurysm dissection and bowel ischemia can mimic urolithiasis and must be diagnosed clinically or by radiographic study before pain is assumed to be from urolithiasis. Also consider other causes of abdominal pain (see Chapter 15).

E. **Imaging studies.** Noncontrast spiral CT has replaced IVP as the study of choice for the diagnosis of urolithiasis. The sensitivity of CT is 96% vs. 86% for IVP. Additionally, it is faster and requires less radiation and no dye exposure. However, CT will not demonstrate indinavir stones.

III. **Initial Treatment.** Analgesia, adequate hydration, and obtaining a urine specimen for analysis. Antibiotics as indicated for pyelonephritis or concurrent UTI.

A. **Ketorolac 15 to 30 mg IV and narcotics** (such as **morphine** 2 to 10 mg or more IV) are usually required for analgesia. NSAIDs (such as ketorolac) are as effective as if not more effective for renal colic than are narcotics. However, they should be used as supplements to IV narcotics. There is no indication for IM medications in treating renal colic.

B. **IV fluids** should be used to maintain hydration. However, the use of large volumes of fluid is controversial and may increase pain in the patient with an obstructed ureter by increasing hydrostatic pressure behind the stone.

C. **The majority of stones will pass spontaneously within 48 hours.** However, those 6 mm or greater will pass spontaneously only 10% of the time and those 4 to 6 mm 50% of the time. If pain persists or the stone does not pass, consideration of nephrostomy stent placement and urologic intervention (such as basket removal of stone) is suggested. Renal injury from obstruction generally does not occur for at least 72 hours.

IV. **Discharge from the Office or ED.** If the patient is discharged, he or she should be sent home with indomethacin suppositories or other NSAID (reduces need for narcotics, decreases return visits to ED) and oral narcotics (such as hydrocodone). All urine should be strained, and any stones found brought for analysis.

V. **Hospital Admission.** Hospital admission is required if parenteral analgesics are required, if persistent vomiting prevents adequate oral hydration, if pyelonephritis is suspected, or if patient has elevated BUN and creatinine, oliguria, or anuria.

VI. **Continuing Care.** All patients with kidney stones should increase their daily fluid intake regardless of the composition of the stones. Analysis of the stones may identify specific preventive measures. There is good evidence that reducing the dietary intake of animal protein can reduce stone formation.

A. **Uric acid stones.** Represent 10% of stones. Should evaluate for hyperuricosuria. Allopurinol 200 to 300 mg/day inhibits uric acid synthesis and can reduce stone formation. Purines in the diet should be limited. Alkalinization of urine (oral bicarbonate 1.0 to 1.5 mEq/kg/day) will also be of some benefit.

B. **Calcium oxalate stones.** Represent 75% of all stones. Hypercalciuria is often idiopathic, but it may occur in hyperparathyroidism, sarcoidosis, and type I renal tubular acidosis (have associated nonanion gap acidosis, alkaline urine pH). Reducing sodium intake in diet can reduce hy-

8

NEPHROLOGY AND UROLOGY

percalciuria and stone formation. Despite "common wisdom," it is clear that **decreasing calcium intake may actually lead to additional stone formation.** Patients should be instructed to continue a normal calcium intake during meals. This will help bind oxylate and reduce the incidence of stone formation. Thiazide diuretics (25 to 100 mg/day) decrease calcium excretion and lead to a reduction in stone formation within 1 to 2 years. Potassium phosphate also reduces stone formation but is falling out of favor because of need for QID administration.

C. **Magnesium ammonium phosphate stones (struvite stones).** Represent 10% of all stones. Occur in the setting of high urinary pH seen in chronic urinary infections with urease-producing organisms. Antibiotics and acidification of the urine are indicated. Lithotripsy should be used to remove all visible stones from the urinary tract.

ACUTE SCROTAL PAIN AND SCROTAL MASSES

I. **Acute Scrotal Pain.** Must be assessed immediately to exclude testicular torsion.

A. **Evaluation.**
1. **History.** Inquire about trauma; nature, location, and duration of pain; associated symptoms; or recent infection of urethra, bladder, and prostate.
2. **Examination.** Localization of the painful structure is important for diagnosis. Assess for inguinal hernia, urethritis, or possible prostatitis.
3. **Lab tests.** Will be directed by the findings on history and physical. Urinalysis should be obtained to assess for hematuria or evidence of infection.

B. **Causes.**
1. **Trauma.** May be difficult to get accurate history if unusual sexual practices involved. Ultrasonography of scrotum and testicles can be useful in assessing trauma.
2. **Urolithiasis.** Indicated by hematuria. Often there is or has been associated flank pain. Examination will reveal normal scrotal contents.
3. **Hernia.** Incarcerated hernia may cause only scrotal pain. Examination may reveal the presence of bowel sounds in the scrotum. Signs of intestinal obstruction may be present. Ultrasonogram is diagnostic.
4. **Epididymitis.** Often a history of prior urethral symptoms. Commonly occurs in sexually active men. Culture urethral discharge and urine. Will be swelling and tenderness of the epididymis. The pain of epididymitis is often lessened by elevation of the scrotum. See Table 8-1 for treatment.
5. **Torsion of the testicle.** A urologic emergency, torsion present for longer than 4 to 6 hours will result in loss of the testicle. Generally present in young males after physical activity. Frequently complain of abdominal pain and nausea and may not initially notice testicular

pain. Exam may be remarkable for localized tenderness of the testicle, elevated testis, or an abnormal testicular lie. If torsion has been present for some time, epididymis will also be swollen and tender, complicating differentiation. Cremasteric reflex will generally be absent on the affected side. **But no combination of physical findings is sufficiently sensitive to rule out torsion.** Ultrasonography may be useful **but has an 11% false-negative rate. However, in no case should urgent consultation with a urologist be delayed if torsion is clinically suspected.** Manual detorsion may be attempted (if immediate surgical evaluation is not possible) by infiltrating the spermatic cord near the external ring with 5 ml of 2% lidocaine and counterrotating the affected testicle. Viewed from below the patient's scrotum, the patient's right testicle would be detorsed by counterclockwise rotation, the patient's left by clockwise rotation (done in a manner similar to opening a book).

6. **Referred pain** such as from entrapment of a nerve during appendectomy.

II. **Painless Scrotal Masses.**

A. **Possible causes include** tumors of the testicle or spermatic cord, spermatoceles, hydroceles, varicoceles, hernias, or lipomas. Most are painless or associated with only mild pain. Acute, severe pain should prompt an evaluation as discussed above. Occasionally tumors will cause acute pain, possibly from hemorrhage.

B. **Varicocele.** Common. Usual clinical presentation is adolescent or young adult male with incidentally noted swelling in (usually) the left scrotum. Physical examination is generally diagnostic with varicosities (typically described as a feeling of "a bag of worms") palpated above and separate from testicle. Varicosities enlarge with Valsalva maneuver.

1. **Treatment.** Firm scrotal support if symptomatic.

2. **Further evaluation or referral is indicated for the following:**

   a. Large or bilateral varicocele in young adolescent. May result in inhibited growth of left or both testicles, possibly resulting in decreased function (testosterone production, spermatogenesis).

   b. Male adult who is a member of an infertile couple.

   c. New-onset varicocele in man older than 30 years (may indicate intra-abdominal process that is impeding blood return).

   d. Right-sided varicocele without concomitant left-sided varicocele.

C. **Hydrocele.** Typically manifests as a gradually enlarging painless cystic structure. Can be transilluminated. Communicating hydroceles usually resolve before age 1 year. Ultrasonography may be advisable in older age group because a hydrocele can be secondary to tumor.

D. **Spermatocele.** Usually asymptomatic. Firm but somewhat compressible mass located superior to and separate from the testicle in the spermatic cord. Ultrasonography can aid in diagnosis. Requires no treatment for small spermatoceles. Larger ones may cause discomfort and may require exploration and surgical excision.

E. **Testicular tumor.** Generally occurs in a young adult. Usually painless. Firm, nontender mass will be found on the testicle. Cannot be transilluminated. Ultrasonography will confirm location of mass. Urologic consultation required for evaluation.

URINARY INCONTINENCE

I. **General.** Defined as involuntary loss of urine.
II. **Causes.** Causes of transient incontinence include delirium, infection, atrophic vaginitis or urethritis, drugs, including sedatives, hypnotics, diuretics, opiates, calcium-channel blockers, anticholinergics (antidepressants, antihistamines), decongestants, and others. Less common causes include depression, excess urine production (diabetes, diabetes insipidus), restricted mobility (i.e., patient cannot get to the bathroom), and stool impaction.
III. **Types of Incontinence and Their Specific Causes.**
A. **Urge incontinence.** Involuntary loss of urine associated with a sudden urge and desire to void. Associated with detrusor overactivity. Causes include neurologic disorders (such as stroke, multiple sclerosis), urinary tract infections, and uroepithelial cancer.
B. **Stress incontinence.** Involuntary loss of urine during coughing, sneezing, laughing, or other increases in intra-abdominal pressure. Most commonly seen in women after middle age (especially with repeated pregnancies and vaginal deliveries), stress incontinence is often a result of weakness of the pelvic floor and poor support of the vesicourethral sphincteric unit. Another cause is intrinsic urethral sphincter weakness such as that from myelomeningocele, epispadias, prostatectomy, trauma, radiation, or sacral cord lesion.
C. **Overflow incontinence.** Involuntary loss of urine associated with overdistension of the bladder. May have frequent dribbling or present as urge or stress incontinence. May be attributable to underactive bladder, bladder outlet obstruction (such as tumor, prostatic hypertrophy), drugs (such as diuretics), fecal impaction, diabetic neuropathy, or vitamin B_{12} deficiency.
D. **Functional incontinence.** Immobility, cognitive deficits, paraplegia, or poor bladder compliance.
IV. **Evaluation.** Confirm urinary incontinence and identify factors that might contribute:
A. **History,** including medications and provoking factors.
B. **Physical,** including abdominal exam, pelvic exam, rectal exam, sensation in the rectal and perineal area, edema, drugs.
C. **Do stress testing.** Have patient cough or sneeze.
D. **UA** and microscopic examination of urine. Urine culture, if warranted.
E. **Check postvoid residual;** will be increased by outlet obstruction, neurogenic bladder, etc.
F. **Follow timing** of incontinence. Observe patient urinating and watch for signs of straining, etc.

G. **Cystometry** with flow rates, etc., may be needed if cause clinically inapparent.

V. **Treatment.** Set goals and scoring system ahead of time. Most patients will respond to behavioral techniques. Most require structured input from nursing personnel.

A. **Bladder training.** Need education, scheduled voiding, and rewards. Must inhibit urinating until a set time, and this set amount of time should be progressively increased. Start at 2 to 3 hours and progress upward. 12% may become entirely continent, and 75% may have a 50% reduction in incontinent episodes. Works best in urge incontinence but also may help stress incontinence.

B. **Habit training.** Teach patients to void when they normally would (e.g., morning, before bed, after meals).

C. **Prompted voiding.** Especially good in cognitively impaired individuals. Reduced incontinent episodes by about 50%.

D. **Pelvic floor exercises (Kegel exercises).** Especially useful in stress incontinence; 16% cure rate and 54% improve.

E. Intermittent catheterization may also be used.

F. **Drugs.**
   1. **For urge incontinence, bladder spasms, detrusor instability.** Oxybutynin (Ditropan, Ditropan XL), tolterodine (Detrol) (low incidence of dry mouth). Tolterodine is expensive and no more efficacious than is oxybutynin. Second-line drugs include propantheline (may affect smooth muscle in the small bowel), flavoxate (Urispas), hyoscyamine sulfate (Levsin, Levsinex), and tricyclic antidepressants.
   2. **For stress incontinence.** Agents that increase bladder outlet resistance (e.g., pseudoephedrine).
   3. **For men.** Treating obstructive prostatic symptoms may help (see section on BPH).
   4. **In women.** Estrogen may be useful for stress and urge incontinence (start with half applicator of estrogen cream every other day and increase to 1 applicator QHS if needed or used orally as for postmenopausal use). The efficacy of estrogen has been questioned by double-blind studies. May need surgical repair.
   5. **Newer products** include Introl bladder neck support prosthesis (similar to pessary and assists women with incontinence secondary to urethral hypermobility), Reliance urinary control insert, magnetic innervation technology.

8

NEPHROLOGY AND UROLOGY

PENILE PROBLEMS

I. **Priapism.** Pathologic prolongation of a penile erection associated with pain. Fever and difficulty voiding can also be present. May result in impotence in 17% to 50% of cases; early intervention is paramount.

A. **Causes.** Idiopathic, sickle cell, trauma, neoplastic disease, drugs (heparin, phenothiazines, ETOH, hydralazine, intracavernous injection of papaverine or PGEL).

B. **Treatment.**
  1. **Medical.** Terbutaline 0.25 to 0.5 mg SQ has been used with limited success. Phenylephrine 0.5 to 1 mg instilled into each corpus followed by irrigation is the treatment of choice. Generally, IV narcotics are required for pain control. However, medical measures should not delay surgical intervention.
  2. **Surgical.** Administer IV narcotics and sedate the patient. Anesthetize the glans with 1% lidocaine and perform aspiration of blood with an 18-gauge needle inserted through the glans into each corpora cavernosa. After aspiration of 30 to 90 ml of blood, irrigate with normal saline. May take multiple irrigations and aspirations to resolve. Therapy is surgical intervention if symptoms persist.

ERECTILE DYSFUNCTION

I. **Evaluation.**
A. **History.** Includes a detailed sexual history on changes of libido, problems with ejaculation or orgasm, and daily stresses. Risk factors: age over 60, type 2 diabetes, hypertension, hyperlipidemia, smoking, renal failure, hyperthyroidism, depression, sickle cell disease, alcohol abuse, medication use (common examples are thiazide diuretics, beta-blockers, alpha-adrenergic blockers, cimetidine, spironolactone, psychotropic medications such as SSRIs, marijuana, morphine, cocaine, and metoclopramide).
B. **Complete physical examination.** Includes signs of vascular and thyroid disease, changes in secondary sex characteristics, perianal sensation, and sphincter tone. Some advise measuring penile blood pressure. Penile:brachial index less than 0.6 indicates significant vascular stenosis.
C. **Laboratory.** Baseline labs, CBC, testosterone, prolactin, glucose, liver function test, fasting lipid profile, and PSA if patient older than 40. Often it is not necessary to find out the cause before starting the treatment. Androgen levels should be checked (serum free testosterone). If androgens are low, FSH, LH, and prolactin levels should be checked. Do Doppler studies to assess blood flow.
D. **Many are psychogenic** (50%). The ability to have an erection with masturbation or REM sleep generally indicates a psychogenic disorder.
II. **Treatment.**
A. **Treat the cause.** Better management of diabetes, remove offending drugs, better control of hypertension and hyperlipidemia. Testosterone injection or transdermal testosterone for hypogonadism. Sexual counseling may be useful.
B. **Pharmacologic and devices.** More than 90% of patients respond to the following interventions regardless of etiology.
  1. **External vacuum device.** Highly effective and acceptable. Side effects include cool penile skin temperature, discomfort, bruising, and impaired ejaculation.

2. **Intracavernosal therapy.** Alprostadil is the only agent approved for this purpose. Dose has to be adjusted in office. Side effects include priapism. Only 30% of individuals respond, and it can only be used three times per week. Constriction band has to be used concomitantly in veno-occlusive deficits.

3. **Intraurethral suppository of prostaglandin** (alprostadil). Effective in two thirds of patients. Side effects include penile pain, hypotension. Cost is also a factor.

4. **Sildenafil** (Viagra). Type V phosphodiesterase enzyme inhibitor. Doses of 25 to 100 mg have been effective. It is taken orally 1 hour before anticipated sexual activity and is effective for about 4 hours. Response rates range from 43% to 68%. Side effects include headache, flushing, dyspepsia, rhinitis, and visual disturbances. Cost is also a factor. It is contraindicated in patients on nitrates because it potentiates the hypotensive effects of these agents.

5. **Apomorphine** (Uprima, Zydis) is FDA approved for male impotence. Vomiting and nausea are major side effects.

6. Surgical implants. Popular in 1970s and 1980s. Patients with cavernous veno-occlusive disease are not good candidates for this operation.

RENAL FAILURE

I. **Acute Renal Failure.** Sudden loss of renal function as evidenced by oliguria or anuria, increase in BUN or serum creatinine.

II. About 75% of cases of acute renal failure are secondary to diminished renal perfusion (prerenal causes) or ATN.

A. **Prerenal cause.** Diminished renal perfusion because of volume depletion, inadequate cardiac output, or volume redistribution ("third spacing" from cirrhosis, burns, nephrotic syndrome, etc.). Kidney retains sodium and fluid in attempt to increase circulating volume (and therefore renal perfusion). BUN-to-creatinine ratio generally >20:1.

B. **Renal causes.** Glomerular (rapidly progressive glomerulonephritis), vascular (renal artery or vein thrombosis, vasculitis), or tubulointerstitial (ATN most common; see below).

C. **Postrenal causes.** Obstruction of the urinary tract from prostate disease or retroperitoneal disease.

III. **Diagnosis.** May have urine output less than 400 ml per 24 hours, elevated BUN and creatinine, or decreased creatinine clearance. A progressive daily increase in serum creatinine is diagnostic of acute renal failure.

A. Estimated creatinine clearance = [(140 − Age) × (body weight [kg])] divided by 72 × Serum creatinine). For women, multiply this figure by 0.85.

B. May not reflect early renal damage because of compensatory hypertrophy of remaining glomeruli.

C. Normal for healthy adult is 94 to 140 ml/min for men and 72 to 110 ml/min for women.

8

NEPHROLOGY AND UROLOGY

IV. **Differentiating the Causes of Renal Failure** (Table 8-2).
A. **Formulas.** These formulas apply best when there is oliguria (<500 ml/day). Factors such as diuretic use may invalidate the results.
   1. U/P = Urine osmolality to plasma osmolality ratio.
   2. FE_{Na} = Fractional excretion of Na = (Urine sodium/Plasma sodium)/(Urine creatinine/Plasma creatinine) × 100.
B. **Urinalysis in renal failure.** If prerenal cause, generally normal UA with only hyaline casts. If ATN, may have smoky urine with dark granular casts (however, 20% may be normal). In glomerulonephritis, hematuria and proteinuria will be present.
V. **Acute Tubular Necrosis (ATN).**
A. Acute renal failure resulting from renal ischemia or toxic insult. Renal function generally returns to adequate level if patient survives. Sepsis is a major cause of death in ATN.
B. May progress from oliguric renal failure (urine output <400 ml/day) to nonoliguric renal failure, which may be manifested by massive urine output. The duration of renal failure is generally 1 day to 6 weeks (average 10 to 14 days). There is no prognostic difference between oliguric and nonoliguric renal failure.
C. **Laboratory findings.** Progressive hyponatremia, hyperkalemia, azotemia (creatinine increase by 0.5 to 2.5 mg/dl/day) and acidosis.
D. **Causes of ATN.**
   1. **Ischemic and hypoperfusion injury.** Shock, sepsis, hypoxia, hypotension, cardiac arrest, or surgery.
   2. **Toxic sources.** Radiologic contrast media, heavy metals, aminoglycosides, myoglobinuria from burns, trauma, polymyositis, cisplatin, IV acyclovir, and many other drugs.
E. **Evaluation.** Diagnosis often apparent because of clinical history. Rule out obstructive process (ultrasonography of kidneys and ureters helpful).

TABLE 8-2

DIFFERENTIATING CAUSES OF RENAL FAILURE

	BUN/Cr	Urine Na (meq/L)	Fractional excretion of sodium	Urine osmolality (mOsm/kg)	Urine Findings
Prerenal	>20:1	<20	<1	>500	Hyaline casts
Renal azotemia,	<20:1	>20	>1	250-300	Granular cast, renal tubular cells
Postrenal	>20:1	Variable	>1	<400	Normal, RBC, WBC, crystals
Glomerulonephritis	>20:1	<20	<1	>500	Nephritic urine

Urinalysis may reveal renal epithelial cells or cellular casts, or may be normal. See Table 8-2 for differentiation from other causes.

F. **Treatment.** Maintain fluid balance and blood pressure. Dopamine, mannitol, and diuretics have not been shown to have any renal-sparing effect. See treatment of acute renal failure below for details.

VI. **Prerenal Azotemia.**

A. **Cause and diagnosis.** Commonly caused by dehydration (often attributable to excessive diuretic therapy). May be secondary to decreased renal perfusion as with cardiac dysfunction or liver failure. Labs reveal evidence of decreased renal function with BUN elevated out of proportion to serum creatinine, often greater than 20:1.

B. **Treatment.**

1. **Adequate intravascular volume** will prevent progression to oliguric or anuric failure if it is secondary to inadequate volume. There is no evidence that albumin is superior to crystalloids in restoring plasma volume.

2. **Treat cardiac failure** as per CHF in Chapter 3. In those with CHF, consider also prerenal azotemia secondary to excessive diuretic use, ACE inhibitor–induced renal failure, and use of NSAIDs.

3. **If prerenal azotemia is secondary to liver failure,** outcome is poor unless patient is transplant candidate.

VII. **Postrenal Azotemia.** Usually caused in males by bladder outlet obstruction and is rapidly treatable with a Foley catheter. Other causes include pelvic tumors and surgical injury.

VIII. **Glomerulonephritis.**

A. **Causes** include poststreptococcal glomerulonephritis, hemolytic uremic syndrome, Henoch-Schönlein purpura, collagen vascular diseases, and others.

B. **Clinical presentation.** Sudden or gradual onset of renal failure, hematuria, proteinuria, azotemia, and edema.

C. **Diagnosis.** See section on nephrotic syndrome and nephritis below.

IX. **Treatment of Acute Renal Failure.**

A. **Careful monitoring** of fluid and electrolyte status. Fluids should be restricted to replacement of losses (urine output, other losses [GI], and approximately 500 ml/day for insensible loss). Dietary intake of K^+ and phosphates should be severely restricted. Hyperphosphatemia may be prevented by use of oral calcium carbonate or calcium acetate antacids to absorb dietary phosphates and maintain PO_4 <5.5 mg/dl. Calcium should be monitored, because it will tend to fall if phosphorus rises. Hyperkalemia should be treated as noted in Chapter 6. Fluid overload may require dialysis or diuretics, such as furosemide 20 mg IV or more. Adding a thiazide diuretic (e.g., metolazone, hydrochlorothiazide) may improve the diuresis. Dopamine can be used for pressure support.

B. **Monitor acidosis.** Mild to moderate metabolic acidosis should be anticipated and may be well tolerated. Severe acidosis may require oral bicarbonate solution, which contains significant quantities of sodium.

8

NEPHROLOGY AND UROLOGY

C. **Monitor carefully for signs of infection** (a common cause of death during acute renal failure).

D. **Dialysis** is indicated for uremic pericarditis, severe hyperkalemia or other unmanageable electrolyte abnormality, severe acidosis, significant fluid overload, and other uremic symptoms (especially neurologic). **Hemodialysis has been shown to improve survival.**

CHRONIC RENAL FAILURE

I. **Definition.** Clinical syndrome of chronic compromise of renal function, which can be categorized into three major groups:

A. **Inadequate renal reserve,** characterized by inability to compensate for extreme water or solute loading or deprivation.

B. **Renal insufficiency,** characterized by elevated BUN and greatly diminished capacity for dealing with water solute fluctuations, but otherwise can maintain homeostasis.

C. **Renal failure,** characterized by progressive increase in BUN to the point of causing uremia, fluid, and electrolyte imbalance (GFR <6 mg/min/m^2).

II. **Causes** Common causes include diabetes, hypertension, glomerulonephritis, polycystic kidney disease, obstructive uropathy, and amyloidosis. See section on nephritis and nephrotic syndrome for differential diagnosis. Unfortunately, deterioration may continue even after initial insult resolves, perhaps because of a change in intrarenal hemodynamics.

III. **Clinical manifestation.** Early manifestations may include only nocturia because of inability to concentrate urine (therefore mobilize fluid at nighttime when recumbent). Fatigue, altered mental status, peripheral neuropathy, anorexia, N&V, and pruritus may indicate uremia. Hypertension is common. Fluid and electrolyte imbalances result in varying signs and symptoms. Loss of erythropoietin and vitamin D function results in anemia and osteodystrophy. Patients may remain asymptomatic until GFR is less than 10% of normal.

IV. **Laboratory diagnosis.** Generally reflected in an elevated BUN and creatinine. A 24-hour urine study will show a decreased creatinine clearance. Acidosis is usually present, as is a normochromic-normocytic anemia. Hyperkalemia and hyponatremia are often present.

V. **Preventive methods.** ACE inhibitors have been shown to decrease progression to renal failure in both diabetic and nondiabetic patients. Protein restriction may reduce progression of chronic renal disease, although the data are conflicting. It seems reasonable to limit patients with early renal insufficiency to 0.8 g/kg/day of high-biologic-value protein, those with GFR below 55 ml/min to 0.7 to 0.8 g/kg/day, and those with GFR <25 ml/min to 0.6 g/kg/day. Blood pressure should be controlled to below 130/80 mm Hg if with proteinuria and those without to below 135/85.

VI. **Treatment.**

A. **Sodium and fluid hemostasis.** Generally not a problem. The kidney maintains ability to regulate sodium until extremely late in course. Use diuretics (such as furosemide) to remove excess free water.

B. **Potassium.** May require potassium restriction to 2 g/day late in the course of renal failure. May develop aldosterone resistance (and therefore hyperkalemia) requiring more aggressive therapy such as fludrocortisone and potassium-binding resins. See Chapter 6 for details.

C. **Acidosis.** Can be treated with oral sodium bicarbonate (1.2 to 2.4 g/day) if symptomatic (lethargy, fatigue, tachypnea) or if serum bicarbonate levels <17 mEq/L. This will give a sodium load; therefore be careful in setting of CHF and similar conditions.

D. **Dietary restrictions.** Required to maintain appropriate fluid and electrolyte balance. Protein restriction as above in preventive methods section.

E. **Phosphate and calcium ions.** Phosphate intake should be limited, and hyperphosphatemia should be treated with phosphate binders such as oral calcium acetate or calcium carbonate to prevent the development of renal osteodystrophy (elevated parathyroid and calcium mobilization). Avoid magnesium- and aluminum-containing preparations. Supplements of vitamin D will eventually be needed. Calcitriol 0.25 to 1 μg/day is generally a good choice.

F. **Anemia.** Generally attributable to decreased erythropoietin production in kidney. Rule out other causes such as slow GI bleed, etc. Give erythropoietin 30 to 50 U/kg SQ three times per week (up to 150 U/kg has been used in some studies, and dose should be adjusted to response). Several factors, including adequate dialysis and control of renal failure related to hyperparathyroidism, will improve the response to erythropoietin. Iron supplementation is also important.

G. **Bleeding.** Can be treated with FFP or cryoprecipitate.

H. **Dialysis.** Hemodialysis and chronic ambulatory peritoneal dialysis. Absolutely indicated for uremic pericarditis, progressive motor impairment, fluid overload not responsive to other interventions or producing CHF, severe acidosis, and hyperkalemia. Early consultation with nephrologist should be considered.

I. **Transplantation.** An alternative to dialysis. Decision to proceed with dialysis or transplantation requires the assistance of a nephrologist.

8

NEPHROLOGY AND UROLOGY

PROTEINURIA, NEPHROTIC SYNDROME, AND NEPHRITIC URINE

I. **Nephrotic Urine versus Nephritic Urine.** The **nephrotic** urine contains a large amount of protein but does not contain elements indicating active inflammation such as WBCs and RBC casts. In contrast, the **nephritic** urine is suggestive of acute renal inflammation and will contain protein, RBC casts, blood by dipstick, and WBCs. The differential diagnosis can be narrowed based on whether a nephritic or nephrotic urine is present.

II. **Nephrotic Syndrome.**

A. **General.** Nephrotic syndrome is not a disease but rather the renal manifestation of multiple underlying causes. The primary disease may be renal in origin, such as minimal-change disease, or may be a systemic illness with renal manifestations, such as diabetes mellitus with
nephropathy. Nephrotic syndrome may be related to glomerulonephritis
and other causes of nephritis. Once active renal disease (nephritis) is no
longer ongoing (that is, burned out), the patient may end up with
nephrotic syndrome and a nephrotic urine.

B. **Definition.** Nephrotic syndrome manifests as proteinuria of >2 to
3 g/day, hypoalbuminemia, edema, and hyperlipidemia. Thrombotic
events may also occur. Nephrotic syndrome may occur at any age, including in children ("nil disease" most common in children).

C. **Presentation.**
   1. Anorexia, malaise, edema, anasarca, or pleural effusions.
   2. Focal edema, especially ankles and genitalia.
   3. May be hypertensive, especially in those with collagen-vascular
      disease.
   4. Thrombotic phenomenon including renal vein thrombosis. Mostly
      caused by decreased fibrinolytic activity.
   5. Frothy urine secondary to proteinuria, nocturia secondary to in-
      creased vascular volume at night from fluid mobilization.

D. **Laboratory findings.**
   1. **Urine:** Pronounced *proteinuria* (excretion >2 g/day); *urinary protein-
      to-creatinine ratio:* >2; *casts:* hyaline, granular, waxy, or epithelial;
      urine Na: low (<1 mmol/L); *K:Na ratio:* >1.
   2. **Blood.**
      a. Hypoalbuminemia.
      b. Globulins, adrenocortical hormones, or thyroid hormones may
         be low.
      c. BUN and creatinine are variable depending on progression of re-
         nal disease.
      d. Aldosterone initially high (aldosterone causes K excretion, Na re-
         tention, and hypertension).
      e. Lipemia including elevated cholesterol and triglycerides. May have
         lipiduria.
      f. Microcytic anemia from urinary loss of transferrin or poor erythro-
         poietin production.
      g. Coagulation disorders may be from loss of factor IX, factor XII, and
         thrombolytic factors (urokinase and antithrombin III) in the urine
         and increased serum levels of factor VIII, fibrinogen, and platelets.

E. **Diagnosis.** Focused on determining underlying cause (Table 8-3).
   History and associated clinical findings go a long way in making the diagnosis. Family history is important, because many causes may be
   familial.

TABLE 8-3

**DISEASES ASSOCIATED WITH THE NEPHROTIC SYNDROME
OR NEPHRITIC URINE OR PROTEINURIA**

	Approximate Incidence	
	Children	Adults
PRIMARY RENAL DISEASE	90%	75%
Minimal-change disease (MCD)	65	15
Focal glomerulosclerosis	10	15
Membranous glomerulonephritis	5	30
Membranoproliferative glomerulonephritis	10	7
Others: mesangial proliferative glomerulonephritis, IgA nephropathy, rapidly progressive glomerulonephritis	10	3
SECONDARY DISEASE	10%	25%

Metabolic: Diabetes mellitus, amyloidosis

Immunogenic: Systemic lupus erythematosus, Henoch-Schönlein purpura, polyarteritis nodosa, Sjögren's syndrome, sarcoidosis, serum sickness, erythema multiforme

Neoplastic: Leukemias, lymphomas, Hodgkin's lymphoma, multiple myeloma, carcinoma (bronchus, breast, colon, stomach, kidney), melanoma

Nephrotoxic and drugs: Gold salts, penicillamine, NSAIDs, lithium carbonate, street heroin

Allergenic: Insect stings, snake venoms, antitoxins, poison ivy, poison oak

Infective: Bacterial—postinfective glomerulonephritis, vascular prosthetic nephritis, infective endocarditis, leprosy, syphilis

Viral—hepatitis B and C, Epstein-Barr, herpes zoster, HIV

Protozoal—malaria

Helminthic—schistosomiasis, filariasis

Congenital nephrotic syndrome: Finnish type

Heredofamilial: Alport's syndrome, Fabry's disease

Miscellaneous: Toxemia of pregnancy, malignant hypertension

8

NEPHROLOGY AND UROLOGY

F. **Work-up.** Overlaps with that of glomerulonephritis. See below.
G. **In children.** Orthostatic proteinuria, a benign condition, is frequently found in children. In orthostatic proteinuria, protein is found only in the urine after the child has been upright, so a first morning void should be free of protein (if the bladder was emptied just before bedtime). A 24-hour urine analysis can be done in two containers—one that collects the first morning void and another that collects the urine while the patient is awake and upright. Diagnostic criteria include the following: (1) no or little protein in the first morning void; (2) not greater than a total of 1.5 g of protein in a 24-hour urine; and (3) 80% to 100% of the protein in the specimen collected while the child is upright (fractionate

collection into two 12-hour periods in separate containers). However, many physicians make the diagnosis with only the absence of protein in the urine from the morning void.

H. **Prognosis and treatment. All patients with proteinuria should be considered for ACE inhibitor therapy. ACE inhibitors will slow the progression to renal failure even in the nondiabetic patient with proteinuria.** Treat hyperlipidemia with HMG-CoA reductase inhibitors. Indomethacin or another NSAID may reduce proteinuria; it may take several weeks to see a response. Treatment of specific syndromes is beyond the scope of this manual and is frequently inadequate. The exception is minimal-change disease or "nil disease." Minimal-change disease has the best prognosis, with 90% of children and 50% of adults responding to steroid therapy. A nephrology consult should be obtained.

GLOMERULONEPHRITIS AND NEPHRITIS

I. **General.** Discussion of specific entities is beyond the scope of this manual. However, diagnostic work-up should proceed as noted below.

II. **Diagnosis and work-up for nephrotic syndrome, nephritis, or suspected glomerulonephritis.** Use clinical judgment in ordering appropriate tests. This work-up may also be appropriate for those with nephrotic syndrome and proteinuria when looking for an underlying cause. Work-up may include the following:

A. **Minimum:** CXR, CBC, screening cancer tests (as appropriate for age and symptoms), pursue cancer diagnosis in appropriate clinical setting (weight loss, elderly, adenopathy, back pain, etc.), other "routine" chemical analyses.

B. **Serum and urine protein electrophoresis and immunoelectrophoresis** to detect Bence Jones protein and monoclonal gammopathy.

C. **Check for diabetes mellitus, amyloid, and SLE.**

D. **Check for hepatitis B** surface antigen (HBsAg). This causes up to 22% of nephrotic syndrome depending on the population. Also, hepatitis C and HIV.

E. **Family history** of renal failure or deafness (Alport's nephropathy).

F. **Sexual history** (syphilis, hepatitis B, or HIV).

G. **Hemoptysis** (Wegener's granulomatosis or Goodpasture syndrome).

H. **Paresthesias** or neurologic deficits (Fabry's disease).

I. **ANA or ANCA,** or both (Wegener's granulomatosis, other vasculitides).

J. **C3, C4** (low in endocarditis, post-streptococcal glomerulonephritis, lupus, membranoproliferative glomerulonephritis, or cryoglobulinemia).

K. **ASO** and other detection for recent streptococcal infection (status post-streptococcal glomerulonephritis).

L. **Anti–glomerular basement membrane antibodies:** positive in Goodpasture syndrome.

M. **Cryoglobulins.**

N. **Evaluation for sarcoid** (see Chapter 4).

O. **Biopsy.**

BIBLIOGRAPHY

AHCPR clinical practice guideline: update guideline for urinary incontinence, Rockville, Md, 1996, Agency for Health Care Policy and Research.

Andersen JT et al: Can finasteride reverse the progress of benign prostatic hyperplasia? A two-year placebo-controlled study, *Urology* 46(5):631, 1995.

Avorn JL et al: Reduction of bacteriuria and pyuria after ingestion of cranberry juice, *JAMA* 271(10):751, 1994.

Benson G: *Priapism,* AUA Update Series, vol 15, lesson 11, Baltimore, 1996, American Urological Association.

Berkow Z et al, editors: *The Merck manual of diagnosis and therapy,* Rahway, NJ, 1999, Merck.

Burgher SW. Acute scrotal pain, *Emerg Med Clin North Am* 16(4): 1998.

Burns-Cox N, Gingell C: Medical treatment of erectile dysfunction, *Postgrad Med J* 74:336, 1998.

Cardamakis E et al: Comparative study of systemic interferon alfa-2a plus isotretinoin versus isotretinoin in the treatment of recurrent condyloma acuminatum in men, *Urology* 45(5):857, 1995.

Chen J, Koontz W: *Inflammatory lesions of the kidney,* AUA Update Series, vol 14, lesson 26, Baltimore, 1996, American Urological Association.

Cordell WH et al: Indomethacin suppositories versus intravenously titrated morphine for the treatment of ureteral colic, *Ann Emerg Med* 23(2):262, 1994.

Curhan GC et al: A prospective study of dietary calcium and other nutrients and the risk of symptomatic kidney stones, *N Engl J Med* 328(12):833, 1993.

Dale DC, Federman DD, editors: *Scientific American medicine,* New York, 2000, Scientific American.

Dinsmore W, Evans C: ABC of sexual health. Erectile dysfunction, *BMJ* 318:387, 1999.

Gilbert DN et al: *The Sanford guide to antimicrobial therapy,* Dallas, 2000, Antimicrobial Therapy.

Hannedouche T et al: Randomised controlled trial of enalapril and beta blockers in nondiabetic chronic renal failure, *BMJ* 309:833, 1994.

Hooton TM et al: Randomized comparative trial and cost analysis of 3-day antimicrobial regimens for treatment of acute cystitis in women, *JAMA* 273(1):41, 1995.

Ifudu O et al: The intensity of hemodialysis and the response to erythropoietin in patients with end-stage renal disease, *N Engl J Med* 334(7):420, 1996.

Kass EJ, Lundak B: The acute scrotum, *Pediatr Clin North Am* 44(5):1251, 1997.

Kinkaid T, Menon M: *Renal tubular acidosis,* AUA Update Series, vol 14, lesson 7, Baltimore, 1995, American Urological Association.

Kuritzky L, Ahmed O, Kosch S: Management of impotence in primary care, *Comp Ther* 24(3):137, 1998.

Licht MR: Use of oral sildenafil (Viagra) in the treatment of erectile dysfunction, *Comp Ther* 25(2):90, 1999.

Linet OI et al: Efficacy and safety of intracavernosal alprostadil in men with erectile dysfunction, *N Engl J Med* 334:873, 1996.

Low FC, Fagleman E: Phytotherapy in the treatment of benign prostatic hyperplasia: an update, *Urology* 53:671, 1999.

Maschio G et al: Effect of the angiotensin converting enzyme inhibitor benazepril on the progression of chronic renal failure, *N Engl J Med* 334:939, 1996.

Mcconnell J: *Clinical practice guideline N8. Benign prostatic hyperplasia: diagnosis and treatment,* Feb 1994, US Department of Health and Human Services, Public Health Service, Agency of Health Care Policy and Research.

Millar LK et al: Outpatient treatment of pyelonephritis in pregnancy: a randomized controlled trial, *Obstet Gynecol* 86(4 pt 1):560, 1995.

Nairn SJ et al: Adequacy of follow-up in children diagnosed with urinary tract infections in a pediatric emergency department, *Pediatr Emerg Care* 11(3):156, 1995.

Pedrini MT et al: The effect of dietary protein restriction on the progression of diabetic and non-diabetic renal diseases: a meta-analysis, *Ann Intern Med* 124:627, 1996.

Preminger G: *Medical management of urinary calculus disease. Part 1: Pathogenesis and evaluation. Part 2: Classification of metabolic disorders and selective medical management,* AUA Update Series, vol 14, lesson 5, Baltimore, 1995, American Urological Association.

Schlager TA et al: Explanation for false-positive urine cultures obtained by bag technique, *Arch Pediatr Adolesc Med* 149(2):170, 1995.

Sharlip ID: Evaluation and nonsurgical management of erectile dysfunction, *Urol Clin North Am* 25(4):647, 1998.

Skoog S: Benign and malignant pediatric scrotal masses, *Pediatr Clin North Am* 44(5):1229, 1997.

Turner GM et al: Fever can cause pyuria in children, *BMJ* 311(7010):924, 1995.

Walsh P et al: *Campbell's urology,* ed 6, Philadelphia, 1992, Saunders.

Ziada A, Rosenblum M, Crawford DE: Benign prostatic hyperplasia: an overview, *Urology* 531, 1999.

NEUROLOGY

Coleman O. Martin

HEADACHE

I. **Overview.** Headaches (HAs) are a common problem and are often responsible for visits to primary care physicians. Although most headaches are benign, it is the responsibility of the health care provider to obtain a history and a careful examination to rule out other causes of pain. The ability to properly classify a particular headache syndrome allows specific treatment.

II. **Approach to the Headache Patient.**

A. **History** contributes most to the diagnostic process in assessing headaches. Pertinent are when the headaches first started, rapidity of onset, time to maximal pain, HA duration, frequency, location, quality, triggers (such as chocolate or red wine), aura, associated symptoms, and response to previous medications.

B. **Physical exam.** Mental status should be normal during a benign headache. Delirium raises the specter of CNS infection, hemorrhage, or vasculitis (e.g., lupus). Check cranial nerves with special attention to visual fields, extraocular movements, corneal reflexes, gag reflexes, and fundi. Screen for abnormalities of strength, coordination, reflexes, and gait. Palpate the temples (for temporal arteritis, TMJ syndrome, and muscle-tension headache) and occipital region (for occipital neuralgia), apply pressure over the sinuses, and visualize the tympanic membranes.

C. **Neuroimaging.**
   1. **Who to image.** It is not necessary for every patient with a headache to have an imaging study. However, those with a headache pattern suggestive of an intracranial lesion (e.g., SAH, abscess, tumor); those with the "worst headache of their life"; and those with any focal signs or symptoms or persistent, nonmigrainous headache should be imaged. The yield in those with a migraine type of headache is 0.4%. Remember, however, that only 30% of those with an SAH will have an initially focal neurologic exam.
   2. **CT:** sensitive for hemorrhagic strokes and subarachnoid hemorrhages.
   3. **MRI** is the test of choice to rule out brain tumors. Consider an MRI when patients have focal neurologic signs or a daily headache for more than 1 month.

D. **Laboratory studies** are generally unnecessary. In the proper clinical setting consider sedimentation rate for temporal arteritis; consider an LP when subarachnoid hemorrhage, CNS infection, or pseudotumor cerebri is suspected.

E. Remember simple causes such as sinusitis, toothache, TMJ syndrome.

III. **Characteristics of Various Types of Headaches.** It is sometimes difficult to classify a patient into any one headache type based on the definitions below. *The headache characteristics defined by the Headache Classification Committee of the International Headache Society are meant as guidelines to the diagnosis rather than absolute diagnostic criteria.* See Table 9-1 for a comparison of headache characteristics.

TABLE 9-1

CHARACTERISTICS OF VARIOUS TYPES OF PRIMARY HEADACHES

Headache	Patient Population	Family History	Aura	Quality	Location	Duration	Behavior During Headache	Associated Symptoms
Migraine without aura	Onset age: 6-25 yrs Female-to-male 3:1 but 1:1 at extremes of age	Positive	No	Begin as a dull penetrating pain that progresses to moderate or severe throbbing pain	Unilateral or bilateral	6-48 hrs	Reclusive, supine in darkened room	Nausea, vomiting, photophobia, phonophobia
Migraine with aura	As above	As above	Yes	Throbbing	Unilateral	3-12 hrs	As above	Visual prodrome, nausea, vomiting, photophobia, phonophobia
Tension-type	Any age or gender	No	Dull, squeezing, nonthrobbing and not exacerbated by routine activity	Diffuse bilateral	30 min to 7 days			Depression

					Quality	Location	Duration	Behavior	Associated features
Cluster	Age 20-40 Male-to-female 9:1	Occasionally positive	Uncommon (6%)	Boring	Unilateral, especially orbit, severe, boring, tearing like a "hot poker in the eye"	15-120 min	Agitated, pacing, rocking, moaning, crying	Ipsilateral tearing, Horner's syndrome, nasal stuffiness, hemifacial sweating
Subarachnoid hemorrhage				Throbbing, severe	Variable	Variable		May have focal neurologic symptoms or decreased level of consciousness but may be alert with nonfocal exam
Chronic paroxysmal hemicrania	33 years Female-to-male 2:1	Absent	No	Severe	Severe, sharp, boring, throbbing, unilateral, supraorbital, or temporal pain always on the same side; unilateral, orbital, or temporal	1-40 attacks a day lasting 2-25 min No periods of remission		Conjunctival injection, ptosis, lacrimation, rhinorrhea, and relieved with Indocin

A. **Primary headaches.**

  1. **Migraine.** Migraine HA is a common problem in the United States, affecting nearly 18% of women and 6% of men.

    a. Onset is gradual, escalating to maximum intensity over 1 to 2 hours. Headache may last from a few hours to 3 days. Frequency of attacks varies widely. *Status migrainosis* indicates a continuous migraine headache lasting more than 3 days. Because of the unilateral nature, occipital neuralgia (see below) is frequently mistaken for a migraine headache.

    b. **Migraine without aura (common migraine)** makes up 80% of migraine headaches (Box 9-1).

    c. **Migraine with aura (classical migraine)** makes up 20% of migraine headaches (Box 9-2).

    d. **Treatment for migraine.**

      (1) **Abortive therapies** are most effective when taken during the aura phase or early in the headache. With the exception of

---

BOX 9-1

CRITERIA FOR MIGRAINE WITHOUT AURA

Migraine without aura must have at least five attacks meeting the following criteria:

Headache attacks last 4 to 72 hours

Headache has at least two of the following:

- Unilateral location
- Pulsating quality
- Moderate or severe intensity (inhibits daily activity)
- Aggravation by routine physical activity

During the headache, at least one of the following:

- Nausea or vomiting
- Photophobia and phonophobia

No organic etiology found by history, physical, or neurologic exam.

BOX 9-2

CRITERIA FOR MIGRAINE WITH AURA

Migraine with aura must have at least two attacks fulfilling the following criteria:

At least three of the following are present:

- One or more fully reversible aura symptoms indicating focal cerebral cortical or brainstem dysfunction.
- At least one aura symptom develops gradually over more than 4 minutes.
- No aura symptom lasts more than 60 minutes (duration proportionally increases if more than one aura symptom present).
- HA follows the aura within 60 minutes (but HA may begin before or with the aura). HA usually lasts 4 to 72 hours but may have only the aura.
- No organic etiology found by history, physical, or neurologic exam.

Note: Common aura types include scintillating scotomata, multiple small dots, homonymous visual disturbance, hemisensory disturbance, difficulty communicating, and occasionally vertigo.

antihistamines and antiemetics, all abortive therapies can lead to rebound headaches. Ergotamine derivatives, triptans, and isometheptene combinations are contraindicated in coronary disease, peripheral vascular disease, uncontrolled hypertension, and migraines with other neurologic signs such as alteration of consciousness, weakness, and diplopia.

(2) **Narcotics** are for occasional use only and should not be considered first-line treatment in the migraineur.

(3) **NSAIDs** are effective for many patients with migraines. Ibuprofen (400 to 800 mg) and aspirin (650 to 975 mg) have the advantage of rapid onset. Naproxen (500 mg) has a longer duration and when taken twice daily for 2 weeks can terminate status migrainosus. Over-the-counter preparations with caffeine are also effective. The use of metoclopramide 10 mg PO enhances the efficacy of oral medication by promoting gastric emptying and decreasing vomiting. Consider **dexamethasone** 4 mg IM or a short course of prednisone (40 to 60 mg PO QD), combined with analgesics, if migraine continues >24 hours **and** is unresponsive to standard therapy.

(4) **Antiemetics** do not lead to analgesic rebound headaches, combat nausea, and also provide adequate analgesia for many patients. IV preparations are more effective than rectal, which are more effective than PO.
  - Prochlorperazine (Compazine) 10 mg PO/IV or 25 mg PR.
  - Droperidol 1.25 to 2.5 mg IV/IM (may use up to 5 mg).
  - Promethazine (Phenergan) 25 mg PO/IM/PR.

(5) **Isometheptene combinations** are well tolerated. Midrin (isometheptene/dichloralphenazone/acetaminophen 65/100/325 mg) 2 tabs at onset followed by 1 tab per hour until relief. Max 5 tabs per 12-hour period.

(6) **Ergotamine derivatives.**
  - Ergotamine/caffeine (Cafergot, Wigraine) 1/100 mg each, 2 tabs at onset and 1 Q30min up to 6 per 24 hours.
  - Dihydroergotamine (DHE-45, Migranal). Highly effective. Advisable to premedicate with metoclopramide or prochlorperazine before administering IV to avoid nausea. May not be used within 24 hours of a triptan medication. Injectable: 1 mg IV/IM/SC. May repeat in 1 hour if necessary for max dose of 2 mg per 24 hours. Intranasal: 1 spray in each nostril, repeat after 15 minutes. Max dose 6 sprays in 24 hours or 8 sprays in 1 week.
  - **Triptans.** May not be used within 24 hours of an ergotamine derivative. Primary drawback is cost (>$15 per dose). Lack of effectiveness of one triptan generally not predictive of efficacy of other triptans.

9

NEUROLOGY

- Sumatriptan (Imitrex). Efficacy: subcutaneous > intranasal > oral. Efficacy is 80% SQ and 50% PO in properly selected patients. **However, because it is short acting, up to 50% require rescue medication.** Subcutaneous: 6 mg at onset, may repeat once after an hour to a max dose of 12 mg/24 hours. Intranasal: 20 mg at onset, may repeat once after 2 hours to a max dose of 40 mg/ 24 hours. Oral: 25 mg at onset; if no response, additional 25 to 100 mg Q2h to a max dose of 300 mg/24 hours.
- Naratriptan (Amerge) 2.5mg PO. May repeat after 4 hours. Max dose 5 mg/24 hours.
- Rizatriptan (Maxalt, Maxalt MLT) 5 to 10 mg PO. May repeat at 2 and 4 hours if needed. MLT form placed on tongue for oral absorption (superior with prominent nausea). Use 5 mg dose only for patients also taking propranolol. Max dose 30 mg/24 hours or 15 mg/24 hours in patients taking propranolol.
- Zolmitriptan (Zomig) 1.25 to 2.5mg PO. May repeat after 2 hours. Max dose 10 mg/24 hours.

(7) Valproic acid IV has been used to abort migraines with success.

e. **Prophylactic therapies** of migraine are appropriate when headaches occur more than twice a month or they lead to significant loss of productivity or quality of life. Consider other medical problems when choosing a prophylactic (e.g., use a beta-blocker if patient is also hypertensive or a tricyclic if patient is also depressed.)

(1) **Beta-blockers.** Contraindicated in asthma, depression, and heart block. Options include propranolol (Inderal) 30 to 80 mg BID or sustained-release 60 to 160 mg QD; atenolol (Tenormin) 50 to 100 mg QD; nadolol (Corgard) 40 to 120 mg QD; sustained-release metoprolol 50 to 200 mg per day. If one beta-blocker fails after an adequate trial (6 to 8 weeks), consider switching to an alternative beta-blocker.

(2) **Calcium-channel blockers.** Less effective for migraine than beta-blockers but fewer side effects. Contraindicated in heart block and systolic CHF. Verapamil sustained release (Isoptin SR, Calan SR) 180 to 480 mg QD. Trial should be >2 months. Other calcium-channel blockers are less effective.

(3) **Tricyclic antidepressants.** Start at low dose and titrate to efficacy over a few months; this is a good choice because will also help tension-type headaches and sleep. Side effects include sedation, dry mouth, urinary retention, and other anticholinergic side effects. Contraindicated in cardiac arrhythmias, prolonged QT etc. Options include amitriptyline (Elavil) 10 to 200 mg QHS; nortriptyline (Pamelor) 10 to 200 mg QHS; doxepin (Sinequan) 10 to 200 mg QHS; desipramine (Norpramin) 10 to 200 mg QHS.

(4) **SSRI antidepressants.** Less effective but well tolerated.

Options include paroxetine (Paxil) 20 to 60 mg QAM; fluoxetine (Prozac) 20 to 80 mg QAM.

(5) **Anticonvulsants.**
  - Valproic acid (Depakote, Depakene) 250 mg BID to 500 mg TID. Effective and FDA approved for migraine prophylaxis. Can adjust dose by blood level if control difficult or sedation problematic. Possible side effects include increased appetite, sedation, transient alopecia, and hepatotoxicity. Check AST at onset, 1 mo, 3 mo, and then Q6mo.
  - Gabapentin (Neurontin) 300 mg BID to 800 mg TID. Less effective but well tolerated. No monitoring required.
  - Antihistamines can be effective and with the exception of mild sedation are well tolerated. Cyproheptadine (Periactin) 4 mg BID, may increase to maximum dose of 8 mg TID.

(6) Riboflavin (vitamin B$_2$) 400 mg QD. Safe and effective.

(7) **Methysergide** (Sansert) 2 mg QD to 2 mg QID. Effective but difficult to use; 2-month drug holiday required for every 6 months of therapy. Chronic use mandates periodic monitoring with echocardiogram, chest x-ray, and IVP to monitor for retroperitoneal fibrosis.

(8) **ACE inhibitors** have had some efficacy in a double-blind trial.

f. **Nonpharmacologic therapies.**
  (1) **Diet.** Avoid monosodium glutamate, nitrates, and alcohol. Spread out caffeine evenly. Keeping a log can identify foods that trigger headaches.
  (2) **Lifestyle changes.** Regular eating, sleeping, and exercise.
  (3) **Behavioral therapies.** Biofeedback, stress management, and self-help groups.

2. **Tension-type headaches.** The most common type of headache (Box 9-3). May be episodic or chronic. Although they affect quality of life, these headaches are rarely debilitating. Nearly everyone experiences tension headaches from time to time.

a. Tension-type headache is separated into two subtypes based on frequency:
  (1) Episodic type.
    - Headache lasts 30 min to 7 days.
    - No nausea or vomiting with headache.

BOX 9-3

CRITERIA FOR TENSION-TYPE HEADACHE

Headache with at least two of the following:
- Pressing or tightening quality
- Mild or moderate intensity
- Bilateral location
- No aggravation by routine physical activity

No organic etiology found by history, physical, or neurologic exam

- Photophobia and phonophobia are absent, or one but not the other is present.
- At least 10 previous headaches as above, with number of headache days less than 180 per year and less than 15 per month.

(2) Chronic type.
- Headache averages 15 days per month (180 days per year), for at least 6 months.
- No vomiting.
- No more than one of the following: nausea, photophobia, or phonophobia.

d. **Treatment.**
(1) **Abortive therapy.** Simple analgesics, NSAIDs, and dihydroergotamine as per migraine section above. Overuse may lead to rebound headaches. Encourage nonpharmacologic therapies.
(2) **Prophylactic therapy.** TCAs, beta-blockers, or calcium-channel blockers as per migraine section above.

3. **Cluster (episodic or chronic).** Cluster headaches (Box 9-4) are uncommon, occurring in 0.1% to 0.4% of the general population. They are named by their curious periodicity, typically occurring up to several times a day for weeks or months, then spontaneously remitting. Additionally, their unique head pain profile and autonomic features set them apart from other headache syndromes. Headaches are so severe that patients may threaten suicide. Indeed, suicide rates in this population are increased.

BOX 9-4

CRITERIA FOR CLUSTER HEADACHE

Severe unilateral orbital, supraorbital, or temporal pain peaking in 10 to 15 minutes an lasting 30 to 45 minutes (occasionally up to 180 minutes). Pain rapidly resolves. Cluster headaches have a propensity to occur at night and may lead to sleep deprivation. Cycles generally last for a few weeks or months but may last for more than 1 year.

Headache is associated with at least one of the following on the painful side:
- Conjunctival injection
- Rhinorrhea
- Lacrimation
- Miosis
- Nasal congestion
- Ptosis
- Forehead and facial sweating
- Eyelid edema

Additionally:
- Frequency of attacks ranges from one to eight daily.
- There have been at least five episodes of headache.

a. **Abortive therapies.** Usefulness is limited by the high frequency and short duration of the headaches.
   (1) **Oxygen.** 7 L/min by face mask relieves headache in 60% to 70% of patients. Effect occurs in approximately 5 minutes.
   (2) **Sumatriptan** (Imitrex) 6 mg SQ is rapidly effective and appears to be safe up to twice daily. Intranasal may also be effective. Because, by definition, cluster headaches are short lived, sumatriptan is an excellent choice for these patients.
   (3) **Lidocaine** 4% on a long cotton swab placed intranasally against the sphenopalatine ganglion is helpful for some patients.

b. **Prophylactic therapies.** Most patients with daily cluster headaches should also be treated with a prophylactic medication. This medication is continued for a few weeks beyond the termination of the headaches. For patients who relapse, chronic prophylactic therapy can be considered. If patients are unresponsive to standard therapy, consider the diagnosis of chronic paroxysmal hemicrania.
   (1) **Prednisone** 60 mg QD for 3 days followed by a taper to 0 mg over 15 days is a rapid and effective short-term treatment.
   (2) **Ergotamine tartrate** 1 mg BID. Contraindicated in coronary disease, peripheral vascular disease, uncontrolled hypertension.
   (3) **Lithium carbonate.** Start 300 mg BID and titrate to level of 0.4 to 0.8 mEq/L. More effective in chronic cluster headaches.
   (4) **Verapamil, methysergide, or valproic acid** as per migraine headache above.

4. **Chronic paroxysmal hemicrania** (Box 9-5). A severe unilateral orbital, throbbing supraorbital, or temporal pain always on the same

---

BOX 9-5

CHRONIC PAROXYSMAL HEMICRANIA

1. Attack frequency is generally 1 to 40 per day (periods of lower frequency may occur, but there is rarely a total remission).
2. Headache is associated with at least one of the following on the pain side:
   • Conjunctival injection.
   • Eyelid edema.
   • Lacrimation.
   • Nasal congestion.
   • Ptosis.
   • Rhinorrhea.
3. Absolute effectiveness of indomethacin (150 mg/day or less).
4. At least 50 attacks occur as above.
5. No organic etiology found by history, physical, or neurologic exam

side, lasting 2 to 45 min. The average age of onset is 33 years with female-to-male ratio of 2:1. No aura.

   a. Therapy is indomethacin, up to 150 mg/day.

5. **Analgesic rebound headache.** Produced by the overzealous use of analgesics. Often coexists with migraine or tension headaches that prompted the analgesic overuse.

   a. **Patient population.** All patients who use analgesics two or more times per week in the symptomatic treatment of headache are at risk for this syndrome. Occurs most commonly when analgesics are used daily.

   b. **Causal medications.** NSAIDs, acetaminophen, ergotamine derivatives, triptans, isometheptene combinations, and narcotics.

   c. **Pain characteristics.** Similar to tension headache pain.

   d. **Time course.** Daily or near-daily headache that is dulled or relieved by analgesics only to return when the analgesic wears off.

   e. **Treatment.** Most effective therapy is to stop analgesics. Hydroxyzine 25 to 50 mg Q6h PRN may be used to dull the rebound headache. Warn patients that they will probably experience a constant headache for 1 to 2 weeks. Sometimes a long-acting NSAID (such as naproxen) can be scheduled daily for 2 weeks and then discontinued without recurrence of the headache. Consider use of a prophylactic headache medication targeted at the primary headache syndrome that precipitated the analgesic overuse.

6. **Occipital neuralgia.** Occipital headache with retro-orbital or frontal component. Occurs secondary to entrapment of the occipital nerve, especially after cervical strain or secondary to muscle tension. Frequently misdiagnosed as migraine headache because of the hemicranial nature. Pain can be reproduced by pressure to occipital notch and is treated by either NSAIDs and muscle relaxants or injection with bupivacaine and triamcinolone.

B. **Secondary headaches.** HA accompanied by systemic illness, neurologic deficits, or mental status changes are likely to be secondary to other cranial pathology. **Patients with benign headache syndromes are equally at risk for secondary headaches, mandating that a patient with a new type of headache be reevaluated.**

1. **Increased intracranial pressure (pseudotumor cerebri).** Idiopathic, occurs in 19 per 100,000 with a predilection for obese females (although may occur in others). Has been associated with tetracycline and ibuprofen use. Often manifests as chronic retrobulbar HA exacerbated by eye movements. Loss of peripheral vision, diplopia, meningeal signs, and paresthesias may occur. Exam may reveal papilledema and CN VI palsy. CSF is normal except for elevated opening pressure (250 to 450 mm H_2O). **Treatment:** weight loss, serial LPs each removing 20 to 40 ml of CSF, diuretics (e.g., furosemide), acetazolamide 500 to 1000 mg QD (reduces CSF pro-

duction as well as being a diuretic), prednisone 40 to 60 mg QD, optic nerve fenestration, and rarely a shunt.

2. **Brain tumor.** HA is the most common isolated complaint, although only 50% of tumors cause HA. A classic tumor headache (worse in morning, exacerbated by bending over, and associated with nausea and vomiting) only occurs in 17%. Most have only symptoms of a typical tension-type headache. Other neurologic signs or symptoms may help localize tumor but may be absent.

3. **Temporal (giant cell) arteritis** should be considered in people over age 55 (although rarely in younger patients). Tenderness at the temples, jaw claudication, vision changes, and constitutional symptoms all suggest the diagnosis. Sedimentation rate is usually elevated but is normal in 15%. Referral to an ophthalmologist for a detailed retinal exam; a temporal artery biopsy is suggested. Blindness may rapidly occur if treatment is delayed. See rheumatology chapter for further details.

4. **Meningitis and herpes encephalitis.** See CNS infections, this chapter.

5. **Carbon monoxide poisoning.** See Chapter 2.

6. **Subarachnoid hemorrhage.** Patients generally have the acute onset of the "worst headache of their life." May have nausea, vomiting, mental status changes, or loss of consciousness. Most (59%) have a "warning leak" before severe event and may have antecedent headaches for weeks. Mortality rate is 60% for each bleed; therefore diagnosis of a warning leak can prevent death and morbidity.

   a. May have mental status changes and meningeal signs but may not (39% initially free of CNS symptoms and signs).

   b. Only 10% have initially focal exam.

   c. May have fever and leukocytosis from meningeal irritation.

   d. CT should be done on those with a sudden-onset severe headache and in those with a severe headache that is different from their usual headache. In one study, 33% of those with new onset of severe headache **and no CNS signs or symptoms and no other obvious cause of headache** had SAH. CT scan will find only about 90% of SAH (98% in third-generation scanners). **All those who need a CT also need an LP.**

   e. Response to nonnarcotic and narcotic analgesia does not rule out SAH.

7. **Miscellaneous headaches (benign).** Postcoital headache, cold-induced headache (e.g., from ice cream), jolts and jabs (also known as ice-pick headache—stabbing, sharp, headache in temple or retro-orbital area lasting seconds), cough- or Valsalva-related headache (benign in 80% to 90%). Arnold-Chiari malformation may cause headache and can be diagnosed by MRI. Arnold-Chiari malformation may lead to permanent disability.

DEMENTIA

I. **Overview.**

A. **Definition** (DSM-IV diagnostic criteria). Acquired memory impairment and with at least one additional acquired cognitive deficit such as aphasia, apraxia (difficulty in carrying out motor activities despite intact motor function), agnosia (difficulty recognizing objects despite intact sensory function), or disturbance in executive function (as in organizing, planning). To be considered dementia, symptoms must represent a decline from the patient's prior baseline and must not be better accounted for by delirium or mental illness.

B. **Prevalence.** At age 65, 1% of the population has dementia. This percentage doubles with every 5 years of age. Fifty percent of individuals living to their tenth decade have some degrees of dementia.

C. **Potentially reversible causes.** The primary goal of a dementia workup is to uncover potentially reversible etiologies. Overall, 3% to 15% of dementia cases are reversible. Causes include Wernicke encephalopathy, vitamin B_{12} deficiency, subdural hematoma, normal-pressure hydrocephalus (see below), CNS infections (such as syphilis), depression (pseudodementia, see below), and resectable brain tumors. Subacute delirium (see below) is frequently mistaken for dementia and can arise from: medication side effects, systemic infections, malignant hypertension, dehydration, uremia, liver failure, hypothyroidism, hyponatremia, hypercalcemia, and hypoglycemia.

D. **Irreversible causes.** Alzheimer's disease, vascular dementia, frontotemporal dementias (e.g., Pick's disease), dementia with Lewy bodies, Huntington's chorea, Creutzfeldt-Jakob disease, AIDS-related dementia, bovine-spongiform encephalopathy, Parkinson's-related dementia, and heavy-metal poisoning (including lead, mercury, arsenic, manganese, and thallium).

II. **Diagnostic Evaluation.**

A. **History and physical** with a complete neurologic exam are essential. Babinski's sign, asymmetry of reflexes, and visual-field deficits are suggestive of multi-infarct dementia or focal CNS abnormality rather than Alzheimer's disease.

B. **Mini-Mental State examination** is a useful office screening tool for a quick assessment and serial exams (Box 9-6). A score <25 increases odds of dementia. Dementia can still be present despite a "normal" MMSE score (more likely in younger or well-educated patients).

C. **Initial lab tests.** Should include CBC, ESR, chemistry panel (with electrolytes, BUN, creatinine LFTs, calcium, glucose), thyroid function tests, RPR, vitamin B_{12}, and folate. A brain CT without contrast is the minimum neuroimaging required to screen for subdural hematoma, brain tumor, normal-pressure hydrocephalus, and multi-infarct dementia.

D. **Additional tests.** May be obtained if indicated by history, PE, or initial lab tests. These additional tests include UA, TSH, HIV, 24-hour urine

---

BOX 9-6

FOLSTEIN MINI-MENTAL STATE INVENTORY

SCORE

( ) 1. What is the year_____, season_____, date_____,
      day_____, month_____?

( ) 2. Where are we: state_____, county_____,
      town_____, place_____, floor_____?

( ) 3. Name 3 objects: orange_____ airplane_____ tobacco_____
         (trials)_____

( ) 4. Serial 7's:_____
           93   86   79   72   65
      or spell "world" backwards_____
                       d   l   r   o   w

( ) 5. Recall 3 objects: orange_____ airplane_____ tobacco_____

( ) 6. Name a pencil_____, and a watch_____.

( ) 7. Read and obey_____ ⟶ | CLOSE YOUR EYES |

( ) 8. Copy design_____(below).

     9. Write a sentence_____(below).

    10. Repeat the following: "No if, and, or buts"_____

    11. Follow a 3-stage command: (a) Take a paper in your
                                      right hand._____
                                  (b) Fold it in half._____
                                  (c) Put it on the floor._____

Level of consciousness_____(check)
                       alert   drowsy   stupor   coma

(One point for each blank. Maximum = 30)

9

NEUROLOGY

heavy-metal screen, ECG, chest radiograph, EEG, MRI, blood gas, serum ammonia, lumber puncture, and drug levels.

E. **Neuropsychologic testing.** Useful for the assessment of cases that are atypical such as onset at a young age (<60), rapidly progressing, early loss of language, or possible psychiatric component. Testing allows the progression of the dementia to be accurately monitored and can help address important issues such as driving, cooking, independence, and financial independence management.

F. **Memory in normal aging.** The perception of memory impairment is common among the elderly with between one quarter and one third of nondemented healthy elderly complaining of memory difficulty. Cognitive performance is reduced somewhat with advancing age, with speed of processing being most affected. As a rule, accuracy of responses should not suffer significantly. Formal neuropsychologic testing can be especially helpful both for patient reassurance and to establish a baseline for future testing.

III. **General Management of Dementia.** Management varies by etiology and is discussed separately under each entity. However, some general management principles are common to all patients with dementia. Provide a supportive environment with frequent cues for orientation to the day, date, place, and time. As functioning decreases, nursing home placement may be necessary. Provide the family with supportive therapy and referral to community support groups. For agitation, try behavior modification first such as a low stimulus environment that facilitates safe wandering. Low-dose haloperidol (Haldol) may be useful in patients other than those with dementia with Lewy bodies (DLB). New atypical antipsychotics such as quetiapine (Seroquel), risperidone, and olanzapine have fewer side effects and may be tolerated well. Quetiapine may cause leukopenia. Lorazepam is also used for agitation. However, any drug therapy is fraught with side effects in this population.

IV. **Common Types of Dementia.**

A. **Alzheimer's dementia (AD).** Most common dementing illness representing up to 60% of dementia. AD is of enormous medical and social importance.

  1. **Characteristics.** In addition to meeting the above definition of a dementia, AD is typified by the following. **Onset.** Is gradual with relentless progression and rarely begins before age 60. **Memory impairment** is most severe for recent events. Spacial disorientation is common early in the disease, and patients may become lost or disoriented when performing simple tasks (e.g., driving to the store). **Social graces** are relatively preserved, but there may be incontinence of urine and stool. **Anosognosia.** Patients are often unaware of their deficits. **Psychiatric disturbances** (hallucinations and delusions) can occur, typically later in the course. However, depression is common early in the course. **Sundowning.** Nocturnal hallucinations, wandering, and confusion are common later in the course.

  2. **Diagnosis.** It is vitally important to exclude other treatable causes of dementia. Brain CT may initially be normal; later, diffuse atrophy is evident. Disturbances of gait, sudden onset of dementia, focal neurologic exam, or new onset of seizures should call the diagnosis into question.

  3. **Treatment.**

    a. **Donepezil (Aricept)** is indicated for the treatment of mild to moderate AD. Initial dose is 5 mg PO QHS for 4 to 6 weeks. Then the dose may be increased to 10 mg PO QHS if needed. Side effects are common and include cholinergic manifestations such as salivation, nausea, seizures, etc.

    b. **Rivastigmine** (Exelon) is indicated for the treatment of AD. The initial dose is 1.5 mg BID and advance to 3 to 6 mg BID over 2 months. Side effects are similar to donepezil.

    c. **Vitamin E,** 2000 IU PO QD. Limited efficacy. Does not reverse but may slow the progression of AD.

B. **Vascular dementia (formerly multi-infarct dementia).** Accounts for up to 20% of dementia in the elderly.
   1. **Characteristics. Onset** is often discrete and progresses in a step-wise deteriorating manner. **Risk factors.** Male, smoking, history of TIAs, strokes, hypertension, coronary artery disease, and atrial fibrillation. **Associated symptoms** include disturbances of gait and early incontinence.
   2. **Diagnosis.** Requires evidence of strokes, such as focal neurologic deficits and neuroimaging showing evidence of multiple hemispheric infarcts. Dementia should not be better accounted for by AD or other illness.
   3. **Treatment.** Reduce modifiable risks for stroke. See section on stroke below.
C. **Frontotemporal dementias** (FTDs). Represents a heterologous group of neurodegenerative diseases including **Pick's disease.** They are important to differentiate from AD because of differences in management.
   1. **Characteristics. Onset** is insidious and course is slowly progressive. **Psychiatric manifestations** occur early and include social inappropriateness, disinhibition, delusions, ritualistic behavior, and mood disorders. **Language.** Progressive reduction in speech with overuse of stock phrases and sometimes echolalia. **Loss of personal awareness.** Neglect of hygiene and grooming. **Spatial orientation and praxis** are often preserved. **Other signs** include incontinence, late rigidity, akinesia, and tremor.
   2. **Diagnosis.** MRI reveals relative atrophy of the frontal lobes and the anterior temporal lobes.
   3. **Management.** Unfortunately, no specific medications have proven beneficial. Treatment is symptomatic with behavior-modifying environment and medications (short-acting benzodiazepines, antipsychotics, and SSRIs).
D. **Dementia with Lewy bodies (DLB).** Representing as much as 25% of dementia cases, DLB is an interesting crossroads of dementia and parkinsonism. The extrapyramidal symptoms tend to be mild with rigidity, bradykinesia, and frequent falls. Sometimes syncope occurs. Tremor is not prominent.
   1. **Characteristics. Fluctuations** of attention and alertness with patients having good and bad days. **Visual hallucinations.** Often detailed and recurrent. Hallucinations in other modalities can also occur. **Memory disturbance.** Typified by inefficient memory retrieval. With prompting memory can be surprisingly intact. **Visual spatial ability** may be particularly impaired.
   2. **Treatment.**
      a. **AVOID ANTIPSYCHOTICS.** Patients with DLB are markedly sensitive to antipsychotics, which exacerbate their parkinsonism. New "atypical" antipsychotics may be of benefit but may still have extrapyramidal side effects.

9

NEUROLOGY

      b. **Donepezil (Aricept)** may be helpful for both the memory and psychiatric disturbances.

      c. **Dopamine agonists** may improve parkinsonism. Monitor for worsening hallucinations.

E. **Normal-pressure hydrocephalus.**

  1. **Characterized** by triad of gradual onset of dementia, gait disturbance, and urinary incontinence.

  2. **Diagnosis.** CT scan shows enlarged ventricles with preserved cortical ribbon. MRI reveals transependymal flow.

  3. **Treatment.** Surgical ventriculoperitoneal CSF shunting may greatly improve symptoms or even be curative.

F. **Pseudodementia.** So named for depression masquerading as dementia. Often patients indicate depression directly when asked. Other clues include patients having the ability to pinpoint the onset of symptoms and give detailed accounts of their impairments. Remote memory may be sketchy when interviewed, unlike other dementias where remote memory is relatively intact. Neuropsychologic testing shows poor effort and improvement on coaxing. Treatment is directed at the underlying depression (see psychiatry chapter).

DELIRIUM

I. **Overview.**

A. **Prevalence.** Affects 10% of all hospitalized patients, 20% of burn patients, 30% of ICU patients, and 30% of hospitalized AIDS patients.

B. **Predisposing factors.** Extremes of age (young and elderly) and patients with a history of brain damage, dementia, or prior delirium.

C. **Delirium is a medical emergency** and requires a prompt, thorough evaluation.

II. **Diagnosis by DSM-IV Criteria.** The three following criteria must be met.

A. **Disturbance of consciousness** with reduced ability to focus, shift, or sustain attention.

B. **A change in cognition** (such as memory deficit, disorientation) or development of a perceptual disturbance not better accounted for by dementia.

C. **Symptoms develop over a short period of time** and tend to fluctuate during the day.

III. **Common Causes of Delirium.**

A. **Organ failure.** Renal (uremia), hepatic (hyperammonemia), pulmonary (hypoxia), cardiac (hypotension, low perfusion states).

B. **Nutritional.** Vitamin B_{12}, folate, and thiamine deficiencies; hypoglycemia.

C. **Endocrine.** Hypothyroidism, hyperthyroidism, hypercorticism, hypopituitarism, and hyperparathyroidism.

D. **Trauma.** Burns, fractures (especially of hips).

E. **Infectious.** Pneumonia, sepsis, cystitis, pyelonephritis.

F. **Drugs.** Anticonvulsants, antidepressants, antihypertensive drugs, antiparkinsonian drugs, corticosteroids, digitalis, antihistamines, narcotics, phenothiazines, drugs with anticholinergic side effects, H2 blockers, and alcohol or sedative-hypnotic intoxication or withdrawal.

G. **Electrolyte and acid-base disturbances.** Hypernatremia, hyponatremia, hyperkalemia, hypokalemia, hypermagnesemia, hypomagnesemia, hypercalcemia, hypocalcemia, acidosis, alkalosis.

H. **Urinary retention or fecal impaction.**

I. **Primary brain disorder.**
   1. **Structural.** Trauma, tumor, subdural hematoma, subarachnoid hemorrhage, stroke, concussion.
   2. **Seizure.** Postictal state, nonconvulsive status epilepticus.
   3. **Infection.** Meningitis, encephalitis.

J. **Change in environment.** Demented patients are susceptible to confusion and disorientation with changes in location and sleep as commonly occurs with travel.

IV. **Diagnostic Evaluation.**

A. **Bystander effect.** Most commonly the brain is an "innocent bystander" to a serious process elsewhere in the body. Workup should proceed from immediately life-threatening conditions to more indolent medical and neurologic causes.

B. **See Table 9-2** to differentiate delirium, dementia, and acute psychosis.

C. **History.** Ask family or nurse regarding patient's baseline level of function, any recent medication changes, systemic illnesses, or a history of mental illness.

D. **Physical examination.** Perform a thorough physical exam paying attention to signs of the causes listed above. Assess for neck stiffness. If possible, perform Folstein's mental status exam (Box 9-5). A score of 24 or lower indicates significant cognitive disturbance). Neurologic exam should include a careful cranial nerve assessment and sensory, motor, and reflex screening to detect a brainstem or hemispheric process.

E. **Laboratory tests.** Basic lab tests include CBC, electrolytes, blood chemistry panel, UA, ECG, oxygen saturation, CXR, and abdominal film. If cause not rapidly apparent obtain ABG, cultures, and brain CT. Other labs as indicated by patient's history, PE, and clinical situation: cardiac isoenzymes, vitamin B_{12}, folate, cortisol, ammonia, ANA, RPR, TSH, toxicologic analysis, drug levels, MRI, lumbar puncture, EEG, and HIV serology.

V. **Management.**

A. **Treat the underlying medical conditions** promptly to decrease risk of death (10% to 65%) from the cause of delirium.

B. **Minimize any aggravating medications.**

C. **Optimize nutrition and hydration.**

D. **Create a supportive environment.**

E. **Reassurance.** Family members provide reassurance. Procure familiar items from home to reorient patient.

F. **Sleep** should be regular and uninterrupted. Avoid naps during the day.

G. **Location.** Place patient near a nursing station for easier monitoring.

TABLE 9-2

CLINICAL FEATURES OF DELIRIUM, DEMENTIA, AND ACUTE FUNCTIONAL PSYCHOSIS

Clinical Feature	Delirium	Dementia	Psychosis
Onset	Sudden	Insidious	Sudden
Course over 24 hours	Fluctuating, with nocturnal exacerbation	Stable	Stable
Consciousness	Reduced	Clear	Clear
Attention	Globally disordered	Normal, except in severe cases	May be disordered
Cognition	Globally disordered	Globally impaired	May be selectively impaired
Hallucinations	Usually visual or visual and auditory	Usually absent	Predominantly auditory
Delusions	Fleeting, poorly systematized	Usually absent	Sustained, systematized
Orientation	Usually impaired, at least to time	Often impaired	May be impaired
Psychomotor activity	Increased, reduced, or shifting unpredictably	Often normal	Varies from psychomotor retardation to severe hyperactivity, depending on the type of psychosis
Speech	Often incoherent; slow or rapid	Patient has difficulty finding words; perseveration	Normal, slow, or rapid
Involuntary movements	Often asterixis or coarse tremor	None	Usually absent
Physical illness or drug toxicity	One or both are present	Often absent	Usually absent

Adapted from Bross MH, Tatum NO: Am Fam Physician 50(6):1325, 1994.

H. **Agitation.** Treatment of associated agitation is difficult because sedatives prolong the delirium and cloud the diagnostic process. If absolutely necessary, treat with haloperidol (Haldol) initial dose of 0.5 to 1 mg IM or IV. Orally, try haloperidol or one of the new atypical antipsychotics such as olanzapine (Zyprexa). If antipsychotics are not effective, consider adjunctive lorazepam (Ativan) 0.5 to 1.0 mg IM or IV. Soft restraints may be necessary for safety.

I. **Bed rails** are not protective and increase the number and severity of falls.

SEIZURES

I. **Overview.**

A. **Epidemiology.** Prevalence of epilepsy in the United States is 0.5% to 1%. Approximately 2% to 5% of children have febrile seizures with an age range of 3 months to 5 years.

B. **Definition. Epilepsy** refers to recurrent seizures that reflect aberrant electrical activity of cerebral cortical neurons. **Convulsion** applies to a seizure in which motor manifestations predominate. **Note:** A single seizure is not sufficient to warrant a diagnosis of epilepsy.

II. **Classification.**

A. **Primary generalized seizures.** Bilateral and symmetric without focal onset and usually idiopathic.

1. **Absence (petit mal).** Brief (2- to 10-second) lapse of consciousness. Onset 4 to 12 years of age, and decreased frequency of attacks in adolescence. No aura. Manifested by staring, eye blinking, lip smacking. EEG characteristically shows a diffuse 3 Hz spike-and-wave pattern.

2. **Myoclonic.** Quick paroxysmal contractions of part of a muscle, whole muscle, or groups of muscles. Can occur as single jerk or intermittently in the same or different part of the body. Note: not all myoclonus is epileptic.

3. **Clonic, tonic, and tonic-clonic (grand mal).** With or without aura, the patient abruptly loses consciousness and has a tonic, clonic, or tonic-clonic convulsion, followed by postictal confusion.

4. **Infantile spasms with hypoarrhythmic EEG.** Begin in the first year of life and manifest as a series of myoclonic spasms (also known as salaam seizures). These are generally from underlying brain or neurologic disease and mandate a complete evaluation.

B. **Partial (focal) seizures.**

1. **Simple.** Consciousness *is not* impaired. Subjectively, patients are likely to experience déjà vu and sensory, motor, or autonomic symptoms. For example, patients may note vague abdominal or thoracic sensations. With motor involvement, patients are likely to exhibit hemifacial or hemibody twitching.

2. **Complex.** Consciousness *is* impaired. May have automatic behaviors such as lip smacking, fumbling with clothes, or even walking. Patients are amnestic for part or all of the episode.

III. **Causes.** Seizures result from electrical irritability of gray matter through many possible mechanisms, including CNS infection, inborn errors of metabolism, congenital malformations, acquired metabolic disorders (hypoglycemia, uremia, hepatic encephalopathy, disturbances of Na, Cl, Mg, Ca, pH), structural lesions (stroke, trauma, subarachnoid hemorrhage, subdural hematoma, tumors), gliosis from old brain injuries, new medications or medication withdrawal, drug or alcohol use or withdraw, and familial epilepsy. Common causes based on age are shown in Table 9-3.

IV. **Diagnosis.**

A. **History.** Direct questions to accurately characterize the beginning, middle, and end of the spell. Collateral information from witnesses is essential. Ask about prior seizures, medications, fever, headache, circumstances precipitating events, history of drug abuse, ingestions, and trauma.

B. **Physical examination.** Assess neurologic (responsiveness, fontanelles, pupils, fundi, cranial nerves, sensory, motor, and reflex asymmetry); cardiovascular (BP, perfusion); pulmonary (cyanosis, irregular breathing). Check for breath odor (fruity indicates DKA, fetor hepaticus), rash, signs and symptoms of infection (sepsis, meningitis), signs of trauma, and cirrhosis.

C. **Laboratory tests.** Electrolytes, Ca, Mg, glucose, BUN, CBC, anticonvulsant levels (if applicable), toxicology screen, sepsis workup including LP if indicated; consider LFTs, Pb, NH_4^+, CT scan.

D. **EEG.** Supports diagnosis of seizures. Abnormal neuronal discharges are more frequent in the first few days following a seizure. Obtaining an EEG during this period improves sensitivity and the chances of electrically localizing a seizure focus. A normal EEG does not rule out a seizure disorder, and an abnormal EEG does not always mean epilepsy because the EEG will generally be positive after a seizure but may revert to normal in 3 to 4 weeks. Nasopharyngeal leads can increase the sensitivity of the EEG.

TABLE 9-3

CAUSES OF EPILEPSY IN DIFFERENT AGE GROUPS

Age of Onset	Probable Cause
Infancy and childhood	Congenital malformation, inborn errors of metabolism, idiopathic, birth trauma
Adolescence	Idiopathic, trauma
Early adulthood	Idiopathic, trauma, tumor, alcohol or other hypnotic drug withdrawal
Middle age	Trauma, tumor, vascular disease, alcohol or other drug withdrawal
Late life	Vascular disease, tumor, degenerative disease

F. **Video EEG monitoring.** In patients with frequent spells, video EEG is helpful to differentiate epileptic seizures from other types of spells (see below).

G. **MRI.** Sensitive for structural brain lesions, including tumors, strokes, and hippocampal sclerosis.

V. **Differential Diagnosis of Seizures.**

A. **Syncope.** Global brain hypoperfusion secondary to decreased cardiac output or vasodilation. Convulsions are common if a syncopal patient is not immediately moved to a supine position. Patients often report that syncopal spells are preceded by light-headedness, and postevent confusion is minimal. These patients do not need an EEG or seizure workup if there is simple syncope followed by a brief tonic-clonic seizure (but should be evaluated for syncope). See Chapter 2 for details.

B. **Pseudoseizures.** Often a manifestation of psychologic illness, pseudoseizures are usually poorly stereotyped, varying in form and duration. Most epileptic seizures last less than 3 minutes, but pseudoseizures may have a much longer duration. They are much more likely to occur during times of stress and do not typically occur while alone or during dangerous activities such as cooking or drinking. Without capturing a spell on EEG, it can be difficult to differentiate pseudoseizures from epileptic seizures. Comparing a prolactin level drawn within 15 minutes of a spell to another drawn 24 hours later can be informative. Epileptic seizures are usually accompanied by a significant rise in prolactin level over that of the normal circadian variation. However, a normal prolactin is not helpful because not all seizures are associated with a rise in prolactin level.

C. **Transient ischemic attack.** Like a seizure, they are usually of relatively short duration, although TIAs are characterized by *loss* of neurologic function and only rarely cause motor activity.

D. **Migraine aura.** Also a cause of transient neurologic dysfunction, these spells do not manifest as motor activity. They can cause alteration in sensation, dexterity, balance, vision, and alertness (see migraine headache earlier this chapter).

E. **Breath-holding spells.** Seen in infants and small children. During crying, the infant voluntarily holds breath during expiration, becomes cyanotic, loses consciousness, and may have a few convulsive limb movements. Breath-holding spells are distinguished from seizures by (1) occurring only during emotional outbursts and by (2) the cyanosis preceding (not following) the convulsive movements. Resolves with maturity (usually by 5 years of age).

VI. **Treatment.**

A. **Principles.** Optimally use single-drug therapy because polypharmacy impairs drug effectiveness and side effects accumulate. Drugs of choice are (1) carbamazepine, valproic acid, and phenytoin for most simple partial, complex partial, and generalized seizures; and (2) ethosuximide and valproic acid for absence seizures. Many anticonvulsants elevate hepatic enzymes. Some are also associated with anemias. Baseline, 3-month, and yearly LFTs and CBCs may be necessary. Anticonvulsant levels are useful for monitoring compliance and adjusting dosages when seizures are uncontrolled or side effects occur. Many anticonvulsants are notoriously nonlinear in their pharmacokinetics, making it useful to recheck anticonvulsant levels after a dosage adjustment or changing some other

TABLE 9-4

COMMON ANTIEPILEPTIC DRUGS

Drug	Adult Dose (mg/day)	Principal Therapeutic Indications	Monitoring	Effective Levels (mg/L)
Carbamazepine (Tegretol)	600-1200	Generalized tonic-clonic, complex partial seizures	LFTs, CBC	4-12
Clonazepam (Klonopin)	1.5-20	Myoclonic seizures	None	NA
Ethosuximide (Zarontin)	750-1500	Absence seizures only	CBC	40-100
Gabapentin (Neurontin)	900-3600	Adjunct therapy in partial seizures age >12 years	None	NA
Lamotrigine (Lamictal)	200-500	Adjunct in partial onset seizures	None	NA
Levetiracetam (Keppra)	1000-3000	Adjunctive therapy for partial onset seizures in adults	None	NA
Oxcarbazepine (Trileptal)	600-2400	Adjunctive therapy of partial onset seizures in adults	None	NA
Phenobarbital (Luminal)	60-200	Generalized tonic-clonic, simple, and complex partial seizures	LFTs, CBC	10-30
Phenytoin (Dilantin)	300-400	Generalized tonic-clonic, simple, and complex partial seizures	LFTs	10-20
Primidone (Mysoline)	750-1500	Generalized tonic-clonic, simple, and complex partial seizures	LFTs, CBC	5-15
Tiagabine (Gabatril)	32-56	Adjunctive therapy in partial onset seizures, age >12	None	NA
Topiramate (Topamax)	200-400	Adjunctive therapy in partial onset seizures, age >3	None	NA
Zonisamide (Zonegran	200-600	Adjunctive therapy of partial onset seizures in adults	None	NA
Valproic acid (Depakene)	1000-3000	Generalized tonic clonic, absence, complex partial seizures	LFTs	50-100

drug with a known anticonvulsant interaction. Otherwise, checking levels when the patient is doing well is unnecessary. **Note:** Most antiepileptic drugs decrease the effectiveness of oral contraceptives. This should be discussed with the patient. See Table 9-4.

B. **Surgical treatment** is becoming increasingly useful in modern epilepsy management.

  1. **Temporal lobectomy.** Most effective method for patients with focal onset intractable epilepsy. Consider a patient to be a surgical candidate if seizures are socially disabling and refractory to maximal dose of standard medications. Moreover, certain epilepsy syndromes (mesial temporal-lobe epilepsy and discrete neocortical lesion) have a poor prognosis with purely medical treatment but respond well to surgical treatment.

  2. **Vagus nerve simulator.** Implanted device that intermittently stimulates the left vagus nerve. Well-tolerated, effective adjuvant therapy for refractory partial onset seizures.

C. **Treatment of status epilepticus.** *Status epilepticus* is defined as a seizure (convulsive or otherwise) persisting more than 30 minutes or when a patient fails to return to normal consciousness between seizures. A seizure lasting more than 5 minutes is at increased risk to develop into status epilepticus. Because permanent brain damage starts in as little as 30 minutes, a rapid systematic approach is necessary. See Chapter 2 for treatment.

PARKINSON'S DISEASE

I. **Overview.** Parkinson's disease (PD) is a slowly progressive movement disorder of unknown etiology that primarily affects the pigmented dopamine-containing neurons of the pars compacta of the substantia nigra. Usually appears late in adult life but occasionally as early as the forth decade. Family history is present in 5% to 10% of cases. Epidemiologic studies have identified the following risk factors: rural living, agrochemical exposure, well-water consumption, and living near wood pulp mills.

II. **Diagnosis.** Diagnosis is made clinically. **Onset** is insidious and asymmetric. **Cardinal symptoms** are gross resting tremor (often pill rolling) of the hands and sometimes feet, bradykinesia, rigidity (described as lead pipe with cogwheeling), and postural instability (e.g., unable to maintain balance when pulled from behind). The parkinsonian **gait** is classically festinating (rapid small steps); turning requires several steps, and propulsion, retropulsion, and falling are common. **Other features** include masked facies, decreased blinking, stooped posture, and salivation. **Depression and dementia** can also accompany the disease. A favorable response to dopaminergic drugs helps confirm the diagnosis.

III. **Differential Diagnosis.**

A. **Essential tremor.** Symmetric, fine, rapid, action tremor intensified by a sustained posture such as holding the hands extended at arms length. It is relieved by alcohol, is usually familial, and a head and voice tremor may be prominent. Exam is otherwise normal without other signs of PD. Treatments include propranolol 20 to 60 mg TID, primidone (Mysoline) 50 mg QHS increased slowly to 250 mg TID, gabapentin (Neurontin) 300 to 600 mg TID, implanted brain stimulator.

B. **Parkinsonism from drugs** such as antipsychotics, metoclopramide (Reglan), or carbon monoxide poisoning is usually apparent from the history.

C. **Multiple system atrophy.** A catch term for several degenerative disorders, including Shy-Drager syndrome. Patients have parkinsonism **without tremor** plus any of the following: autonomic dysfunction (including incontinence and severe orthostasis), ataxia, and rarely anterior horn cell loss leading to amyotrophy. Course is aggressive with progressive debilitation. Levodopa response is poor and may result in dystonias.

D. **Progressive supranuclear palsy.** Manifests similarly to PD, but tremor is mild (if present) and rigidity is worse in the neck than the extremities. Dementia is common. Patients develop paresis of voluntary downward gaze. Course is aggressive, and response to levodopa is disappointing.

E. **Normal-pressure hydrocephalus.** Characterized by triad of incontinence, dementia, and ataxia that typically manifests with falling. Tremor and rigidity are absent (see above for details).

IV. **Treatment.**

A. **Nonpharmacologic strategies.**

1. **Support.** Because of the debilitating nature of PD, caregivers often suffer from stress, sleep deprivation, depression, and financial hardship. It is important to discuss these issues openly and be prepared to make referrals to social workers and counselors who specialize in chronic illnesses.

2. **Nutrition.** PD patients often suffer from malnutrition. Establishing good eating habits early in the disease course with ample fiber and calcium is important. Dietary restriction of protein is useful only for patients taking levodopa who experience motor fluctuations (see below).

3. **Exercise.** Although exercise does not alter disease progression, it slows the development of comorbid deterioration.

B. **Pharmacologic therapy.** Medications should be initiated when patients experience functional impairment such as difficulty with activities of daily living, danger of falling, or losing employment. Which medication(s) to start is controversial and depends on such factors as the severity of disease, age, cognitive status, projected life span, and risk of developing complications of levodopa therapy. Medications should be chosen based on the potency needed and a patient's predicted sensitivity to side effects. With the exception of tolcapone, entacapone, and selegiline, all drugs must be started at low dose and titrated to a therapeutic effect over a few weeks. Similarly, drugs must be slowly withdrawn. Precipitously stopping dopaminergic drugs can lead to neuroleptic malignant syndrome.

1. **Selegiline (Eldepryl).** Selective MAO-B inhibitor. It has mild dopaminergic effects and possible neuroprotective effects making it a good choice for early, mild disease. Taking with an SSRI or tricyclic antidepressants can cause a hypertensive crisis, so selegiline must be stopped 2 weeks before starting these drugs. Other side effects include dry mouth, dizziness, syncope, and confusion (especially in the elderly).

2. **Anticholinergics.** Useful for improving resting tremor in younger (<70) cognitively intact patients. Trihexyphenidyl (Artane) and benztropine (Cogentin) starting dose: 0.5 mg BID. Slowly titrate to efficacy or a maximum dose of 2 mg TID. Side effects are numerous, including urinary retention, confusion, exacerbation of closed-angle glaucoma, and memory and psychiatric disturbances.

3. **Amantadine (Symmetrel).** Antiviral drug incidentally discovered to have antiparkinson benefits. Sometimes used in early disease with transient benefit ranging from 2 months to 1 year. Late in the disease, amantadine can help reduce dyskinesias. Start 100 mg QOD for 1 week and then increase slowly to 100 mg BID to TID. Side effects are similar to other dopamine agonists. Livedo reticularis and ankle edema can also occur but rarely mandate stopping this drug. Avoid in the elderly because of CNS side effects, and discontinue by taper.

4. **Dopamine agonists** work by directly stimulating dopamine receptors. They have a longer duration of action than immediate-release levodopa and offer several therapeutic advantages in the right patient. (1) They may be neuroprotective for dopaminergic neurons for a variety of theoretic reasons. (2) Earlier in the disease course, they allow symptomatic relief while sparing the patient the dyskinesia risks of levodopa. (3) Later in the disease course, agonists can be added to levodopa to minimize "off time." Consequently many neurologists avoid levodopa by using agonists in early to mid disease, particularly in patients younger than 70. Later in the disease course, levodopa can be started and the agonist slowly tapered. In advanced disease it may be necessary to add the agonist back to avoid levodopa dosages greater than 600 mg/day and reduce motor fluctuations (see below). Side effects of agonists are similar to those of levodopa: nausea, orthostatic hypotension, and hallucinations. Note that although agonists do not appear to cause dyskinesias in patients naive to levodopa, they may exacerbate them in patients already taking levodopa. Additionally, the ergot derivatives bromocriptine and pergolide can lead to erythromelalgia, Raynaud's syndrome, and pulmonary and retroperitoneal fibrosis.

5. **Nonergot agonists** have more specific binding at the dopamine receptors and are rapidly being embraced by neurologists for early and late PD therapy. Sleep attacks are a rare idiosyncratic reaction to these drugs.

9

NEUROLOGY

      a. **Ropinirol (Requip).** Start 0.25 mg TID, slowly taper to efficacy or a maximum of 8 mg TID.

      b. **Pramipexole (Mirapex).** Start 0.125 mg TID, slowly taper to efficacy or a maximum of 1.5 mg TID.

6. Ergot-derivative agonists.

      a. **Bromocriptine (Parlodel).** Start 1.25 mg BID, slowly taper to efficacy or a maximum of 20 mg BID.

      b. **Pergolide (Permax).** Start 0.1 mg QD, slowly taper to efficacy or a maximum of 2.5 mg BID.

7. **Levodopa (Sinemet).** The most effective antiparkinson drug. Sinemet is a combination of carbidopa, which minimizes the gastrointestinal side effects, and levodopa, the neurologically active drug. Initially start with Sinemet 25/100 (carbidopa/levodopa) 1/2 tablet QD advancing over a few weeks to a clinically effective dose, typically 1 tablet TID to QID. Alternatively, Sinemet CR (controlled-release Sinemet) offers several advantages: convenient dosing, fewer motor fluctuations, and potentially fewer dyskinesias. Start 50/200 (carbidopa/levodopa) 1/2 tablet QD advancing slowly to 1 tablet BID. Bioavailability of Sinemet CR is 30% less than immediate-release Sinemet, and switching between drugs may require a dosage adjustment. Patients who fail to respond to high-dose levodopa (1000 mg/day) may not have PD and are unlikely to respond to other dopaminergic drugs. Levodopa has the following important **side effects.**

      a. **Nausea and vomiting** usually occur from insufficient carbidopa, particularly when taking small doses of Sinemet. Adding more carbidopa (available directly from Dupont Pharmaceuticals at no charge) or increasing the total dose of Sinemet can treat GI symptoms. Antiemetics such as promethazine (Phenergan) can be useful. Avoid phenothiazines (e.g., prochlorperazine [Compazine]) and metoclopramide (Reglan).

      b. **Orthostatic hypotension** is common late in the disease. It may also respond to additional carbidopa. If present early in the disease course, the patient may have multiple-system atrophy (Shy-Drager syndrome; see above).

      c. **Motor fluctuations** are problematic later in the disease course. First, patients develop "wearing off" of the benefits of levodopa before their next dose; later they may develop "on/off phenomena" (unpredictable freezing up). May respond to changing to Sinemet CR or adding a catechol O-methyltransferase (COMT) inhibitor that decreases the destruction of dopamine peripherally (see below).

      d. **Dyskinesias** develop in 50% to 90% of patients on levodopa for 5 to 10 years. They typically occur at peak dose and are involuntary choreiform movements involving the neck or proximal arm or legs. Dyskinesias may respond to lowering the dose or switching to Sinemet CR.

e. **Psychosis.** Visual hallucinations and delusions are common in the elderly taking dopaminergic drugs. Try to taper off any unnecessary drugs, and consider lowering levodopa dose. Avoid the standard neuroleptics because they worsen PD. Olanzapine (Zyprexa) 1 to 15 mg QHS, risperidone (Risperdal) 1 to 8 mg QHS, and quetiapine (Seroquel) 25 mg BID can all be effective. Clozapine (Clozaril) 12.5 mg QHS increased to 25 to 75 mg QHS can have remarkable effects but requires weekly CBCs.

8. **COMT inhibitors** can reduce "off time" in patients with advanced PD by prolonging the half-life of levodopa. Be prepared to reduce the dose of levodopa by 30% if the patient develops worsened dyskinesias.

a. **Entacapone (Comtan).** 200 mg must be taken with each dose of levodopa up to 1200 mg per day. A combined levodopa, carbidopa, entacapone formulation is under development. No monitoring is required.

b. **Tolcapone (Tasmar).** Requires monitoring of liver enzymes weekly for the first 6 months of therapy, then every other week for the duration of therapy because of a small risk of hepatic necrosis. Dose at 200 mg TID. Diarrhea develops in 5% of patients taking tolcapone.

9. **Surgical Therapy.** Pallidotomy can provide relief for refractory dyskinesias, and brain stimulators are effective for refractory tremor. Fetal tissue transplantation continues to be an area of research.

V. **When to Refer.** It is useful to refer the patient to a neurologist at the disease onset to assess for other causes of parkinsonism and confirm the diagnosis. Also, patients may need periodic follow-up, especially if complications of therapy arise.

BENIGN NOCTURNAL LEG CRAMPS

I. **Definition and Overview.**

A. **Definition.** A benign muscle cramp is an involuntary, localized, visible, and usually painful skeletal muscle contraction (calf muscles most commonly affected). Cramps are believed to arise from irritability of the motor neuron. The source of the irritability is unknown. Cramps typically occur at night, are sporadic and random, and usually last seconds to minutes.

B. **Lifetime incidence.** 35% to 95%. Most common in older adults.

C. **Precipitating factors.** Muscle fatigue and passive plantar flexion.

II. **Diagnosis.**

A. **Predisposing factors** may include the following: **lower motor neuron disease**—polyneuropathy, peripheral nerve injury, radiculopathy, amyotrophic lateral sclerosis (starts with weakness and fasciculations); **altered fluid and electrolyte levels**—hypoglycemia, severe hyponatremia, hypocalcemia, respiratory alkalosis, hypermagnesemia, hypokalemia, hyperkalemia; **drugs**—nifedipine (Procardia), beta-agonists (terbutaline sulfate), clofibrate (Atromid-S), penicillamine (Cuprimine); **miscella-**

9

NEUROLOGY

neous—alcohol ingestion, thyroid disease, tetany, heat cramps, hemodialysis, dystonias, peripheral vascular disease, and pregnancy.

B. **Physical examination.** Generally unrevealing unless a cramp is observed. Look for evidence of peripheral vascular disease, polyneuropathy, nerve injury, muscle wasting, weakness, and fasciculations.

III. **Treatment.**

A. **Acute muscle cramp.** Stretching of the affected muscle (as in walking).

B. **Mechanical prevention.** Advise to stretch calf muscles intermittently throughout the day, use a footboard during sleep, and dangle feet over the edge of bed when lying supine.

C. **Pharmacologic prevention.**

1. **Quinine.** The efficacy of quinine sulfate at low doses (such as 300 mg PO QHS) has been supported by several recent analyses. Its use is controversial because of potential side effects, including fatal thrombocytopenia, hypersensitivity reactions, and cardiac arrhythmias.

2. Other reportedly helpful medications include vitamin E (800 U/day), verapamil (Calan), carbamazepine (Tegretol), diphenhydramine (Benadryl), phenytoin (Dilantin), methocarbamol (Robaxin), and riboflavin; however, no randomized, controlled studies are found in the literature.

RESTLESS LEGS SYNDROME

I. **Overview.** Restless legs syndrome (RLS) is a common condition afflicting between 5% and 15% of the population. It is characterized by dysesthesias and restlessness of the legs and may be associated with other medical conditions. RLS is treatable, although therapy must be individually tailored.

II. **Signs and Symptoms.**

A. **Unpleasant limb sensations.** Sensations are described as crawling, creeping, aching, jittery, or fidgety in nature. Legs are much more commonly effected than the arms (hence the name).

B. **Sensations are precipitated by rest.**

C. **Compelling motor restlessness.** Movement of the limb may briefly relieve the sensation.

D. **Worse at night.** Sometimes occurs in the evening or while riding in a car.

E. **Periodic limb movements of sleep.** Patients with RLS often have semirhythmic flexion/extension movements of the foot, which occur every 20 to 40 seconds during non-REM sleep.

III. **Etiology.** The etiology of RLS is unknown; however, familial cases clearly exist. Although no causative link has been established, several medical conditions are known to occur in high frequency in patients with RLS. Symptoms may respond to treatment of the underlying conditions. Among the potential causes are **iron deficiency anemia, diabetes mellitus, uremia, pregnancy, rheumatoid arthritis, vitamin deficiencies** (e.g., B_{12}, folate), **peripheral nerve injury** (e.g., polyneuropathy or radiculopathy), and **Parkinson's disease. Medications** that may contribute to RLS symptomatology include lithium, beta-blockers, tricyclic antidepressants, caffeine, alcohol, and histamine blockers. Neuroleptics deserve special mention because they can lead to akathisia, which resembles RLS.

IV. **Diagnosis.** Diagnosis is by history. Consider other conditions that cause nocturnal limb discomfort: benign nocturnal leg cramps (see above), peripheral vascular disease, polyneuropathy, fibromyalgia, meralgia paresthetica (burning in the thigh/upper leg secondary to lateral cutaneous nerve entrapment), and drug-induced akathisia. Lab tests detect associated conditions and should include BUN, creatinine, glucose, ferritin, folate, and CBC. Consider ankle brachial indices, EMG, and a sleep study.

V. **Treatment.**

A. **General measures.** Limit smoking, alcohol, and caffeine. Discontinue aggravating medications.

B. **Treatment of associated conditions.** May improve RLS.

C. **Pharmacologic treatment options.**

1. **Levodopa (Sinemet).** A proven and effective treatment for RLS. Dose 25/100 mg (carbidopa/levodopa) 1 hour before bedtime. If breakthrough symptoms develop in the middle of the night, switch to Sinemet CR 50/200 mg. Commonly, patients taking levodopa begin to develop RLS during the day. If this occurs, switch to a dopamine agonist (2, 3, or 4 below).

2. **Pergolide (Permax)** 0.5 mg 1 hour before bedtime. Efficacy supported by placebo-controlled study. Start at 0.1 mg and increase to target dose over 2 weeks. Higher doses may be used if necessary.

3. **Pramipexole (Mirapex)** 0.125 mg Q8h increasing to 0.25 mg Q8h. Efficacy supported by placebo-controlled study. Higher doses may be used if necessary.

4. **Ropinirol (Requip).** Starting dose 0.25 mg QHS. Increase dose by 2.5 mg per week up to 4 mg QHS. If symptoms are present during the day, ropinirol may be advanced to a maximum dose of 4 mg TID. Efficacy is supported by an open-label trial. Mean effective dose was 2.8 mg/day.

5. **Clonidine (Catapres)** 0.1 to 0.3 mg 1/2 hour before bedtime. Efficacy supported by a placebo-controlled study. Higher doses may be used if necessary.

6. **Gabapentin (Neurontin)** 300 mg QHS. May increase to 800 QHS and give additional doses for daytime symptoms to a maximum dose of 800 mg QID. Open-label trials suggest less efficacy than dopamine agonists, but gabapentin is well tolerated and lacks drug interactions.

7. **Clonazepam (Klonopin)** 0.5 to 4.0 mg 1/2 hour before bedtime is effective in some patients. Can contribute to nighttime falling and worsening of sleep apnea and is addictive.

8. **Opiates.** Codeine and oxycodone are both effective but can cause nighttime confusion and constipation and are addictive. May be beneficial in patients who failed other therapies.

9

NEUROLOGY

CNS INFECTION

I. **Overview.** Infections of the CNS are broadly classified as meningitis, encephalitis, and abscess. Patients can have more than one type simultaneously (e.g., meningoencephalitis). CNS infections can be difficult to diagnose, and sometimes the survival of the patient relies on a high index of suspicion by the health care provider.

II. **Meningitis.**

A. **Bacterial meningitis** is a true medical emergency. Despite our best care, the overall mortality rate is approximately 25%. The goal is to have IV antibiotics infusing within 30 minutes of presentation. If the LP is going to be delayed (e.g., for CT), administer antibiotics before CT and LP. It is far better for a patient to receive an unnecessary dose of antibiotics than to allow the infection to progress while awaiting test results.

1. **Organisms** (Table 9-5). Common organisms include *Streptococcus pneumoniae, Neisseria meningitidis, Streptococcus agalactiae, Listeria monocytogenes,* and *Haemophilus influenzae. S. agalactiae* primarily affects neonates. *L. monocytogenes* affects people at both extremes of age.

2. **Presentation.** At presentation, the classic triad of headache, fever, and stiff neck is present in only two thirds of cases. However, at least one part of the triad is reliably present. Symptoms generally develop in less than 2 days but in some cases may progress over 7 to 10 days. Nausea, vomiting, and photophobia are common. Seizure, decreased mental status, or focal neurologic deficits may also occur.

3. **Examination** should include assessment for papilledema, middle ear and sinus infections, petechiae (common with *N. meningitidis*), nuchal rigidity, and Kernig's sign (knee cannot be extended beyond 135 degrees with hip flexed at 90 degrees). Kernig's and Brudzinski's signs are present in only 9%.

4. **Laboratory exam.** Always draw blood cultures. A spinal fluid exam should be performed as soon as possible. A brain CT before LP is not necessary if the patient is alert, has no papilledema, has no focal neurologic finding, is HIV negative, and a subarachnoid hemorrhage is not suspected. If neuroimaging is necessary, draw blood cultures

TABLE 9-5		
AGENTS CAUSING BACTERIAL MENINGITIS		
Organism	Percentage of Meningitis Cases	Gram Stain
Streptococcus pneumoniae	47%	Positive cocci
Neisseria meningitidis	25%	Negative cocci in pairs
Streptococcus agalactiae	12%	Positive cocci
Listeria monocytogenes	8%	Positive bacilli
Haemophilus influenzae	7%	Negative bacilli

and begin antibiotics before the study. Spinal fluid should be sent for cell count, WBC differential, glucose, protein, culture, and Gram stain. Acid-fast bacilli stain and cryptococcal antigen may be obtained when indicated. If subarachnoid hemorrhage is also suspected, xanthochromia should be looked for and cell counts should be sent on tubes 1 and 4. As soon as spinal fluid is obtained, start antibiotics. CSF results are listed in Table 9-6. Latex agglutination studies (for *H. influenzae* type b, *S. pneumoniae*, *N. meningitidis*, *E. coli* K1, and the group B streptococci) have good specificity but limited sensitivity, so do not defer treatment based on a negative latex agglutination study.

5. **Treatment.** Treatment of bacterial meningitis generally must begin before the causative organism is identified. Other factors affecting treatment are the patient's age and immunocompetency and the local prevalence of cephalosporin-resistant strains of *S. pneumoniae*. Often, a phone call to the hospital's infectious disease specialist is helpful.

   a. **Antibiotics** (Table 9-7). As information about Gram stain, species identification, and resistance becomes available, the therapy should be narrowed in scope.

   b. **Steroids.** Children who have not been vaccinated against *H. influenzae* should receive dexamethasone. Controversy exists as to whether steroids have any place in the treatment of adults with meningitis. Dose: 0.15 mg/kg IV Q6h for 4 days. The first dose should precede antibiotics by 20 minutes. If dexamethasone is used, substitute rifampin for vancomycin.

TABLE 9-6

CEREBROSPINAL FLUID FINDINGS IN LUMBAR PUNCTURE

Condition	Protein (mg/dl)	Glucose (mg/dl)	WBC (number/mm^3)
Normal	15-45	45-80	Up to 5 lymphocytes
Bacterial meningitis	100-500	0-40	50 to 10,000 chiefly neutrophils
Herpes encephalitis	15-150	Normal	50 to 200 chiefly lymphocytes (also up to 10,000 RBC)
Viral meningitis or encephalitis	20-200	Normal	10 to 500 chiefly lymphocytes; neutrophils may dominate in acute phase
Tuberculous meningitis	45-500	10-45	25 to 1000 chiefly lymphocytes
Cryptococcal meningitis	<500 in 90%	Moderately decreased in 55%	<800 chiefly lymphocytes

TABLE 9-7

EMPIRICAL TREATMENT OF BACTERIAL MENINGITIS

Clinical Setting	Antimicrobial Therapy
0 to 4 weeks of age	Ampicillin + cefotaxime; or ampicillin + amino-glycoside
4 to 12 weeks of age	Ampicillin + ceftriaxone
3 months to 18 years of age	Ceftriaxone (± vancomycin) or ampicillin plus chloramphenicol
18 to 50 years of age	Ceftriaxone (± vancomycin)
>50 years of age	Ampicillin + ceftriaxone (± vancomycin)
Immunocompromised state	Vancomycin + ampicillin + ceftazidime
Basilar skull fracture	Ceftriaxone (± vancomycin)
Head trauma; after neurosurgery	Vancomycin + ceftazidime
Cerebrospinal fluid shunt	Vancomycin + ceftazidime
GRAM STAIN (MOST LIKELY AGENT)	
Positive cocci (*S. pneumoniae*)	Ceftriaxone (± vancomycin)
Positive bacilli (*L. monocytogenes*)	Ampicillin or penicillin G + aminoglycoside
Negative cocci (*N. meningitidis*)	Penicillin G
Negative bacilli (*H. influenzae*)	Ceftazidime

Note: Many authors recommend adding vancomycin to initial therapy given the prevalence of resistant *Pneumococcus*.

    c. **Prophylaxis.** Direct contacts to cases of *N. meningitidis* should receive rifampin 20 mg/kg not to exceed 600 mg BID for 2 days **or** ciprofloxacin 500 mg as a single dose **or** ceftriaxone 250 mg IM as a single dose. For those exposed to *H. influenzae* meningitis, use rifampin 20 mg/kg not to exceed 600 mg QD for 4 days.

B. **Viral meningitis.** Viral meningitis manifests similarly to bacterial meningitis, although its course is rarely aggressive. The diagnostic process and exam is similar to that for bacterial meningitis.

    1. **Organisms.** The most common causes of viral meningitis are enteroviruses, herpes simplex virus, and HIV.

    2. **Presentation.** In addition to fever, photophobia, headache, myalgias, and nausea, the diagnosis of viral meningitis may be suggested by associated signs, including genital lesions (herpes simplex type 2), diarrhea, or a maculopapular rash (enteroviruses).

    3. **Diagnosis** is made by the history, exam, and spinal fluid results. Early in the course, the CSF may show a predominantly neutrophilic inflammatory response. This necessitates hospitalization and IV antibiotics until cultures return negative. Consider HIV testing.

    4. **Treatment** is symptomatic. If genital lesions are also present, consider acyclovir.

III. **Encephalitis** is characterized by prominent changes in mental status, headache, seizures, and sometimes focal neurologic deficits.

A. **Bacterial encephalitis** is rare and usually occurs in the setting of menin-goencephalitis. Agents known to invade brain parenchyma include *Listeria monocytogenes, Rickettsia rickettsii* (Rocky Mountain spotted fever from ticks), leptospirosis (from animal urine), and the ameba *Naegleria fowleri* (from swimming). Treatment is directed at the causative agent.

B. **Viral encephalitis.**

1. **Mosquito-borne.** St. Louis, Eastern Equine, and Western Equine are all encephalitides native to the United States. They are characterized by a decreased mental status, fever, seizures, and sometimes other focal neurologic deficits. Treatment is symptomatic.

2. **Herpes simplex.** Accounting for 10% of encephalitis cases, herpes simplex is a devastating but often treatable CNS infection.

3. **Presentation.** Acute onset of decreased mental status, headache, possibly seizures and disturbances of language, memory, or behavior.

4. **Diagnosis.** CSF usually shows a lymphocytic pleocytosis. Occasionally CSF WBC is normal. RBC is often dramatically elevated and misinterpreted as a traumatic tap. PCR of the CSF has replaced brain biopsy and is now the standard test for the diagnosis of HSV encephalitis. MRI shows inflammation of the temporal lobes and is the best means of early diagnosis. EEG may be helpful. CT with contrast is less sensitive than MRI but will be positive in most cases of HSV encephalitis.

5. **Treatment.** Begin acyclovir immediately in all patients with encephalitis until the diagnosis of HSV is either confirmed or excluded. Dose: 10 mg/kg IV Q8h for 14 days. Monitor renal function during treatment.

IV. **Brain Abscess.** Most commonly, brain abscesses arise from traumatic or hematogenous spread of infection. They can also occur from contiguous spread of a suppurative process such as sinusitis or otitis media.

A. **Presentation** is variable and may include focal neurologic signs, seizures, headache, and indicators of systemic infection.

B. **Diagnosis** is made by neuroimaging with contrast. Needle aspiration confirms the diagnosis. Lumbar puncture is contraindicated and can lead to abscess rupture. The diagnosis of brain abscess mandates other studies seeking the etiology, which may include HIV serology, sinus studies, and transesophageal echocardiogram.

C. **Treatment.** Directed by the clinical setting and includes IV antibiotics and sometimes neurosurgical evacuation.

CEREBROVASCULAR DISEASE

I. **Overview.** Cerebrovascular disease annually affects 750,000 Americans, killing 30% of those afflicted, making it the third most common cause of death. The surviving 70% of stroke patients often suffer significant disability, further underscoring the importance of proper medical treatment and prevention of cerebrovascular disease.

9

NEUROLOGY

II. **Classification.**

A. **Transient ischemic attacks (TIAs).** Focal neurologic deficits arising from interruption of perfusion in a vascular territory typically lasting between 2 and 20 minutes. Risk of ischemic stroke increases markedly after a TIA. Thus a prompt evaluation is required.

B. **Ischemic stroke.** Accounts for 70% of strokes. Can be secondary to a large number of diseases resulting in thrombosis or embolic occlusion of a cerebral artery.

C. **Hemorrhagic stroke.** Fifteen percent to 20% of all strokes result from a breach in the vascular tree allowing a hematoma to form in the brain tissue. Hemorrhagic transformation of an ischemic stroke can occur after large infarctions or with heparin or tPA therapy.

D. **Subarachnoid hemorrhage (SAH).** Typically results from aneurysmal bleeding in the subarachnoid space. Accounts for 5% to 10% of strokes, with a 40% overall mortality rate and a 60% mortality rate with recurrent bleeding. Approximately 40% of survivors are disabled. Early diagnosis is critical. See also section on headaches earlier in this chapter.

III. **Presentation.**

A. **TIAs and ischemic stroke.** All cerebrovascular events are characterized by sudden onset over seconds to minutes. TIAs and strokes are typified by loss of neurologic function such as weakness, anesthesia, incoordination, loss of vision, aphasia, and dysarthria. Occasionally, headache or vertigo may occur.

B. **Hemorrhagic stroke.** Also typified by loss of function, but headache, nausea, and vomiting are common. **Hemorrhagic stroke cannot be accurately differentiated from ischemic stroke without CT scanning.**

C. **SAH.** Sudden onset of severe headache usually without focal neurologic deficits such as paralysis. Nausea, vomiting, and alterations in consciousness are often prominent.

IV. **Differential Diagnosis.**

A. **TIAs.** Episodes without abrupt onset and termination are rarely TIAs. Other considerations include hypoglycemia, hypotension, delirium, postictal state, and migraine aura.

B. **Stroke.** Hypoglycemia, head trauma, subdural and epidural hematomas, MS, postictal state, delirium, tumor, brain abscess, radiculopathy.

C. **SAH.** Main differential diagnoses are migraine headache and meningitis. In migraine there is usually a prior history. The consequences of missing SAH and CNS infection are so grave that the clinician should err on the side of performing a diagnostic workup (including CT and lumbar puncture) in all questionable headaches.

V. **Emergency Evaluation and Treatment.**

A. **TIAs.** Patients with TIAs should generally be admitted for observation. Brain CT without contrast should be performed (see etiology and prevention below). Deficits lasting beyond 20 minutes are likely to progress to infarction and should be approached as strokes. The use of IV heparin in TIAs is unproven and is contraindicated.

B. **Ischemic stroke.**
   1. **Acute treatment.** History, examination, and brain CT are essential components of the initial stroke evaluation. Patients being treated within 3 hours of symptom onset should be emergently considered for tPA. Organize the health care team early. A neurologist should be contacted when a possible tPA candidate arrives. A radiologist or neurologist should be available to read the CT because of limited sensitivity in detecting hemorrhages among physicians who do not routinely read these studies. A systematic approach is essential for a prompt, thorough evaluation. The **tPA checklist** is recommended (Figure 9-1). **Most studies of thrombolytics in stroke are negative, and tPA is not without substantial risk, however, it has gained a wide acceptance as a treatment.**
      a. **Heparin.** Few therapies are more controversial in neurology than IV heparin in acute ischemic stroke. No definitive studies have shown a clear benefit to using IV heparin, and adverse effects such as hemorrhagic transformation of stroke are common. For this reason, the use of IV heparin in stroke is not recommended. It certainly should not be used with tPA. Subcutaneous heparin (5000 U SQ Q12h) is clearly beneficial for the prevention of DVTs in patients with ischemic stroke.
      b. **Intraarterial thrombolysis** is a promising experimental therapy that may allow intervention beyond the 3-hour time window of tPA.
      c. **Aspirin** (325 mg) should be started in those with ischemic stroke within 24 hours of the event.
C. **Hemorrhagic stroke.** The diagnosis is confirmed by brain CT. If the hemorrhage exerts significant mass effect or extends into the ventricular system, or if there is a clotting deficiency, a neurosurgical consultation should be obtained. Blood pressure should be monitored closely and treated somewhat more aggressively than with ischemic stroke. If the patient is taking warfarin, reverse anticoagulation with fresh frozen plasma. Avoid anticoagulants, including subcutaneous heparin. See discussion of prophylactic antiepileptics below.
D. **SAH.** Usually evident on CT as blood surrounding the midbrain. If CT is negative but there is a clinical suspicion, an LP is required to exclude SAH. If the diagnosis is confirmed, an emergent neurosurgical consultation is necessary. Pending this evaluation, blood pressure should be aggressively controlled (see below). See previous section on headache for further details. **Prophylactic measures to prevent seizures** (e.g., IV phenytoin) are frequently recommended. This reduces seizure occurrence in the first week following the event but has no effect on long-term outcome. Screening of asymptomatic relatives of patients with SAH for an aneurysm is not generally helpful because the rate of morbidity and mortality from surgical repair is the same as that of watchful waiting.
IV. **Supportive Care of Stroke.**
A. **Blood pressure.** Acutely, a target of a systolic BP of 185 and a diastolic BP of 110 should be the goal. Use IV labetalol to lower BP to these

9

NEUROLOGY

tPA Checklist

☐ **Onset <3 hours.** Time of onset must be definitively known. Strokes recognized when waking are assumed to have occurred at onset of sleep.

☐ **Labs.** Several parameters must be normal before thrombolytic therapy. When patient arrives, send stat glucose, INR, aPTT, electrolytes, and CBC. Note that coagulation studies take a minimum of 30 minutes to complete.

☐ **Exam.** Initially should be brief and pertinent. NIH stroke scale (NIHSS) provides a quick, reliable means of classifying a stroke's severity. See http://www.vh.org/Providers/ClinGuide/Stroke/Scaledef.html. Also assess for meningeal signs, evidence of head trauma, fractures, and dislocations.

☐ **Head CT without contrast.** Allows the exclusion of hemorrhagic strokes and subdural and epidural hematomas.

☐ **ECG.** Assess for concurrent myocardial infarction.

☐ **Blood pressure control.** Use IV labetalol to reduce systolic BP <185 and diastolic BP <110. Be judicious with blood pressure control. Suddenly lowering the blood pressure below 185/110 is risky and can be associated with stroke progression secondary to decreased perfusion.

☐ **Informed consent.** Often stroke patients are aphasic. Do not lose contact with the next of kin. Overall the risk of serious hemorrhagic transformation of ischemic stroke is approximately 1 in 16 patients.

☐ **Other exclusion criteria.** Glucose <50; platelet count <100,000; INR >1.4; aPTT >2 seconds above upper limit; trauma, surgery, myocardial infarction, or GI bleed within 2 weeks; head trauma or other stroke within 6 weeks; suspicion of SAH; CT demonstrating acute stroke involving more than one third of a hemisphere; NIHSS <3 or >22.

☐ **tPA dose.** 0.9 mg/kg up to total of 80 mg. 10% IV is bolus over 5 min followed by infusion of the remaining drug over 1 hour.

☐ **If on-site neurosurgical support is not available,** arrange for fastest possible travel to tertiary care facility immediately after tPA infusion is completed.

FIGURE 9-1

tPA checklist.

levels. In the first 48 hours, BP should *not* be more aggressively controlled to prevent widening of an ischemic infarct. After 48 hours, BP can be gently lowered by PO medications.

B. **Free water** should be limited to 1200 ml in the first 48 hours of stroke. If IV fluids are needed, use isotonic saline.

C. **Ancillary services.** Physical therapy, speech pathology, occupational therapy, and a social worker should be involved early in care.

D. **Prevention of complications.** Frequent turning in bed may be necessary to prevent skin ulcers. A **swallowing study** should be done to evaluate for aspiration. Feeding tube may be necessary to safely deliver medications and nutrition. Compression stockings or subcutaneous heparin should be employed to prevent DVTs.

V. **Uncovering the Etiology.** Determining the etiology of the stroke is helpful for guiding future stroke prevention. Studies are tailored to the case in question.

A. **Chest x-ray** assesses cardiac size and screens for pulmonary complications.

B. **ECG** is useful for the diagnosis of atrial fibrillation, atrial enlargement, and myocardial infarction. Telemetry may be necessary, especially among patients with hemorrhages, because there is a direct myocardial depressant effect from CNS illness and arrhythmias may occur.

C. **Echocardiogram.** Transesophageal echocardiogram is useful to exclude vegetations, shunts, and intracardiac thrombi. This should be performed on most patients without other clear risk factors for ischemic stroke.

D. **Carotid duplex** should be performed in all patients with ischemic stroke who would potentially be candidates for carotid endarterectomy.

E. **Fasting lipid profile** should be checked in all stroke patients 3 months after the event.

F. **Coagulation studies** should be undertaken in patients younger than 55 without other clear risk factors for stroke. In the acute setting draw activated protein C resistance, prothrombin gene rearrangement, factor V Lyden, dilute Russel viper venom test, and anticardiolipin antibodies. Draw protein C, protein S, and antithrombin III after 3 months, because these will be falsely depressed in the acute period.

G. **MRI.** Helpful for the diagnosis of small strokes, tumors, and lesions in the posterior fossa.

H. **Cerebral angiogram** is reserved for subarachnoid hemorrhage, nonhypertensive cerebral hemorrhages, cases of suspected vasculitis, and perhaps in the setting of young patients without other known etiology.

VI. **Prevention of Future Events.**

A. **TIAs and stroke.**

1. **Aspirin** 81 or 325 mg is the primary first-line therapy for prevention of TIAs and noncardioembolic ischemic strokes.

2. **Ticlopidine (Ticlid)** 250 mg BID and clopidogrel (Plavix) 75 mg QD are suitable for patients who failed or are intolerant of aspirin. Ticlopidine requires CBCs twice monthly for 3 months because of a

0.5% risk of neutropenia. Thrombotic thrombocytopenic purpura is also a potential complication of both medications.

3. **Aggrenox (aspirin 25 mg/sustained-release dipyridamole 200 mg) BID** is also suitable for patients who failed aspirin alone. The principle side effect is headache. Patients may require supplemental ASA. Dipyridamole is considered second line after ASA and clopidogrel.

4. **Ramipril (Altace) 5 mg BID.** Independent of their effect on blood pressure, ACE inhibitors are emerging as an important class of drugs to lower the risk of stroke. Other ACE inhibitors probably have the same effect as ramipril.

5. **Warfarin** anticoagulation should be considered in patients with known cardioembolic sources.

6. **Lipid-lowering drugs** and dietary modifications should be aggressively pursued in stroke patients with elevated lipids (see Chapter 3).

7. **Hypertension** requires careful control in the outpatient setting to lower the risk of future strokes. Unless otherwise indicated, preferentially use an ACE inhibitor (see Chapter 3).

8. **Carotid endarterectomy** is appropriate for good surgical candidates with >50% stenosis in a symptomatic arterial distribution or >60% in an asymptomatic distribution, provided the surgeon has a documented track record of less than a 3% complication rate.

9. **Tobacco consumption** is a strong risk factor for stroke and should be stopped.

NEUROPATHY

I. **Overview.** *Neuropathy* is an umbrella term for nonradicular diseases of the peripheral nerves. Neuropathy can be acute and life threatening as in Guillain-Barré syndrome or chronic as in diabetic neuropathy. Assessment of the patient seeks to define the time course of the disease, identify which nerves are involved, and, if possible, determine the underlying cause.

II. **Classification.**

A. **Anatomic classification.**

1. **Mononeuropathy.** Involvement of a single nerve (e.g., carpal tunnel syndrome, meralgia paresthetica).

2. **Polyneuropathy.** Diffuse involvement of the peripheral nerves (e.g., diabetic neuropathy).

3. **Mononeuritis multiplex.** Seemingly random involvement of multiple isolated nerves. Can occur in vasculitis, porphyria, diabetes, HIV, and others.

B. **Cellular classification.**

1. **Axonal neuropathy.** Loss of function from loss of nerve cells. Typically affects longest nerves first with patients describing loss of sensation or paresthesias of the feet. Axonal neuropathy is usually symmetric, although it may be asymmetric early in the course. Weakness occurs late and tends to involve the most distal muscles.

    2. **Demyelinating neuropathy.** Damage to the Schwann cells leads to impairment of nerve conduction. Weakness tends to involve both proximal and distal muscles.

C. **Time course.**

    1. **Acute neuropathy.** Sudden onset of dysfunction from an injury or immunologic attack.

    2. **Chronic neuropathy.** Usually insidious onset with slow progression from low-level ongoing nerve injury.

III. **Diagnosis.**

A. **Careful history** should elicit the onset and rate of progression of symptoms. Assess for other medical problems, medications, and toxic exposures (see below for details). Inquire about weakness and autonomic dysfunction (erectile dysfunction, bladder disturbances, and orthostasis). Ask what sensory modalities are involved. Have the patient draw a line on the skin to separate areas of normal and abnormal sensation.

B. **Physical exam.** Includes cranial nerves, proximal and distal strength, reflexes, gait, Romberg's sign and sensation to pin, monofilament nylon (see under diabetes in Chapter 5), 128 Hz vibration, and position.

C. **Laboratory testing.**

    1. **Tests for all patients with unexplained neuropathy.** CBC, glucose tolerance test, Vitamin B_{12}, rheumatoid factor, TSH, free T4, sedimentation rate, ANA, serum protein electrophoresis with immunofixation. If monoclonal gammopathy is present, obtain quantitative immunoglobulins, urine protein electrophoresis, and skeletal x-ray survey.

    2. **Other tests to consider strongly.** HIV antibody, VDRL, Lyme titer, lumbar puncture.

    3. **Tests useful in proper clinical setting.** Folate, urine heavy-metal screen, ganglioside antibodies (GM1, anti-MAG, antisulfatide), and paraneoplastic antibodies (anti-Hu).

    4. **Ganglioside antibodies** may be found in multifocal motor neuropathy (positive in 80% to 90%). These neuropathies are characterized by slowly progressive, asymmetric neuropathy that generally begin in the hands and the distal musculature rather than the proximal musculature. There are generally no or few sensory findings, and they can be differentiated from ALS by the absence of hyperreflexia and spasticity.

    5. **Paraneoplastic syndromes** are associated with a neoplasm (especially ovarian, lung, breast) and include Eaton-Lambert syndrome, which is manifested by weakness that improves with muscle use; patients may have anti–presynaptic calcium-channel (anti-PCC) antibodies. Some paraneoplastic syndromes are sensory neuropathies associated with anti-Hu antibodies; others are related to CNS injury (especially cerebellar degeneration associated with anti-Yo, anti-Hu, and anti-Ri antibodies). Some paraneoplastic syndromes are indistinguishable from Guillain-Barré syndrome.

9

NEUROLOGY

D. **Electromyography (EMG) and nerve conduction studies** are helpful to confirm a clinical impression. They can often differentiate a radiculopathy from a neuropathy and can classify a primarily axonal from a primarily demyelinating process. Electromyographers function best when asked specific questions; for example, "Is this carpal tunnel syndrome, C6 radiculopathy, or asymmetric polyneuropathy?"

E. **Nerve biopsy** is undertaken only when etiology remains unknown after electrodiagnostic and other laboratory tests have been completed.

IV. **Common and Important Neuropathies.**

A. **Guillain-Barré syndrome (GBS).** GBS can be immediately life threatening and deserves special attention. GBS is an acute immune-mediated demyelinating polyneuropathy. It manifests with progressive, usually symmetric, weakness over a span of 2 days to 4 weeks. Weakness progresses from distal to proximal. Sensory disturbances are variable. Frequently a history of a recent respiratory or GI illness (especially *Campylobacter*) can be elicited. In addition to weakness, physical exam is remarkable for absent reflexes. Electrodiagnostic studies confirm the clinical impression. LP showing elevated CSF protein provides additional evidence. Some patients may also be anti-GM1 positive (see above). **Patients with GBS can undergo acute pulmonary decompensation,** and overall 33% require ventilatory support. Even patients with mild symptoms should be admitted for a minimum of 24 hours. Forced vital capacity (FVC) or negative inspiratory force (NIF) should be assessed every 2 to 4 hours until patients prove pulmonary stability. Patients with a FVC of less than 1 liter or NIF less forceful than -30 should be transferred to the ICU. ABG and pulse oxymetry are insensitive to impending decompensation. IVIG and plasma exchanges shorten the course of GBS.

B. **Diabetic neuropathy.** This is the most common cause of diffuse polyneuropathy. It arises in one half of all diabetics, and the neuropathy is primarily axonal. The mechanism of the axonal loss is under debate and may be a combination of vascular, metabolic, and immunologic stress on the nerve fibers. Tight glucose control reduces the risk of developing neuropathy and may help halt progression. Some patients continue to progress despite tight control. Immunologic therapy is under investigation.

C. **Carpal tunnel syndrome.** See Chapter 16.

D. **Hereditary neuropathies.** Charcot-Marie-Tooth (CMT) encompasses a group of largely autosomal dominant neuropathies. Both axonal (CMT type 2) and demyelinating (CMT type 1 and CMT X-linked) forms exist. Onset frequently occurs during adulthood. Patients have a stocking-glove sensory loss and distal weakness. Slender hands and feet and high foot arches (pes cavus) typify the physical exam. In addition to electrodiagnostic tests, genetic testing is available. Treatment is symptomatic.

E. **Drug-induced neuropathies.** Nitrofurantoin, dapsone, metronidazole, isoniazid, disulfiram, amiodarone, vincristine, cisplatin, Taxol, phenytoin, chloramphenicol, hydralazine, and high-dose pyridoxine can all lead to neuropathies.

F. **Environmental toxins.** Lead is the most common environmental toxin and is usually associated with gastric distress, anemia, and weakness of finger and wrist extension. Inquire about recent work in radiator shops, battery factories, etc. Remote exposure to lead is rarely responsible for a neuropathy. Diagnosis is confirmed by 24-hour urine heavy-metal testing.

G. **Malnutrition.** Vitamin B_{12} deficiency leads to dysfunction in several areas of the nervous system, including a predominantly axonal neuropathy, dementia, and spasticity. A macrocytic anemia may or may not be present. Serum B_{12} testing usually confirms the diagnosis. If results are low-normal, consider a Schilling test. Deficiencies of vitamin B_6 (pyridoxine), vitamin E, niacin, and folate are rare causes of neuropathy.

H. **Alcoholic neuropathy.** Controversy exists as to whether isolated alcoholism is sufficient to lead to a neuropathy. Usually there is comorbid malnutrition. The neuropathy is predominately axonal and characterized by distal weakness, stocking-glove sensory loss, and unsteadiness of gait.

I. **Collagen vascular diseases** can lead to a vasculitic neuropathy. Nerves infarct, resulting in an axonal neuropathy. Mononeuritis multiplex may lead to a confluent stocking-glove neuropathy. Screen with an ANA and rheumatoid factor. Consider a referral to a neuromuscular specialist for possible nerve biopsy.

J. **Infectious causes.** Lyme, HIV, syphilis, and leprosy can all lead to neuropathy. Consider testing in the appropriate setting.

K. **Chronic inflammatory demyelinating polyradiculoneuropathy (CIDP)** is a progressive neuropathy with prominent weakness of the proximal and distal musculature leading to difficulty arising from a chair and an unsteady gait. Diagnosis is made by electrodiagnostic studies and LP, which shows an elevated total protein and a normal cell count. CIDP can herald a plasma cell dyscrasia, and the workup should include a skeletal survey and both urine and serum protein electrophoresis with immunofixation. Consider a hematologic consultation. Treatment is with IVIG or prednisone.

L. **Other metabolic neuropathies** include symptomatic thyroid disease, porphyria, and renal or hepatic failure.

V. **Symptomatic treatment** of neuropathy pain and paresthesias is directed at reducing the pain. Possible treatments include amitriptyline (Elavil) 10 to 75 mg HS, nortriptyline (Pamelor) 10 to 100 mg HS, gabapentin (Neurontin) 400 mg HS to 800 mg TID, or carbamazepine (Tegretol) 200 to 400 mg TID. Capsaicin cream has also been used with some success.

MULTIPLE SCLEROSIS

I. **Overview.** Multiple sclerosis (MS) typically begin in early adulthood and is characterized by multiple areas of demyelination and sclerosis of the brain, spinal cord, or both. The cause is unknown and the fa-

9

NEUROLOGY

milial incidence is low. Whites are more susceptible than Blacks and Asians. Pregnancy decreases the risk of exacerbations, but exacerbations increase immediately postpartum. Infection or trauma may trigger exacerbations.

II. **Clinical Manifestations.** MS is characterized by episodes of focal neurologic dysfunction separated in both space and time. Onset of symptoms is usually acute and worsens over a few days. Symptoms may last up to several weeks followed by either partial or full resolution. Later, other deficits appear, which again show a waxing and waning course.

Common symptoms include weakness or numbness of a limb, monocular visual loss, diplopia, vertigo, facial weakness or numbness, sphincter disturbances, ataxia, and nystagmus. A history of symptoms aggravated by a hot bath is sometimes obtained. MS is classically divided into two forms:

A. **Relapsing remitting MS.** Episodes fully resolve with good neurologic function between exacerbations. Accumulation of deficits is slow over decades, if at all.

B. **Chronic progressive MS.** Episodes fail to fully resolve, and deficits accumulate steadily. Relapsing remitting MS can convert to chronic progressive MS.

III. **Laboratory Tests.** About 90% of patients have abnormal findings in CSF that include a mild mononuclear pleocytosis, a modest increase in total protein, a greatly increased gamma-globulin fraction, a high IgG index, presence of oligoclonal bands, and an increase in myelin basic protein. MRI with gadolinium enhancement is highly sensitive and differentiates old from new lesions. Visual-evoked responses are abnormal in 80% of patients with definite MS.

IV. **Differential Diagnosis.** Behçet's disease, SLE, metastatic tumors, vascular malformations, Arnold-Chiari malformation, herniated intervertebral disk, spinocerebellar degeneration, CNS vasculitis, primary CNS lymphoma, HIV encephalitis and progressive multifocal leukoencephalopathy, and multiple strokes.

V. **Prognosis.** One study showed that a 25-year mortality rate was about 26% compared with 14% in the general population. After 25 years two thirds of the survivors were still ambulatory. 60% of those with optic neuritis will develop MS over 40 years. Unfortunately, it is not possible to accurately predict which patients will progress.

VI. **Treatment.**

A. **Acute exacerbations.**

1. **Triggers.** Urinary tract or other infections can precipitate MS exacerbation. Treating a UTI often leads to resolution of the neurologic symptoms without the use of steroids.

2. **Methylprednisolone (Solu-Medrol)** is often used to shorten the duration of acute exacerbations, although its utility in preventing long-term disability is unproven. A typical regimen is 250 mg IV QID for 3 days or 1000 mg IV QD for 3 days. Infusions are followed by a ta-

per of prednisone 1 mg/kg/day for 11 days followed by a rapid taper of 5 days. The use of high-dose oral steroids is controversial and needs further study.

B. **Maintenance immunomodulatory.**

1. **Interferon β-1b (Betaseron)** 250 μg SQ QOD. Has been shown to significantly reduce frequency of exacerbations and long-term disability in relapsing remitting MS.
2. **Interferon β-1a (Avonex).** 30 μg IM Q week. Similar efficacy to interferon β-1b but administered weekly.
3. **Glatiramer acetate (Copaxone)** 20 mg SQ QD. Different mechanism of action, but similar efficacy to the above agents.
4. **Methotrexate** 7.5 mg PO Qwk. May be effective in reducing the rate of progression in chronic progressive MS. Monitor CBC and AST monthly for the duration of therapy.
5. **Mitoxentrone** (Novantrone), a potent immunosuppressive, has been used with success but is not FDA-approved for this indication.

VERTIGO AND DIZZINESS

I. **Overview.** Disturbances of balance are common. Frustrating the evaluation is the poor vocabulary patients use to describe their symptoms. *Dizziness* is a general term indicating spatial disorientation and can be avoided by asking patients to describe their symptoms without using the word "dizzy." When dizziness is categorized as vertigo, presyncope, or dysequilibrium, the evaluation becomes much more straightforward.

II. **Classification with Signs and Symptoms.**

A. **Vertigo.** Defined as the hallucination of movement, a sense that the environment is spinning, a sensation of feeling impelled forward, backward, or to either side. Others describe "tilting" of their environment or a "back-and-forth" feeling. The evaluation of vertigo centers around two questions: (1) Is it a single episode or is it recurrent? (2) Is it likely to be of central or peripheral origin?

B. **Single episode or recurrent.** Careful questioning is required to define the symptoms over time. In vertiginous patients, motion exacerbates the symptoms, making it difficult to differentiate discrete episodes of movement-induced vertigo from mild baseline vertigo with movement-induced exacerbations. The questions "When are the symptoms present?" and "When are the symptoms absent?" are equally important.

C. **Central or peripheral** (Table 9-8).

1. **Central causes** arise from damage or dysfunction of the pons or cerebellum. With the exception of TIAs they manifest as single (though often prolonged) episodes of vertigo. Other neurologic deficits such as dysarthria, numbness, weakness, or diplopia may accompany the vertigo. Nystagmus may be prominent. Difficulty walking is usually more severe with central causes.

TABLE 9-8

COMPARISON OF PERIPHERAL AND CENTRAL VERTIGO

Feature	Peripheral	Central
Occurrence of vertigo	Episodic	May be constant
Vertigo severity	+ +	+
Exacerbated by motion	+ +	+
Nausea/vomiting	++	+
Hearing loss	Possible	—
Tinnitus	Possible	—
Central compensation	Good	Fair
Loss of consciousness	No	Possible
Other neurologic signs/symptoms	No	Possible
DIX-HALLPIKE TEST		
Nystagmus latency	10-30 seconds	None
Nystagmus duration	Brief	Long
Nystagmus fatigue with multiple trials	Yes	No
Vertigo improves with multiple trials	Yes	No

2. **Peripheral causes** arise from damage or dysfunction of the labyrinth or VIII nerve. Nausea and vomiting are typically more prominent with peripheral vertigo. Other symptoms referable to the ear, including hearing loss, pain, ear fullness, and tinnitus, are common. Episodes can be single or recurrent, depending on the etiology. Compensation is more rapid and complete with peripheral vertigo.

D. **Other types of dizziness that must be differentiated from true vertigo.**

1. **Presyncope.** Vertigo is distinctly different from presyncope. Presyncope is a feeling of light-headedness or faintness. It is often associated with generalized weakness, visual blurring, a sense of impending blacking out, diaphoresis, SOB, or palpitations. Typically it is episodic and caused by a transient decrease in cerebral perfusion.

2. **Disequilibrium** is primarily experienced when one is standing or walking and is absent when lying or sitting. Crowds and difficult walkways (such as stairs, ramps, and escalators) exacerbate the patient's symptoms. There is no clear hallucination of movement but rather a vague feeling of being off balance.

III. **Vertigo Syndromes.**

A. **Vertigo by time frame.**

1. **Benign positional vertigo.** Each episode lasts seconds to minutes.

2. **Ménière's disease.** Each episode lasts hours to days.

3. **Toxic damage to labyrinth** (e.g., salicylates, ETOH). Variable depending on etiology.

4. **Labyrinthitis (e.g., viral).** Each episode of vertigo lasts days.
B. **Causes of recurrent episodes of vertigo.**
   1. **Benign paroxysmal positional vertigo (BPPV).** Most common cause of recurrent vertigo. Historical characteristics: change in head position precipitates brief episodes of vertigo; not associated with tinnitus; may be associated with nausea but rarely emesis. Follows a waxing and waning course over months to years, but most cases resolve with time. Most common age of onset is between 60 and 70. Women with BPPV outnumber men by 2:1. This condition is caused by calcium carbonate crystals displaced within the posterior semicircular canal. Confirm by the Dix-Hallpike test, which is performed by rapidly laying down the patient from sitting position, allowing the head to hang over the edge of the bed while simultaneously turning the head to the left or right. A positive test manifests as vertigo and the observation of rotatory nystagmus within 30 seconds of the maneuver. With the diagnosis confirmed, a positioning procedure can be performed that relocates the offending crystal (see Furman JM: *N Engl J Med* 4(21): 590-596, 1999). Literature cites success rates in excess of 85% for patients treated in this manner. For refractory cases, brief therapy with benzodiazepines (e.g., diazepam 2 to 5 mg TID to QID) or vestibular rehabilitation exercises may be of use. Meclizine (Antivert) is an alternative. Dimenhydrinate (Dramamine) may be superior to the benzodiazepines at least acutely.
   2. **Ménière's disease.** Syndrome with recurrent attacks of vertigo and tinnitus lasting hours to days and associated hearing loss (low frequencies lost first; discrimination is maintained). Generally have a feeling of ear fullness that resolves after episodes of vertigo. **Brief, transient vertigo is not Ménière's disease.** May have nausea, vomiting, and ataxia. Onset age 30 to 60 years. Patients with newly suspected cases should be evaluated with MRI and audiometry. 60% resolve spontaneously without treatment. Treatment includes bed rest, IV fluids (if unable to maintain hydration), antihistamines, and phenothiazines or diazepam (as above). Salt restriction and diuretics (such as hydrochlorothiazide or furosemide) may be helpful. Data are poor, but two thirds are reported to respond to either sodium restriction or diuretics. If severe symptoms, surgical ablation may be performed (labyrinthectomy if hearing is lost; vestibular nerve section if hearing is preserved). See BPPV above for symptom control.
   3. **Migraine aura.** Vertigo can arise as an aura to migraine. Other symptoms may include scintillating scotoma, homonymous hemianopsia, cortical blindness, diplopia, dysarthria, ataxia, and paresthesias. Patients are typically young women and adolescents. Symptoms last up to 30 minutes, and migraine headache occurs after the vertigo. Treatment of basilar migraines should avoid vasoconstrictors, other-

9

NEUROLOGY

wise standard abortive and prophylactic migraine medications are appropriate.

4. **Perilymph fistula** occurs from a perilymph leak. Vertigo is often precipitated by prolonged standing, change in head position, coughing, sneezing, swallowing, straining, barotrauma, air travel, or loud noises. There is often an antecedent history of head trauma that results in a small tear in the oval or round window leading to a perilymph leak. Tends to be better in the morning and worse after being upright for a time. May be associated tinnitus and hearing loss. **Diagnosis:** pneumatic otoscopy reproduces symptoms. Often heals spontaneously. Surgical correction if ongoing symptoms.

B. **Causes of a single acute episode of vertigo.**

1. **Acute peripheral vestibulopathy (viral labyrinthitis).** Acute onset of severe vertigo, nausea, and vomiting that lasts days and slowly returns to normal. Hearing loss and tinnitus are not typical. Nystagmus may be present in the first 48 hours. Occurs in all ages. Cause unclear but may be viral (45% cluster around viral infections). Consider performing audiogram and brainstem auditory evoked potentials to screen for structural causes of the symptoms. MRI is necessary if screening test abnormal or if >60 years of age with history or risk factors for vascular disease. **Treatment:** bed rest, antiemetics, IV fluids, diazepam, and antihistamines per BPPV. Some have used steroids (32 mg on day 1, 16 mg BID on days 2 to 4, taper to 4 mg on day 8) with success.

2. **Vertebrobasilar stroke.** Sudden vertigo often with symptoms less severe than other syndromes. Nausea and vomiting may be seen. Hearing loss and tinnitus are not seen. Nystagmus is often prominent. Other neurologic deficits such as dysarthria, numbness, weakness, ataxia, and diplopia may accompany the vertigo. Weakness or numbness affecting one side of the face and the opposite side of the body may be seen. Often there is a history of risk factors for cerebrovascular disease. Any patient at risk for stroke should have posterior fossa imaging (MRI preferred; CT if MRI unavailable). Consider neurology consultation for further workup.

3. **Cerebellar hemorrhage.** Produces acute onset of vertigo, headache, inability to walk, nausea, and vomiting. Physical signs include horizontal nystagmus, ipsilateral limb ataxia, and facial palsy. Any patient with acute-onset headache and vertigo should be considered for an emergent head CT. **Patients with cerebellar hemorrhage may deteriorate rapidly. Neurosurgical consult for the question of posterior fossa decompression is recommended.**

4. **Multiple sclerosis.** Vertigo less severe than in peripheral disorders. Nausea, vomiting, and ataxia may be seen. Hearing loss is rare.

Usually associated with other neurologic symptoms of demyelination in CNS. Most common in young women.

5. **Head trauma.** Dizziness usually attributable to postconcussion syndrome (that is, disequilibrium dizziness). Less common: BPPV, perilymph fistula, or basilar skull fracture.

6. **Toxic damage to labyrinth.** Antibiotics (especially aminoglycosides), salicylates, ethanol, phenytoin, quinine, benzene, and arsenic can all cause damage or dysfunction to the labyrinth.

7. **Acoustic neuroma.** Benign tumor arising from cranial nerve VIII. May have tinnitus and hearing loss, **but discrimination is lost long before hearing loss is complete.** May have associated facial palsy. Auditory brainstem evoked potentials and MRI with contrast are the most sensitive tests.

IV. **Presyncope and Syncope.** See Chapter 3.

V. **Disequilibrium.**

A. **Processes that disturb equilibrium.** Disequilibrium typically arises from dysfunction of multiple sensory channels with or without impaired higher cortical processing or motor responsiveness.

B. **Abnormalities of sensory input** can result from diseases that decrease or distort vision, impair the vestibular system, or interfere with proprioception. Cumulatively, these impairments result in disorientation while ambulating. This may result in falling, especially in dark environments. This problem is an especially common cause of falls in the elderly.

C. **Abnormalities of central integration.** Dementia, metabolic encephalopathy, and sedative medications can all contribute.

D. **Abnormalities of motor response.** Disturbance in pyramidal, extrapyramidal (such as Parkinson's disease), or cerebellar function (such as alcohol-related, degenerative, or neoplastic disease) may further impair ambulation.

E. **Diagnostic evaluation of disequilibrium.** Review medications. Ask about visual problems, hearing loss, sensory loss, paresthesias, and a history of vertigo. Check for hyporeflexia or hyperreflexia, Romberg's sign, and signs of Parkinson's disease. If hearing loss, obtain audiometry or brainstem auditory evoked potentials. Consider MRI and neurologic consultation.

F. **Therapy for disequilibrium.** Discontinue aggravating medications. Correct metabolic derangements. If visual symptoms present, refer to ophthalmologist. If bilateral hearing abnormality on audiometry or BAER, refer to ENT. Treat peripheral neuropathy or Parkinson's disease as discussed earlier. Patients may benefit from use of a light cane, a soft cervical collar, vestibular exercises, or environmental improvements (e.g., lights at night) to their home.

VI. **Non-stroke Weakness.** Table 9-9 lists some differential diagnoses of weakness that are not related to stroke.

TABLE 9-9

PARTIAL DIFFERENTIAL DIAGNOSIS OF WEAKNESS

Illness	Autonomic Involvement	Sensory Changes	Fever	Fasciculations/ Muscle Cramps	Cranial Nerve Involvement
Myasthenia gravis	No	No	No	No	Yes
Guillain-Barré	Possible	Yes	No	No	Rare, pupil reactivity maintained
Botulism	Dry mouth	No	No	No	Yes, early
Tick paralysis	No	Paresthesias	No	No	No
Diphtheria	No	Occasional	Yes	No	Pharyngeal followed by other cranial nerves; may resolve before generalized weakness
Eaton-Lambert	No	No	No	No	Yes

Reflexes	GI Symptoms	CSF	Pattern of Paralysis	Notes
Present until muscle strength lost	No	Normal	Diplopia and facial muscle commonly first, then extremities; fatigable muscle strength	EMG, anti-ACh receptor antibody positive (85%)
Absent	No	Elevated CSF protein, possibly anti-GM1 antibody	Lower extremity involvement first preceding cephalad	Antecedent URI or diarrhea (weeks), especially *Campylobacter*
Not lost until complete paralysis of muscle group	Nausea, diarrhea, constipation in children (unless wound related)	Normal	Face and upper extremities first	Not all who eat same food will be symptomatic
Early loss	No	Normal	Lower extremity then ascending	Tick should be present, especially on head
Absent when patient has generalized weakness	No	Normal	Starts distally and progresses proximally (like GB); 10 days to 3 months after sore throat	Pharyngitis prominent, may have cardiac involvement (heart block, myocarditis)
Present	No	Anti-PCC antibody	Strength may improve with repeated stimulation	A paraneoplastic syndrome especially with small cell carcinoma of the lung

Continued

TABLE 9-9

PARTIAL DIFFERENTIAL DIAGNOSIS OF WEAKNESS—cont'd

Illness	Autonomic Involvement	Sensory Changes	Fever	Fasciculations/ Muscle Cramps	Cranial Nerve Involvement
Organophosphate poisoning (or pyridostigmine overdose)	Prominent sweating, bradycardia, other cholinergic signs	No	No	Yes	Yes
Subacute multifocal motor neuropathy	No	Occasionally	No	No	No
ALS	No	No	No	Prominent but disappear in advanced disease	Early
Polymyositis/ dermatomyositis	No	No	No	No	Pharyngeal only; ocular usually intact

Reflexes	GI Symptoms	CSF	Pattern of Paralysis	Notes
Present	Diarrhea, salivation			
Hyporeflexia	No	Paraproteins (IgG and IgM)	Hands and distal first	Positive ganglioside antibody in 80%-90% (anti-GM1, MAG, and sulfatide)
Hyperreflexia	No	Normal	Intrinsics of hand first, then upper extremity, then bulbar	Life expectancy <3years; muscle biopsy, EMG helpful; consider cervical cord compression
Present	Absent	Normal	Proximal musculature primarily involved	Elevated CPK, muscle tenderness; biopsy helpful

9

NEUROLOGY

BIBLIOGRAPHY

Adams HP Jr et al: Guidelines for the management of patients with acute ischemic stroke: a statement for healthcare professionals from a special writing group of the Stroke Council, *Stroke* 25:1901, 1994.

Adams HP Jr, Zoppo GJ, von Kummer R: *Management of stroke: a practical guide for the prevention, evaluation and treatment of acute stroke,* ed 1, Caddo, OK, 1998, Professional Communications.

Adler CH: Treatment of restless legs syndrome with gabapentin, *Clin Neruopharmacol* 20(2):148, 1997.

American Psychiatric Association: *Diagnostic and statistical manual of mental disorders,* ed 4, Washington, DC, 1994, American Psychiatric Association.

Aul EA, Davis BJ, Rodnitzki RL: The importance of formal serum iron studies in the assessment of restless legs syndrome, *Neurology* 51:912, 1998.

Baloh RW: Vertigo, *Lancet* 352:1841, 1998.

Barohn RJ: Approach to peripheral neuropathy and neuronopathy, *Semin Neurol* 18(1):7, 1998.

Brodeur C, Montplaisir J, Godbout R, et al: Treatment of restless legs syndrome and periodic movements during sleep with L-dopa: a double-blind controlled study, *Neurology* 38:1845, 1988.

Bromberg MB: Nondiabetic peripheral neuropathies, *Comp Ther* 24(11/12):545, 1998.

Bross MH, Tatum NO: Delirium in the elderly patient, *Am Fam Physician* 50(6):1325, 1994.

Cramer JA, Fisher R, Ben-Menachem E, et al: New antiepileptic drugs: comparison of key clinical trials, *Epilepsia* 40(5):590, 1999.

Cummings JL, Vinters HV, Cole GM, et al: Alzheimer's disease: etiologies, pathophysiology, cognitive reserve, and treatment opportunities, *Neurology* 51(suppl 1):S2, 1998.

DeToledo JC, Ramsay RE: Patterns of involvement of facial muscles during epileptic and nonepileptic events: review of 654 events, *Neurology* 47:621, 1996.

Diener H, Cunha L, Forbes C, et al: European stroke prevention study 2. Dipyridamole and acetylsalicylic acid in the secondary prevention of stroke, *J Neurol Sci* 143:1, 1996.

Epley JM: The canalith repositioning procedure: for treatment of benign paroxysmal positional vertigo, *Otolaryngol Head Neck Surg* 107(3):399, 1992.

Fisher RS: Emerging antiepileptic drugs, *Neurology* 43(suppl 5):S12, 1993.

Folstein MF et al: "Mini-Mental State": a practical method for grading the cognitive state of patients for the clinician, *J Psychiatr Res* 12:189, 1975.

Forsyth PA et al: Headaches in patients with brain tumors: a study of 111 patients, *Neurology* 43(9):1678, 1993.

Hahn AF: Guillain-Barré syndrome, *Lancet* 352(9128):635, 1998.

Haskell SG, Fiebach NH: Clinical epidemiology of nocturnal leg cramps in male veterans, *Am J Med Sci* 313(4):210, 1997.

Headache Classification Committee of the International Headache Society: Classification and diagnostic criteria for headache disorders, cranial neuralgias, and facial pain, *Cephalalgia* 8(suppl 7):1, 1988.

Heart Outcome Prevention Evaluation Study Investigators: Effects of an angiotensin-converting-enzyme inhibitor, ramipril, on cardiovascular events in high risk patients, *N Engl J Med* 432(3):145, 2000.

Kaye JA: Diagnostic challenges in dementia, *Neurology* 51(suppl 1):S45, 1998.

Lauerma H, Markkula J: Treatment of restless legs syndrome with tramadol: an open study, *J Clin Psychiatry* 60:241, 1999.

Lowenstein DH, Alldredge BK: Status epilepticus, *N Engl J Med* 338(14):970, 1998.

Man-Son-Hing M, Wells G, Lau A: Quinine for nocturnal leg cramps: a meta-analysis including unpublished data, *J Gen Intern Med* 13:600, 1998.

Marks DR, Rapport AM: Diagnosis of migraine, *Semin Neurol* 17(4):303, 1997.

Mathew NT: Cluster headache, *Semin Neurol* 17(4):313, 1997.

Mellick GA, Mellick LB: management of restless legs syndrome with gabapentin (Neurontin), *Sleep* 19(3):224, 1996.

Miller A, Bourdette D, Cohen JA, et al: Multiple sclerosis, *Continuum* 5(5):100, 1999.

Montplaisir J, Nicolas A, Deneslie R, et al: Restless legs syndrome improved by pramipexole: a double-blind randomized trial, *Neurology* 52:938, 1999.

O'Keefe ST: Restless legs syndrome: a review, *Arch Intern Med* 156:243, 1996.

Ondo W: Ropinirole for restless legs syndrome, *Movement Disorders* 14(1):138, 1999.

Pruitt AA: Infections of the nervous system, *Neurol Clin North Am* 16(2):419, 1998.

Silber MH: Restless legs syndrome, *Mayo Clin Proc* 72:261, 1997.

Silberstein SD, Niknam R, Rozen TD, et al: Cluster headache with aura, *Neurology* 54:219, 2000.

Tunkel AR, Scheld WM: Acute meningitis. In *Mandell, Douglas and Bennett's principles and practice of infectious diseases,* Philadelphia, 2000, Churchill Livingstone.

Wetter TC, Stiasny K, Winkelmann J, et al: A randomized controlled study of pergolide in patients with restless legs syndrome, *Neurology* 52:944, 1999.

Young WB, Silberstein SD, Dayno JM: Migraine treatment, *Semin Neurol* 17(4):325, 1997.

Younger DS, Rosoklija G, Hays AP: Diabetic peripheral neuropathy, *Semin Neurol* 18(1):95, 1998.

9

NEUROLOGY

INFECTIOUS DISEASES

Philip M. Polgreen

A word on antibiotics: The overuse of antibiotics has led to a problem with microbial resistance. Be judicious in your use of antibiotics. Reserve newer agents (linezolid for gram-positive organisms and quinupristin-dalfopristin) for cases in which they are the only alternative. **Gram stain results are interpreted in Table 10-1.**

PRINCIPLES OF CULTURING

I. **Blood cultures.** Volume of blood is the most important factor in determining rate of positive cultures. Anaerobic cultures are most likely to be useful in those with underlying immunosuppression (e.g., steroids), those with a suspected abdominal source of infection, and those with suspected endocarditis. There is no need to change the needle before inoculating the culture bottle. There is a slightly increased risk of contamination, but it is safer and prevents needle sticks.

A. **Adults.** How much? How often?
    1. Before antibiotics, 20 to 40 ml from two separate sites to eliminate possibility of skin contaminant. Cultures can be drawn at the same time. There is no advantage to waiting 20 minutes. Drawing from an IV site is acceptable for one set.
    2. For fever of unknown origin, a second set should be drawn on a different day. See section on fever of unknown origin later in this chapter.
    3. First two cultures will detect 92% to 99.3% of septicemias and 98% of endocarditis; 20% of patients hospitalized for pneumonia will have positive blood culture.
    4. If the patient has received antibiotics, blood should be drawn for a resin-containing medium in addition to the aerobic and anaerobic bottles (30 ml/site).

B. **Pediatrics.** How much? How often?
    1. From 1 to 5 ml is adequate to detect serious disease because pediatric patients generally have higher bacterial loads.
    2. Multiple sites are unnecessary and do not increase yield.

C. **Interpreting results.** *Staphylococcus epidermidis, Corynebacterium,* and *Propionibacterium acnes* are likely contaminants unless multiple cultures are positive.

D. **Sputum cultures.** Specific etiology for pneumonia is determined in only about 50% of cases even with extensive noninvasive testing. The correlation between Gram stain and culture is only about 30%, and Gram stain is usually more helpful. Sputum is always contaminated by upper respiratory tract secretions unless obtained invasively. If the patient is unable to produce sputum, consider an induced sputum with assistance from respiratory therapy.

TABLE 10-1
MICROBIOLOGIC CHARACTERISTICS OF BACTERIA BASED ON GRAM STAINING

		Microbiologic Characteristic	
	Organism		
GRAM-POSITIVE BACTERIA			
		CATALASE	MISCELLANEOUS	AEROBIC?
Cocci				
	Streptococcus	Negative		Yes
	Enterococcus	Negative		Yes
	Aerococcus	Negative		Yes
	Lactococcus	Negative		Yes
	Staphylococcus aureus	Positive	Coagulase positive	Yes
	Staphylococcus epidermidis	Positive	Coagulase negative	Yes
	Micrococcus	Positive	Coagulase negative	Yes
	Peptostreptococcus			Anaerobic
Bacilli				
	Bacillus		Spore forming	Yes
	Nocardia		Branching	Yes
	Actinomyces	Negative		Yes
	Lactobacillus	Negative		Yes
	Corynebacterium	Positive		Yes
	Listeria	Positive		Yes
	Clostridium		Spore-forming	Yes
	Actinomyces		Spore-forming	Anaerobic
	Propionibacterium		Non–spore forming	Anaerobic
	Eubacterium		Non–spore forming	Anaerobic
			Non–spore forming	Anaerobic

GRAM-NEGATIVE BACTERIA	OXIDASE	MISCELLANEOUS	AEROBIC?
Bacilli			
Haemophilus		No growth on sheep blood agar	Yes
Campylobacter		No growth on sheep blood agar	Yes
Legionella	Negative	No growth on sheep blood agar	Yes
Enterobacter, including:		Ferments glucose	Yes
Escherichia coli, Salmonella, Shigella, Klebsiella, Serratia, Proteus, Yersinia			
Actinobacillus	Negative		
Gardnerella	Negative	Ferments glucose	Yes
Acinetobacter	Negative	Ferments glucose	Yes
Pseudomonas	Negative	No glucose fermentation	Yes
Vibrio	Positive	No glucose fermentation	Yes
Pasteurella	Positive	Ferments glucose	Yes
Brucella	Positive	Ferments glucose	Yes
Campylobacter	Positive	No glucose fermentation	Yes
Helicobacter pylori	Positive	No glucose fermentation	Yes
Bordetella	Positive	Urease producing	Yes
Pseudomonas	Positive	No glucose fermentation	Yes

Continued

10

INFECTIOUS DISEASES

TABLE 10-1

MICROBIOLOGIC CHARACTERISTICS OF BACTERIA BASED ON GRAM STAINING—cont'd

	Organism	Microbiologic Characteristic		
		OXIDASE	MISCELLANEOUS	AEROBIC?
GRAM-NEGATIVE BACTERIA				
Bacilli—cont'd				
	Bacteroides fragilis		No glucose fermentation	Yes
	Bacteroides ureolyticus		Bile resistant	Anaerobic
	Fusobacterium		No bile resistance	Anaerobic
			No bile resistance	Anaerobic
Cocci				
	Neisseria	Positive		Yes
	Moraxella		No glucose fermentation	Yes
Acid-fast				
	Mycobacterium tuberculosis	Positive		Yes
	Mycobacterium marinum	Positive		Yes
	Cryptosporidium			
Weakly acid-fast				
	Nocardia			

INFESTATIONS

I. **Parasitic Infestation by Pinworms.**
A. **Presentation.** *Enterobius vermicularis* is a small 2 to 5 mm yellow-white worm that inhabits the lower GI tract and migrates out the anus at night causing pruritus, vulvitis, and restless sleep. May cause acute nocturnal vaginal pain in girls. Often whole families are affected.
B. **Examination.** Sometimes worms can be seen in the perianal area about an hour after the child goes to sleep. The definitive diagnostic test is to stick cellophane tape onto the perianal area in the morning before bathing. Then place the tape on a slide and examine under a microscope for the characteristic oval ova. Ask the patient to obtain specimens over three to five mornings and store them in the refrigerator before bringing them to the office.
C. **Treatment.** All members of the household should be treated simultaneously along with daily laundering of the affected child's underclothes and bedding.
　　1. **Mebendazole** (Vermox) 100 mg PO in one dose for adults and children >2 years. Repeat in 2 weeks.
　　2. **Pyrantel pamoate** (Antiminth) 11 mg/kg (up to 1 g PO in one dose). Repeat in 2 weeks.
D. **Prevention.** Good hand washing, keeping affected child's fingernails short, and tight-fitting pajamas to prevent perianal scratching.

II. **Scabies.**
A. **Presentation.** Caused by mite, *Sarcoptes scabiei,* that burrows in the skin. Most common in children, but found in all ages. Usually transmitted by person-to-person transmission, but may be picked up from bedding, clothes, etc. Causes an intensely pruritic, papular eruption that is especially pruritic at night. Areas most affected are interdigital folds, flexor aspect of wrists, extensor aspect of elbows, belt line, thighs, navel, penis, areola, abdomen, inter gluteal fold.
B. **Examination.** Look for pruritic papules, vesicles, and linear burrows. May also see excoriations, crusting, and secondary infection. See above for the most common locations. A high percentage of children who are found to have scabies have persistent reddish brown nodules. These are caused by a hypersensitivity reaction to the scabies mite and can make diagnosis difficult. Confirm with scraping of lesion with scalpel blade placed on slide with mineral oil and look for mites, ova, or fecal pellets.
C. **Treatment.**
　　1. **Permethrin 5% (Elimite).** Permethrin is the preferred treatment. Apply from head to toes; 8 to 14 hours later rinse off. May be used on infants >2 months old, children, and pregnant women.
　　2. **Lindane (Kwell).** Use with caution on patients less than 2 years of age. Apply from neck to toes. For children leave on for 6 to 8 hours and then rinse off. If used in infants, rinse off after 6 hours.

3. **Crotamiton 10% (Eurax).** Apply thin layer of medication from head to toe. Reapply 24 hours later. Do not bathe between applications. Take a cleansing bath 48 hours after the final application.

4. Ivermectin 100 to 200 µg/kg PO can be given in the treatment of severe scabies.

5. Precipitated sulfur (6%) in petroleum applied for three consecutive nights is an alternative in those <2 months of age and in pregnancy.

6. Family members should be treated even if asymptomatic. Bed linens and clothing should be washed in hot water (>120° F) or stored in tightly sealed bags for 1 week.

III. **Pediculosis.** Two species of lice affect humans: *Pediculus humanus* (*capitis* and *corporis*) and *Phthirus pubis.* Sensitization to louse saliva and antigens results in clinical manifestations.

A. *Pediculus humanus capitis* (head lice). Seen primarily in preschoolers and early elementary school ages but occurs in all ages and socioeconomic groups (however, low incidence in African-Americans). Spread by direct contact or on fomites (helmets, combs, etc.). Signs and symptoms: pruritus; erythematous papules usually on occiput, postauricular region, and nape of the neck; lice; and nits (eggs firmly attached to hair shaft about 1 cm from scalp). Differential diagnosis includes seborrhea, psoriasis, tinea capitis, and impetigo.

B. *Pediculus humanus corporis* (body lice). Live in clothing or bedding and not on humans. Seen primarily in lower socioeconomic groups. The louse bites at night and leaves pruritic vesicles or papules (especially in the axillae, groin, and truncal areas). Diagnosis is by examination of clothes to find nits or lice.

C. *Phthirus pubis* (pubic lice). Transmitted by intimate contact. Diagnosis is by pubic or anogenital pruritus and by lice or nits found especially in the pubic hair, but also trunk, beard, eyelashes, or axilla. Often associated with additional STDs.

D. **Treatment for all of the above involves a pediculicide.**

1. Treat all sexual partners and household members simultaneously.

2. Wash all bedding, clothes, towels, and hats in hot water and use a hot dryer.

3. If eyelashes or eyebrows are infested, avoid a pediculicide in those areas. Instead apply petrolatum five times per day until clear. Remove nits with forceps.

4. Pruritus may last for several weeks after successful treatment.

5. **For head lice or crabs:** permethrin (Nix) 1% cream rinse is drug of choice, applied to scalp after shampooing, left on 10 minutes, then rinsed off. Should be examined in 1 week and if nits still present retreat. Alternative: lindane 1% shampoo (Kwell, Scabene). Avoid in infants because may be neurotoxic.

6. For body lice, use pyrethrum with piperonyl butoxide (RID) lotion over the whole body and wash off after 10 minutes. Re-treat in 7 to 10 days.

TUBERCULOSIS

I. **TB Screening.** Recommended for:
A. **Close contacts** of those with known or suspected TB.
B. **Persons infected with HIV.**
C. **IV drug users** or users of other illicit drugs.
D. **Chronically ill patients** with conditions or diseases that increase the risk of progressing from latent to active TB: DM, high-dose steroids, immunosuppressive therapy, chronic renal failure, lymphoma, leukemia, other cancer, weight loss to more than 10% below ideal weight, silicosis, gastrectomy, and jejunoileal bypass.
E. **Foreign-born persons** and those arriving within the last 5 years from countries that have had a high incidence of TB.
F. **Residents and employees of high-risk institutions:** correctional facilities, nursing homes, mental institutions, and homeless shelters.
G. **Health care workers** serving high-risk patients.
H. **Medically underserved** and low-income populations.
I. **Infants, children, and adolescents** exposed to high-risk adults.

II. **Screening Methods.**
A. **Protein purified derivative (PPD).** Use 5 tuberculin units of PPD in 0.1 ml injected intradermally; read in 48 to 72 hours. In the elderly, if the PPD is initially negative, administer a second dose 1 month later to boost latent positive reactions. (This process identifies positive PPD that is the result of a distant exposure to TB, instead of a true, new conversion.)
   1. **False-positive results.** Nontuberculotic mycobacteria; BCG-induced reactivity (decreases with time, frequently gone after 1 year and is unlikely to persist for more than 10 years).
   2. **False-negative results.** Impaired immunity. Place mumps and *Candida* controls. If immunity is impaired, the controls will also be negative.

III. **Interpretation of PPD. The PPD should be interpreted in the same way in those who have had BCG and those who have not.**
A. **Measure induration** (the elevated and firm area, not the area of erythema).
B. **5 to 10 mm induration is considered positive among:**
   1. **Recent close contact** of patients with active TB.
   2. **HIV positive** or those with HIV risk factors with an unknown HIV status.
   3. **Chest radiograph** consistent with healed TB.
C. **10 mm or greater: 90% of reactors are infected with TB.** 10 mm or greater induration is considered positive among:
   1. **IV drug abusers** known to be HIV seronegative.

2. **Medical conditions with increased risk** for progressing from latent to active TB: DM, high-dose steroids, immunosuppressive therapy, chronic renal failure, lymphoma, leukemia, other cancer, weight loss to more than 10% below ideal, silicosis, gastrectomy, jejunoileal bypass.

3. **Residents and employees of prisons,** nursing homes, residential mental health facilities, or homeless shelters.

4. **Foreign-born** and arrived from countries with high incidence of TB within last 5 years.

5. **Medically underserved,** low-income populations.

6. **Children** less than 4 years old.

7. **A child or adolescent** exposed to high-risk adult.

D. **Greater than 15 mm is positive for patients with no risk factors** (e.g., they meet none of the above criteria).

IV. **Prevention. Isolation** is indicated for any patient known or suspected to have TB. Isolation should consist of a single-patient room with negative-pressure ventilation. Persons entering the room should wear appropriate respiratory protection.

V. **Indications for Preventive Therapy after a Positive PPD.**

A. Approximately 5% of patients with a new PPD conversion will develop active TB within 2 years of their conversions if untreated, and another 5% will develop active TB later in life. Chemoprophylaxis reduces the risk of active TB dramatically. Chemoprophylaxis is given only after active disease is ruled out with a negative CXR or sputums for acid-fast bacilli.

B. **Prophylaxis is given to patients less than 35 years of age** regardless of when the patient may have converted.

C. **No age limit exists for prophylaxis in the following groups:**

1. **PPD conversion** from negative to positive within 2 years (5% risk of active disease in first year; must have had a negative PPD within last 2 years).

2. **All HIV-positive** reactors (risk of conversion to active disease 5% to 10% per year).

3. **Household contacts** of those with **active TB even if their screening PPD was negative.** Therapy can be stopped if they have a negative repeat PPD 12 weeks after exposure.

4. **Those with past TB** who have not had adequate treatment **but who have no active disease.**

5. **Positive reactors with underlying illness** or other factors, such as DM, high-dose steroids, immunosuppressive therapy, chronic renal failure, lymphoma, leukemia, other cancer, weight loss to more than 10% below ideal, silicosis, gastrectomy, jejunoileal bypass, IV drug abuse, malnutrition.

6. **Those who have evidence on radiography** of nonprogressive TB disease **but who have no active disease.**

D. **No prophylaxis** is given to PPD-positive patients older than age 35 years unless they are in one of the high-risk groups mentioned above.

E. **Weigh the risk of INH-hepatitis against benefits.** Initial reports 20 years ago suggested that the incidence of INH-hepatitis is less than 1% under age 35 and 1% to 3% over age 35 years. More recent data suggest that the rate is about 0.1% and almost all occur within the first 3 months (Nolan CM et al: *JAMA* 281:1014, 1999.).

VI. **Preventive Therapy.**

A. **Adults.** Isoniazid (INH) 300 mg PO QD for 6 to 12 months (12 if HIV positive or if the chest x-ray is consistent with previous TB infection). Add pyridoxine 10 to 50 mg PO per day to prevent development of peripheral neuropathy.

B. **Children.** INH 10 mg/kg/day PO QD for 9 months (up to 300 mg/day total).

C. **If multidrug-resistant TB is likely** (Southeast Asia, Korea, New York, New Jersey, California, Florida), consider multidrug preventive therapy. Check with your local health department about resistance in your area. Rifampin alone for an INH-resistant exposure is a good choice with PZA and a quinolone a good choice if resistance to INH and rifampin if suspected.

D. For those who are unreliable, consider therapy that is directly observed (INH 15 mg/kg twice per week).

E. **Obtain baseline liver function enzymes and continue to monitor, especially in older patients.** Check every 2 weeks for the first month then every month for months 2 and 3. If transaminase levels increase greater than five times normal, discontinue the INH.

VII. **Therapy for Active Pulmonary TB.**

A. **Patients should be initially be treated with four-drug therapy, unless there is only a slight chance of a drug-resistant infection** (less than 4% of primary resistance to INH in the community, no known exposure to drug-resistant infections, and the patient is not from a high-prevalence region). Contact the local health department for recommendations.

B. **The initial treatment should include INH, rifampin, pyrazinamide, and ethambutol or streptomycin QD for 8 weeks.** The fourth drug may be discontinued if the susceptibility testing shows sensitivity to the first three drugs. Complete a 16-week course.

C. **Treat for at least 9 months if HIV positive** (6 months beyond culture conversion to negative).

D. Contact the local health department for the identification of contacts.

E. Directly observed therapy is preferred for all patients.

IMMUNOSUPPRESSED HOST

I. **Factors that predispose patients to infection include** neutropenia, diabetes, alcoholism, AIDS, lymphomas, leukemia, malnutrition, cirrhosis, skin breakdown, therapy with steroids or cytotic drugs, solid organ and bone marrow transplants, complement deficiencies, splenectomies, and renal failure.

II. **Elderly.** Acute confusion or change in mental status often indicates an infection in an elderly patient. The presentation may be otherwise non-

10

INFECTIOUS DISEASES

specific, lacking fever and localizing signs and symptoms. Sepsis should be strongly suspected in any elderly person with vomiting, mental status changes, or an elevated WBC and band count. Hospital admission and a septic work-up are advisable for such a patient.

III. **Infections in the immunosuppressed patient may not manifest the usual signs or symptoms** even when they are septic. Specifically, the patient may not mount a fever or white blood cell response. Localizing symptoms may be absent. The patient may not manifest lymphadenopathy. Urinary tract infections may exist in the absence of pyuria (especially in a neutropenic patient).

IV. **Neutropenic fever is defined** as one temperature of greater than 38.3° C or multiple temperatures greater than 38.0° C and an absolute neutrophil count less than 500 cells/μl. The risk for an infection in a neutropenic patient is greatest when the neutrophil count is less than 100 cells/μl. The risk also increases with the duration of the patient's neutropenia. Start empiric antibiotics as soon after taking cultures as possible.

V. **Work-up** for all immunosuppressed patients should include a UA, blood and urine cultures, a chest x-ray, and a biopsy or aspirate from sites that may be infected. A microbiologic diagnosis is usually not made initially; thus initial therapy is usually empiric.

VI. **Treatment** should be directed against gram-negative bacilli. Options include an anti-*Pseudomonas* beta-lactam antibiotic and an aminoglycoside. Monotherapy with ceftazidime, imipenem, meropenem, and cefepime are other options for initial therapy. Consider adding vancomycin if patients have central lines that may be infected, extensive mucositis, or if patients fail to respond after 48 hours of therapy directed toward gram-negative organisms. After 3 to 7 days, if the patient is still febrile, amphotericin B is often added. Continue the antimicrobial therapy at least until the neutropenia has resolved.

VII. **With neutropenia, treatment with granulocyte colony–stimulating factor (G-CSF)** and granulocyte-macrophage colony–stimulating factor (GM-CSF) reduces the length of neutropenia but has not improved survival rates.

SEPSIS

I. **Definitions.**

A. **Bacteremia.** The presence of bacteria in the bloodstream detected by blood cultures. Transient bacteremias occur daily in healthy patients.

B. **Systemic inflammatory response syndrome (SIRS).** A response to an inflammation or injury that can be infectious or noninfectious (e.g., pancreatitis), defined by having two of the following:

1. Temperature above 38° C or less than 36° C.
2. Heart rate >90.
3. Respiration rate >20 or $Paco_2$ <32 torr.
4. WBC >12,000/mm³ or <4000, or >10% bands.

C. **Sepsis.** SIRS thought to be caused by an infectious process.

D. **Septic shock.** Sepsis with a systolic BP <90 mm or drop of 40 mm Hg from baseline value in absence of other causes. Severe sepsis may cause organ dysfunction (altered mental status, acute oliguria, lactic acidosis, elevated liver enzymes).

II. **Causes.** Historically, gram-negative bacteria have been the most common cause of sepsis, but they are now surpassed by gram-positive organisms. The reasons for this include the increased use of intravascular catheters, empirical antibiotic regimens designed for gram-negative pathogens, increased use of indwelling prosthetic devices, and emerging antibiotic resistance among gram-positive organisms.

A. **Gram-negative bacteria.** *Escherichia coli, Klebsiella pneumoniae, Pseudomonas aeruginosa, Proteus* spp., *Serratia* spp., *Neisseria meningitidis.*

B. **Gram-positive bacteria.** *Staphylococcus aureus,* coagulase-negative *Staphylococcus, Streptococcus pneumoniae, Streptococcus pyogenes,* enterococci.

C. **Other causes.** Opportunistic fungi (2% to 3%), viral, rickettsia, and protozoa.

III. **Risk Factors.** Include hospitalization, illness, or invasive procedures.

A. **Risk for gram-negative septicemia increases with** diabetes, cirrhosis, alcoholism, lymphoproliferative diseases, burns, cancer, iatrogenic immunosuppression (e.g., chemotherapy, steroids), total parenteral nutrition, and urinary, biliary, or GI infections. Additionally, neonates and the elderly with urinary dysfunction are at very high risk.

B. **Risk for gram-positive septicemia increases with** indwelling IV catheters, indwelling mechanical devices, IV drug use, and burns.

C. **Higher risk of fungal septicemia.** Immunosuppressed, neutropenic, prolonged use of broad-spectrum antibiotics.

D. **Splenectomized patients.** *Streptococcus pneumoniae, Haemophilus influenzae, Neisseria meningitidis.*

IV. **Clinical Manifestations.** Presentation may vary greatly between patients and is often subtle at the extremes of age. Early signs and symptoms include fever, chills, and tachypnea. Later, they include mental status changes, cold and clammy extremities, and oliguria.

V. **Work-up.**

A. **History and chart review with special attention directed toward:**
   1. Medications (especially antibiotics, immunosuppressive drugs).
   2. Recent surgeries or dental procedures.
   3. Previous illnesses and surgeries (splenectomy).
   4. HIV risk factors.
   5. IV drug use.

B. **Physical exam.**

C. **Diagnostic tests.**
   1. CBC with a differential.
      a. Leukocytosis with left shift or leukopenia.

10

INFECTIOUS DISEASES

b. Toxic granulations, Döhle bodies, or intracytoplasmic vacuolization in PMNs.

c. Thrombocytopenia is suggestive of DIC, as are an increase in fibrin degradation products, a decrease in fibrinogen, and an increase in PT.

d. RBC morphology is generally normal unless DIC; then microangiopathic hemolytic anemia with schistocytes is a possibility.

2. Blood cultures. Obtain at least two sets from two sites (blood cultures are often negative).

3. Culture all possible sources for the infection. Sputum, urine, skin lesions, CSF.

4. Urinalysis with micro. UTIs are a common cause of sepsis in the elderly.

5. Electrolytes, glucose, BUN/creatinine, Liver function tests, PT/PTT, CXR, ABG. Patients generally have a respiratory alkalosis followed by a metabolic acidosis.

6. Lumbar punctures if patient has a headache or meningeal signs.

7. Abdominal ultrasound or CT if the abdomen is possible source (e.g., bowel perforation, ischemic bowel, cholecystitis, diverticulitis).

VI. **Common Primary Infections.** Pneumonia, UTIs, wounds, cellulitis, abscesses, IV line infection, sinusitis, meningitis.

VII. **Differential Diagnosis.** Other causes of shock include myocardial infarction, pulmonary embolus, drug overdose (especially salicylates, which may mimic sepsis), bleeding, cardiac tamponade, rupture of aortic aneurysm, aortic dissection, and toxic shock syndrome.

VIII. **Treatment.** See Table 10-2 for **empiric antibiotics** in sepsis.

A. **Respiratory and hemodynamic support.** Keep oxygen saturation greater than 92%. Consider ventilator support for progressive hypoxia or respiratory muscle failure.

B. **Fluid management.** IV normal saline fluid boluses with the goal of a mean arterial BP >60 mm Hg. To avoid pulmonary edema, keep the CVP between 10 and 12 cm H_2O and the PCWP between 14 and 18 mm Hg. Colloid solutions have no proven benefits over crystalloid solutions.

1. **Adults,** 1 to 1.5 L in first 1 to 2 hours; probably will need more (about 4 to 6 L on average).

2. **Children,** 20 ml/kg over 2 to 5 minutes (neonates over 20 minutes) repeated twice in first hour if needed to maintain good perfusion.

3. **Continuing support.**

a. Transfuse as needed.

b. Try to keep urine output between 30 and 60 ml/hr in adults and 0.5 to 1.5 ml/kg/hr in pediatric patients.

D. **If a patient has failed volume resuscitation with normal saline,** start dopamine and titrate up to 20 μg/kg. In dopamine-unresponsive patients use norepinephrine infusion. Dobutamine may be added later to keep cardiac output greater than 4 L/m². These drugs should be used in an intensive care unit usually in conjunction with intra-arterial and pulmonary artery catheters. **However, pulmonary artery catheters may increase mortality rates.**

TABLE 10-2

EMPIRIC ANTIBIOTICS IN SEPSIS

Likely Source of Sepsis	Likely Organisms	Antibiotics
Urosepsis	Gram-negative rods, enterococci	Third-generation cephalosporin ± an aminoglycoside
		Ticarcillin/clavulanic acid ± an aminoglycoside
		Piperacillin/tazobactam ± an aminoglycoside
		Imipenem or meropenem ± an aminoglycoside
Intraabdominal infection	Polymicrobial, anaerobes	Ampicillin/sulbactum ± an aminoglycoside
		Cefoxitin ± an aminoglycoside
		Cefotetan ± an aminoglycoside
		Ticarcillin/clavulanic acid ± an aminoglycoside
		Piperacillin/tazobactam ± an aminoglycoside
		Imipenem or meropenem ± an aminoglycoside
Nosocomial pneumonia	Resistant gram-negative rods	Aminoglycoside (gentamicin or tobramycin with an antipseudomonal (ticarcillin, piperacillin, ceftazidime)
		If resistant to aminoglycosides, third-generation cephalosporins, and aztreonam, may be susceptible to imipenem or meropenem
Neutropenia		Ceftazidime ± an aminoglycoside
		Imipenem or meropenem ± an aminoglycoside
		Cefepime ± an aminoglycoside
Intravenous catheter	*Staphylococcus aureus, S. epidermidis* (methicillin-resistant *S. aureus*)	Vancomycin
Unknown primary site		Third- or fourth-generation cephalosporin + an aminoglycoside
		Ticarcillin/clavulanic acid + an aminoglycoside
		Piperacillin/tazobactam + an aminoglycoside
		Imipenem or meropenem + an aminoglycoside

10

INFECTIOUS DISEASES

IX. **Adrenal insufficiency** should be considered in any patient with refractory hypotension who has taken steroids for longer than 2 weeks within the last year or is infected with either TB or *N. meningitidis.*

X. **Other modalities.** Monoclonal antibodies against gram-negative endotoxin, steroids, and anti-TNF antibodies have not demonstrated significant reduction in mortality. Recent study suggests low-dose steroids may help in septic shock, but this is not yet standard of care. **Activated protein C has been shown to be effective with an absolute mortality reduction of 6%. It should only be used in patients with end-organ failure.** (See Bernard GR: *NEJM* 344(10), 2001.)

XI. **Treat the infectious agent (surgical drainage may be needed in some cases). Start antibiotics as soon as possible,** preferably after cultures are obtained; tailor to most likely source until culture results are available.

FEVER OF UNKNOWN ORIGIN

I. **Definition.** *Fever of unknown origin* (FUO) is an illness of longer than 3 weeks' duration with a fever >38.3° C for which a diagnosis has not been found after 1 week of inpatient or outpatient investigation.

II. **Evaluation.** The diagnosis is usually made clinically with supporting evidence found on lab and radiographic studies. There is no substitute for a good history and physical exam. Patients who do not have a diagnosis made actually have the best outcomes, and fever will generally resolve in 4 to 5 weeks. The minimal work-up is listed in Box 10-1.

III. See comprehensive list of illnesses known to cause an FUO in Box 10-2.

BOX 10-1

MINIMUM WORK-UP FOR FEVER OF UNKNOWN ORIGIN

- Comprehensive history
- Repeated physical examination
- CBC, including differential and platelet count
- Routine blood chemistry, including LDH, bilirubin, and liver enzymes
- UA, including microscopic examination
- CXR
- ESR
- ANA, Rheumatoid factor
- ACE
- Routine blood cultures (×3) while not receiving antibiotics
- CMV IgM antibodies or virus detection in blood, heterophil antibody test in children and young adults
- Tuberculin skin test
- CT of abdomen or radionuclide scan
- HIV antibodies or virus detection assay
- Further evaluation of any abnormalities detected by above tests

Adapted from Arnow P, Flaherty J: *Lancet* 350(9077):575, 1997.

BOX 10-2

ILLNESSES KNOWN TO CAUSE FUO

INFECTION

- Intraabdominal abscess (e.g., periappendiceal, diverticular, subphrenic): liver, splenic. Pancreatic, perinephric, psoas, or placental abscess. Appendicitis, cholecystitis, cholangitis aortoenteric fistula, mesenteric lymphadenitis, toboovarian abscess, pyometra
- Intracranial abscess, sinusitis, mastoiditis, otitis media, dental abscess
- Chronic pharyngitis, tracheobronchitis, lung abscess
- Septic jugular phlebitis, mycotic aneurysm, endocarditis, intravenous catheter infection, vascular graft infection
- Wound infection, osteomyelitis, infected joint prosthesis, pyelonephritis, prostatitis
- Tuberculosis, *Mycobacterium avium* complex, leprosy, Lyme disease, relapsing fever, *Borrelia recurrentis*, syphilis, Q fever, legionellosis, yersiniosis
- Salmonellosis (including typhoid fever), listeriosis, *Campylobacter,* brucellosis tularemia, bartonellosis, ehrlichiosis, psittacosis, *Chlamydia pneumoniae,* murine typhus, scrub typhus
- Gonococcemia, meningococcemia
- Actinomycosis, nocardiosis, melioidosis, Whipple's disease *(Trophermyma whippleii),* candidemia, cryptococcosis, histoplasmosis, coccidioidomycosis, blastomycosis, sporotrichosis, aspergillosis, mucormycosis, *Malassezia furfur,* Pneumocystis carinii
- Visceral leishmaniasis, malaria, babesiosis, toxoplasmosis, schistosomiasis, fascioliasis, toxocariasis, amebiasis, infected hydatid cyst, trichinosis, trypanosomiasis
- CMV, HIV, herpes simplex, Epstein-Barr virus, parvovirus B19

NEOPLASIA

- FUO has been reported in association with all common malignant diseases and with 46 malignancies altogether

COLLAGEN VASCULAR DISEASE

- Adult Still's disease, SLE, cryoglobulinemia, Reiter's syndrome, rheumatic fever, giant cell arteritis/polymyalgia rheumatica, Wegener's granulomatosis, ankylosing spondylitis, Behçet's syndrome, polyarteritis nodosa
- Hypersensitivity vasculitis, urticarial vasculitis, Sjögren's syndrome, polymyositis, rheumatoid arthritis, erythema multiforme, erythema nodosum, relapsing polychondritis, mixed connective-tissue disease, Takayasu's aortitis, Weber-Christian disease, Felty's syndrome, eosinophilic fasciitis

MISCELLANEOUS

- Hematoma, thrombosis, recurrent pulmonary embolism, aortic dissection, femoral aneurysm, post–myocardial infarction syndrome, atrial myxoma
- Drug fever, Sweet's syndrome, familial Mediterranean fever, familial Hibernian fever, hyperimmunoglobulin D syndrome, Crohn's disease, ulcerative colitis, sarcoidosis, granulomatosis, hepatitis

10

INFECTIOUS DISEASES

Continued

BOX 10-2

ILLNESSES KNOWN TO CAUSE FUO—cont'd

MISCELLANEOUS—cont'd

- Subacute thyroiditis, hyperthyroidism, adrenal insufficiency, primary hyperparathyroidism, hypothalamic hypopituitarism, autoimmune hemolytic anemia
- Gout, pseudogout
- Cirrhosis, chronic active hepatitis, alcoholic hepatitis, shunt nephritis
- Malakoplakia, Kawasaki's syndrome, Kikuchi's syndrome
- Mesenteric fibromatosis, inflammatory pseudotumor
- Castleman's disease, Vogt-Koyanagi-Harada syndrome, Gaucher disease, Schmitzler's syndrome, FAPA syndrome (fever, aphthous stomatitis, pharyngitis, adenitis; found in children, recurs monthly, responds to steroids), Fabry's disease
- Cholesterol emboli, silicone embolization, Teflon embolization
- Lymph node infarction, sickle cell disease, vaso-occlusive crisis, anhidrotic ectodermal dysplasia, cyclic neutropenia, Brewer's yeast ingestion, Hamman-Rich syndrome
- Milk protein allergy, hypersensitivity pneumonitis, extrinsic allergic alveolitis, metal fume fever, polymer fume fever, idiopathic hypereosinophilic syndrome
- Complex partial status epilepticus, cerebrovascular accident, brain tumor, encephalitis
- Anomalous thoracic duct, psychogenic fever, habitual hyperthermia, factitious illness

From Arnow P, Flaherty J: *Lancet* 350(9077):575, 1997.

LYME DISEASE

I. **Epidemiology.**
A. Worldwide distribution. Three foci in the United States.
    1. Northeast: Massachusetts to Maryland.
    2. Upper Midwest, especially Wisconsin and Minnesota.
    3. Coastal California and Oregon.
B. Onset of illness is usually May to November, peaking in June and July.
II. **Pathogenesis.**
A. **Cause.** *Borrelia burgdorferi,* a spirochete.
B. **Transmission.** Bite from deer tick, *Ixodes scapularis* or *Ixodes pacificus* during spring nymph stage.
C. An infected tick that is attached for less than 24 hours is unlikely to transmit infection, but almost 100% transmission occurs when greater than 72 hours has elapsed.
III. **Clinical Characteristics.**
A. Stage I (first weeks to months).
    1. **Erythema chronicum migrans.** Red macules with central clearing start 3 to 32 days after infection at the site of the bite and enlarge

centrifugally to >5 cm. Erythema chronicum migrans is seen in 60% to 70% of patients with Lyme disease.

2. **Flulike illness.** Myalgia, arthralgia, fatigue, headache, neck pain and stiffness, fever, chills, and sore throat.

3. **Borrelia lymphocytoma.** Red, firm nodule on ear pinna in children, on nipple and areola in adults.

B. **Stage II** (begins weeks to months after bite/rash).

1. **Neurologic involvement** in 15%, including lymphocytic meningitis, encephalitis, chorea, unilateral or bilateral facial nerve palsy or any cranial nerve palsy, radiculoneuritis, mononeuritis multiplex, diffuse peripheral sensorimotor neuropathy.

2. **Cardiac involvement** in 5%, including fluctuating AV block (can be first, second, or third degree), myopericarditis with ST-segment changes, arrhythmias, syncope, presyncope, or palpitations. Valvular involvement rare.

C. **Stage III** (weeks to years after tick bite).

1. **Varies** from migratory musculoskeletal pain to overt inflammatory arthritis. Asymmetric oligoarticular intermittent pain and swelling, usually of large joints (most commonly the knee). Other chronic neurologic syndromes can also occur.

IV. **Diagnosis.**

A. Usually based on clinical and epidemiologic evidence. **Diagnosis requires a positive ELISA confirmed by Western blot.** A positive Western blot by itself is not specific enough and will have false positives.

1. **False-negative** results occur in the first 3 to 4 weeks of illness (no significant antibody response) and because of variable assay sensitivities between labs.

2. **False-positive** results can occur with *Treponema pallidum,* oral treponemes, *Escherichia coli,* juvenile rheumatoid arthritis, SLE, mononucleosis, and bacterial endocarditis.

B. **Differential diagnosis.**

1. **Dermatologic manifestations can mimic** erythema multiforme, systemic lupus erythematosus, prodromal phase of hepatitis B, erythema marginatum, aseptic meningitis, infectious mononucleosis, and lymphoproliferative disorder.

2. **Rheumatologic manifestations can mimic** rheumatic fever, reactive arthritis, and juvenile rheumatoid arthritis.

3. **Neurologic manifestations can mimic** Bell's palsy, multiple sclerosis, Guillain-Barré syndrome, and brain tumor.

V. **Treatment.**

A. **Early disease.** Doxycycline 100 mg PO BID for 10 to 21 days **or** amoxicillin 500 mg TID (if <9 years of age, 40 to 50 mg/kg/day) for 10 to 21 days **or** erythromycin 500 mg/QID (if <9 years of age, 30 to 40 mg/kg/day) for 10 to 21 days.

1. **Jarisch-Herxheimer**–like reaction (fever, chills, rash, lymphadenopathy within 6 hours of beginning treatment) is seen in 15%.

10

INFECTIOUS DISEASES

    2. **Constitutional symptoms** may continue for extended periods despite adequate treatment.

    3. **Facial palsy** alone (even bilateral) may be treated the same as early disease.

B. **Late disease.**

    1. Lyme meningitis, serious carditis, or persistent arthritis. Treat with ceftriaxone 1 g IV BID (children 75 to 100 mg/kg/day) **or** penicillin G 20 to 24 million U/day (children 300,000 U/kg/day) IV divided Q4h for 10 days.

VI. **Prevention.**

A. Protective clothing: long sleeves, long pants tucked into socks, insect repellent, check for ticks BID when in endemic areas.

B. Prophylaxis after a tick bite is not recommended.

C. Vaccine.

    1. Appears to be 85% effective and well tolerated.

    2. The length of the immunity conferred is unknown.

    3. The vaccine is currently recommended only for adults over age 15 who live, work, or recreate in areas of high to moderate risk.

    4. Three doses of the vaccine are needed. The initial dose is followed by a second dose 1 month later and a third dose 12 months after the first dose. The third dose should be administered several weeks before April for maximal efficacy. An accelerated schedule with yearly boosters may soon be recommended.

EHRLICHIOSIS

I. **Epidemiology.**

A. **Onset.** April to September, peaking in June and July; two thirds are rural residents.

B. **Human monocytic ehrlichiosis** (HME) is more common in southeast and southcentral United States (Oklahoma, Georgia, Arkansas).

C. **Human granulocytic ehrlichiosis** (HGE) is more common in Minnesota, Wisconsin, New York, and Maryland.

II. **Pathogenesis.**

A. HME caused by *Ehrlichia chaffeensis.*

B. HGE caused by *Ehrlichia equi.*

C. Transmitted by *Ixodes scapularis* and *Dermacentor variabilis.*

III. **Clinical Characteristics.**

A. Fever, diaphoresis, myalgias, arthralgias, malaise, headache, nausea, vomiting.

B. About 15% have severe complications: renal failure, DIC, pulmonary hemorrhage, interstitial pneumonitis, bronchiolitis obliterans with organizing pneumonia (BOOP), seizures, coma.

C. **Lab findings include** leukopenia, anemia, thrombocytopenia, and elevations of AST, ALT, LDH. May see morulae in circulating peripheral WBCs.

IV. **Diagnosis.**

A. Usually clinical, because therapy should be started before lab results are obtained.
B. Can be confirmed by serum antibody acute and convalescent titers or PCR testing.
V. **Treatment.** Doxycycline 100 mg BID for adults (3 mg/kg/day divided BID for children) until 3 days after defervescence (minimum 5 to 7 days).
VI. **Prevention.**
A. When outdoors in tick-infested areas wear light-colored clothing, use insect repellent, and check thoroughly for ticks afterwards.
B. Antibiotic prophylaxis is not recommended after a tick bite.

BABESIOSIS

I. **Epidemiology.**
A. Most cases in New England, Wisconsin, and California.
B. Transmission by *Ixodes dammini,* the same vector as for Lyme disease.
C. Rodents act as reservoirs.
II. **Causes.** *Babesia microti* and *B. divergens,* which are intraerythrocytic protozoan parasite.
III. **Clinical Features.**
A. Malaria-like illness, but unlike malaria, fevers are irregular.
B. Fever chills, drenching sweats, lethargy, malaise, myalgias, arthralgias, and darkened or red urine.
C. The most severe cases occur in the splenectomized patients and the elderly.
IV. **Laboratory Findings.** Elevated liver enzymes, leukopenia, and hemolytic anemia, as well as hemoglobinuria.
V. **Diagnosis.** Can find the intracellular organisms with Giemsa stain.
A. **Multiple parasites per RBC,** with pronounced pleomorphism. Often 4% to 7% RBCs infected (rarely up to 40%).
B. **Serologic** characteristics may also be diagnostic (ELISA, IFA).
C. **PCR** appears most specific.
VI. **Treatment.** The illness is generally self-limited except in the splenectomized and elderly. Treatment consists of clindamycin 12 to 2400 mg/day IV divided TID or QID plus oral quinine 650 mg Q6-8h for 7 to 10 days. *Children:* clindamycin 20 mg/kg/day, quinine 25 mg/kg/day.

LEPTOSPIROSIS

I. **Epidemiology.**
A. Uncommon in United States; many domestic and wild animal carriers.
B. Transmission via direct contact with animal tissue or urine or indirect through contaminated water, soil, or vegetation (usually via conjunctivae, broken skin).
C. More common in teenagers and young adults; July through October. Also common in those with occupational exposure such as farmers, veterinarians, and abattoir workers.

II. **Pathogenesis.**

A. Caused by spirochetes of *Leptospira interrogans* complex.

B. *Leptospira icterohaemorrhagiae* associated with hepatic and renal dysfunction.

III. **Clinical Characteristics.**

A. Fever, chills, headache, conjunctivitis, myalgias.

B. Anorexia, nausea, vomiting in 50%, diarrhea less common.

C. Symptom complex may resemble pneumonia, hepatitis, nephritis, and gastroenteritis.

D. Children tend to get acalculous cholecystitis, pancreatitis, abdominal causalgia, hypertension, and severe peripheral desquamation of a rash (life threatening).

IV. **Clinical Syndromes.**

A. Weil's syndrome: leptospirosis with jaundice, often with azotemia, ATN, hemorrhages, anemia, altered mentation, or fever.

B. Atypical pneumonia syndrome: bilateral bronchopneumonia may progress to ARDS.

C. Aseptic meningitis: CSF with 10 to $100/mm^3$ WBCs, normal glucose, high protein.

D. Myocarditis: arrhythmias usually not clinically significant, rarely causes CHF.

V. **Diagnosis.**

A. Blood or CSF culture positive for *Leptospira* (needs special medium).

B. Detection of antibodies by ELISA in 6 to 12 days of illness, with fourfold rise in titers.

VI. **Treatment.**

A. IV penicillin 1.5 million U every 6 hours for 7 days.

B. Jarisch-Herxheimer reaction (JHR) seen in 15% to 80% after penicillin treatment.

C. Disease seems to worsen within hours of first penicillin dose. Body temperature rises, then falls, and hypertension is followed by hypotension.

D. Doxycycline 100 mg PO BID for 7 days if allergic to penicillin. Other options include amoxicillin 500 mg PO QID and ampicillin 500 to 750 mg Q6h.

VII. **Prognosis.** Mortality rate 7%, primarily among those with hepatorenal syndrome.

ROCKY MOUNTAIN SPOTTED FEVER

I. **Epidemiology.**

A. All states except Maine and Alaska; more common in South Atlantic states than in the Rocky Mountain states.

B. Peak incidence between April and October 1.

C. Most cases are in children ages 5 to 9 years.

II. **Etiology.** A tick-borne illness caused by *Rickettsia rickettsii,* an intracellular organism. The tick has to be attached for at least 4 hours for transmission to occur; disease can also be transmitted when a tick is crushed during removal.

III. **Physical Findings.** After an incubation period of 2 to 7 days, there is sudden onset of spiking fever, headache, confusion, myalgias, and weakness. The disease may progress to obtundation with CSF pleocytosis on LP. Patients may also have nausea, vomiting, diarrhea, and hepatosplenomegaly.

A. **Rash** starting on extremities and spreading to trunk is a hallmark feature of this disease. Generally appears as erythematous macules on wrist and ankle within 24 hours, becomes petechial by day 4 if not treated. **However,** 4% to 10% have no rash, and in others it may be evanescent.

B. Rarely there may be pulmonary involvement or myocardial vasculitis with nonspecific ST-T changes.

IV. **Laboratory Tests.**

A. Slightly decreased WBCs, thrombocytopenia (may develop DIC), anemia, elevated aminotransferases.

B. Serologic testing should be used to confirm the diagnosis. The Weil-Felix reaction is no longer used, and diagnostic titers may not be elevated until 10 to 14 days into the course.

C. Immunohistologic examination of a cutaneous biopsy is both relatively sensitive and highly specific.

V. **Treatment.**

A. **In adults,** doxycycline 100 mg PO BID or tetracycline 500 mg PO QID.

B. **In children,** doxycycline 2.2 mg/kg PO BID for 1 day, and then 2.2 mg/kg QD.

C. Chloramphenicol 50 to 75 mg/kg/day divided QID is another alternative.

D. Treat both children and adults for 5 to 7 days or until afebrile for 2 to 5 days.

BACTERIAL ENDOCARDITIS

I. **General.** Bacterial endocarditis is an infection of the endothelial lining of the heart caused by direct invasion of bacteria, usually on valvular surfaces. The disease occurs most commonly in patients with underlying structural heart disease. Bacterial endocarditis can be classified as either acute or subacute, or by certain etiologic factors such as prosthetic valves versus native valves.

II. **Risk Factors.**

A. **Underlying heart disease.** Rheumatic valvular damage, congenital heart disease, mitral valve prolapse, prosthetic valves, hypertrophic cardiomyopathy, and previous bacterial endocarditis are predisposing factors for endocarditis. With more virulent organisms, such as *Staphylococcus aureus,* previous valvular damage is present in only about 50% of the cases.

B. **Events predisposing patients to bacteremia** such as intravenous drug use, intravenous catheters, dental and genitourinary procedures.

10

INFECTIOUS DISEASES

C. **Age greater than 50 years.**
III. **Etiology of Bacterial Endocarditis.**
A. **Native valve endocarditis.** *Streptococcus viridans,* enterococci, *S. aureus,* HACEK *(Haemophilus, Actinobacillus, Cardiobacterium, Eikenella, and Kingella).*
B. **Prosthetic valve endocarditis.** Coagulase-negative staphylococci, *Staphylococcus aureus,* enterococci, gram-negative bacilli, fungi.
C. **Endocarditis in IV drug users.** *S. aureus,* streptococci, gram-negative bacillus, enterococci, fungi, polymicrobial.
D. **Culture negative (marantic endocarditis).** A nonbacterial thrombotic endocarditis. About 5%.
E. **Acute bacterial endocarditis.** *S. aureus,* pneumococcus, group A streptococcus.
IV. **Clinical Manifestations.**
A. **Acute bacterial endocarditis.** Acute onset of fever, chills, arthralgias, and myalgias. Patients appear systemically ill and often develop sepsis. CNS symptoms occur in about 30% of patients from systemic emboli causing cerebral infarctions, brain abscesses, mycotic aneurysms, cerebrovascular hemorrhages, and aseptic meningitis. Septic emboli to the kidneys, coronary arteries, and mesenteric arteries can also occur. Cardiac valvular destruction can lead to rapid ventricular failure and heart block. Peripherally, Janeway lesions occur, but other peripheral stigmata of subacute endocarditis are uncommon.
B. **Subacute bacterial endocarditis.** Fever and chills are almost always present, but the onset of the disease is insidious. Symptoms can be present from weeks to months before they are brought to medical attention. Patients complain of night sweats, weakness, fatigue, arthralgias, and myalgias. Complications included septic emboli, heart failure from valvular destruction, and heart block. Sepsis is less common than in acute bacterial endocarditis. On exam, heart murmurs are usually found. Physical exam findings also include splinter hemorrhages, Roth spots, Osler nodes, and splenomegaly.
V. **Diagnosis.**
A. **Blood cultures** should be obtained in any patient suspected to have the diagnosis. Blood cultures are positive in greater than 90% of the cases but can be negative if the patient has recently been given antimicrobial therapy. The bacteremia is usually continuous. Three sets during a 1-hour period usually suffice. The cultures should be obtained before starting empiric antibiotic therapy if at all possible. In the acutely ill patient, cultures should be drawn (two or three sets) and empiric antibiotic treatment should be given without delay. Antimicrobial treatment can be refined when the culture results are available. In suspected cases with a subacute onset, the cultures can be obtained over a 24-hour period before starting antibiotic therapy. If the blood cultures remain negative over several days and endocarditis is still suspected, the lab should be notified to hold the blood cultures for 3 weeks.

B. **Echocardiograph** is not absolutely essential to make the diagnosis, and absence of vegetation on echocardiography does not rule out the diagnosis. Transthoracic and transesophageal echos have a sensitivity of about 65% and 90%, respectively.

VI. **Treatment.** For culture-positive endocarditis, refer to lab susceptibilities and *JAMA* 274:1706, 1995.

A. **Empiric therapy** awaiting culture results.

   1. **Native valve.**
      a. Nafcillin 2 g IV Q4h plus gentamicin 1 mg/kg IV Q8h plus penicillin G 20 million U IV Q24h or ampicillin 12 g IV Q24h, **or**
      b. Vancomycin 15 mg IV Q12h plus gentamicin 1 mg/kg IV Q8h.
   2. **Prosthetic valve.** Vancomycin 15 mg IV Q12h plus gentamicin 1 mg/kg IV Q8h plus rifampin 600 mg PO Q24h.

C. **Duration of therapy** varies from 2 to 6 weeks depending on the organism. Indications for surgery include progressive CHF, multiple embolic events, fungal endocarditis, persistent bacteremia, extension of infection into the conducting system (new heart block on ECG), relapse of infection, abscess on echo, and sometimes large vegetations.

MALARIA

I. **General.** Malaria is a systemic illness manifested by recurrent fever and chills occurring weeks to months after exposure to areas of the world in which the disease is endemic.

II. **Epidemiology.** Endemic in most of the tropical and subtropical world, including South and Central America, the Caribbean, Africa, the Middle East, Southeast Asia, and Oceania.

III. **Pathogenesis.** Four species of intraerythrocytic parasites transmitted by the female anopheline mosquito.

A. *Plasmodium falciparum* is the most serious and is responsible for most deaths. No relapses.

B. *Plasmodium vivax,* relapses.

C. *Plasmodium ovale,* relapses.

D. *Plasmodium malariae,* no relapses.

IV. **Clinical Characteristics.**

A. **Recurrent fevers and chills:** *P. vivax* and *P. ovale* typically occur at 48-hour intervals, *P. malariae* at 72-hour intervals, *P. falciparum* at irregular intervals.

B. **Headaches,** arthralgias, myalgias, nausea, vomiting, and diarrhea are common. Patients may be free of symptoms between episodes of fevers and chills.

C. Severe cases of *P. falciparum* can cause **mental status changes,** including coma, renal failure, hypoglycemia, pulmonary edema, and anemia.

D. Severity of cases are proportional to the degree of parasitemia.

V. **Laboratory findings.** WBC counts are almost always within normal limits, liver function tests are elevated in 50% of patients, thrombocythemia and anemia occur less commonly.

VI. **Diagnosis.** A definitive diagnosis depends on the identification of the parasites in a peripheral blood smear, preferably stained with Giemsa stain. Multiple smears are usually not needed to detect parasitemia, but if clinical suspicion is high obtain multiple smears over a 48-hour period.

VII. **Treatment.** Treatment is heavily dependent on the level of drug resistance in the area of exposure. For CDC malaria treatment information, see www.cdc.gov or call (770)488-7788.

VIII. **Prevention.**

A. **Avoid outdoor exposures** between dusk and dawn in endemic areas.

B. **Use insect repellent** with DEET.

C. **Dress to minimize exposure** of skin.

D. **Use mosquito nets** sprayed with permethrin when possible.

E. **Chemoprophylaxis** depends on level of drug resistance; see www.cdc.gov or call (888)232-3228.

BIBLIOGRAPHY

Advice for travelers, *Med Lett* 41(1051):39, 1999.

American Thoracic Society and CDC recommendations, *Am J Respir Crit Care Med* 49:1359, 1994.

Arnow P, Flaherty J: Fever of unknown origin, *Lancet* 350(9077):575, 1997.

Astiz ME, Rackow EC: Septic shock, *Lancet* 351:1501, 2000.

Bone R: Important new findings in sepsis, *JAMA* 278(3):249, 1997.

Centers for Disease Control and Prevention: Human granulocytic ehrlichiosis—New York, 1995, *MMWR* 44(32):593, 1995.

Centers for Disease Control and Prevention: Screening for tuberculosis and tuberculosis infection in high-risk populations: recommendations of the Advisory Council for the Elimination of Tuberculosis, *MMWR* 44(RR-11):19, 1995.

Cunha B: Fever of unknown origin, *Infect Dis Clin North Am* 10(1):111, 1996.

Dumler JS, Bakken JS: Ehrlichial diseases of humans: emerging tick-borne infections, *Clin Infect Dis* 20:1102, 1995.

Fowler VG et al: Outcome of *Staphylococcus aureus* bacteremia according to compliance with recommendations of infectious disease specialists: experience with 244 patients, *Clin Infect Dis* 27:478, 1998.

Freedman D, Woodall J: Emerging infectious diseases and risk to the traveler, *Med Clin North Am* 83(4):865, 1999.

Giesel BE et al: Management of bacterial endocarditis, *Am Fam Physician* 61(6):1725, 2000.

Gordin FM et al: A controlled trial of isoniazid in persons with anergy and human immunodeficiency virus infection who are at high risk for tuberculosis, *N Engl J Med* 337:315, 1997.

Hamilton J: Zoonotic diseases in Canada: an interdisciplinary challenge, *Can Med Assoc J* 155(4):413, 1996.

Harkess JR: Ehrlichiosis, *Infect Dis Clin North Am* 5(1):37, 1991.

Hughes WT et al: 1997 guidelines for the use of antimicrobial agents in neutropenic patients with unexplained fever, *Clin Infect Dis* 25:551, 1997.

Humar A, Keystone J: Fortnightly review: evaluating fever in travelers returning from tropical countries, *BMJ* 312(7036):953, 1996.

Kirkland KB et al: Therapeutic delay and mortality in cases of Rocky Mountain spotted fever, *Clin Infect Dis* 20(5):1118, 1995.

Laszlo A: Tuberculosis: 7 laboratory aspects of diagnosis, *Can Med Assoc J* 160(12):1725, 1999.

Lefering R et al: Steroid controversy in sepsis and septic shock: a meta-analysis, *Crit Care Med* 23(7):1294, 1995.

Lobel HO, Kozarsky PE: Update on prevention of malaria for travelers, *JAMA* 278:1767, 1997.

Magnarelli LA: Current status of laboratory diagnosis of Lyme disease, *Am J Med* 98(4A):10S, 1995.

Mandell GL, Bennett JE, Colin R: *Mandell, Douglas, and Bennett's principles and practice of infectious disease CD-ROM,* ed 4, New York, 1996, Churchill Livingstone.

McCray E et al: The epidemiology of tuberculosis in the United States, *Clin Chest Med* 18(1):99, 1997.

Moore M: Trends in drug-resistent tuberculosis in the United States, 1993-6, *JAMA* 278:833, 1997.

Murray HW et al: Recent advances: tropical medicine, *BMJ* 320:490, 2000.

Nadelman RB, Wormser GP: Erythema migrans and early Lyme disease, *Am J Med* 98(4A):15S, 1995.

Nolan CM et al: Hepatotoxicity associated with isoniazid preventive therapy: a 7-year survey from a public heath tuberculosis clinic, *JAMA* 281:1014, 1999.

O'Grady NP et al: Practice guidelines for evaluating new fever in critically ill adult patients, *Clin Infect Dis* 26:1042, 1998.

Pablos-Mendez A et al: Global surveillance for antituberculosis-drug resistance, 1994-1997, *N Engl J Med* 338:1641, 1998.

Parsons LM et al: Drug resistance in tuberculosis, *Infect Dis Clin North Am* 1(4):905, 1997.

Prevention of malaria, *Med Lett* 42(1070):8, 2000.

Pruthi RK et al: Human babesiosis, *Mayo Clin Proc* 70:853, 1995.

Rangel-Frausto M et al: The natural history of the systemic inflammatory response syndrome: a prospective study, *JAMA* 273(2):117, 1995.

Reese RE, Betts RF: *A practical approach to infectious disease,* Boston, 1996, Little, Brown.

Salpeter SR et al: Monitored isoniazid prophylaxis for low-risk tuberculin reactors older than 35 years of age; a risk-benefit and cost-effectiveness analysis, *Ann Intern Med* 127:1051, 1997.

Sands K et al: Epidemiology of sepsis syndrome in 8 academic medical centers, *JAMA* 278(3):234, 1997.

Sanford JP: *A guide to antimicrobial therapy,* Dallas, 1996, Antimicrobial Therapy, Inc.

The choice of antibacterial drugs, *Med Lett* 41(1064):95, 1999.

Tuberculosis morbidity—United States, 1997, *MMWR* 47:253, 1998.

Venkatarama KR et al: Delays in the suspicion and treatment of tuberculosis among hospitalized patients, *Ann Intern Med* 130:404, 1999.

Villanova PA, Root RK, Jacobs R: Septicemia and septic shock. In Wilson JD et al, editors: *Harrison's principles of internal medicine,* ed 12, New York, 1991, McGraw-Hill.

Vlessis AA et al: New concepts in the pathophysiology of oxygen metabolism during sepsis, *Br J Surg* 82:870, 1995.

Walker D et al: Emerging bacterial zoonotic and vector-borne diseases: ecological and epidemiological factors, *JAMA* 275(6):463, 1996.

Wheeler A, Bernard G: Current concepts: treating patients with severe sepsis, *N Engl J Med* 340(3):207, 1999.

Williamson Z et al: Multiple drug-resistant tuberculosis, *Infect Dis Clin North Am* 12(1):157, 1998.

Zumia A: Science, medicine and the future: tuberculosis, *BMJ* 316(7149):1962, 1998.

10

INFECTIOUS DISEASES

HIV/AIDS

Rudolf J. Kotula

11

DEFINITION AND TRANSMISSION OF HIV/AIDS

I. For purposes of this chapter, the terms *HIV* and *AIDS* will be used synonymously except when the term *HIV* is used to refer to the virus.

II. The treatment of AIDS and related illnesses is a rapidly changing field. Although the recommendations below were current at the time of writing, changes in the treatment regimens may have occurred since then.

III. **AIDS is a spectrum of disease manifestations,** ranging from asymptomatic to life-threatening conditions characterized by severe immunodeficiency, opportunistic infections, and cancers that occur in individuals not receiving immunosuppressive drugs and with no other immunosuppressive disease. AIDS is caused by the human immunodeficiency virus (HIV). There are two recognized subtypes of HIV: HIV-1 causes AIDS worldwide, and HIV-2 produces an AIDS-like illness, but progression to immunodeficiency occurs more slowly than with HIV-1. These retroviruses cause a progressive loss of helper T cells (also known as T4 lymphocytes, or CD4+ lymphocytes), leading to a progressive loss of immune competence and subsequent opportunistic infections. Viral replication tends to be highly dynamic at all stages of the infection with HIV. See diagnosis of AIDS for the list of AIDS-defining conditions.

IV. **High-Risk Behaviors and Modes of Transmission.** The HIV virus is transmitted by the exchange of infected body fluids including blood and semen. High-risk behaviors include:

A. **Unprotected sexual intercourse** with multiple partners, a high-risk partner (commercial sex worker, IV drug user), or an infected partner.

B. **IV drug use,** or exchanging sexual intercourse for drugs.

C. **Persons receiving blood products before 1985.**

D. Transmission has occurred in women who were artificially inseminated.

V. **Perinatal and Vertical Transmission.**

A. **Perinatal.** Whether in utero, intrapartum, or by breast-feeding, there is a perinatal transmission rate of 15% to 30%. Risk factors include advanced maternal disease status, low maternal CD4+ cell count, infant exposure to maternal blood, prolonged duration of ruptured membranes, maternal vitamin A deficiency, and an increased quantity of HIV in maternal blood at delivery (as with acute infection). Breast-feeding is not recommended for HIV-seropositive mothers in the US. See below for details of perinatal diagnosis and prophylaxis of HIV transmission.

B. There is no evidence implicating an insect vector in the transmission of HIV. Likewise, living with an HIV-infected person or even sharing the same toothbrush is not considered high-risk behavior for contracting the AIDS virus.

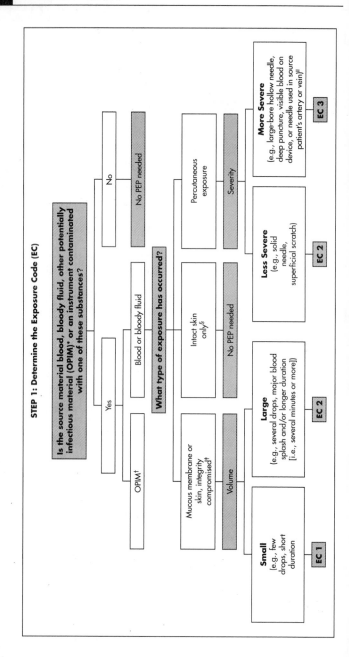

STEP 1: Determine the Exposure Code (EC)

Is the source material blood, bloody fluid, other potentially infectious material (OPIM)* or an instrument contaminated with one of these substances?

Yes — No

No → No PEP needed

OPIM† — Blood or bloody fluid

What type of exposure has occurred?

Mucous membrane or skin, integrity compromised‡ — Intact skin only§ — Percutaneous exposure

Intact skin only§ → No PEP needed

Volume — Severity

Small (e.g., few drops, short duration) → EC 1

Large (e.g., several drops, major blood splash and/or longer duration [i.e., several minutes or more]) → EC 2

Less Severe (e.g., solid needle, superficial scratch) → EC 2

More Severe (e.g., large-bore hollow needle, deep puncture, visible blood on device, or needle used in source patient's artery or vein)‖ → EC 3

FIGURE 11-1

STEP 1 in determining the need for PEP. *OPIM,* Semen or vaginal secretions; cerebrospinal, synovial, pleural, peritoneal, pericardial, or amniotic fluids; or tissue. †Exposures to OPIM must be evaluated on a case-by-case basis. In general, these body substances are considered a low risk for transmission in health-care settings. Any unprotected contact to concentrated HIV in a research laboratory or production facility is considered an occupational exposure that requires clinical evaluation to determine the need for PEP. ‡Skin integrity is considered compromised if there is evidence of chapped skin, dermatitis, abrasion, or open wound. §Contact with intact skin is not normally considered a risk for HIV transmission. However, if the exposure was to blood, and the circumstance suggests a higher volume exposure (e.g., an extensive area of skin was exposed or there was prolonged contact with blood), the risk for HIV transmission should be considered. ¶The combination of these severity factors (e.g., large-bore hollow needle *and* deep puncture) contribute to an elevated risk for transmission, if the source person is HIV positive. *Adapted from* MMWR 47 *(No. RR-7): 14-15, May 15, 1998.*

11

HIV/AIDS

POSTEXPOSURE PROPHYLAXIS RESOURCES AND REGISTRIES

I. Although infected transfusions are almost 100% effective in transmitting HIV, seroconversion after a "routine" exposure to infected blood in health care workers (such as a splash or a needle stick) occurs in only 4 per 1000. The risk of transmission is increased if the needle stick is deep or directly enters a vein or a large volume of blood is involved.

II. **Postexposure Prophylaxis (PEP) can potentially reduce the rate of conversion by 81%. PEP should be regarded as urgent and should be started as soon as possible after the exposure. The interval after which there is no benefit for PEP for humans is undefined.**

III. See Figure 11-1, 11-2, and 11-3 for CDC recommendations for determining the need for PEP. The National Clinician's Postexposure Hotline number is (888) 448-4911 and the HIV Postexposure Prophylaxis Registry number is (888) 737-4448.

IV. PEP should be continued for 4 weeks if the source is known to be or turns out to be HIV positive. PEP has many side affects and is not without risk. Discussions of the pros and cons should be initiated with the prospective recipient.

AIDS BY ORGAN SYSTEM

Use the following list to help to identify an illness in a patient with AIDS who has symptoms referable to a particular organ system.

I. **Pulmonary Disease.** *Pneumocystis carinii* pneumonia, bacterial pneumonia, mycobacterial disease, fungal disease (histoplasmosis, coccidioidomycosis, cryptococcosis, aspergillosis), viral diseases (including

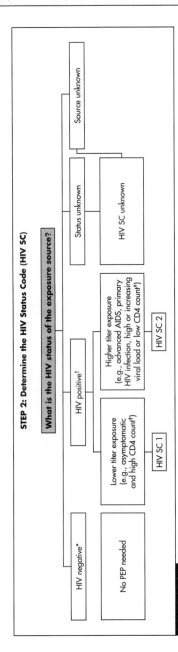

FIGURE 11-2

STEP 2 in determining the need for PEP. *A source is considered negative for HIV infection if there is laboratory documentation of a negative HIV antibody, HIV polymerase chain reaction (PCR), or HIV p24 antigen test result from a specimen collected at or near the time of exposure. †A source is considered infected with HIV (HIV positive) if there has been a positive laboratory result for HIV antibody, HIV PCR, or HIV p24 antigen or physician-diagnosed AIDS. ‡Examples are used as surrogates to estimate the HIV titer in an exposure source for purposes of considering PEP regimens and do not reflect all clinical situations that may be observed. Although a high HIV titer (HIV SC 2) in an exposure source has been associated with an increased risk for transmission, the possibility of transmission from a source with a low HIV titer also must be considered. *Adapted from MMWR 47 (No. RR-7): 14-15, May 15, 1998.*

STEP 3: PEP Recommendations

EC	HIV SC	PEP Recommendation
1	1	PEP may not be warranted. **Exposure type does not pose a known risk for HIV transmission.** Whether the risk for drug toxicity outweighs the benefit of PEP should be decided by the exposed HCW and treating clinician.
1	2	Consider basic regimen.* **Exposure type does not pose a known risk for HIV transmission.** A high HIV titer in the source may justify consideration of PEP. Whether the risk for drug toxicity outweighs the benefit of PEP should be decided by the exposed HCW and treating clinician.
2	1	Recommend basic regimen. Most HIV exposures are in this category; no increased risk for HIV transmission has been observed but, use of PEP is appropriate.
2	2	Recommend expanded regimen.† Exposure type represents an increased HIV transmission risk.
3	1 or 2	Recommend expanded regimen. Exposure type represents an increased HIV transmission risk.
Unknown		If the source or, in the case of an unknown source, the setting where the exposure occurred suggests a possible risk for HIV exposure and the EC is 2 or 3, consider PEP basic regimen.

FIGURE 11-3

STEP 3 in determining the need for PEP. *Basic regimen is four weeks of zidovudine 600 mg per day in two or three divided doses *and* lamivudine 150 mg BID. †Expanded regimen is the basic regimen plus **either** indinavir 800 mg Q8h **or** nelfinavir 750 mg TID. *Adapted from MMWR 47 (No. RR-7): 14-15, May 15, 1998.*

CMV, varicella zoster, influenza), Kaposi's sarcoma, AIDS-related non-Hodgkin's lymphoma, lymphoid interstitial pneumonitis.

II. **Gastrointestinal Disease.**
A. **Esophageal diseases.** Including candidal esophagitis, CMV and HSV esophagitis, rarely Kaposi's sarcoma and AIDS-related non-Hodgkin's lymphoma.
B. **Intestinal disease.**
    1. **Bacteria.** *Salmonella, Shigella,* and *Campylobacter* organisms; *Mycobacterium avium-intracellulare* complex.
    2. **Parasites.** *Cryptosporidium, Isospora, Entamoeba, Giardia* organisms.
    3. **Viruses.** CMV, herpes simplex, HIV enteropathy.
    4. **Neoplasms** including AIDS-Kaposi's sarcoma and AIDS-Non-Hodgkin's lymphoma, anogenital carcinoma, condylomata acuminata.
C. **Hepatobiliary and pancreatic diseases.**
    1. Any AIDS-related infection or neoplasm.
    2. Drugs including DDI, DDC, sulfonamide antibiotics, pentamidine-induced pancreatitis, DDI-induced pancreatitis.
    3. *Mycobacterium avium-intracellulare* complex.
    4. AIDS cholangiopathy. Severe RUQ abdominal pain, spiking fevers, elevated alkaline phosphatase levels. Pathologically sclerosing cholangitis and papillary stenosis. Can be diagnosed by ERCP or HIDA-scan (see Chapter 15).
D. **Ophthalmologic disease.**
    1. **Cornea.** Ulcerative keratitis, dry eye, herpes simplex keratitis, herpes zoster ophthalmicus, Microsporida order.
    2. **Retina and choroid.** Microvasulopathy (cotton-wool spots, retinal hemorrhages), cytomegalovirus retinitis, acute retinal necrosis, progressive outer retinal necrosis, syphilis, toxoplasmosis, *Pneumocystis* choroidopathy, cryptococcosis, mycobacterial infection, intraocular lymphoma, candidiasis, histoplasmosis.
    3. **Drug-associated ocular toxicity.** Didanosine-associated retinal depigmentation or optic neuritis, rifabutin-associated uveitis.
    4. **Neuro-ophthalmic.** Disk edema (papilledema), optic neuropathy, cranial nerve palsies.
    5. **Orbital disorder.** Orbital lymphoma, orbital infection.
E. **Neurologic disease.**
    1. **Primary viral (HIV) syndromes.** HIV encephalopathy, atypical aseptic meningitis, spinal vacuolar myelopathy.
    2. **Opportunistic viral illnesses.** Cytomegalovirus, herpes simplex virus (types 1 and 2), varicella-zoster virus, papovavirus (progressive multifocal leukoencephalopathy), adenovirus (type 2)
    3. **Nonviral infections.** *Toxoplasma gondii, Cryptococcus neoformans, Candida albicans, Aspergillus fumigatus, Coccidioides immitis,* mucormycosis (caused by *Mucor, Absidia,* and *Rhizopus* species). *Acremonium alabamensis, Histoplasma capsulatum, Mycobacterium tuberculosis, Mycobacterium avium-intracellulare, Listeria monocytogenes, Nocardia asteroides.*

4. **Neoplasms.** Primary CNS lymphoma, metastatic systemic lymphoma, metastatic Kaposi's sarcoma.
5. **Cerebrovascular complications.** Infarction, hemorrhage, vasculitis.
6. **Complications of systemic AIDS therapy.**
    a. **Peripheral neuropathic syndromes.** Distal symmetric peripheral neuropathy, inflammatory demyelinating polyradiculoneuropathy, mononeuropathy multiplex, progressive polyradiculopathy.

F. Gynecologic diseases.
1. **Sexually transmitted diseases.** There is a three- to five fold increased risk of HIV transmission with both ulcerative and nonulcerative STD's.
    a. *Neisseria gonorrhoeae, Chlamydia,* and *Trichomonas.* Little data available.
    b. **PID.** Recurrent PID is more common in HIV-seropositive women, who are more likely to require surgical intervention than are women with PID in the general population.
    c. **Genital ulcerative infections.** HSV is more severe and frequent, and has atypical recurrences with progressive immunosuppression. Syphilis also has atypical presentations, abnormally high titers, and more persistent primary lesions with increased risk of treatment failure for secondary disease. Chancroid may present atypically and an increased risk for treatment failure.

2. **HPV, CIN, and cervical cancer.**
    a. Increased diagnosis of HPV with progressive immunosuppression.
    b. Increased proportion of abnormal Pap smears. **There are no firm guidelines on screening HIV positive women for gynecologic cancer. The literature would suggest the following approach, however.**
        (1) If a Pap smear obtained during initial evaluation is normal, a follow-up Pap smear should be obtained in 6 months to rule out false-negative results. With a normal follow-up Pap smear, HIV-infected women should be advised to have a Pap smear every 6 months or annually (recommendations vary). If an HIV-infected woman has a **history** of abnormal Pap smears, she should absolutely have a Pap smear every 6 months.
        (2) If either the initial or follow-up Pap smear reveals severe inflammation with reactive squamous cellular changes, the next follow-up Pap smear should be obtained in 3 months, and management should be guided by the cause of the inflammation. Monitoring with annual or Q6 month Pap smears is advised for HIV-infected women with Pap smears showing only atypical cells of undetermined significance.
        (3) Management for HIV-infected women with Pap smears showing low-grade squamous intraepithelial lesions (SIL) is controversial. Some experts would obtain a follow-up Pap smear at 3 months and then refer the patient for colposcopy if the lesion persisted. Other experts elect to monitor Pap smears at frequent intervals (Q3 months), whereas still other health care providers refer all HIV-infected patients with low-grade SIL for colposcopy.

11

HIV/AIDS

(4) With a Pap smear result showing a high-grade SIL or squamous cell carcinoma, the woman should be referred for colposcopy and biopsy.

(5) Colposcopy is not indicated for HIV-infected women with normal Pap smears.

c. CIN tends to be more severe and multifocal and may involve the vagina, vulva, and perianal area. Rapid progression occurs; recurrence rates are higher and lesions tend to be more refractory to treatment as the patient becomes more immunocompromised.

3. **Amenorrhea and menstrual disorders.** Associated with weight loss and wasting. Often secondary to anemia, which may be a direct result of HIV, marrow infection, malignancy, or drug treatment and prophylaxis regimens.

G. **Hematologic disease.** Early stage HIV-associated thrombocytopenia (ITP). Platelet counts increases as HIV infection progresses.

H. **Kidney disease.** HIV nephropathy, including HIV-associated glomerulosclerosis, IgA nephropathy, amyloidosis and nephrotoxic drug related , e.g. pentamidine, foscarnet, amphotericin B.

HOW TO DIAGNOSE HIV INFECTION

I. **Background.** While obtaining informed consent to test for the HIV virus, it is important to discuss with the patient the implications of a positive test including insurance and work or school ramifications. Many HIV-infected persons still face substantial public intolerance. Confidentiality in diagnosis and treatment are therefore useful for HIV-infected individuals. Currently, 31 states in the U.S. regard HIV infection as a reportable disease. Posttest counseling is also recommended to include information on high-risk behaviors and re-testing for seronegative individuals, behaviors to prevent transmission, strategies for health protection with an immunocompromised system, and the necessity of contact tracing for HIV-seropositive individuals.

II. **Seroconversion to HIV positive usually occurs within 9 to 12 weeks** of exposure to the HIV virus, but patients may remain antibody seronegative for up to 36 months. Sequential testing may be required. CDC recommends testing high-risk individuals every 6 months.

III. **The criteria for HIV infection in persons greater than or equal to 13 years of age.**

A. **Reactive screening test for HIV antibody** by ELISA (sensitivity > 99.9 %) with specific antibody identified by the use of supplemental tests. Western blot is a confirmatory test for the diagnosis of HIV (specificity when combined with ELISA >99.9%) With an intermediate result, may want to retest at a later date if high clinical suspicion or use another test. RNA testing is *not* recommended since there are a high number of false positives and false negatives.

B. **Direct identification of virus** in host tissues by virus isolation.

C. **HIV <u>DNA</u> detection by Polymerase Chain Reaction** (PCR) in the blood is the most sensitive test for diagnosing an acute infection with this virus. The p24 antigen, which indicates active HIV replication, is also positive before seroconversion but is less sensitive.

D. HIV <u>RNA</u> quantitative **PCR** or branched <u>DNA</u> (bDNA) tends to be the most useful tests for determining the prognosis and monitoring the therapy for HIV. The most ultrasensitive assays are able to detect less than 40 copies of viral <u>RNA/ml.</u>

E. Genotyping and phenotyping are newer methods using molecular biology that detect resistance to HIV therapy and assist in drug selection.

F. A positive result on any other highly specific licensed test for HIV.

IV. **The diagnosis in the neonatal period is more complicated** because, although transmission rates for the virus from mother to child are 15% to 30%, a high percentage of the children born to HIV positive mothers will test positive using the Western blot and ELISA tests because of the passive transmission of maternal antibody transplacentally. This antibody will be present for up to 18 months.

A. **For a child <18 months of age who is known to be HIV seropositive (ELISA + Western Blot) or born to an HIV-infected mother,** the diagnosis is confirmed with positive results on 2 separate determinations with one or more of the following tests:

1. **Culture, very good but expensive.** 48% sensitive at birth and 75% sensitive at 3 months.

2. **PCR or other technique for demonstrating viral RNA** in the blood. This is highly sensitive and specific, is reasonably priced, and requires a small sample of whole blood. Accuracy is 84% at birth and 98% to 100% at 1 month of age.

3. **Could check for the p24 antigen** (a major core protein of the HIV virus). However, this is only 18% sensitive at birth.

4. Or meets criteria for acquired immunodeficiency syndrome diagnosis based on the 1987 AIDS surveillance case definition. (see section on AIDS in the pediatric patient).

B. **For a child greater than or equal to 18 months of age born to an HIV-infected mother or any child infected by blood, blood products, or other known modes of transmission,** the diagnosis of HIV is confirmed under the following conditions:

1. **HIV-antibody positive** by repeatedly reactive enzyme immunoassay (EIA) and confirmatory test (Western blot or immunofluorescence assay [IFA]) or meets any of the criteria listed above (IV-A-1-4).

THE INITIAL EVALUATION OF THE HIV-POSITIVE PATIENT

I. **Initial laboratory data** should include (1) HepB core antibody, (2) HepB surface antigen, (3) CD4+ count and viral RNA load, (4) CBC with differential, platelet count, (5) VDRL or RPR and FTA if VDRL positive, (6) PPD (some authors consider >5 mm positive in HIV patients), (7) mumps and *Candida* skin tests (documents anergy, control for PPD), (8) liver and renal function studies, electrolytes, (9) UA, (10) GC culture (genital, rectal, and oral) and *Chlamydia* testing, (11) stool for ova and parasites × 3, (12) stool for culture, (13) toxoplasmosis and cytomegalovirus titers,

11

HIV/AIDS

(14) Varicella IgG if negative history, (15) chest x-ray, (16) G6PD if indicated, and (17) Pap smear and wet mount in women.

NATURAL HISTORY

I. **The acute phase** occurs soon after exposure and may present as an influenza or a mononucleosis-like illness with fever, sweats, fatigue, adenopathy, diarrhea, arthralgias, rash, headache, and occasionally thrombocytopenia (HIV infection may present with epistaxis or even seborrheic dermatitis). There may also be an acute drop in the CD4+ lymphocyte count with an occasional opportunistic infection.

II. **Ongoing HIV replication leads to immune system damage** and progression to AIDS. Disease progression tends to differ among HIV infected individuals. Contraction of this virus is always harmful, and true long term disease free survival without clinically significant immune dysfunction is unusual. Asymptomatic phase is characterized by gradual decline of CD4+ count with persistent lymphadenopathy.

III. **Antigenic stimulation** (intercurrent infections, parasites, etc.) of CD4+ cells hastens viral replication and cell death.

IV. There is some evidence that repeated exposure to different strains of the HIV virus shortens the time to the development of AIDS. Therefore it is important to practice safe sex even if one's partner is also HIV positive.

V. **AIDS-Related Complex (ARC)** comprises lymphadenopathy, fever, and malaise in the absence of opportunistic infections. Biopsy specimens of lymph nodes show a nonspecific hyperplasia. Normal lymph node architecture is gradually destroyed with time. HIV infected persons are no longer capable of generating effective immune response and replace CD4+ cells already lost to this infection.

MANAGEMENT OF HIV INFECTION

I. **Immunize.** Should fully immunize including pneumococcal vaccine, tetanus and influenza vaccine, hepatitis B if not already immune **but do not give live, attenuated vaccines to these patients.** The following vaccines are live: BCG, measles, MMR, MR, mumps, OPV (oral poliovirus), rubella, oral typhoid, varicella, and yellow fever. If foreign travel is being considered, practitioners should consult the CDC web page.

II. **Ongoing evaluation should include the following:**

A. A follow-up at 2 to 4 weeks to discuss questions, lifestyle changes, and support systems and to deal with emotional issues and suicidal ideation (rates of suicide are increased in HIV-positive patients).

B. Therapy based on CD4+ counts, clinical manifestations, and viral RNA counts. Draw CD4+ counts at the same time each visit, due to diurnal variation. Table 11-1 lists monitoring and indications for HIV therapy.

III. **Recommended antiretroviral (ARV) agents for treatment of established HIV infection based on strong evidence of clinical benefit and/or sustained suppression of plasma viral loads (Box 11-1).**

IV. Use of laboratory testing in initiation and monitoring of ARV therapy.

TABLE 11-1

INDICATIONS FOR THE INITIATION OF ARV IN THE CHRONICALLY
HIV-INFECTED PATIENT

Clinical Category	CD4 Count and HIV RNA	Recommendation
Symptomatic (e.g., AIDS, thrush, unexplained fever, other opportunistic infection)	Any value	Treat
Asymptomatic	CD4 <500/mm³ or HIV RNA >10,000 (bDNA)	Treatment should be offered. Strength of recommendation is based on prognosis for disease-free survival and willingness of the patient to accept therapy.*
Asymptomatic	CD4 >500/mm³ and HIV RNA <10,000 (bDNA)	Many experts would delay therapy and observe; however, some experts would treat.

Adapted from *MMWR* 47:1-32, 1998.

*Some experts would observe patients whose CD4 counts are between 350-500/mm³ and HIV RNA levels <10,000 (bDNA).

11

HIV/AIDS

BOX 11-1

RECOMMENDED THERAPY FOR HIV

One choice each from column A and column B. Drugs are listed in random, not priority order:

Column A	Column B
Indinavir	ZDV+ddI
Nelfinavir	d4T+ddI
Ritonavir	ZDV+ddC
Saquinavir	ZDV+3TC
Ritonavir + Saquinavir	d4T+3TC

Alternative (less likely to provide sustained virus suppression):

1 NNRTI (Nevirapine) + 2 NRTIs (Column B)

Saquinavir + 2 NRTIs (Column B)

Not Recommended:

2 NRTIs (viral suppression not sustained)

Monotherapies (except ZDV therapy in pregnancy)

Combinations of d4T + ZDV, ddC + ddI, ddC + d4T, ddC + 3TC (virologically undesirable or overlapping toxicities)

NNRTI, Nonnucleoside reverse transcriptase inhibitors; *NRTI*, nucleoside reverse transcriptase inhibitors.

A. Viral RNA measures the magnitude of HIV replication and is associated with the rate of CD4+ depletion. It is correlated with the risk for disease progression and can be followed as a measure of response to antiretroviral therapy. Viral RNA should be obtained at the time of diagnosis of HIV and every 3-4 months in an untreated patient. It should be measured immediately prior to and every 4-8 weeks after initiation of ARV, then every 3-4 months to monitor the success of therapy. Avoid measurements within 4 weeks of systemic infection or immunization since these may transiently increase the viral RNA. See Table 11-2 for details on ARV.

B. CD4+ count indicates the extent of immune damage. It helps to establish the risk for developing opportunistic infections (OIs) and should be measured at the time of diagnosis and every 3-4 months.

V. **Criteria for changing Antiretroviral (ARV) Therapy.**

A. **Less than 0.5-0.75 log reduction in HIV RNA** by 4-8 weeks following initiation of therapy.

B. **Failure to suppress HIV RNA to undetectable levels within 4-6 months** of initiating the therapy.

C. **Repeated detection of virus in plasma after initial suppression** to undetectable levels, suggesting the development of resistance.

D. Any reproducible significant increase from the nadir of plasma HIV RNA not attributable to intercurrent infection, vaccination, or test methodology.

E. **Persistently declining CD4+,** measured on at least two separate occasions

F. Clinical deterioration.

INFECTIONS IN AIDS PATIENTS

I. Remember, AIDS patients get the usual organisms too and have an increased incidence of *Haemophilus influenzae, Streptococcus pneumoniae, Salmonella* sepsis, etc. Do not focus only on the opportunistic organisms. Always pursue a definitive diagnosis but treat broadly in life-threatening conditions until you have isolated an organism. AIDS patients may not mount a white blood cell count response and may not run a fever with infections. Maintain a high clinical suspicion.

II. **Infection Prophylaxis in the HIV-Positive Patient.** Primary prophylaxis (Table 11-3) is indicated against certain OIs and is indicated based on the CD4+ count. Secondary prophylaxis or chronic suppression is required after the initial episode of certain diseases (Table 11-4).

III. **Occurrence of OIs and conditions based on decreasing CD4+ count.**

A. **CD4+ count of >500:** Recurrent vaginal candidiasis, lymphadenopathy.

B. **CD4+ count of 200-500:** Herpes zoster, oral candidiasis, cervical intraepithelial neoplasia, anemia, Kaposi sarcoma, non-Hodgkin's lymphoma.

C. **CD4+ count of 100-200:** *Pneumocystis carinii* pneumonia, AIDS dementia complex, AIDS related wasting.

D. **CD4+ count of <50:** CMV retinitis, MAC, Cryptosporidiosis, primary multifocal leukoencephalopathy, primary CNS lymphoma.

IV. **Prophylactic Therapy.** See Tables 11-3 and 11-4.

A. **Pneumocystis:** Get 60% recurrence in first year without prophylaxis. Recent data suggest that it is safe to discontinue TMP-SMX if CD4+ >200 and the patient tolerates ARV. This is not yet routinely done for all patients and should be considered on a case by case basis.
B. **CMV retinitis.** Recent European data suggest the option of discontinuing chronic suppression for CMV retinitis if the CD4+ count >150-200 and the patient tolerates ARV therapy *and* if the patient has visual loss related to the return of immune competence (e.g., proven immune reconstitution). This is not yet standard of care, however. Sustained-release ganciclovir disk implants in the vitreous cavity (lasting 6 to 8 months) or intravitreal injections can be used with PO ganciclovir to prevent disease progression with fewer systemic side effects.
C. **Routinely recommended prophylaxis by CD4+ count** (see notes in Table 11-3 for mitigating factors).
    1. CD4+ <200: Pneumocystis
    2. CD4+ <100: Toxoplasmosis
    3. CD4+ <50: MAC
D. Not routinely recommended but may be considered depending on circumstances (see Table 11-3).
    1. CD4+ <100: Histoplasmosis
    2. CD4+ <50: CMV, cryptococcus
V. **Treatment and Chronic Suppression of OIs in the HIV-Positive Patient.**
A. *Pneumocystis carinii.*
    1. **Diagnosis.**
        a. Presenting infection in 50% of those with AIDS.
        b. Clinically have subacute, nonproductive cough, tachypnea, and hypoxia (cardinal signs). May have clear lungs or only wheezes.
        c. An interstitial pneumonitis pattern is common on radiograph, but the patient may have a normal radiograph. Occasionally, cavitary lesions are seen.
        d. Diagnosis is by seeing the organism in the sputum especially by immunofluorescent techniques. The patient may require bronchoscopy and biopsy if the diagnosis is suspected, but the sputum is normal.
    2. **Management of pneumocystis.**
        a. **If not acutely ill with PO$_2$ >60 mm Hg.**
            (1) Trimethoprim/sulfamethoxazole (TMP/SMX) 10 to 15 mg/kg PO BID-TID based on the TMP component for 21 days. Frequently get rash and fever in AIDS patients taking TMP/SMX; can continue drug if not severe.
            (2) Alternatives for mild or moderate disease.
                • TMP 5mg/kg PO TID + dapsone 100 mg PO QD or pyrimethamine 50 to 75 PO QD.
                • Atovaquone 750 mg PO BID-TID + pyrimethamine.
                • Clindamycin 600 mg PO or IV TID + primaquine 30 mg base PO QD for 21 days.

TABLE 11-2

ANTI-HIV DRUGS*

Name, Dosage Forms	Dosage (oral)	Adjust Dose for Renal/Hepatic Insufficiency†	Dietary Restriction
NUCLEOSIDE REVERSE TRANSCRIPTASE INHIBITORS (NRTIS)			
Zidovudine (AZT, Retrovir) 100 mg capsule, 300 mg tablet, 10 mg/ml oral syrup	300 mg Q12h	Renal, hepatic	None
Lamivudine (3TC, Epivir) 10 mg/ml oral solution, 150 mg tablet	150 mg Q12h <50 kg: 2 mg/kg Q12h	Renal	None
Stavudine (d4T, Zerit) 15 mg, 20 mg, 30 mg, 40 mg capsules	>60 kg: 40 mg q12h <60 kg: 30 mg Q12h	Renal, hepatic	None
Didanosine (ddl, Videx) 25 mg, 50 mg, 100 mg, 150 mg, 200 mg tablets 10 mg/ml suspension w/ Maalox	>60 kg: 200 mg Q12h or 400 mg Qd <60 kg: 125 mg Q12h or 250 mg qd	Renal; consider hepatic	Empty stomach; contains buffer; separate from some other meds
Zalcitabine (ddC, Hivid) 0.375 mg, 0.75 mg tablets	0.75 mg Q8h	Renal; consider hepatic	Avoid Al- and Mg-containing antacids.
Abacavir (Ziagen) 300 mg tablets, 20 mg/ml oral solution	300 mg Q12h	Possibly hepatic; insufficient data are available to recommend a hepatic dosage	None

Table compiled by Dena Behm Dillon, Pharm.D., Clinical Pharmacy Specialist-Infectious Diseases, and Tracy Jepson, Pharm.D., Pharmacy Practice Resident, both at University of Iowa Hospitals and Clinics.
AWP, Average wholesale price (for 30-day supply).
*This chart is not all-inclusive. Please refer to manufacturer labeling for additional information.
†Contact pharmacist for specific dosing requirements.

Adverse Effects	Monitoring	Comments
Nausea, vomiting, headache, anemia, low WBC, bone marrow suppression, loss of muscle tissue	CBC with differential, LFTs	Also available as Combivir (3TC/AZT 150 mg/ 300 mg): 1 tablet Q12h
Nausea, headache, low WBC, peripheral neuropathy, hair loss (rare)	CBC, SCr, LFTs	Also available as Combivir (3TC/AZT 150 mg/ 300 mg): 1 tablet Q12h
Peripheral neuropathy, stomach upset, pancreatitis, liver damage	Serum amylase and lipase, SCr, LFTs	
Peripheral neuropathy, pancreatitis, diarrhea, nausea	Serum amylase and lipase, LFTs, Electrolytes	Chew or crush tablets before swallowing. Must have two tablets for each dose to get adequate buffer for absorption. Alcohol may exacerbate toxicity.
Peripheral neuropathy, pancreatitis, stomatitis	CBC, serum amylase and lipase, LFTs, glucose, SCr	
Nausea, vomiting, diarrhea, loss of appetite/anorexia, insomnia; increase in blood glucose, triglycerides, LFTs, creatinine phosphokinase	LFTs, glucose, triglycerides	If hypersensitivity reaction occurs, stop immediately. DO NOT rechallenge. Criteria: skin rash or 2 or more of the following: • Fever • Nausea, vomiting, or abdominal pain • Severe tiredness, achiness, or general ill feeling

Continued

TABLE 11-2
ANTI-HIV DRUGS—cont'd

Name, Dosage Forms	Dosage (oral)	Adjust Dose for Renal/Hepatic Insufficiency	Dietary Restriction
NONNUCLEOSIDE REVERSE TRANSCRIPTASE INHIBITORS (NNRTIS)			
Nevirapine (viramune) 200 mg tablet	200 mg QD × 14 days, then 200 mg Q12h	Hepatic	None
Delavirdine (Rescriptor) 100 mg tablet	400 mg Q8h	Consider hepatic	1 hour apart from antacids. Take with acidic beverage if have achlorhydria.
Efavirenz (Sustiva) 100 mg, 200 mg tablets	600 mg QD	Caution with hepatic, no specific dose recommendations	Avoid high fat meal.
PROTEASE INHIBITORS (PIS)			
Indinavir (Crixivan) 200 mg, 400 mg capsules	800 mg Q8h	Hepatic	Best on empty stomach; however, may take with low fat, low calorie, low carbohydrate snack.
Ritonavir (Norvir) 100 mg capsule 80 mg/ml oral solution	600 mg Q12h	Caution with hepatic, no specific dose recommendations	Take with food, if possible.

Table compiled by Dena Behm Dillon, Pharm.D., Clinical Pharmacy Specialist-Infectious Diseases, and Tracy Jepson, Pharm.D., Pharmacy Practice Resident, both at University of Iowa Hospitals and Clinics.

Adverse Effects	Monitoring	Comments
Rash, increased AST/ALT, hepatitis	LFTs	Dose escalation to lower risk of rash. Experimental: 400 mg qd
Rash (less frequently than with nevirapine), headaches	LFTs, Scr, CBC	Slurry may be made in ≥3 oz water and patient should drink immediately. Experimental: 600 mg Q12h
Difficulty sleeping and concentrating, dizziness, drowsiness, unusual dreams, rash, nausea, vomiting, diarrhea	LFTs, Scr, CBC	CNS effects less noticeable if taken at bedtime. Patient should avoid becoming pregnant.
Nausea, rash, nephrolithiasis, headache, asthenia, blurred vision, dizziness, metallic taste, hyperglycemia, thrombocytopenia, hyperlipidemia	Lipids, LFTs, bilirubin, glucose	Drink at least 48 ounces of water per day.
Nausea, vomiting, diarrhea, asthenia, paresthesias, taste perversion, hepatitis, triglyceride increase >200%, AST/ALT elevation, elevated CPK and uric acid, hyperglycemia, hyperlipidemia	Lipids, LFTs, bilirubin, CPK, glucose	Dose escalation: Day 1-2: 300 mg Q12h Day 3-5: 400 mg Q12h Day 6-13: 500 mg Q12h Day 14: 600 mg Q12h Refrigeration of capsules is recommended, but not required if stored below 77° F and used within 30 days.

11

HIV/AIDS

Continued

TABLE 11-2

ANTI-HIV DRUGS—cont'd

Name, Dosage Forms	Dosage (oral)	Adjust Dose for Renal/Hepatic Insufficiency	Dietary Restriction
PROTEASE INHIBITORS (PIS)—cont'd			
Saquinavir (Fortovase soft-gel capsule) 200 mg capsule	1200 mg Q8h	Caution with hepatic, no specific dose recommendations	Take with full meal (high-fat preferred).
Nelfinavir (Viracept) 250 mg tablet, Powder: 50 mg/scoop	750 mg Q8h	Caution with hepatic, no specific dose recommendations	Take with food (meal or light snack)
Amprenavir (Agenerase) 150 mg capsule, 15 mg/ml oral solution	Capsule: 1200 mg BID; solution dose is not equivalent	Hepatic	Avoid high fat meal; separate at least 1 hour from antacids. Avoid large quantity vitamin E
RIBONUCLEOTIDE REDUCTASE INHIBITORS			
Hydroxyurea (Hydrea) 500 mg capsule	500 mg Q12h	Renal	None

Table compiled by Dena Behm Dillon, Pharm.D., Clinical Pharmacy Specialist-Infectious Diseases, and Tracy Jepson, Pharm.D., Pharmacy Practice Resident, both at University of Iowa Hospitals and Clinics.

b. **If unable to take PO or acutely ill or PO$_2$ <60 mm Hg,** take TMP/SMX 20 mg/kg based on the TMP component divided Q6h.

c. **Should start prednisone** 40 mg PO BID × 5 days (15-30 minutes before TMP/SMX does) and then 40 mg QD × 5 days, followed by 20 mg PO QD × 11 days, and then taper off to zero. This reduces the rate of respiratory failure and mortality, although it increases the rate of herpes zoster. Important to get definitive diagnosis if going to use steroids because prednisone may worsen TB.

d. May get clinical and radiographic worsening during the first 3 to 5 days of therapy but usually get improvement within 7 to 10 days.

e. **Alternative therapy includes** pentamidine 4 mg/kg/day IV or isethionate for 21 days or trimetrexate 45 mg/m^2 IV QD + leucovorin 20 mg/m^2 IV or PO Q6h + dapsone 100 mg PO QD. **Must use leucovorin with trimetrexate or it can induce fatal toxicity.**

Adverse Effects	Monitoring	Comments
Stomach upset, gas, abdominal pain, nausea, diarrhea, headache, elevated AST/ALT, hyperglycemia, hyperlipidemia	Lipids, LFTs, bilirubin, glucose	If used in combination with ritonavir a lower dose of 400 mg Q12h for both agents is given. Invirase hard-gel capsule has lower bioavailability (soon to be phased out).
Diarrhea, hyperglycemia	Lipids, LFTs, bilirubin, glucose	Experimental: 1250 mg Q12h
Nausea, vomiting, rash, fatigue, depression, oral/perioral paresthesias, headache, hyperglycemia, hyperlipidemia	Lipids, LFTs, bilirubin, glucose	Potential for sulfa cross allergy.
Pancytopenia, fever, nausea, vomiting, renal dysfunction, pancreatitis, rash, carcinogenic	CBC, BUN/SCr, LFTs, serum amylase	Experimental agent for HIV; patient should avoid becoming pregnant.

11

HIV/AIDS

B. **Mucosal candidiasis/esophagitis.**
   1. Presents with oral curd like lesions or dysphagia, odynophagia.
   2. May have esophageal disease without oral disease.
   3. **Therapy.**
      a. Orally may use nystatin (100,000 units/ml swish and swallow 5 ml or 500,000 U tablets PO Q6h) or clotrimazole (troches 10 mg 5 × day or vaginal suppositories 100 mg QD or BID) dissolved in mouth, or fluconazole 100 to 200 mg PO QD for 2 weeks or itraconazole 100-200 mg oral solution PO QD or fluconazole 200mg day 1 then 100mg PO × 14 days.
      b. **For esophageal candidiasis:**
         (1) Fluconazole 200 to 400 mg PO or IV daily for 14 to 28 days or itraconazole 200 mg PO QD or fluconazole 400-800mg PO QD-BID or amphotericin B oral solution 500mg PO QID.

Text continued on p. 443

TABLE 11-3

PROPHYLAXIS TO PREVENT FIRST EPISODE OF OPPORTUNISTIC DISEASE IN ADULTS AND ADOLESCENTS INFECTED WITH HIV

Pathogen	Indication	Preventive Regimens	
		First Choice	Alternatives
I. STRONGLY RECOMMENDED AS STANDARD OF CARE			
Pneumocystis carinii*	CD4+ count <200/ml or oropharyngeal candidiasis	TMP-SMZ 1 DS PO QD (AI) TMP-SMZ 1 SS PO QD (AI)	Dapsone 50 mg PO BID or 100 mg PO QD (BI); dapsone 50 mg PO QD. *plus* pyrimethamine 50 mg PO q. week *plus* leucovorin 25 mg PO q. week. (BI); dapsone 200 mg PO *plus* pyrimethamine 75 mg PO *plus* leucovorin 25 mg PO q. week. (BI); aerosolized pentamidine 300 mg q. mo via Respirgard II nebulizer (BI); atovaquone 1500 mg PO QD (BI); TMP-SMZ 1 DS PO t.i.w. (BI)
Mycobacterium tuberculosis Isoniazid-sensitive†	TST reaction ≥5mm *or* prior positive TST result without treatment *or* contact with case of active tuberculosis	Isoniazid 300 mg PO *plus* pyridoxine, 50 mg PO QD × 9 mo (AII) or isoniazid 900 mg PO *plus* pyridoxine, 100 mg PO b.i.w. × 9 mo (BI); rifampin 600 mg PO *plus* pyrazinamide 20 mg/kg PO QD × 2 mo (AI)	Rifabutin 300 mg PO QD *plus* pyrazinamide 20 mg/kg PO QD × 2 mo (BIII); rifampin 600 mg PO QD × 4 mo (BIII)
Isoniazid-resistant	Same; high probability of exposure to isoniazid-resistant tuberculosis	Rifampin 600 mg PO *plus* pyrazinamide 20 mg/kg PO QD × 2 mo (AI)	Rifabutin 300 mg *plus* pyrazinamide 20 mg/kg PO QD × 2 mo (BIII); rifampin 600 mg PO QD × 4 mo (BIII); Rifabutin 300 mg PO QD × 4 mo (CIII)

		Choice of drugs requires consultation with public health authorities	None
Multidrug-(isoniazid and rifampin) resistant *Toxoplasma gondii*‡	Same; high probability of exposure to multidrug-resistant tuberculosis IgG antibody to *Toxoplasma* and CD4+ count <100/ml	TMP-SMZ 1 DS PO QD (AII)	TMP-SMZ 1 SS PO QD (BIII): dapsone 50 mg PO QD *plus* pyrimethamine 50 mg PO q. week *plus* leucovorin 25 mg PO q. week. (BI); atovaquone 1500 mg PO QD with or without pyrimethamine 25 mg PO QD *plus* leucovorin 10 mg PO QD (CIII)
Mycobacterium avium complex (MAC)§	CD4+ count <50/ml	Azithromycin 1200 mg PO q week (AI) or clarithromycin 500 mg PO BID (AI)	Rifabutin 300 mg PO QD (BI); azithromycin 1200 mg PO q. week *plus* rifabutin, 300 mg PO QD (CI)

Modified from *MMWR* 48 (No. RR-10): 1-59, 1999.

b.i.w., twice a week; *DS*, double-strength tablet; *PO*, by mouth; *QD*, daily; *q. mo*, monthly; *q. week*, weekly; *SS*, single-strength tablet; *t.i.w.*, three times a week; *TMP-SMZ*, trimethoprim-sulfamethoxazole; *TST*, tuberculin skin test.

*Prophylaxis should also be considered for persons with a CD4+ percentage of <14%, for persons with a history of an AIDS-defining illness, and possibly for those with CD4+ counts >200 but <250 cells/μl. TMP-SMZ also reduces the frequency of toxoplasmosis and some bacterial infections. Patients receiving dapsone should be tested for glucose-6 phosphate dehydrogenase deficiency. A dosage of 50 mg QD is probably less effective than that of 100 mg QD. The efficacy of parenteral pentamidine (e.g., 4 mg/kg/month) is uncertain. Fansidar (sulfadoxine-pyrimethamine) is rarely used because of severe hypersensitivity reactions. Patients who are being administered therapy for toxoplasmosis with sulfadiazine-pyrimethamine are protected against *Pneumocystis carinii* pneumonia and do not need additional prophylaxis against PCP.

†Directly observed therapy is recommended for isoniazid, 900 mg b.i.w.; isoniazid regimens should include pyridoxine to prevent peripheral neuropathy. Rifampin should not be administered concurrently with protease inhibitors or nonnucleoside reverse transcriptase inhibitors. Rifabutin should not be given with hard-gel saquinavir or delavirdine; caution is also advised when the drug is coadministered with soft-gel saquinavir. Rifabutin may be administered at a reduced dose (150 mg QD) with indinavir, nelfinavir, or amprenavir; at a reduced dose of 150 mg QOD (or 150 mg t.i.w.) with ritonavir; or at an increased dose (450 mg QD) with efavirenz; information is lacking regarding coadministration of rifabutin with nevirapine. Exposure to multidrug-resistant tuberculosis might require prophylaxis with two drugs; consult public health authorities. Possible regimens include pyrazinamide plus either ethambutol or a fluoroquinolone.

‡Protection against toxoplasmosis is provided by TMP-SMZ, dapsone plus pyrimethamine, and possibly by atovaquone. Atovaquone may be used with or without pyrimethamine. Pyrimethamine alone probably provides little, if any, protection.

§See footnote † regarding use of rifabutin with protease inhibitors or nonnucleoside reverse transcriptase inhibitors.

Continued

TABLE 11-3

PROPHYLAXIS TO PREVENT FIRST EPISODE OF OPPORTUNISTIC DISEASE IN ADULTS AND ADOLESCENTS INFECTED WITH HIV—cont'd

Pathogen	Indication	Preventive Regimens First Choice	Alternatives
I. STRONGLY RECOMMENDED AS STANDARD OF CARE—cont'd			
Varicella zoster virus (VZV)	Significant exposure to chicken-pox or shingles for patients who have no history of either condition or, if available, neg-ative antibody to VZV	Varicella zoster immune globulin (VZIG) 5 vials (1.25 ml each) im, administered 96 hrs after expo-sure, ideally within 48 hrs (AIII)	
II. GENERALLY RECOMMENDED			
Streptococcus pneumoniae¶	All patients	Pneumococcal vaccine 0.5 ml IM (CD4+ 200/ml [BII]; CD4+ <200/ml [CIII])—might reimmu-nize if initial immunization was given when CD4+ <200/ml and if CD4+ increases to >200/ml on HAART(CII)	None
HBV#	All susceptible (anti-HBc-negative) patients	Hepatitis B vaccine: 3 doses (BII)	None
Influenza virus#	All patients (annually, before in-fluenza season)	Whole or split virus, 0.5 ml IM/yr (BIII)	Rimantadine 100 mg PO BID (CIII), or amantadine 100 mg PO BID (CIII)
HAV#	All susceptible (anti-HAV-negative) patients with chronic hepatitis C	Hepatitis A vaccine: two doses (BIII)	None

III. NOT ROUTINELY INDICATED

Bacteria	Neutropenia	G-CSF 5-10 mg/kg SQ QD × 2-4 week or GM-CSF 250 mg/m² iv over 2 hr QD × 2-4 week (CII)	None
		None	Itraconazole 200 mg PO QD (CIII)
*Cryptococcus neoformans***	CD4+ count <50/ml	Fluconazole 100-200 mg PO QD (CI)	None
*Histoplasma capsulatum***	CD4+ count <100/ml, endemic geographic area	Itraconazole capsule 200 mg PO QD(CI)	None
Cytomegalovirus (CMV)††	CD4+ count <50/ml and CMV antibody positive	Oral ganciclovir 1 g PO TID (CI)	None

Modified from *MMWR* 48 (No. RR-10): 1-59, 1999.

Anti-HBc, Antibody to hepatitis B core antigen; *HAART,* highly active antiretroviral therapy; *HAV,* hepatitis A virus; *HBV,* hepatitis B virus; *HIV,* human immunodeficiency virus; *IM,* intramuscular; *IV,* intravenous; *PO,* by mouth; *QD,* daily; *SQ,* subcutaneous; *G-CSF,* granulocyte-colony-stimulating factor, *GM-CSF,* granulocyte-macrophage colony-stimulating factor.

¶Vaccination should be offered to persons who have a CD4+ T-lymphocyte count <200 cells/μl, although the efficacy might be diminished. Revaccination 5 years after the first dose or sooner if the initial immunization was given when the CD4+ count was <200 cells/μl and the CD4+ count has increased to >200 cells/μl on HAART is considered optional. Some authorities are concerned that immunizations might stimulate the replication of HIV. However, one study showed no adverse effect of pneumococcal vaccination on patient survival.

#These immunizations or chemoprophylactic regimens do not target pathogens traditionally classified as opportunistic but should be considered for use in HIV-infected patients as indicated. Data are inadequate concerning clinical benefit of these vaccines in this population, although it is logical to assume that those patients who develop antibody responses will derive some protection. Some authorities are concerned that immunizations might stimulate HIV replication, although for influenza vaccination, a large observational study of HIV-infected persons in clinical care showed no adverse effect of this vaccine, including multiple doses, on patient survival (J. Ward, CDC, personal communication). Hepatitis B vaccine has been recommended for all children and adolescents and for all adults with risk factors for HBV. Rimantadine and amantadine are appropriate during outbreaks of influenza A. Because of the theoretical concern that increases in HIV plasma RNA following vaccination during pregnancy might increase the risk of perinatal transmission of HIV, providers may wish to defer vaccination until after antiretroviral therapy is initiated.

**In a few unusual occupational or other circumstances, prophylaxis should be considered; consult a specialist.

††Acyclovir is not protective against CMV. Valacyclovir is not recommended because of an unexplained trend toward increased mortality observed in persons with AIDS who were being administered this drug for prevention of CMV disease.

11

HIV/AIDS

TABLE 11-4

PROPHYLAXIS TO PREVENT RECURRENCE OF OPPORTUNISTIC DISEASE (AFTER TREATMENT OF ACUTE DISEASE) IN ADULTS AND ADOLESCENTS INFECTED WITH HIV

Pathogen	Indication	Preventive Regimens	
		First Choice	Alternatives
I. RECOMMENDED FOR LIFE AS STANDARD OF CARE			
Pneumocystis carinii	Prior *P. carinii* pneumonia	TMP-SMZ 1 DS PO QD (AI) TMP-SMZ 1 SS PO QD (AI)	Dapsone 50 mg PO BID *or* 100 mg PO QD (BI); dapsone 50 mg PO QD *plus* pyrimethamine 50 mg PO q. week. *plus* leucovorin 25 mg PO q. week. (BI); dapsone, 200 mg PO *plus* pyrimethamine, 75 mg PO *plus* leuco-vorin 25 mg PO q. week. (BI); aerosolized pentamidine 300 mg q. mo via Respirgard IIO nebulizer (BI); atovaquone 1500 mg PO QD (BI); TMP-SMZ, 1 DS PO t.i.w. (CI)
Toxoplasma gondii*	Prior toxoplasmic encephalitis	Sulfadiazine 500-1000 mg PO QID *plus* pyrimethamine 25-75 mg PO QD *plus* leucovorin, 10-25 mg PO QD (AI)	Clindamycin 300-450 mg PO Q6-8h *plus* pyrimethamine 25-75 mg PO QD *plus* leucovorin, 10-25 mg PO QD (BI); ato-vaquone 750 mg PO Q6-12h with or without pyrimeth-amine 25 mg PO QD *plus* leucovorin 10 mg PO QD (CIII)
Mycobacterium avium complex (MAC)†	Documented disseminated disease	Clarithromycin 500 mg PO BID (AI) *plus* ethambutol 15 mg/kg PO QD(AII); with or without rifabutin 300 mg PO QD (CI)	Azithromycin 500 mg PO QD (AII) *plus* ethambutol, 15 mg/kg PO QD(AII); with or without rifabutin 300 mg PO QD (CI)

Cytomegalovirus (CMV)	Prior end-organ disease	Ganciclovir 5-6 mg/kg IV 5-7 days/wk or 1000 mg PO TID (AI); or foscarnet 90-120 mg/kg IV QD (AI); or (for retinitis) ganciclovir sustained-release implant Q6-9 mo *plus* ganciclovir 1.0-1.5 g PO TID (AI)	Cidofovir 5 mg/kg IV q.o.w. with probenecid 2 g PO 3 hrs before the dose followed by 1 g PO given 2 hours after the dose, and 1 g PO 8 hrs after the dose (total of 4 g) (AI); fomivirsen 1 vial (330 mg) injected into the vitreous, then repeated every 2-4 wks (AI)
Cryptococcus neoformans	Documented disease	Fluconazole 200 mg PO QD (AI)	Amphotericin B 0.6-1.0 mg/kg IV q. week-t.i.w. (AI); itraconazole 200 mg PO QD (BI)
Histoplasma capsulatum	Documented disease	Itraconazole capsule 200 mg PO BID (AI)	Amphotericin B 1.0 mg/kg IV q. week (AI)
Coccidioides immitis	Documented disease	Fluconazole 400 mg PO QD (AII)	Amphotericin B 1.0 mg/kg IV q. week (AI); itraconazole 200 mg PO BID (AII)
Salmonella species, (non-*typhi*)‡	Bacteremia	Ciprofloxacin 500 mg PO BID for several months (BII)	Antibiotic chemoprophylaxis with another active agent (CIII)

From *MMWR* 48 (No. RR-10): 1-59, 1999.

b.i.w., Twice a week; *DS*, double-strength tablet; *PO*, by mouth; *QD*, daily; *q. mo*, monthly; *q. week*, weekly; *SS*, single-strength tablet; *t.i.w.*, three times a week; *TMP-SMZ*, trimethoprim-sulfamethoxazole.

*Pyrimethamine-sulfadiazine confers protection against *P.carinii* pneumonia, as well as toxoplasmosis; clindamycin-pyrimethamine does not.

†Many multiple-drug regimens are poorly tolerated. Drug interactions (e.g., those seen with clarithromycin and rifabutin) can be problematic; rifabutin has been associated with uveitis, especially when administered at daily doses of >300 mg or concurrently with fluconazole or clarithromycin. Rifabutin should not be administered concurrently with hard-gel saquinavir or delavirdine; caution is also advised when the drug is coadministered with soft-gel saquinavir. Rifabutin may be administered at reduced dose (150 mg QD with indinavir, nelfinavir, or amprenavir, or 150 mg QOD with ritonavir) or at increased dose (450 mg QD) with efavirenz (*MMWR* 47[RR-20]: 1998.). Information is lacking regarding coadministration of rifabutin with nevirapine.

‡Efficacy of eradication of *Salmonella* has been demonstrated only for ciprofloxacin.

Continued

TABLE 11-4

PROPHYLAXIS TO PREVENT RECURRENCE OF OPPORTUNISTIC DISEASE (AFTER TREATMENT OF ACUTE DISEASE) IN ADULTS AND ADOLESCENTS INFECTED WITH HIV—cont'd

Pathogen	Indication	Preventive Regimens	
		First Choice	Alternatives
II. RECOMMENDED ONLY IF SUBSEQUENT EPISODES ARE FREQUENT OR SEVERE			
Herpes simplex virus	Frequent/severe recurrences	Acyclovir 200 mg PO TID or 400 mg PO BID (AI) Famciclovir 500 mg PO BID (AI)	Valacyclovir 500 mg PO BID (CIII)
Candida (oropharyngeal or vaginal)	Frequent/severe recurrences	Fluconazole 100-200 mg PO QD (CI)	Itraconazole solution 200 mg PO QD (CI); ketoconazole 200 mg PO QD (CIII)
Candida (esophageal)	Frequent/severe recurrences	Fluconazole 100-200 mg PO QD (BI)	Itraconazole solution 200 mg PO QD (BI); ketoconazole 200 mg PO QD (CIII)

From *MMWR* 48 (No. RR-10): 1-59, 1999.

†Many multiple-drug regimens are poorly tolerated. Drug interactions (e.g., those seen with clarithromycin and rifabutin) can be problematic; rifabutin has been associated with uveitis, especially when administered at daily doses of >300 mg or concurrently with fluconazole or clarithromycin. Rifabutin should not be administered concurrently with hard-gel saquinavir or delavirdine; caution is also advised when the drug is coadministered with soft-gel saquinavir. Rifabutin may be administered at reduced dose (150 mg QD with indinavir, nelfinavir, or amprenavir, or 150 mg QOD with ritonavir) or at increased dose (450 mg QD) with efavirenz (*MMWR* 47[RR-20]: 1998.). Information is lacking regarding coadministration of rifabutin with nevirapine.

‡Efficacy of eradication of *Salmonella* has been demonstrated only for ciprofloxacin.

(2) If no response in 1 week, change to amphotericin B 0.3 to 0.4 mg/kg IV QD.

(3) Secondary prophylaxis for chronic suppression indicated.

C. **Cytomegalovirus (CMV).**

1. **Retinitis.** Presents with visual changes, decreased vision, floaters, flashes of light, blind spots, and blurred vision. Diagnosed by funduscopic exam. Fluffy white infiltrates associated with central pallor, surrounding retinal hemorrhage, and perivascular sheathing are seen.

2. **CNS infection, mononeuritis, esophagitis, colitis.** Same treatment as for retinitis, but efficacy is not as good.

3. **Hepatitis.** No treatment recommended.

4. **Treatment.** Both ganciclovir and foscarnet are fairly toxic. (Ganciclovir is associated with myelosuppression and foscarnet is associated with nephrotoxicity and hypocalcemia.)

   a. **Ganciclovir** 5 mg/kg IV over 1 hour Q12h for 14-21 days (induction) followed by 5 mg/kg/day. May be given with granulocyte-macrophage colony-stimulating factor.

   b. **Foscarnet** 90 mg/kg IV over 2 hours Q8-12h for 14 to 21 days (induction) followed by 90 to 120 mg/kg/day in 1 dose IV daily.

   c. Must continue lifelong suppression for CMV retinitis (see above, however).

D. **Toxoplasmosis.**

1. Most common cause of CNS mass lesion in AIDS; 47% of patients with AIDS develop CNS toxoplasmosis.

2. Presents with frequent headache, lateralizing signs, altered mentation, fever, and seizures.

3. CT shows "ring"-enhancing lesions, usually bilateral.

4. **Treatment.**

   a. **Pyrimethamine** 200mg PO induction × 1 then 75-100 mg PO QD **and** sulfadiazine 1 to 1.5 PO Q6h + leucovorin 10 mg/day. Use this regimen for 4 to 6 weeks. Alternatively, may use clindamycin 600 PO or IV Q6h + pyrimethamine 50 to 100 mg/day and leucovorin 10 mg PO QD. Alternative regimens include atovaquone 750 mg PO QID or azithromycin 1200 mg PO QD or clarithromycin 1 g PO BID plus pyrimethamine 50-100 PO QD and leucovorin 10 mg PO QD.

   b. Must use chronic suppression for life (see Table 11-4).

E. **Herpes zoster (varicella zoster).**

1. Presents with grouped vesicles over one or more dermatomes and consider immunosuppression in any patient that presents with zoster in greater than one dermatome.

2. **Treatment.** Acyclovir 800 mg PO 5 × a day or 10 mg/kg IV Q8h for 7 to 10 days.

   a. Resistance may develop and so if the patient has been treated previously with acyclovir, may have to use foscarnet 40 mg/kg IV

11

HIV/AIDS

Q8h for 14 to 26 days, or famciclovir 500 mg PO TID or valacy-clovir HCl 1000 mg PO TID for 5 days.

   b. Must begin antiviral therapy within 72 hours of the development of lesions in order to be effective.

F. **Cryptococcal meningitis.**

   1. Presents with headache, fever, delirium, nausea, and vomiting. Only 20% have meningismus and photophobia. Rarely patients present with seizures.

   2. Only 21% have CSF WBC counts >20 WBC/mm^3.

   3. Diagnose with India ink or CSF cryptococcal antigen.

   4. Do head CT before LP because of high incidence of mass lesions in AIDS patients to avoid transtentorial herniation.

   5. **Treatment.**

      a. Amphotericin B 0.7 to 1 mg/kg/day IV with or without flucytosine 25 mg/kg PO Q6h for 2 to 4 weeks. Follow with fluconazole 400 mg PO QD or itraconazole 200 mg PO BID for 10 weeks.

      b. Must continue suppression (see Table 11-4).

G. **Bacterial infections (only in selected patients).** For neutropenia, start granulocyte colony-stimulating factor 5 to 10 μg/kg SQ QD for 2 to 4 weeks or granulocyte-macrophage colony-stimulating factor 250 μg/m^2 IV over 2 hours QD for 2 to 4 weeks.

VI. **AIDS-Associated Diarrhea**

A. **General.** 30% to 50% of AIDS patients in the United States have diarrhea at some point during their illness. Since the causes of diarrhea in these patients are protean, empiric therapy is almost never indicated. It is important to try to identify the organism. A general approach includes good history, physical exam, and stool for (1) culture and sensitivity (need to culture for *Salmonella* species, which is 100 times more common than in "normal" population, *Shigella flexneri,* and *Campylobacter jejuni*); (2) ova and parasites × 3 and *Giardia* antigen; (3) *Clostridium difficile* toxin; (4) acid-fast stains and in advanced disease chromotrope-based stains × 2 (see below for details). It may be necessary to proceed to colonoscopy (culture and biopsy for CMV, *Mycobacterium,* adenovirus, and herpes simplex) or esophagogastroduodenoscopy (culture for CMV and *Mycobacterium*). General supportive measures are also indicated including fluids and antimotility drugs **unless** the patient has fecal leukocytes or abdominal pain.

B. **Dietary and drinking water precautions.**

   1. Avoid raw meat (sushi, etc.) and raw eggs. Cook meat thoroughly. Do not use cracked eggs. Thaw frozen meat in the refrigerator or microwave, not at room temperature.

   2. Listeriosis is a rare disease; however, it may be contracted by eating hot dogs and cold cuts from delicatessen counters. These foods should be reheated before consumption.

3. Avoid drinking water from lakes or rivers because of the risk of cryptosporidiosis and giardiasis. Even accidental ingestion while swimming carries a risk.

C. Specific causes of AIDS-associated diarrhea.

1. *Cryptosporidium.*
   a. Transmitted by fecal-oral route.
   b. Presents with chronic voluminous diarrhea and abdominal pain, anorexia, nausea, and malabsorption.
   c. The most sensitive test is a direct immunofluorescence antibody done on the stool; ELISA has also been used. Diagnosis can also be made by biopsy of colon or small bowel or by acid-fast stain of the stool.
   d. Treatment includes paromomycin 750 mg PO TID with or without Azithromycin 600 mg PO QD. Nitrazoxamide 2 gm PO QD promising, not approved yet by FDA. Supplemental benefit from octreotide 50 μg SQ Q8h × 48 hours and then increased by 100 to 200 μg Q8h every 1-2 weeks to maximum dose of 500 μg Q8h.
   e. Treatment outcome for *Cryptosporidium* is not good with only a 42% response rate.

2. *Giardia lamblia.*
   a. Transmitted by water and fecal-oral route.
   b. The diagnosis is made by detecting *Giardia* antigen in the stool by immunofluorescence (most common) or ELISA. This is from 85%-98% sensitive. *Giardia* can also be diagnosed by duodenal biopsy (90% sensitivity) or stool for O & P with a 50% sensitivity.
   c. Treatment is metronidazole 250 mg PO TID for 5 days **or** quinacrine 100 mg PO TID after meals for 5 days (see Chapter 5 for further information).

3. *Isospora.*
   a. Constitutes 1% to 3% of AIDS diarrhea in the United States (higher elsewhere).
   b. Symptoms are similar to those of *Cryptosporidium,* but the patient gets an associated eosinophilia.
   c. Diagnosed by acid-fast stain of stool.
   d. Treatment is by TMP/SMX DS 1 PO QID for 21 days. Maintain on TMP/SMX DS 1 PO QOD or sulfadoxine-pyrimethamine (Fansidar) once weekly. Alternatively, Pyrimethamine 75 mg PO QD + Leucovorin 10 mg PO QD for 14 days can be used. Chronic suppression needed.

4. *Microsporida* order: *Enterocytozoon bieneusi, Septata intestinalis.*
   a. An excellent screening test is fluorescence with calcofluor. Diagnose by duodenal biopsy and electron microscopy **or** stain formalin fixed stool with giemsa or chromotrope-based technique and use light microscopy.

  b. No standard treatment. However, albendazole 400 mg PO BID
     for 1 month has been used with a good response in 50% to
     100% of treated patients.

5. **CMV.**
   a. Culture biopsy of colon.
   b. No good treatment for CMV diarrhea but can try ganciclovir or
      foscarnet (see protocol above).
   c. May cause necrosis and perforation.

6. **Histoplasma capsulatum.**

7. **Mycobacterium avium-intracellulare (MAC).** Diarrhea is usually associated with disseminated disease. See section below on mycobacterial disease.

8. **AIDS-associated enteropathy.** Comprising villous atrophy, malabsorption, and lactase deficiency in the absence of an identifiable
   pathogen after extensive work-up. Antiretroviral drugs may improve
   symptoms.

9. **Bacterial disease.**
   a. Diagnosed by culture.
   b. Treatment is by ciprofloxacin 500 mg PO BID empirically once
      cultures are done. However, should base on culture sensitivities
      when known.

10. **Herpes Simplex Virus proctitis.**
    a. May have proctitis, esophagitis, or genital and perianal
       lesions.
    b. Presents with tenesmus, constipation, dysphagia, and anorectal
       pain.
    c. Treatment is acyclovir 400 mg 5 × per day for 7 days. Alter-
       natively, famciclovir HCl 500 mg BID × 7 days.
    d. Chronic suppression with acyclovir 400 mg BID if there is
       recurrence.

D. **Suppression.** Suppression indicated for *Salmonella, Shigella,* HSV, and
   Candida if there is recurrent disease frequently. Must suppress CMV; see
   Table 11-4.

VII. **Tuberculosis in HIV Infection**

A. Because *Mycobacterium tuberculosis* is more virulent than *Pneumocystis* species, it will often present at an earlier stage of HIV infection
   than will *Pneumocystis.*

B. Of those with TB, extrapulmonary disease develops in 70% of those patients with preexisting AIDS and 45% of those with HIV infection.

C. Incidence is inversely associated with baseline CD4+ count. Among
   those who have disease, it is most likely reactivation rather than from a
   recent exposure.

D. **Clinical presentation.** Persistent cough >2 weeks, dyspnea, hemoptysis, fever, night sweats, and significant weight loss >10% of body
   weight.

E. **Diagnosis.**

1. **Positive PPD.** Must do controls for *Candida* and mumps to rule out false negative from anergy.
   a. 5 mm result is considered a positive test in those with HIV infection.
   b. Must do at least 3 sputa for AFB.
   c. Can diagnose by CXR with perihilar adenopathy and cavitary lesions. May have effusions. Miliary TB may mimic *Pneumocystis* on CXR.

F. **Treatment.**
   1. Treat prophylactically in all HIV positive patients with positive PPD regardless of age, since 8% will develop active disease every year. Treat prophylactically for 12 months. See Table 11-3.
   2. Treat active disease as per the protocol recommended in your area. Pockets of drug-resistant TB make blanket recommendations unwise at this time.

G. **Precautions.** Do not use nebulized pentamidine in those with TB because of the possibility of transmission of the disease to others.

VIII. **Mycobacterium Avium-Intracellulare (MAC/MAI)**

A. May present as diarrhea, fever, night sweats, and generalized wasting.

B. Can generally culture from blood or stool.

C. Treatment regimens include clarithromycin 500 to 1000 mg PO BID or azithromycin 500 mg PO QD plus ethambutol 15-25 mg/kg/day ± rifabutin 300 mg PO QD. Alternative regimen includes clarithromycin or azithromycin + ethambutol ± rifabutin and ciprofloxacin 750 mg PO BID or ofloxacin 400 mg PO BID or amikacin 7.5-15 mg/kg IV QD.

IX. **Syphilis in AIDS.**

A. **Penicillin is recommended for treatment in all HIV-infected patients** in all stages of syphilis. Skin testing is advised to confirm allergy though the utility in immunocompromised patients is questionable. For HIV-infected patients who are penicillin allergic, the CDC recommends desensitization and then treatment with PCN. Alternative treatments are suboptimal.

B. **For primary and secondary syphilis** among HIV-infected individuals, the treatment is benzathine penicillin G 2.4 million units IM as one dose. However, these patients may have CSF abnormalities of unknown prognostic significance, and therefore some experts elect to obtain an LP before treatment and modify therapy accordingly. If have positive CSF pleocytosis **or** positive CSF VDRL test, treat for neurosyphilis. May also have elevated CSF total protein.

C. **For latent syphilis** among HIV-infected individuals, the treatment is benzathine penicillin G 2.4 million units as 3 weekly doses of 2.4 million units each. CSF examination is mandatory in HIV infected individuals.

D. **For treatment failure,** evaluation of CSF is indicated. If the CSF is normal, the penicillin dose is the same as that for latent syphilis. Follow-up study for treatment failure includes clinical and serologic evaluation at 1 month and then 2, 3, 6, 9, and 12 months after treatment.

11

HIV/AIDS

E. **Treatment for neurosyphilis** is aqueous penicillin G 12-24 million units IV/QD × 10-14 days or procaine penicillin G 2.4 million units IM QD + probenecid 500 mg PO BID × 14 days.

AIDS-ASSOCIATED WEIGHT LOSS AND WASTING

I. **Weight loss and malnutrition are major problems** in the AIDS patient for several reasons, including increased metabolic demand, loss of appetite, eating difficulties from oral and esophageal disease, as well as diarrhea and malabsorption.

II. **Dronabinol** (Marinol), one of the active ingredients in marijuana, is widely used by patients with AIDS to improve their appetite; some evidence indicates that it may be effective. Marijuana is also used by HIV-positive patients (and is medically legal in some states).

III. **The use of megestrol acetate** has been associated with a significant weight gain and improved feeling of well-being in patients with AIDS-associated wasting. Megestrol may be associated with adrenal suppression and should not be discontinued abruptly.

IV. **Anabolic steroids** (fluoxymestrone, oxymetholone, nandrolene, testosterone, and oxandrolone) have demonstrated a significant weight gain in AIDS patients.

V. Exercise with weightlifting provides a substantial benefit with weight gain.

VI. Some less frequently used appetite stimulants include thalidomide, recombinant human growth hormone, insulin-like growth factor-1 and N-3 fatty acid (omega-3 fatty acid-fish oil) supplementation.

NEUROPSYCHIATRIC DISEASE

I. **General.** About 60% of individuals with AIDS have some neuropsychiatric manifestations of the illness. This may be because macrophages and monocytes carry the HIV into the CNS. The virus may also gain direct access because many CNS components are CD4+. It is critical to ascertain that neurologic manifestations are not attributable to infectious causes (other than HIV) or CNS lymphoma before attributing symptoms to the direct effects of the AIDS virus. Individuals with AIDS or HIV infection are undergoing a major stress, and psychologic support is critical to the successful management of their illness. Drug therapies are helpful, but social and psychologic support is important to their overall care.

II. **Terminology.** Subacute encephalitis (AIDS encephalopathy, AIDS dementia complex).

A. Defined by progressive dementia, psychomotor retardation, focal motor abnormalities, behavioral changes, and short-term memory deficits.

B. May manifest headache with problems of coordination, apathy, and affective blunting. Later manifestations include inappropriate behavior, emotional lability, seizures, aphasia, and psychotic manifestations.

C. Advanced cases develop global cognitive deterioration, incontinence, sensory loss, and visual disturbances.

D. 75% of AIDS patients manifest these symptoms, but 90% show pathologic changes on autopsy.

III. **Testing.**

A. Useful tests include the Symbol Digit Modalities Test and Parts A & B of the Trail Making Test, which test psychomotor function. A newly developed screening instrument, the HIV Dementia Scale, is a reliable and quantitative scale superior to the Minimental Status Exam and the Grooved Pegboard in identifying HIV dementia.

B. Double-dose contrast-enhanced CT alone cannot provide a definitive diagnosis. The most common abnormality reported on CT scans of these patients is cerebral atrophy. Radiographically, MRI is best at demonstrating degeneration. The most common white matter lesions are diffuse over a wide area, typically in the centrum semiovale and periventricular white matter. Less commonly, there is localized involvement with patchy or punctate lesions.

C. In atypical aseptic meningitis, there is an increase in the ICP and in the CSF mononuclear pleocytosis, multinucleated giant cells, protein content, and oligoclonal bands.

D. EEG is not particularly helpful.

IV. **Differential diagnosis of neuropsychiatric disorders in HIV disease once one has excluded infectious and other medical causes.**

A. Most common are affective disorders.

B. **Dementia.**
   1. Responds to some degree to high doses of ARV therapy (especially AZT).
   2. Some experimental agents are being investigated to treat AIDS dementia, including nimodipine, pentoxyphylline, memantine, delavirdine and peptide-T.
      a. Do not use in patients with florid psychosis.
      b. Document changes with tests noted above.

C. **Agitation** secondary to delirium may be treated by lorazepam 0.5 mg IV slow push.

D. **Treat psychotic symptoms** with haloperidol 0.5 to 1 mg PO QID.

E. **Depression** can be treated with standard antidepressants. Some patients respond rapidly to methylphenidate 5mg Q AM up to 20-60 mg divided TID. Patients may be sensitive to anticholinergic side effects late in HIV illness. MAO inhibitors are contraindicated.

F. **AIDS patients can get a manic syndrome** related to the use of ganciclovir, zidovudine, and fluoxetine, which may respond to lithium. Treat agitation as above.

G. **Anxiety** can be treated with standard drugs. See Chapter 18.

DERMATOLOGIC MANIFESTATIONS

I. Cutaneous Infections.

A. **Viral.** Herpesviruses produce disseminated, extensive, or chronic herpetic ulcers. Treat with acyclovir 400 mg PO 5 × a day or 5 mg/kg IV

Q8h × 7 to 14 days if severe. Maintenance dose acyclovir 400 mg
PO BID.

B. **Fungal.**
  1. **Dermatophytosis (tinea) by fungi of the genera** *Trichophyton,*
     Microsporum, **and** *Epidermophyton.* For treatment, see Chapter 17.
  2. **Yeasts and mucosal candidiasis.** Treat with systemic antifungals (see
     section on candidiasis above).
  3. **Rarely: histoplasmosis and cryptococcosis.**
C. **Bacterial.**
  1. **Bacterial folliculitis, impetigo.** For treatment, see Chapter 17.
     a. **Mycobacteriosis.** Treatment involves systemic antibiotics; see pre-
        vious section on *Mycobacterium.*
     b. **Bacillary angiomatosis.** Treat with erythromycin 250 to 500 mg
        PO QID until lesions resolve or doxycycline 100 mg PO BID.
II. **Cutaneous Neoplasms**
A. **Kaposi's sarcoma.** Human herpes virus-8 (HHV-8) has been implicated
   as the probable agent of this skin neoplasm. Clinically appear as purplish macules, papules, plaques, nodules, tumors. Histopathologic
   analysis reveals immunostain to type IV collagen. Therapy includes observation, cryotherapy, laser surgery, excisional surgery, radiation therapy or systemic chemotherapy. Anecdotal reports of remissions have
   been reported with foscarnet.
B. **Lymphoma cutis.** Skin is rarely involved, usually B cell in origin.
C. **Possible increased incidence of melanoma,** basal cell carcinoma, and
   squamous cell carcinoma
D. **Oral hairy leukoplakia.** Well-demarcated verrucous plaque with an irregular, corrugated, or hairy surface, most commonly on the lateral or inferior surface of the tongue, or on the buccal and soft palatal mucosa.
III. **Inflammatory Dermatitides**
A. **Seborrheic dermatitis, psoriasis, eczematous dermatitis, and folliculitis.** See Chapter 17 for treatment options. Avoid the use of methotrexate.
B. **Pruritus, prurigo, eosinophilic folliculitis.**
  1. Extremely common and extremely debilitating with 3 to 5 mm edem-
     atous, follicular papules, and pustules.
  2. Treatment is often unsatisfactory. Antihistamines, potent topical fluo-
     rinated corticosteroids (such as clobetasol propionate BID), photo-
     therapy with natural sunlight or UVB radiation.
C. **Cutaneous eruption of HIV.** Presents as erythematous non-pruritic macules soon after infection.

PREGNANCY IN AIDS

I. In a well-designed clinical trial of HIV-seropositive pregnant women with
    a CD4+ count >200, AZT that was given during pregnancy, intra-
    partum, and to the newborn for 6 weeks after birth significantly de-
    creased the vertical HIV transmission rate from 25% to 8% (a 67% re-
    duction). These women had no antiviral therapy before pregnancy and

no clinical indication for AZT. Follow-up testing at 6 months also showed no significant difference in CD4+ counts.

A. **To start AZT begin** with a dose of 100 mg 5 × PO QD at 14 to 34 weeks of gestation and continue throughout the remainder of the pregnancy. The side effects of AZT when given during the first trimester are unknown. In the ACTG 076 trial, the rates of congenital anomalies were equal in the treatment and control groups, an indication that AZT may not be teratogenic.

B. **IV AZT** during labor should be given as 2 mg/kg over 1 hour and then followed by a continuous infusion of 1 mg/kg/hour until delivery

C. **Recent clinical trials with lamivudine (3TC)** with and without AZT administered to women after 38 weeks of gestation have demonstrated good patient tolerance, no major side effects and no short term adverse effects on neonates.

II. Studies from Africa indicate that a single dose of **nevirapine** at the onset of labor and a second dose to the neonates within 72 hours of delivery yielded 50% decrease in transmission of HIV.

III. **HIV-seropositive women have a higher miscarriage rate.** In a prospective study, 124 HIV-seropositive women were followed over a 4-year period; 14 (11%) had spontaneous abortions with half of the miscarried fetuses testing positive (by culture) for HIV. HIV-seropositive women should be counseled about their options regarding pregnancy. Information about contraception, prenatal care, and abortion services should be provided.

IV. **Procedures that increase the likelihood of direct fetal exposure to maternal blood** should be minimized during the antepartum and intrapartum periods. Examples include amniocentesis, fetal scalp electrode placement, and fetal scalp pH measurements. **Although more data are needed,** C-sections may actually reduce the incidence of perinatal infection.

V. **Prophylaxis of opportunistic infections during pregnancy** HIV in pregnancy presents a special dilemma in which the health care provider must carefully weight the risks and benefits. Unfortunately, there are very few data in this area of medicine. Listed below are generally accepted guidelines.

A. Try to limit drug exposures during the first trimester, the most critical period for organogenesis.

B. PCP prophylaxis is important with CD4+ <200. Although animal studies have shown TMP-SMZ to be associated with cleft palate, retrospective human studies have shown no increased risk of congenital malformations. Aerosolized pentamidine and dapsone are believed to be safe during pregnancy; however, pyrimethamine should be used with caution.

C. Preventive therapy should be instituted in pregnant women who have a positive tuberculin skin test or who are exposed to persons with infectious tuberculosis. Treatment with isoniazid should be deferred until after the first trimester and, when started, should be given with pyridoxine 25 to 50 mg PO BID secondary to the risk of peripheral neuropathy. Experience with rifampin and rifabutin is limited.

11

HIV/AIDS

AIDS IN THE PEDIATRIC PATIENT

I. Perinatal transmission accounts for >85% of HIV infection in children in the United States. For infants who are born to HIV-seropositive mothers, AZT should be given for the first 6 weeks of life beginning 8 to 12 hours after birth. The AZT syrup is 2 mg/kg PO Q6h. Anemia (Hb <8 g/dl) should be corrected before the initiation of AZT treatment. There are several case reports of infants being "cured" of HIV with prompt perinatal AZT treatment. 3TC is an alternative; the dose is 2 mg/kg body weight PO BID. Breast-feeding should be discouraged. Additionally, all infants born to an HIV-positive mother should have PCP prophylaxis started at 4 to 6 weeks and continued until 12 months of age unless the child is proved to be HIV negative.

BIBLIOGRAPHY

Armstrong WS et al: Human immunodeficiency virus-associated fever of unknown origin: A study of 70 patients in the United States and review, *Clin Inf Dis* 28:41-345, 1999.

Berger JR: How to distinguish HIV dementia from progressive multifocal leukoencephalopathy, *HIV Newsline* 1(1):11-13, 1995.

Blanche S et al: Relation of the course of HIV infection in children to the severity of the disease in their mothers at delivery, *N Engl J Med* 330(5):308-812, 1994.

Bryson YJ et al: Clearance of HIV infection in a perinatally infected infant, *N Engl J Med* 332(13):833-838, 1995.

Carpenter CCJ et al: Antiretroviral therapy for HIV infection in 1998:Updated recommendations of the the International AIDS Society-USA panel, *JAMA* 280:78-86, 1998.

Center for Disease Control and Prevention: Public Health Service guidelines for the management of health-care worker exposures to HIV and recommendations for postexposure prophylaxis, *MMWR* 47(No. RR-7):1-33, 1998.

Center for Disease Control and Prevention: Public Health Service Task Force recommendations for the use of ARV drugs in pregnant women infected with HIV-1 for maternal health and reducing perinatal HIV-1 transmission in the United States, *MMWR* 47(No. RR-2):1-26, 1998.

Dale DC, Federman DD, editors: *Scientific American Medicine,* New York, 1999, Scientific American, Inc.

Dickover RE et al: Identification of levels of maternal HIV-1 RNA associated with risk of perinatal transmission: effect of maternal zidovudine treatment on viral load, *JAMA* 275(8):599-610, 1996.

Furrer HJ et al: Discontinuation of primary prophylaxis against *Pneumocystis carinii* pneumonia in HIV-1 infected adults treated with combination antiretroviral therapy, *N Engl J Med* 340(17):1301-1306, 1999.

Isada CM et al: *Infectious diseases handbook,* ed 3, 1999, Lexi-Comp Inc.

1999 IDSA/USPHS: Guidelines for the prevention of opportunistic infections in persons infected with HIV, *MMWR* 48(RR-10), 1999

Kahn ME et al: Cost effectiveness of single dose Nevirapine regimen for mothers and babies to decrease vertical transmission in sub-saharan Africa, *Lancet* 354(9181):803-809, 1999

Leinung MC et al: Induction of adrenal suppression by megestrol acetate in patients with AIDS, *Ann Intern Med* 122(11):843-845, 1995.

Martin DF et al: Oral Ganciclovir for patients with Cytomegalovirus retinitis treated with ganciclovir implant, *N Engl J Med* 340(14):1063-1070, 1999.

Medical News and Perspectives: New anti-HIV drugs and treatment strategies buoy AIDS researchers, *JAMA* 275(8):579-580, 1996.

MMWR 44(50):933, 1995.

Musoke GL et al: Intrapartum and neonatal single dose nevirapine compared with zidovudine for prevention of mother-to-child transmission of HIV-1 in Kampala, Uganda, *Lancet* 354(9181):795-802, 1999.

Power C et al: HIV Dementia Scale: a rapid screening test, *J Acquir Immune Defic Syndr Hum Retrovirol* 8(3):273-279, 1995.

Sanford JP: *Guide to antimicrobial therapy,* Dallas, 1999, Antimicrobial Therapy, Inc.

Schacker TW et al: Biological and virological characteristics of primary HIV infection, *Ann Intern Med* 128(8): 613-620, 1998

Whitcup SM: Ocular manifestations of AIDS, *JAMA* 275(2):142-150, 1996.

11

HIV/AIDS

PEDIATRICS

Heidi Koch
Mark A. Graber

NEWBORN NURSERY

I. **Normal Body Temperature.**
A. Observe and maintain a normal body temperature. Normal axillary temperature of a newborn infant is 36.7° to 37.4° C taken for at least 5 minutes. Hyperthermia or hypothermia warrants further investigation.
B. Rectal temperatures provide the only accurate noninvasive method of measuring temperature.
C. If hyperthermia, consider sepsis or intracranial bleed.
D. If hypothermia, consider sepsis, hypoglycemia, hypothyroidism, and heat loss caused by environmental conditions.

II. **Initial Gastrointestinal and Genitourinary Function.**
A. Approximately 70% of newborns pass meconium and urine in the first 12 hours of life, 25% in 24 hours, and the remainder by 2 days.
B. If meconium is delayed, look for meconium plug, sepsis, narcotic exposure, Hirschsprung's disease, hypothyroidism, cystic fibrosis, or imperforate anus.
C. If infant is anuric or oliguric, think about dehydration, sepsis, renal abnormalities, or obstruction.

III. **Monitor weight and head circumference.** Weight initially drops (not >10%) and is usually regained by 2 weeks. Head circumference may decrease or increase (not >1 cm) as a result of initial trauma or molding of labor, or both.

IV. **Red Reflex.** The pupil should be black on direct examination, and red when examined through an ophthalmoscope. If the red reflex looks pale or white, suspect retinoblastoma.

V. **Newborn Prophylaxis.**
A. **Eyes.** Erythromycin 0.5% ointment to prevent gonorrheal conjunctivitis or *Chlamydia trachomatis* ophthalmia neonatorum.
B. **Vitamin K.** 0.5 to 1 mg IM to prevent hemorrhagic disease. Avoid products containing benzyl alcohol because they can be toxic to the newborn.
C. **Hepatitis.**
   1. **For those born of a hepatitis B-negative mother.** Give hepatitis B vaccine 10 μg IM routinely at birth and at 1 and 6 months. Use thimerosal free vaccine (released in late 1999).
   2. **If mother hepatitis B positive (positive HBsAg).**
      a. Clean newborn of hepatitis BsAg-positive mother thoroughly (use alcohol).
      b. Give hepatitis B immune globulin 0.5 ml IM and hepatitis B vaccine 10 μg IM, ASAP.
      c. Repeat hepatitis B vaccine 10 μg IM at 1 and 6 months.
      d. Do a hepatitis B screen at 9 months; if negative, give fourth dose of vaccine; if positive, monitor for chronic active or carrier state.

D. **AIDS.** See Chapter 11 for information about diagnosis, treatment, and prophylaxis of the newborn born to an HIV-positive mother.

VI. **Bathing.** Once the body temperature is stabilized, the infant may be bathed with warm standing water. Avoid running water to avoid burns. Immersion above the umbilicus should be avoided until the umbilical stump has fallen off.

VII. **Umbilical Cord Care.** Keep dry. Apply an antiseptic agent such as triple dye (Brilliant Green, Crystal Violet, and proflavine hemisulfate) or alcohol to avoid colonization and infection with *Streptococcus, Staphylococcus,* and *Clostridium* species and coliforms. The cord generally separates by the end of the second week but may not do so until the third week of life. Delayed separation may be normal or may be attributable to sepsis or poorly functioning leukocytes.

VIII. **Screening Laboratory Tests.**

A. **Metabolic.** Should be done at 24 hours of age or later. Phenylketonuria, hypothyroidism, galactosemia, etc., as required by state law or indicated (such as cystic fibrosis if no meconium stool). If screening is done before 24 hours of age, it may miss some diseases, and screening should be repeated at 1 week to 10 days. Antibiotics may also interfere with screening, and screening should be repeated when patient is no longer using antibiotics. Newer tests obviate the need for repeat screening after antibiotics. Check your state's recommendations.

B. **Hematologic.** Hemoglobin and hematocrit at birth and at 12 months. Screening for glucose-6-phosphate dehydrogenase deficiency is best done when the infant is a couple of months of age. Sickle cell screening in blacks and thalassemia in those of Mediterranean descent will be detected on the hemoglobinopathy portion of the Neonatal Screen (some states may not have a hemoglobinopathy test)

C. **Urinary and meconium drug screening.** If there is maternal history of drug abuse or if a baby's clinical exam could be consistent with withdrawal.

D. **Glucose screening—screen all babies who are LGA, SGA, IDM, or any baby who has signs of possible hypoglycemia.** Repeat regularly until stable (>40 mg/dl). Warm the infant's heel, and draw capillary blood samples from the side of the heel using finger stick test strips for glucose. See section on hypoglycemia, below, for further information on diagnosis and management.

E. **Bilirubin.** Transcutaneous bilirubinometry should be used for screening suspect neonates for jaundice. If value is above 17 mg/dl, serum bilirubin should be measured. The transcutaneous jaundice meter is affected by factors such as gestational age, birth weight, and skin pigmentation.

F. **ABO incompatibility.** Perform blood type and direct Coombs' test (use cord blood) on every infant born to a mother with type O blood or those with Rh-negative mothers.

IX. **Neonatal Nutrition.** See section on pediatric wellness.

NEONATAL JAUNDICE

I. **Jaundice** is visible when a baby has a serum bilirubin level that exceeds 5 mg/dl. Generally jaundice is visible first on the head and progresses to the feet. It resolves with the opposite pattern, the feet clearing first.

II. **Physiologic Hyperbilirubinemia.**

A. Usually not present in first 24 hours.

B. Rarely increases by more than 5 mg/dl in 1 day.

C. Peaks at 48 to 72 hours in full-term infants and 4 to 5 days in the premature ones.

D. **Serum bilirubin does not exceed 13 mg/dl in the full-term infant and 15 mg/dl in the preterm infant.**
   1. Direct bilirubin fraction is generally <2 mg/dl.
   2. Physiologic jaundice disappears by 1 week in full-term infants and by 2 weeks in premature infants.

E. **Any infant that does not meet the above description has nonphysiologic hyperbilirubinemia and should be worked up.**

III. **Nonphysiologic Hyperbilirubinemia.**

A. Those with primarily elevated direct bilirubin. Direct bilirubin >15% of total and therefore conjugated by the liver.
   1. **Infections** including sepsis, perinatally acquired viral infections including hepatitis, and intrauterine viral infections (hepatitis B, TORCHS).
   2. **Metabolic abnormalities** including Rotor syndrome and Dubin-Johnson syndrome, alpha-1 antitrypsin deficiency, galactosemia, tyrosinosis, cystic fibrosis, hereditary fructose deficiency.
   3. **Anatomic abnormalities,** including biliary atresia and Alagille syndrome (ductopenia) and obstructions as with a choledochal cyst.
   4. **Cholestasis** from CVN/TPN, antibiotics (especially ceftriaxone).

B. Those with primarily elevated indirect bilirubin. Therefore not conjugated by liver. Two basic mechanisms:
   1. **From increased production of bilirubin (therefore hemolysis or hematoma breakdown).**
      a. **With positive direct Coombs' test (mother's antibodies on child's cells).** Isoimmunization (Rh, ABO, minor blood group), erythroblastosis fetalis.
      b. **With negative Coombs' test and RBC morphologic abnormalities.** Spherocytosis, thalassemias, G6PD deficiency, elliptocytosis, etc.
      c. **Extravascular blood.** Cephalohematoma, severe bruising, cerebral and pulmonary hemorrhage
      d. **DIC, other hemolytic anemia**
      e. Polycythemia resulting from delayed clamping of cord, twin-twin transfusion, maternal-fetal transfusion.
   2. **From delayed excretion of bilirubin.**
      a. **Inherited disorders** of bilirubin metabolism including Crigler-Najjar syndrome, Gilbert's disease, Dubin-Johnson syndrome, Rotor syndrome.
      b. **Hypothyroidism and prematurity.**

12

PEDIATRICS

IV. **Breast Milk Jaundice.**

A. **General.** One in every 200 infants has prolonged unconjugated hyper-bilirubinemia. Serum bilirubin may reach maximum concentration (15 to 25 mg/dl) during the second to third week. Etiology is unknown. However, one theory is that there is a component in breast milk which can interfere with bilirubin conjugation. Kernicterus has not been reported with breast milk jaundice.

B. **Diagnosis.** Requires the exclusion of all other causes of elevated unconjugated bilirubin in a breast-fed infant.

C. **Treatment options:** (1) Observe, (2) Discontinue breast feeding and substitute formula, (3) Alternate feedings of breast milk and formula, (4) Discontinue breast feeding and start phototherapy, and (5) Continue breast feeding and start phototherapy.

D. **Comment on therapy.** Although any treatment option is reasonable, it is believed that any interruption of breast feeding is undesirable unless very severe hyperbilirubinemia is present (TSB >25). Observe, and continue breast feeding while phototherapy is initiated.

V. **Treatment of hyperbilirubinemia from any cause. (Table 12-1).**

A. Treat the underlying disorder.

B. Ensure adequate hydration, caloric intake, stooling (bilirubin is excreted in stool).

C. **Prophylactic phototherapy.** Indicated for infants showing a rapid rise in bilirubin (>1 mg/dl per hour) and as a temporizing measure when one is contemplating exchange transfusion.

D. Conjugated bilirubin does not cause kernicterus.

TABLE 12-1

MANAGEMENT HYPERBILIRUBINEMIA IN THE HEALTHY TERM NEWBORN

Age (hrs)	Consider Phototherapy (mg/dl)*	Total Bilirubin, Phototherapy (mg/dl)	Exchange Transfusion If Phototherapy Fails†	Exchange Transfusion and Intense Phototherapy
<24‡	—	—	—	—
25-48	≥12	≥15	≥20	≥25
49-72	≥15	≥18	≥25	≥30
>72	≥17	≥20	≥25	≥30

Adapted from *Pediatr Rev* 19:3, March 1998.

*Phototherapy at these TSB levels is a clinical option, meaning that the intervention is available and may be used on the basis of individual clinical judgment.

†Intensive phototherapy should produce a decline of TSB of 1 to 2 mg/dl within 4 to 6 hours, and the TSB level should continue to fall and remain below the threshold level for exchange transfusion. If this does not occur, it is considered a failure of phototherapy.

‡Term infants who are clinically jaundiced at 24 hrs old are not considered healthy, require further evaluation, and may require phototherapy or exchange transfusion but **must** be evaluated for underlying illness.

NOTE: Recommendations of level of bilirubin requiring treatment varies by expert. This table is the most conservative and is based on total bilirubin.

E. **Phototherapy.** The number of banks of phototherapy lights used is determined by the infants total bilirubin level, the rate of rise of the total bilirubin, and the anticipated course of the underlying cause of the hyperbilirubinemia. Serum bilirubin usually decreases by 2.5 to 3 mg/dl per day and 1-2 mg/dl in first 4-6 hours of phototherapy. Bilirubin level should be followed every 12 hours. Phototherapy should be discontinued when the bilirubin reaches levels of about 13 mg/dl. Bilirubin levels should be rechecked again 12 hours after discontinuation, to assess for recurrence.

RESPIRATORY DISORDERS IN THE NEWBORN

I. Respiratory Distress Syndrome and Hyaline Membrane Disease.
A. **Characteristics.**
    1. **Most common in preterm infants** because of surfactant deficiency. Higher incidence with maternal diabetes, acute asphyxia, in second twin and meconium aspiration.
    2. **Prevention and diagnosis of preterm labor is paramount;** steroids can be used if delivery is imminent to hasten lung maturity (betamethasone or dexamethasone 12.5 mg IM Q24h for 48 hours). Resuscitate promptly at delivery.
B. **Clinical findings.**
    1. **Shortly after birth.** Tachypnea (respiratory rate >60), grunting, retractions, and cyanosis, flaring.
    2. **Radiographs.** Ground-glass reticulogranular appearance, air bronchograms.
C. **Treatment.**
    1. Rule out infection; use antibiotics as needed.
    2. **Respiratory support** (endotracheal intubation, mechanical ventilatory support) and metabolic support.
    3. **Exogenous surfactant** (doses differ by preparation) is very effective in treating hyaline membrane disease. Currently recommended drugs include Survanta, 4 cc/kg via endotracheal tube (ETT) Q6h for 4 doses or Exosurf, 5 cc/kg via ETT Q12h for 2-4 doses. Nitric oxide has also been used with some success. Pediatric consult suggested.
II. Transient Tachypnea of the Newborn.
A. **Characteristics.** Diagnosis of exclusion. More common in C-section deliveries and precipitous deliveries. Pathophysiology is the delayed clearance of lung fluid.
B. **Presentation.** Tachypnea, minimal respiratory distress.
C. **Radiographs.** Fluid in fissures, pleural effusion, streaky parenchymal changes.
D. **Management.** Short-term oxygen supplementation. This is a self-limited illness that will resolve spontaneously in 24 to 48 hours.
III. Meconium Aspiration Syndrome.
A. **Characteristics.**
    1. Caused by the presence of thick meconium in the distal airways, causing a valvelike mechanism that obstructs air movement.

2. Meconium aspiration can occur in a stressed neonate in utero or at the time of delivery. Deep fetal gasping causes the aspiration of the meconium-mixed amniotic fluid into the lungs.

B. **Radiographs.** Thick infiltrates, air entrapment, pneumothorax.

C. **Preventive management.** At the delivery of the head, the airway should be cleared by DeLee suctioning. Tracheal visualization and suctioning should then follow. If meconium is at or below the vocal cords, intubation must be repeatedly performed until suctioning returns clear fluid.

D. **Treatment.** Management is complex, and a neonatologist should be consulted. Treatment requires pulmonary support, as well as management of asphyxia-related effects on CNS, cardiovascular system, renal and GI systems. High-frequency ventilation, nitrous oxide, and ECMO are being used with good results. Small studies suggest that surfactant may also be helpful.

IV. **Spontaneous Pneumothorax.**

A. Spontaneous pneumothorax occurs in 1% to 2% of live births. Only symptomatic in 1>1500 live births.

B. When symptoms occur, they include tachypnea, minimal retractions, grunting, nasal flaring, cyanosis. May notice diminished air entry on affected side, shifting of cardiac impulse, muffled heart tones.

C. **Radiographs.** Pneumothorax seen on radiograph.

D. **Treatment.** Supportive, spontaneous resolution is common. If not resolving, consider chest tube or pneumocentesis with a needle.

V. **Bradycardia and Apnea Spells.**

A. **Types.** Bradycardia may be a primary cardiac event. The following refers **only** to noncardiogenic bradycardia and apnea spells. Neonates normally have 3 second pauses in respiratory effort (periodic breathing).

1. **Central.** No respiratory effort for 15 seconds because of arrest of respiratory drive. May have secondary bradycardia. May be secondary to CNS disorder.

2. **Obstructive.** Cessation of gas exchange in the lungs because of obstruction to air flow. May be infectious, functional (poor tone or coordination of pharyngeal muscles), or structural.

B. **Causes.** Prematurity, hypoxia, idiopathic, anatomic abnormalities (choanal atresia), maternal drugs (especially narcotics), infections, metabolic imbalances, temperature instability, seizures, hematologic, cardiovascular, genetic, and CNS disorders. GE reflux or trouble coordinating swallow and palate malformations can all contribute to apnea. In the older child consider breath-holding spells.

C. **Clinical characteristics, work-up, and treatment.**

1. **Document** the duration, frequency, state of consciousness, temporal relationship to feeding, sleep, stooling, seizure activity as well as obstetric history (such as maternal fever, meconium). Gestational age is especially important. Apnea and bradycardia from prematurity usually resolves by a corrected gestational age of 35 to 36 week

2. **Physical exam** should include temperature, BP, gestational age, eye position (as an indication of a CNS disorder), pupillary dilatation, muscle tone, dysmorphic features, respiratory effort, murmur, skin changes.

3. **Lab tests.** Blood glucose, electrolytes, differential CBC, drug levels, T_4, TSH, sepsis work-up, CXR, ABGs, head ultrasonogram (for CNS bleed), EEG.

D. **Treatment.**

1. **Apnea monitor and addressing underlying factor.** Teach CPR to parents and caregivers. Any individual spell will generally resolve with stimulation.

2. **Ventilatory support.** Consider low flow O_2, 3-5 cm of CPAP.

3. **For neonatal apnea.** Caffeine citrate 20 mg/kg PO or IV (10 mg caffeine/10 mg citrate) followed by 5-7 mg/kg QD started 24 hours after first dose. Maintain serum levels at 5 to 25 µg/ml. Theophylline has also been used, but caffeine is preferred. **Continue treatment for 5-7 days.** Observe in hospital off treatment for 5-7 days. If the patient has no further episodes of **neonatal apnea,** they may be discharged.

12

PEDIATRICS

NEONATAL INFECTIONS

I. **Thrush.** Oral candidiasis; peaks at 14 days of life.

A. **Clinically.** White plaques on erythematous base over oral mucosa, tongue.

B. **Treatment.** Nystatin suspension 100,000 to 200,000 U swabbed over affected areas QID for 7 days. Mycostatin cream to maternal areola and nipple if breast fed infant. Continue for 2-3 days after visual evidence of candida resolves.

II. **Neonatal Bacterial Sepsis.**

A. **General comments.** Neonatal bacterial sepsis is associated with 10% to 40% mortality and significant morbidity, especially neurologic sequelae of meningitis. Infants <1 month old are immunologically deficient and are predisposed to serious infections.

B. **Predisposing factors.** Premature rupture of membranes (>24 hours), premature labor, maternal fever, UTI, foul lochia, chorioamnionitis, IV catheters (in infant), intrapartum asphyxia, and intrauterine monitoring (pressure catheter or scalp electrode).

C. **Organisms.**

1. **Early infection (0 to 4 days of age).** Group B streptococci and *Escherichia coli* 60% to 70% of infections. Also *Listeria* (rare in United States), *Klebsiella, Enterococcus, Staphylococcus aureus* (uncommon), *Streptococcus pneumoniae,* group A streptococci.

2. **Late infection (>5 days of age).** *Staph. aureus,* group B streptococci, *E. coli, Klebsiella, Pseudomonas, Serratia, Staph. epidermidis, Haemophilus influenzae.*

D. **Signs and symptoms.** Presentation may be subtle; thus any febrile neonate (temp >38° C) must have a septic work-up. Fever may be absent; so watch for symptoms below.

1. **The presentation** may include irritability, vomiting, poor feeding, poor temperature control, lethargy, apneic spells, and hypoglycemia.
2. **May progress** to respiratory distress, poor perfusion, abdominal distension, jaundice, bleeding, petechiae, or seizures.
3. **Bulging fontanel** is a very late sign of neonatal meningitis, and Brudzinski's sign or Kernig's sign is rarely found.

E. **Work-up.**
   1. Includes LP for cell count, protein, glucose, and culture. Consider sending CSF for viral studies.
   2. UA, CBC (remember neutropenia or thrombocytopenia are also suggestive of infection) and repeat in 5 hours, CXR and C-reactive protein.
   3. Cultures of blood, urine, and any other site as indicated. Latex agglutination test for pneumococcus, *E. coli, H. influenzae,* group B streptococci, and meningococcus in blood, urine, and CSF is done even though the usefulness is questionable. Negative latex agglutination tests do not rule out infection, but positive results may help guide therapy.

F. **Associated lab findings.** Hypocalcemia, hypoglycemia, hyponatremia, and DIC.

G. **Treatment.**
   1. Should be tailored to age of onset, clinical setting, and initial findings.
   2. **There should be NO DELAY in antibiotic therapy.** Begin empiric therapy after cultures are obtained or before cultures if any delay is anticipated. There are isolates of *Streptococcus pneumoniae* that are resistant to penicillin and cephalosporins. As of 1997, the American Academy of Pediatrics recommends adding vancomycin with or without rifampin to these regimens when meningitis or pneumococcal sepsis is suspected until sensitivities are known. *Never use rifampin alone since resistance can rapidly develop.*
   3. **Empiric early (0 to 4 days old).** Ampicillin 50 mg/kg/day (100 mg/kg/day in meningitis) divided 12 hours IV and gentamicin 5 mg/kg/day divided 12 hours IV. **Or** cefotaxime 50mg/kg q 12 h + ampicillin as above (preferred by some authors). Ceftriaxone is an alternative to cefotaxime.
   4. **Empiric late (>5 days old).** Depends on cause (for example, methicillin-resistant *Staph. aureus* outbreak requires vancomycin). General guidelines include ampicillin 100 to 200 mg/kg/day divided Q6h plus cefotaxime 150 mg/kg/day IV Q8h), or ampicillin-gentamicin as above usually adequate. Ceftriaxone 100 mg/kg/day IV Q12h is an alternative to cefotaxime.
   5. **Repeat cultures in 24 to 48 hours.** In meningitis, repeat LP every day until clear.
   6. **Other.** Hemodynamic, respiratory, hematologic, metabolic, and nutritional support and surveillance are critical. Shock may require vol-

ume expansion; respiratory depression may require supplemental oxygen or artificial ventilation (see chapter 2, emergency medicine).

CONGENITAL INFECTIONS

I. **Maternal Diagnostic Screening.**

A. Screen early for antibody to rubella, syphilis, and hepatitis B.

B. Offer HIV testing to all pregnant women. Serologic tests as indicated for HSV, CMV, HIV. Viral cultures as indicated for HSV, rubella, CMV, enterovirus.

II. **Congenital Infections.** Congenital infections should be suspected in those infants who are premature or have IUGR, failure to thrive, hepatomegaly (elevated direct bilirubin), lethargy, thrombocytopenia, anemia, rashes, or seizures. See specific entities below.

III. **Laboratory Studies for Suspected Congenital Infections.**

A. **TORCHS** (*toxoplasmosis, rubella, cytomegalovirus, herpes simplex, syphilis*) titers on baby and mother (draw serum before any blood transfusion).

B. **Obtain IgM** antibodies from baby as well as acute and convalescent IgG titers from baby and mother. IgM does not cross the placenta and therefore indicates a reaction of the infant to infection.

C. **Viral cultures** (HSV, rubella, CMV, enterovirus). Culture of CSF or PCR may be useful in HSV.

D. Tzanck test of vesicles in HSV (infant or mother).

E. Urine cytology and culture for CMV.

F. Dark-field exam of lesions or umbilical cord scraping in syphilis.

G. Send placenta to pathology lab for culture and microscopy.

H. General lab screen including liver function tests, electrolytes, glucose, CBC, and clotting studies.

IV. **Specific Agents.**

A. **Toxoplasmosis.**

1. **Epidemiology.** Caused by *Toxoplasma gondii*. Fetus is infected by transplacental passage during maternal parasitemia. Infection occurs through ingestion of sporulated oocysts in cat feces or ingestion of poorly cooked meat. 50% of the infants born to mothers who seroconvert during pregnancy will become infected. Risk of congenital abnormalities low after 20 weeks gestation.

2. **Postnatal diagnosis.** Isolation of organism from placenta. ELISA to detect specific IgG and IgM; comparison with mother's serum is necessary, since maternal IgG will cross the placenta. PCR can also be used to make the diagnosis.

3. **Clinical findings.**

   a. Only 10% are symptomatic. Most of those who acquire toxoplasma in utero are asymptomatic.

   b. Maculopapular rash, generalized lymphadenopathy, hepatosplenomegaly, thrombocytopenia, signs of active central nervous system infection (such as CSF pleocytosis, CSF hypoglycemia, ele-

12

PEDIATRICS

vated CSF protein, and, in some instances, microcephaly, cerebral calcifications, seizures, and motor abnormalities), chorioretinitis, and pneumonitis. Infants with untreated congenital toxoplasmosis and generalized or neurologic abnormalities at presentation almost uniformly develop mental retardation, seizures, and spasticity.

4. **Prevention and treatment.**
   a. Avoid changing cat litter and eating raw and poorly cooked meat during pregnancy.
   b. A recent meta-analysis questions the efficacy of prenatal treatment of the mother in preventing adverse fetal outcomes (Wallon M - *BMJ* - 1999 Jun 5; 318(7197): 1511-4) However, some physicians choose to treat the mother prenatally with spiramycin (available from the FDA). If documented fetal infection is noted in the prenatal period (via amniotic PCR), consider treatment with pyrimethamine and sulfadiazine.
   c. Treat infant for clinically, serologically, or maternally apparent disease with pyrimethamine and sulfadiazine for 1 year. Folinic acid should be given to prevent bone marrow suppression. A year of treatment allows the infant to become immunocompetent and will reduce neurologic sequelae compared to a shorter course of treatment. A pediatric infectious disease (ID) consultation should be obtained.
   d. Corticosteroid for ocular disease and CNS infection (high level of CSF protein), add prednisone 1mg/kg/d divided q 12 hours until CSF protein is normal and/or ocular inflammation resolves.

B. **Cytomegalovirus (CMV).**
   1. **Epidemiology.**
      a. Most common congenital infection (up to 2.5% incidence) with 95% asymptomatic.
      b. Vertical transmission (from maternal primary or reactivated disease) may be acquired transplacentally or at birth in the genital tract. CMV may also be acquired postnatally by ingestion of CMV-positive breast milk. Infected infants are contagious.
   2. **Clinical findings.**
      a. Sensorineural deafness, mental retardation
      b. "Cytomegalic inclusion disease" with jaundice, hepatosplenomegaly, petechial-purpuric rash, microcephaly, and cerebral calcifications.
   3. **Diagnostic tests.** Virus isolated from urine, pharynx, WBC, CSF, human milk, cervical secretions. CMV-IgM titers. PCR has been used to detect virus as well.
   4. **Treatment.** Evidence suggests that ganciclovir given postnatally may reduce incidence of retardation and other sequelae (but efficacy limited). Consider a pediatric infectious disease or neurology consultation.

C. **Herpes simplex.**
   1. **Epidemiology.** Mostly HSV type 2 transmission occurs at birth through direct contact (5% transmission in recurrent lesion, 50% in primary). Probably 20% or more of women have had HSV-2 and carry the virus. Many women are asymptomatic shedders at the time of delivery, and these account for most of the neonatal infections.
   2. **Clinical findings.**
      a. Average incubation 6 days; can be up to 20.
      b. Disseminated disease may mimic fulminate sepsis with seizures, jaundice, hepatitis, encephalitis, DIC, or pneumonia. If untreated, up to 90% mortality.
      c. Local mucocutaneous disease may be mild. Conjunctivitis, keratitis, or chorioretinitis can result in vision loss and blindness.
   3. **Prevention and treatment.**
      a. Any active lesions during pregnancy should be cultured to confirm disease. Active disease at delivery mandates C-section. Routine use of PCR to identify asymptomatic shedders is not yet standard of care.
      b. If vaginal delivery occurs over active lesions or ROM >4 hours, begin acyclovir 30 mg/kg/day IV Q8h for 14 days. Infected mother and infant should be kept in contact isolation.

D. **Rubella.**
   1. **Epidemiology.** Non-vaccinated or rubella-susceptible mother acquires infection while pregnant. Teratogenicity is the greatest in the first trimester, less in second, none in third. Infants may be contagious.
   2. **Presentation.** Retinopathy, cataracts, patent ductus arteriosus, pulmonary artery stenosis, deafness, thrombocytopenia with "blueberry-muffin" skin lesions.
   3. **Treatment.** Supportive only. Immunize children and nonpregnant women of childbearing age. Immune globulin given to mother does not prevent prenatal infection.

E. **Parvovirus B19 (Fifth disease/Erythema infectiosum)**
   1. **Epidemiology.** Transmission from mother infected during pregnancy in ¼ to ⅓ of cases. Second trimester fetus particularly vulnerable.
   2. **Presentation.** Hemolytic anemia or aplastic anemia with hydrops secondary to high output CHF or myocarditis. Generally, if the pregnancy continues to term, the resulting infant is healthy.
   3. **Treatment.** Weekly ultrasound of mother following documented infection looking for evidence of hydrops for 10-12 weeks. Intrauterine transfusions have been used with success.
   4. **Prevention.** Since most pregnant women have had inapparent infection and because of the low risk to the fetus, routine exclusion from schools, day care, etc., is not recommended for pregnant women. Additionally, patients who manifest symptoms are no longer infectious.

F. **Syphilis.**
   1. **Epidemiology.** High probability that infected mother will transmit the disease. Treponemes cross placenta in all trimesters.
   2. **Presentation.**
      a. 50% asymptomatic. Clinical picture can be benign to fatal.
      b. Findings include SGA, jaundice, recurring rashes, anemia, hepatosplenomegaly, "snuffles" (a serous rhinitis), meningitis, condylomata lata, osteochondritis usually of humerus or of tibia.
   3. **Diagnosis and treatment.**
      a. Suspect strongly in infants of mothers who are seropositive and (1) are untreated or inadequately treated, (2) had no decrease in antibody titers after treatment, (3) had poor follow-up during pregnancy, etc.
      b. Evaluate with physical exam, VDRL, RPR, FTA-ABS, CSF analysis, dark-field microscopy of fluids of vesicular lesions or of condylomata lata, long bone radiographs.
      c. **Treat if there is** a fourfold greater titer of antibody in the infant than in the mother, abnormal CSF (reactive VDRL, cells in the CSF, elevated CSF protein), evidence of active disease by exam (such as rash) or radiologic evidence of disease.
      d. **Treatment.** Procaine penicillin G 50,000 units/kg IM QD × 14 days or aqueous penicillin G 50,000 units/kg IV Q8-12h × 14 days.
      e. **Follow-up titers.** At 1, 2, 3, 6, 12 months to ensure that they are falling. Titer should revert to negative at 6 months. HIV testing should be considered.
G. **HIV.** See treatment of newborn and Chapter 11.
H. **Enterovirus.**
   1. **Characteristics.** Enteroviruses (coxsackie virus, hepatitis A virus, echovirus, poliovirus) are prevalent during warmer months and in transplacentally or during the postpartum period.
   2. **Treatment.** Supportive measures for enterovirus infection. Hepatitis A immunoglobulin 0.5 ml at birth if appropriate.
I. **Gonorrhea and chlamydia.**
   1. **Prevention.** Diagnosis and treatment of maternal GC and chlamydial infections will prevent most neonatal infections. Both infections are transmitted intrapartum by direct contact. Culture the mother's endocervix initially and at 36 weeks if indicated.
   2. **Clinical findings.** Both can cause conjunctivitis at 2 to 12 days. Obtain chlamydial, viral, and bacterial cultures of any purulent conjunctival discharge with Gram stain and Giemsa stain of conjunctival scraping for *Chlamydia*. For documented disease obtain blood and CSF cultures and treat for systemic disease.
   3. **Disseminated gonorrhea** typically involves arthritis and meningitis. Treat all infants of culture-positive mothers with a single dose of ceftriaxone 50 mg/kg IM (maximum of 125 mg). If evidence of disease or positive culture of blood or CSF, then ceftriaxone 25 to 50 mg/kg/day

single IM × 7 to 10 days (75 mg/kg/day × 10 to 14 days for meningitis).

4. *Chlamydia* may produce pneumonia at about 3 weeks with the insidious onset of tachypnea, cough, and no fever. Conjunctivitis is often present. Interstitial infiltrate and hyperinflation may be present on CXR. Diagnose *Chlamydia* with nasopharyngeal culture or seropositivity. Topical treatment has minimal efficacy even for isolated conjunctival disease because of colonization of other sites. Treat with oral erythromycin 40 to 50 mg/kg/day Q6h × 2 to 3 weeks. Trials with azithromycin are currently underway.

NEONATAL HEMATOLOGIC DISORDERS

12

PEDIATRICS

I. **Polycythemia.** Hyperviscous blood from increased HCT, which can cause stasis resulting in venous congestion or thrombosis. Increased incidence with IUGR, Down syndrome and other chromosomal abnormalities, congenital hypothyroidism or congenital adrenal hyperplasia, diabetic mothers, or heavy smokers. May also be response to chronic in utero hypoxia with secondary increase in RBC mass. Finally, it may be caused by increased blood volume from cord milking or twin-to-twin transfusion.

A. **Clinical diagnosis.** Usually presents by 2 to 72 hours with plethora, acrocyanosis, poor peripheral perfusion, respiratory distress or irritability. May be confused with cyanotic congenital heart disease, hypoglycemia, seizures.

B. **Lab diagnosis.** Venous HCT >65% (capillary is usually 4% to 7% higher); thrombocytopenia may occur.

C. **Complications.** Majority do well; stroke is usually the only lasting complication, but there can be CHF, oliguria, gangrene, or necrotizing enterocolitis.

D. **Treatment.**
   1. Observe if HCT 65% to 70% and asymptomatic.
   2. If HCT >70% or symptomatic, then partial exchange transfusion through umbilical vein using FFP or 5% albumin in saline with volume of exchange =

$$\frac{(90 \times \text{Weight in kg}) \times (\text{Measured HCT} - 50)}{\text{Measured HCT}}$$

   3. **Do not merely phlebotomize!** This can cause shock and worsen the situation. Watch for hypoglycemia or hypocalcemia.

NEONATAL METABOLIC DISORDERS

I. **Hypoglycemia** Defined as serum glucose <40 mg/dl at term, <30 mg/dl premature. Use a level of 40 mg/dl to begin looking for cause and treating.

A. **Causes.** Neonatal gluconeogenesis is underdeveloped and is easily disrupted. Be aware of hypoglycemia in small-for-gestational-age and postdate infants and infants with a history of asphyxia, hypothermia, sepsis, prematurity, hypermetabolism (such as erythroblastosis), if mother diabetic (hyperinsulinism) or maternal ingestion of oral hypoglycemics or of beta-agonists. May also be secondary to sepsis.

B. **Diagnosis.** Have a high index of suspicion. Clinical signs: pale, cool, irritable, jittery, poor feeding, apnea, seizures, or may be asymptomatic. Routinely screen as described in the "newborn nursery" section above and recheck if any clinical suspicion of hypoglycemia.

C. **Treatment** should be given for 48 hours before tapering with frequent monitoring as follows:

1. **Stable and >34 weeks, blood glucose >30 mg/dl:** 15 to 30 ml D_5W PO or IV and then advance to breast feeding or formula. Check glucose Q2-3h until 3 normal.

2. **Unstable, <34 weeks or blood glucose <30 mg/dl:** $D_{10}W$ 5 ml/kg or $D_{25}W$ 2 ml/kg IV over 10 minutes and then 2 to 4 ml/kg/hour IV. Advance to PO while continuing IV, follow serial glucose level and taper off IV.

3. If no IV access attainable, glucagon 0.1 mg/kg IM SQ IV for <10 kg (up to 1 mg) Q30 min will raise glucose for 2 to 3 hours but depletes glycogen stores and is not effective when stores are not present (such as SGA). NG feeding is another option.

II. **Hypocalcemia.** Serum calcium <8 mg/dl associated with asphyxia, SGA, premature infant, or diabetic mother. Usually is transient.

A. **Diagnosis.** Hypotonia, apnea, poor feeding, jitters, seizures, serum calcium <8 mg/dl.

B. **Treatment.** Usually resolves in a couple of days; no need to treat asymptomatic infant.

1. **If asymptomatic and wish to treat.** Give 5 to 10 ml/kg/24h of 10% solution of **calcium gluconate** either PO in feedings or by continuous IV over 24 hours.

2. **If symptomatic.** Give 1.0 to 1.5 ml/kg of **calcium gluconate** 10% IV with a maximum of 5 ml in premature infants or 10 ml in a full-term infant. Should get a maximum of 1 ml/min. Can repeat if still symptomatic and then initiate treatment as in (1) above.

3. Consider low magnesium level or congenital hypoparathyroidism if persistent.

III. **Neonatal-Withdrawal Syndrome.** Passive addiction of drugs by maternal use. Estimated 10% of urban births. Narcotics, and stimulants (such as cocaine) most common. These infants have an increased risk of SIDS.

A. **Diagnosis.**

1. **Narcotics.** Jittery, irritable, large appetite, vomiting, hypertonicity, and sneezing. Usually presents within first 72 hours of life.

2. **Cocaine.** Lethargy, hypotonia, and poor feeding. Look for IUGR and cerebral infarctions. Usually presents within the first 72 hours.

3. **Methadone.** Poor feeding, seizures, irritability. Presents at 2 to 4 weeks of life.

B. **Treatment.** For all, swaddling and frequent high caloric feedings are helpful. Neonatal Narcotic Abstinence Scales are available. These scales provide an objective system that helps you determine when pharmacologic treatment is necessary. For narcotics use tincture of opium (10 mg/ml morphine) diluted 1:25 in water, 2 drops/kg Q4-6h to control symptoms, monitor closely. Alternatively, may use phenobarbital 5 mg/kg/day divided Q8 or 12 hours IV, IM, or PO. Taper either regiment gradually over 1 to 3 weeks.

NEONATAL GASTROINTESTINAL DISORDERS

I. **Vomiting and Regurgitation.** See section on vomiting, diarrhea, and dehydration later in chapter for additional discussion.

A. **General Comments.** Regurgitation of the first few feedings is common. 80% infants <3 months of age regurgitate formula at least once a day. Bilious vomiting usually represents a surgical cause of obstruction.

B. **Cause.**
   1. **Nonbilious.** Benign overfeeding, gastroenteritis, reflux, necrotizing enterocolitis, CNS lesion with increased intracranial pressure, pyloric stenosis, metabolic or electrolyte disorders, drugs, sepsis, other entities discussed elsewhere.
   2. **Bilious.** Malrotation with or without a volvulus, atresia, stenosis, or other congenial anomalies.

C. **Evaluation.**
   1. **History.** In infants need to determine how much is being fed (overfeeding), relation to position (reflux), choking or coughing with feeding (achalasia, tracheoesophageal fistula), timing of emesis in relationship to feeds.
   2. **Exam and lab tests.** Evaluate state of hydration (see section on dehydration later in chapter). Look for site of infection. Abdominal and rectal exam for obstruction or imperforate anus. Radiologic studies as indicated, including Gastrografin if indicated.
      a. If child less than 2 months, **consider ultrasonography for pyloric stenosis** if the history or exam is compelling. Gastrografin study is alternative.
      b. If neonatal, consider congenital abnormalities such as duodenal or esophageal atresia, Hirschsprung's disease, volvulus, malformation.
      c. **Reye's syndrome.** Generally occurs after viral illness and presents with intractable vomiting, elevated liver enzymes, decreased mental status, prolonged PT, and elevated serum ammonia. See section on vomiting.
      d. Consider elevated intracranial pressure as a cause of isolated vomiting.
   3. **Treatment.** See dehydration section. Also consider antiemetics such as promethazine or trimethobenzamide if cause is benign. If there is bilious vomiting it could be a surgical emergency. Make infant NPO,

12

PEDIATRICS

place a nasogastric tube to suction, obtain abdominal films and consult pediatric surgery.

I. **Meconium Plug Syndrome**

A. **General comments.** Obstruction of the colon with meconium or mucus. More common in premature, infants of diabetic mothers, acute illness. Can be early presentation of cystic fibrosis or Hirschsprung's disease.

B. **Signs and symptoms.** Difficulty passing stools, normal rectal exam.

C. **Management.** Rectal stimulation with digital exam or glycerin suppository. See constipation section.

II. **Necrotizing Enterocolitis**

A. **Causes.** Unclear, more common in premature babies (80%), SGA, maternal preeclampsia, cyanosis, exchange transfusions, umbilical catheterization, polycythemia. Precipitated by enteral feeding, ischemia, and bacteria.

B. **Prognosis.** Mortality of 20% to 40%.

C. **Signs and symptoms.** Baby has abdominal distension, lethargy, bloody stools, ileus, vomiting. It can progress to DIC, apnea, shock, perforation. Onset may be gradual or fulminant.

D. **Diagnosis.** Abdominal radiograph will show distended loops of bowel, air fluid levels, pneumatosis intestinalis, free air. Requires full sepsis work-up including stool and CSF cultures, CBC, electrolytes, and enzymes. INR/PTT, ABG, etc.

E. **Treatment.** (Surgical consult recommended).
1. NPO, nasogastric tube to suction, IV fluids.
2. Supportive treatment of acidosis, shock.
3. Surgery indicated if perforation, peritonitis, acidosis.
4. Begin broad-spectrum antibiotics (such as ampicillin and gentamicin) after cultures done. If resistant organisms known in hospital, cover with other antibiotics as required.

FEEDING AND SUPPLEMENTATIONS

I. **Breast Feeding**

A. **Breast feeding should be recommended to all pregnant and postpartum mothers** (except those who are HIV positive) and should provide adequate nutrition for the first 5 to 9 months. Human colostrum immediately after delivery is the optimal first feeding. Normal, term babies are born fully hydrated, and supplementation of the first breast feeding is not required.

B. **Information and encouragement** must be provided. References such as those to the local chapter of La Leche League may prove to be valuable.

C. **Feeding on demand** should be encouraged, with recognition that there is a large variety in normal feeding patterns. Typically, infant feeding intervals average every 2 to 3 hours in the first few weeks. Newborns should not go longer than 4 to 5 hours between feedings.

D. **The supply of breast milk** is adequate if the infant is satisfied after each nursing period, has 6 to 8 wet diapers a day, sleeps 2- to 4-hour intervals, and gains weight according to the growth chart.

E. **Attention to sore nipples** should be provided early before severe pain with cracking and abrasions occur. Exposing nipples to air and varying the infant feeding position are recommended; avoid drying soaps. Check the infant for thrush and treat both mother's nipples and infant if present.

F. **Engorgement** can be very uncomfortable for the mother. The mother should be encouraged to nurse or pump often, every 2 to 3 hours. If engorgement is severe, it can cause difficulty with the infant latching on. In this case, recommend manual expression before feeding.

G. **Maternal fatigue** and psychosocial factors should be addressed. Mothers should be encouraged to sleep when their infant sleeps.

H. **Mastitis.** Mastitis is an infection of the breast usually secondary to a blocked milk duct.

   1. **Exam.** Reveals a hot, swollen, tender, and erythematous breast; mastitis is most commonly secondary to *Staphylococcus aureus*.

   2. **Treatment.**

      a. Treatment is by use of antistaphylococcal antibiotics such as dicloxacillin, erythromycin, or amoxicillin-clavulanate. Mastitis can usually be treated in an outpatient setting. However, if patient has fever or looks ill, consider admission for IV antibiotics.

      b. The mother should continue to breast feed or use a breast pump. This is critical and will help resolve the infection.

      c. Local care including hot packs may be helpful.

I. **Drugs and breast milk.** Drugs concentrated in breast milk tend to be weak bases (such as metronidazole, antihistamines, erythromycin, or antipsychotics and antidepressants). Check the breast-feeding recommendations of every drug before approving its use in the nursing mother.

J. **Failure to thrive in the breast-fed infant.**

   1. **Infant causes** include inadequate intake or increased caloric need.

   2. **Maternal causes** include poor milk production because of inadequate diet (especially fluids), illness and fatigue, or poor letdown because of smoking, drugs, or psychologic reasons.

II. **Formula Feeding**

A. Recent data indicate that a linkage of formula feeding with an increase in IDDM is doubtful.

B. **In cases of preference or inability to breast feed,** commercial infant formulas are able to provide adequate nutrition. Most are cow's milk based and contain lactose. Lactose-free soybean-based formulas are available for infants with primary lactase deficiency (watery, guaiac-negative stools, gas), galactosemia, secondary lactase deficiency from GI insult (such as from viral gastroenteritis), and cow's milk protein allergy (generally have diarrhea with blood and failure to thrive). However, remember that some children who are allergic to cow milk protein will also be allergic to soy protein.

C. Most formulas contain 20 kcal/oz, osmolality of 300 to 400 mOsm, and calorie breakdown of 7.2% to 18% protein, 30% to 54% fat, and 40% to 50% carbohydrate.

D. An on-demand schedule of feeding should be encouraged. Most newborns will typically take 2 to 3 ounces every 2 to 3 hours and should not be allowed to go greater than 5 hours between feedings. It is important to inform the parents to avoid overfeeding by being aware of satiety clues from the infant.

E. Reflux or occasional diarrhea are not in themselves indications for switching formula.

III. **Dietary Advancement**

A. **Solids** may begin to be added between months 4 and 6, typically occurring when the infant's hunger is no longer satisfied by milk alone or it is convenient in the family's schedule. Infants should have considerable head control before any solid foods are introduced.

1. **New foods** should generally be introduced at the rate of one new food every 5-7 days. In this manner, if an infant has an allergic reaction to a food it will be easier to identify which food is the culprit.

2. **Generally, cereal is started first,** followed by fruits and vegetables and then meats. Infants typically show an interest in self-feeding at 6 to 8 months of age. Zwieback toast and crackers are typically offered first. A spoon can typically be introduced between 10 and 12 months. By the end of the second year of life, infants should not require assistance.

3. The introduction of cow's milk should be delayed until 12 months of age. Cow's milk given as primary food source before 12 months of age is associated with an increased incidence of iron-deficiency anemia believed to be secondary to occult GI blood loss.

IV. **Toddler Feeding.** Toddlers typically eat three meals as well as one or two snacks a day. Many toddlers will resist eating certain foods or insist on eating one or two favorite foods for long periods of time. It is advisable to avoid struggles and offer a variety of foods and leave the choices to the child. Vitamin supplements are rarely necessary. Toddlers typically have varying appetites. They will eat well at some meals and hardly eat anything at other meals. This is to be expected.

VI. **Vitamin Supplementation**

A. **Iron.**

1. Iron supplementation in breast-fed infants is indicated for infants not receiving formula supplementation between 4 and 6 months of age.

TABLE 12-2

RECOMMENDED SUPPLEMENTAL FLUORIDE DOSAGE SCHEDULE (IN MG/DAY)

	Parts Per Million of Fluoride in Water Supply		
Age of child (years)	<0.3	0.3 to 0.7	>0.7
Birth to 2*	0.25	0	0
2 to 3	0.50	0.25	0
3 to 13*	1.00	0.50	0

*Recommended by the Council on Dental Therapeutics of the American Dental Association and the Committee on Nutrition of the American Academy of Pediatrics. The American Academy of Pediatrics recommends providing supplementation from 2 weeks of age through at least 16 years of age.

12

PEDIATRICS

2. Ferrous sulfate drops may be added at a dose of 1 to 2 mg/kg/day. An alternative is iron-fortified cereals, particularly when mixed with juice, since the vitamin C enhances iron absorption.
3. Premature infants should have supplementation with ferrous sulfate drops at a dose of 2 mg/kg/day at 2 months of age.
4. Bottle-fed infants should use an iron-fortified formula throughout the first year of life. Constipation should not be an indication to switch to a low-iron formula because there is no evidence that there is a causal relationship.

B. **Vitamin D.** Vitamin D is needed only when the breast-fed infant's mother's diet is deficient or the infant has limited sun exposure.

C. **Vitamin B_{12}** Be aware of vitamin B_{12} deficiency in the children of strict vegetarian mothers.

D. **Fluoride.**
   1. Dietary fluoride supplements are recommended by the American Academy of Pediatrics and American Dental Association for infants and young children without access to optimally fluoridated water. The following dosage schedule based on age and water fluoride level has been recommended since 1979 (Table 12-2).
   2. Although a new dosage schedule and guidelines have not been agreed upon, there now is a general consensus that breast-fed infants in areas with fluoridated water usually do not need fluoride supplementation, in part because very few infants are exclusively breast fed for extended periods of time.

PEDIATRIC WELLNESS

I. **Immunizations**

A. The measles-mumps-rubella (MMR) vaccine is safe in those with egg allergies and should not be withheld in this group.

B. **Recommended vaccinations. See Figure 23-10 for a schedule of recommended childhood immunizations.** An afebrile URI is not a contraindication to vaccination. Antibody conversion rates are the same in this population as in the well population.

C. **If a patient misses a vaccination,** start up where the patient left off. For example, if a patient had a diphtheria-pertussis-tetanus (DPT) vaccine at 2 months but missed subsequent doses and shows up at 2 years of age, start at what would have been the fourth-month dose and continue the series from there. Therefore, the patient would get a fourth-month, sixth-month, fifteenth-month, and 4- to 6-year dose for a total of 5 doses by 6 years of age.

E. **Immunization side effects.**
  1. **DTP vaccine.** Local reaction common with erythema, tenderness, swelling. Mild systemic symptoms may occur, including low-grade fever, listlessness. Few children develop high fever. The relationship between DPT vaccine and neurologic symptoms has not been substantiated when cases are looked at critically. In any case, the acellular pertussis vaccine should allay any fears.
  2. **MMR vaccine.** May have local reaction. Fever may occur and may be delayed with onset between 5 and 7 days. A morbilliform rash may occur at the same time.
  3. **Haemophilus influenzae vaccine.** Minimal reaction including local reaction and low-grade fever.
  4. **Poliomyelitis vaccine.** Adults may develop polio if given oral immunization, as may the immunosuppressed. For this reason, the IM (killed virus) polio vaccine is now recommended for all patients.

II. **Growth and Development**

A. **The caloric requirements** for full-term infants are 80 to 120 kcal/kg/day for the first few months of life and 100 kcal/kg to the twelfth month of life. There is significant individual variation.

B. The newborn infant can be expected to lose up to 10%-15% of body weight in the neonatal period. The birth weight should be regained by 10-14 days of life. The full-term infant generally doubles its birth weight by 4 months of age and triples it by 1 year.

C. **Fontanelles and sutures.** Principle sutures should fuse by fifth to sixth month. Premature closure is termed *craniosynostosis* and may lead to neurologic abnormalities. Lateral fontanelle closes by week 6 of life and posterior by 4 months of age. Anterior fontanelle should start to shrink after 6 months of life and closes by 9 to 16 months.

D. **Sinuses.** Maxillary and ethmoid sinuses present at birth and enlarge during childhood. Sphenoid sinuses develop by 1 to 2 years and continue to enlarge during childhood, frontal sinuses by 2 to 6 years.

E. See Figures 23-4 to 23-7 for growth charts.

III. **Developmental Screening. See Table 23-4.**

IV. **Developmental Milestones. See Table 23-4.**

V. **Pediatrics: Failure to Thrive**

A. **General Comments** Failure to thrive is a general term used to describe a child who is failing to maintain growth above the third percentile for weight or height. Typically weight for height is the first parameter affected and later height and head circumference are affected. Psychosocial and parental are the most common causes, but many disease states can also prevent adequate growth. There are three major patterns of inadequate growth when one is comparing age to height, weight, and head circumference.

B. **Decreased weight in proportion to height with a normal head circumference** is the pattern most commonly seen. In the majority of these cases, there is inadequate caloric intake for social, economic, or physical reasons. Malabsorption and metabolic abnormalities can also be the cause.

C. **A moderate decrease in weight compared to height with a normal or enlarged head circumference** can signal a structural dystrophy, endocrine disorder, or other congenital reason for low weight and short stature.

D. **Small head circumference with low weight for height** may indicate a CNS defect or IUGR.

E. Evaluation
   1. **A thorough history and physical exam** focusing on diet, feedings, mother-child interaction, signs of neglect, signs of physical abuse, or obvious physical illness such as diarrhea or chronic infection; a complete calorie count should be done.
   2. **Initial screening lab tests** include CBC, UA, electrolytes, sedimentation rate, serum glucose, stool for ova and parasites and for guaiac test. Depending on the clinical situation, serum lead levels, thyroid functions, and evaluation for adrenal disease may be important.
   3. **The hallmark of evaluation** is a period of time (1 to 2 weeks) under careful observation, with appropriate physical stimulation and adequate caloric intake while growth parameters are being monitored. This typically requires hospitalization but may be accomplished elsewhere if close observation with objective data collection is possible. Usually this cannot be accomplished at home. **To determine dietary need:** Caloric requirements = 120 kcal/kg (actual weight)/day × (Ideal weight/Actual weight). This is an approximation of calories required for catch-up growth. Consulting a dietitian may be helpful. An approach to evaluating a period of observation is found in Table 12-3.

12

PEDIATRICS

SHORT STATURE

I. **Definition.** Subnormal height (usually less than third to fifth percentile) relative to other children of the same sex, age, and ethnicity. This contrasts with growth failure, which is a slow rate of growth irrespective of stature.

II. **Short Stature should be defined with parents' height being taken into account.** If the child is on the growth curve to reach projected height based on parents' heights, it is not considered short stature.

TABLE 12-3

POSSIBLE APPROACHES FOR FAILURE TO THRIVE

Adequate Intake?	Weight Gain?	Most Likely Diagnoses	Treatment Plan
Yes	Yes	1. Feeding problem.	1. Counseling and information
		2. Neglect	
		3. Inability to purchase food	2. Social services help
Yes	No	1. Malabsorption, cystic fibrosis, celiac sprue, parasitic infection, milk allergy	1. Stool: Culture O & P, pH, reducing substances, 72-hour stool fat, D-xylose test
		2. Hypermetabolic, chronic infection, malignancy, hyperthyroid	2. Thyroid function tests, CBC, sedimentation rate, C-reactive protein, liver function tests
		3. Metabolic dysfunction, renal acidosis, hypercalcemia, diabetes, others such as inborn errors of metabolism	3. Serum pH, electrolytes, glucose, calcium, UA
No	No	1. Sucking or swallowing difficulties caused by neurologic disease, congenital anomaly	If nonorganic cause is definitely ruled out, begin to do further work-up and obtain appropriate consultation
		2. Regurgitation: GI obstruction (such as pyloric stenosis), CSF pressure elevation, chronic metabolic disease	1. *Neurologic work-up:* Head CT, consultation
			2. *GI work-up:* Barium swallow, consultation; *Endocrine work-up:* TSH, T_4, etc.

A. **For girls. Approximate** projected adult height = (Mother's height + [Father's height − 5″])/2

B. **For boys. Approximate** projected adult height = ([Mother's height + 5″] + Father's height)/2

III. **Causes.** May be a variation of normal (familial or constitutional); endocrine disorders including growth hormone deficiency, diabetes, and hypothyroidism; skeletal dysplasias; genetic syndromes including Turner's syndrome and Prader-Willi syndrome; malnutrition; chronic disease; lysosomal storage disorders; and psychosocial deprivation. Precocious puberty or elevated levels of androgens and estrogens will prematurely mature bones causing epiphyseal closure and short stature.

IV. **History.** Should include a family history (parental heights, relatives with short stature, genetic syndromes), perinatal insults, hypopituitarism, social and nutritional components. Review of systems should include respiratory and gastrointestinal systems.

V. **Physical Exam.** Should include examination of sexual development, nutritional status, disproportionate body segments (seen in chondromalacias), and observation for stigmata of genetic syndromes.

VI. **Laboratory Tests.** Should be considered in those more than 3 standard deviations below the mean and whose history and physical do not reveal a cause. Consider CBC for evidence of anemia, inflammation, infection, malignancy, and bone marrow suppression; electrolytes, BUN, UA to assess renal status; ESR to screen for inflammatory bowel disease and other chronic inflammatory disorders; karyotype, particularly in girls to evaluate for Turner's syndrome; thyroid studies and calcium, phosphorus, and alkaline phosphatase to screen for rickets.

VII. **To Assess Growth Hormone.** Draw insulin-like growth factor I and II (IGF-I, IGF-II) and IGF-binding protein (IGF-BP). Additional studies may include insulin infusion and induced hypoglycemia, which should lead to an increase in serum growth hormone if system is functioning properly. This test should generally be done under the supervision of an endocrinologist.

VIII. **Hand and Wrist Radiographs to determine bone age.** Delay is seen in hypopituitarism, constitutional delay, chronic disease, Turner's syndrome, and hypothyroidism. It may also be delayed in psychosocial dwarfism, gonadal dysgenesis, and primordial dwarfism. The bone age is normal in cases of familial short stature. Delayed bone age is hopeful, since growth potential is still maintained and child may still reach normal adult stature with resolution of the underlying cause.

12

PEDIATRICS

CRYING AND COLIC

I. **General Comments.** About one fifth of infants are described as having colic. This is described as inconsolable crying often accompanied by drawing up of the legs and gaseous distension of the abdomen. It may occur around the clock but more commonly occurs at a predictable time in the evening. Colic starts by 3 weeks of age, and the peak occurs by 6 weeks of age and may include about 3 hours of crying a day. The severity declines and by 3 months of age "normal" crying patterns are reestablished.

II. **Contributing Factors.** Contributing factors may include formula, aerophagia, too small a hole in a bottle nipple, various foods in the diet of the mother of a breast-fed infants.

III. **Treatment.**

A. After an exam to rule out other causes for irritability and crying (especially otitis, another infections cause, intussusception, hairs around the penis, fingers, or toes, etc.) the parents should be advised on the anticipated course and management. The importance of never shaking a baby should be stressed. An alternative caregiver should be identified if the parents feel at the limit of their ability to cope. Additionally there is good evidence that behavioral interventions (beyond simple emotional support) can be of benefit (Wolke et al: *Pediatrics* 94(3):322-332, 1994).

B. Rocking the child, cuddling, swaddling, taking child for a car ride, or using a child swing may be beneficial. Elimination of cruciferous vegetables and chocolate from a breast-feeding mother's diet may be helpful but has not been proved in a blinded study. Changing formulas to soybean milk or a hydrolyzed milk formula may help in some cases.

C. A well-done, blinded study showed that 2 ml of 12% sucrose/distilled water solution helped mitigate colic that did not respond to stimuli reduction, etc. Others have used a 30% solution. Sucrose causes endorphin release in the child and the analgesic effect of sucrose (and glucose) has been demonstrated in other studies as well (Carbajal R: *BMJ* 1999 319:1393-7). Making the solution using Pedialyte or other rehydration solution assures that the infant gets a proper electrolyte balance.

D. **There is no evidence that simethicone works for infantile colic. Dicyclomine has some benefit but also many side effects.**

SAFETY AND ACCIDENT PREVENTION

I. **SIDS Prevention.** SIDS is the leading cause of death in infants 1 to 12 months of age. To reduce risk, infants should be placed to sleep on their back or side on a firm surface with no pillows or other compressible ob-

---

TABLE 12-4

AGE-SPECIFIC SAFETY RECOMMENDATIONS

Age/Developmental Risk	Safety Recommendations
Prenatal/newborn: completely dependent, can squirm into position of suffocation or off a surface	Crib safety, car seat use, smoke detectors in home, water heater set to 120°, SIDS prevention (see text)
4 month: Beginning to reach, roll over, take solids	Need for constant supervision in bathtub, ingestion and aspiration prevention, caretaker need for choking first aid training, toy safety
6 month: Will begin to crawl, pull to stand	Syrup of ipecac, poison control number, walker dangers
12 month: Walking, stair and furniture climbing	Water safety including need for constant supervision when in bathtub, poisoning prevention, continuation of car seat use
Toddler: May learn to climb out of crib	Matches, electrical hazards, knives/kitchen hazards, fall precautions
Preschool: Increased initiative and desire to imitate adults can lead to more accidents	Traffic safety, matches/fire hazards, need for play to be supervised
School age: Increasing autonomy	Water safety, bicycle safety, fire and burn prevention
Preteen/teen	Drugs, alcohol, cigarettes, sports safety, safer sex, driving.

jects in the bed. Avoiding smoking in the house may also be helpful. Sleeping in the same bed with an infant should be discouraged since it, too, can contribute to SIDS.

II. **See Table 12-4 for age-specific safety recommendations.**

INFECTIONS

See Table 12-5 for common childhood illnesses.

I. **Approach to the Febrile Child.** Fever may be a marker of sepsis, localized infection, occult bacteremia, or benign illness.

A. **General considerations.**

1. **Temperature should be taken rectally.** Axillary and tympanic temperatures are not adequate in the small child.

2. The degree of elevation of the temperature does correlate with the likelihood of bacteremia, especially if >40° C. However, those with a low-grade fever can be septic, and those with high temperatures can have a benign course.

3. **The response to antipyretics cannot be used as a guide to differentiate septic children from those with viral illnesses.** Responders to antipyretics may be septic, whereas those who do not respond may have a mild illness.

4. In those greater than 2 to 3 months of age, clinical appearance is the best indicator of severity of illness. Children less than 3 months of age may not manifest signs of systemic illness.

5. Even though they will look ill, children 3 months to 2 years may not manifest the "typical" symptoms of their underlying illness (that is, no meningeal signs with meningitis).

6. Blood cultures are of limited usefulness in determining which patients should be treated, since results are delayed 48 to 72 hours. A single blood culture may miss up to 50% of bacteremic children, and if cultures are appropriate, two cultures should be done with the largest volume of blood possible (at least 6 ml total). Additionally, most bacteremic children will clear the bacteremia spontaneously.

7. Teething is related to fever, but look for other sources in the ill-appearing child.

8. Fever may be treated with acetaminophen 15 mg/kg Q4-6h or ibuprofen 10 mg/kg Q6-8h or both. Rectal acetaminophen must be dosed at 25-35mg/kg q 6 hours to achieve adequate serum levels. Tepid bathing does not add much to the efficacy of these drugs. Sponging with alcohol may lead to toxicity and is never indicated. Aspirin should be avoided because of the risk of Reye's syndrome.

B. **History.** Should focus on the duration and height of the fever; associated symptoms such as vomiting and diarrhea, rash (especially petechiae), behavioral changes and parental estimation of the degree of illness. Known exposures should be reviewed as well as an immunization and travel history.

12

PEDIATRICS

COMMON PEDIATRIC INFECTIOUS DISEASES AND EXANTHEMS

Disease	Etiologic Agent	Incubation	Prodrome
Chickenpox (varicella)	Varicella	10-21 days	Minimal
Fifth disease (erythema infectiosum)	Parvovirus B19	6-14 days	None
Herpangina	Coxsackievirus, herpesvirus	?	None
Kawasaki disease (mucocutaneous aneurysms lymph node syndrome)	Probable infectious agent not yet discovered	?	Unknown
Meningococcal meningitis	Neisseria meningitidis	1-7 days	URI, fever, headache, diarrhea
Mononucleosis	Epstein-Barr virus, CMV, toxoplasmosis, primary HIV	2-8 weeks	None
Roseola infantum (exanthema subitum)	Human herpesvirus type 6 and type 7	1-15 days	3-4 days of sustained high fever, child generally looks well
Rubella, German measles, 3-day measles	Rubivirus	14-21 days	Lymphadenopathy, fever, headache, malaise

Adapted from Driscoll CE et al: *The family practice desk reference,* ed 3, St. Louis, 1996, Mosby.
*Chickenpox: Some authors would treat the second and subsequent children in a family who develop chickenpox with acyclovir. The second and subsequent cases in a family tend to be more severe than the first case because of a higher initial viral load. Acyclovir reduces duration of illness by 24 to 48 hours and must be started within the first 24 hours of the illness to be effective. Adults and adolescents with chickenpox may be better candidates for acyclovir, since they tend to have more consequences.

Signs and Symptoms	Isolation	Treatments and Comments
Mixture of macules, papules, vesicles in all stages of development; spreads from trunk to extremities for 5-20 days	Until all lesions are crusted Infectious 2 days before appearance	Symptomatic or acyclovir*
Maculopapular rash on face with circumoral pallor (slapped cheek) and spreading to extremities; rash lasts a few days to a few weeks and is brought out by warmth	Not needed. See section under congenital infections.	None
May have the development of arthritis, especially in adults		
High fever, vomiting, ulcers of oral mucosa for 5-6 days	2-6 days	Symptomatic
Fever, adenopathy, inflamed mucosa (pharyngitis, cracked lips, etc.), polymorphous maculosquamous rash, conjunctivitis	?	May have cardiac involvement with artery aneurysms.
Most common below 1 year		
Meningitis; purpuric or petechial rash; septic arthritis	Until 24 hours after first antibiotic dose	See meningitis below
Fatigue, anorexia, exudative tonsillitis, lymphadenopathy, splenomegaly	Avoid saliva contact for 3 months	See section on mononucleosis in Chapter 20.
Macular rash not unusual with amoxicillin use		
Fine pink rash begins at fever defervescence and lasts 2 days; seen from 6 months to 3 years of age	Unknown	Fever control, may have aseptic meningitis
Maculopapular discrete rash appears on face and rapidly spreads to trunk and proximal extremities, lasting 1-3 days; postauricular and suboccipital lymphadenopathy	Communicable from 7 days before until 5 days after rash appears	None

12

PEDIATRICS

Continued

TABLE 12-5

COMMON PEDIATRIC INFECTIOUS DISEASES AND EXANTHEMS—cont'd

Disease	Etiologic Agent	Incubation	Prodrome
Rubeola (measles)	Rubeola virus	10-12 days	High fever, cough, coryza, and conjunctivitis for 3 days
Periodic fever, aphthous stomatitis, pharyngitis, adenopathy syndrome	Unknown		
Whooping cough (pertussis)	Bordetella pertussi	5-10 days; 21 days maximum	1-3 weeks of cough, coryza, and occasional emesis

Adapted from Driscoll CE et al: *The family practice desk reference,* ed 3, St. Louis, 1996, Mosby.

C. **Physical exam.** Should begin with a careful consideration of the general appearance. Careful observation and analysis of the vital signs, state of hydration, and peripheral perfusion are required. Attention should be paid to tachypnea out of proportion to fever, which may indicate pneumonia. A complete exam should be performed including a musculoskeletal exam for septic arthritis and osteomyelitis, neurologic exam, and skin exam. An oxygen saturation should be obtained in the ill appearing child.

D. **Approach to the febrile child without an obvious source of infection varies with age:**
   1. **For a child <8 weeks of age with any degree of fever >38° Celsius (100.4° F).**
      a. The exam and clinical signs and symptoms do not correlate well with seriousness of illness in these children and are an unreliable indicator of severity of disease. 3% to 10% of febrile children in this age group will have a bacterial illness, usually transient bacteremia. This may be reduced with the new pneumococcal vaccine.
      b. Any febrile child of this age without an identifiable focus of disease should have a complete septic work-up including CBC, blood cultures, LP with CSF Gram stain, culture, glucose and cell count, UA, and C&S. The white count is an insensitive indicator of bacterial illness but can be used to separate febrile children into "high-risk" and "low-risk" categories. Those with a

Signs and Symptoms	Isolation	Treatments and Comments
Koplik spots appear 1 or 2 days before maculopapular rash; rash is confluent and spreads from hairline to face and then body; lasts 4-5 days	From fifth day of incubation to fifth day after rash appears	Symptomatic care of cough, coryza, conjunctivitis
Recurrent fever, exudative tonsillitis, malaise, cervical adenopathy, ⅔ with aphthous stomatitis. Look well between episodes	Unknown	Prednisone 2mg/kg single dose
Short paroxysmal cough ending with inspiratory "whoop"	5-10 days with treatment	Erythromycin Culture nasopharynx

12

PEDIATRICS

WBC count of <5000 or >15,000 are in the "high-risk" group. Some authors suggest a CXR as well, but in a child without pulmonary or respiratory symptoms the yield is very low. However, 12% of those with isolated rhinorrhea will have a positive CXR.

c. **Decide if patient has a high risk or a low risk.** A "low-risk" infant is considered:

  (1) 28 to 90 days old and previously healthy.

  (2) Nontoxic appearing.

  (3) No apparent site of focal bacterial infection, except for otitis.

  (4) Good social situation.

  (5) WBC count of 5,000 to 15,000 with a band count below 1,500.

  (6) Normal urinalysis with fewer than 5 WBCs/HPF.

  (7) If diarrhea is present, there should be fewer than 5 WBCs/HPF in the stool.

d. **Admit all patients who look toxic or ill or are less than 28 days of age** and cover with ceftriaxone (50 to 75 mg/kg Q24h not >2 g) until cultures available.

e. **Admit and treat patients with an identifiable illness** requiring hospitalization such as meningitis, pneumonia, or UTI (see specific section for treatments).

    f. **Admit all "high-risk" infants** (WBC count of >15,000 or <5000/mm^3, inability to follow up for social reasons, abnormal UA, WBCs in stool) even if no source evident and treat as for sepsis with ceftriaxone while awaiting cultures.

    g. **Patients who are at low risk (see c above) and appear** well can be treated as an outpatient while awaiting culture results with ceftriaxone 75 mg/kg IM (not >2 g) and should be followed up in 24 hours. If cultures are positive, treat as appropriate. If cultures are negative and patient is afebrile and looks well, can follow up closely. If the child remains febrile, cover with ceftriaxone until cultures final.

2. **Children 3 months to 2 years.**

    a. Many authors will treat children up to 3 months of age as above.

    b. 4% of febrile children in this age group will have occult bacteremia with *Streptococcus pneumoniae* or *Haemophilus influenzae,* though most of these children will clear the bacteremia spontaneously and have no sequelae.

    c. Those with a WBC count of >15,000 or <5000 are at a higher risk of sepsis, but this should not be used as an absolute guide, since children with any WBC count can be septic.

    d. **Non–toxic appearing children with a temperature of <39° C** may be observed with lab testing addressed to the clinical picture.

    e. **For those who are toxic appearing but with a temperature of <39° C,** a complete physical exam should be done and lab examination should be addressed to findings. Blood cultures should be done in those considered at high risk for sepsis (generally look ill). Do not forget a UA.

    f. **Those with a temperature of >39° C** should have a CBC, blood culture, urinalysis, and urine culture. LP, etc. should be done if indicated clinically. If WBC >15,000 or <5000, cover with ceftriaxone 50 to 75 mg/kg IM (not >2 g) and see patient back the next day.

II. **Bacterial Meningitis. See Chapter 9 for CSF findings in various CNS infections.**

A. **Bacterial meningitis** must be suspected in any febrile child or any child with mental status changes. Prompt diagnosis and treatment are paramount to successful outcome. Viral (or aseptic) meningitis is more common, seldom needs more than supportive care, and rarely causes significant sequelae. **Antibiotics must be started within ½ hr of presentation if meningitis is suspected.**

B. **Epidemiology.** There is an increased frequency among rural, African-American and Native-American populations. Most common organisms are:

1. **<1 month** = Group B strep, *E. coli, Listeria.*

2. **>1 month** = *H. influenzae,* type B (especially in toddlers), *Neisseria meningitidis, Streptococcus pneumoniae.*

3. *H. influenzae, N. meningitidis,* and *Strep. pneumoniae* are respiratory tract-borne pathogens, *Listeria* species is most commonly food borne (e.g. hot dogs and prepared meats).

C. **Clinical signs and symptoms.**
   1. Triad of nuchal rigidity (may be absent in <2 years of age), fever, and headache is present in only two-thirds of patients. However, one part of the triad is *always* present. Kernig's and Brudzinski's signs are only present in 9%, so meningitis should never be ruled out based only on the absence of these clinical signs.
   2. Nonspecific signs of irritability, lethargy, poor feeding, nausea, and vomiting are more commonly the presentation in younger children. Check for bulging fontanelle in the neonate (a late sign).
   3. Most common neurologic sign is altered mental status. Focal neurologic deficits are uncommon.
   4. Generalized signs include erythematous (early) or petechial (later) rash and endotoxin-mediated hypotension in meningococcal sepsis.

D. **Laboratory findings.**
   1. **Do not delay LP and CSF examination to do a CT scan unless focal neurologic signs or papilledema suggestive of increased intracranial pressure are present.** If any of these is present, get a head CT first **(but start antibiotics before CT).** Send CSF for CBC, glucose, protein, culture, and Gram stain. Look for leukocytosis, high protein, and low glucose. See Table 23-7 for normal CSF fluid analysis. See Chapter 9 for characteristic findings in bacterial versus viral meningitis.
   2. General sepsis work-up including CBC, UA, CXR (if indicated) should be done. Perform latex agglutination on serum and urine and send blood, CSF, and urine cultures. However, a negative latex agglutination does not rule out an infectious disease and should be used only to guide the choice of antibiotics.
   3. Monitor electrolytes, oxygen saturation, serum glucose, C-reactive protein, serum osmolality, and INR/PTT.

E. **Treatment.**
   1. **Stabilize** with proper airway management (if needed) and IV access. Evaluate and institute needed therapy for dehydration, hypotension, hypoxia, electrolyte abnormalities, SIADH, hypoglycemia, or DIC.
   2. **Give empiric IV antibiotics immediately according to most likely organism for age.** Do not await culture results. **However, changing antibiotics to reflect sensitivities once available is prudent.**
      a. Although the data are contradictory, dexamethasone 0.15 mg/kg Q6h for 4 days may improve outcome when given together with antibiotics especially in *H. influenzae* meningitis. To be effective, however, steroids should be started before or just after first dose of antibiotics. **Vancomycin should be added to all of the regimens below in those with LP proven meningitis until cultures and sensitivities are available!!!**

12

PEDIATRICS

b. **<7 days.** Ampicillin 100 mg/kg/day divided Q12h plus genta-micin 5 mg/kg/day Q12h, or ampicillin plus ceftriaxone 100 mg/kg/day either as a single dose or divided Q12h + **vancomycin**

c. **>7 days.** Ampicillin 150 mg/kg/day divided Q8h plus gentamicin 7.5 mg/kg/day divided Q8h, or ampicillin plus cefotaxime 150 mg/kg/day divided Q8h or ceftriaxone 100 mg/kg/day either as a single dose or divided Q12h + **vancomycin**

d. **1 to 3 months.** Ampicillin 300 mg/kg/day divided Q6h plus cefo-taxime 200 mg/kg/day divided Q6h, or ceftriaxone 100 mg/kg as a single dose or divided Q12h + **vancomycin**

e. **>3 months.** Cefotaxime 200 mg/kg/day divided Q6h, or cef-triaxone 100 mg/kg/day as a single dose or divided Q12h, or ampicillin 300 mg/kg/day divided Q6h plus chloramphenicol 100 mg/kg/day divided Q6h + **vancomycin**

f. **>6 years.** Ceftriaxone 100 mg/kg/day as a single dose or divided Q12h + **vancomycin**

g. **Duration of therapy.** 14 to 21 days for group B streptococci or gram-negative bacteria; 10 days for others.

F. **Prophylaxis.**
1. *Neisseria meningitidis.* Vaccine available for acute outbreak; con-sult local public health organization. Rifampin 20 mg/kg/day PO >1 month (not >600 mg) divided Q12h for 2 days is indicated for all intimate contacts, including household members of patient. Other options for adults include ciprofloxacin 500 mg PO or ceftriaxone 250 mg IM. For children less than 15 years of age ceftriaxone 125 mg IM can be used.

2. *Haemophilus influenzae.* Active immunization recommended, given as 3-dose vaccination at 2, 4, and 6 months with a booster at 15 months. When there are other children in the home, rifampin 20 mg/kg/day as single oral dose for 4 days is recommended for all household contacts including adults.

VOMITING, DIARRHEA, AND DEHYDRATION

I. **Vomiting.**

A. **Overview.** Forceful ejection of gastric contents as opposed to passive reflux. Most common cause is gastroenteritis. In infants consider gastro-esophageal reflux, overfeeding, anatomic obstruction, and systemic in-fection. In children, consider systemic infection, toxic ingestion, appen-dicitis, Reye's syndrome, and pertussis. Consider elevated intracranial pressure as a cause of isolated vomiting.

B. **Evaluation.**
1. **History.** Assess pattern and severity as well as accompanying dehy-dration/malnutrition. If neonatal, consider congenital abnormalities such as duodenal or esophageal atresia, Hirschsprung's disease, volvulus, malformation. In infants, assess how much is being fed

(overfeeding), relation to position (reflux), choking or coughing with feeding (achalasia, tracheoesophageal fistula).

2. **Reye's syndrome.** Reye's syndrome generally occurs after viral illness and presents with intractable vomiting, elevated liver enzymes (but normal bilirubin), decreased mental status (encephalopathy), prolonged PT/INR, and elevated serum ammonia and hypoglycemia. Treatment includes glucose (at least 0.4 mg/kg/hour) to maintain normal serum glucose, fluid and electrolytes at one half maintenance (correct shock first), neomycin 100 mg/kg/ day PO Q6h, vitamin K 5 to 10 mg IV for coagulopathy or FFP for acute bleeding, and management of elevated intracranial pressure. Some would add lactulose to this regimen.

3. **Pyloric stenosis.** Occurs at <2 months of age and presents with intractable vomiting after feeds. Most common in first-born males, may have severe electrolyte disturbance depending on duration. Diagnosis is by ultrasonography or "string sign" on upper GI film (barium passing through a narrowed pylorus). Treatment is surgical though recent studies indicate that nitric oxide may be helpful.

C. **Exam and lab tests.** Evaluate state of hydration (see section on dehydration below). Look for site of infection. Abdominal and rectal exam for obstruction or imperforate anus. Radiologic studies as indicated. If child less than 2 months, consider ultrasonography or upper GI for pyloric stenosis.

D. **Treatment.** See dehydration and oral rehydration sections below. Also consider antiemetics such as promethazine, prochlorperazine (Compazine and others), trimethobenzamide.

II. **Diarrhea** (see Chapter 5).

A. **Overview.** There are numerous causes of acute and chronic diarrhea. Infectious causes include viruses (rotavirus most common), bacteria (*Salmonella, Shigella, Campylobacter* most common), parasites (*Giardia* and *Cryptosporidium* most common), localized infection elsewhere, antibiotic-associated (antibiotic side effect, as well as *Clostridium difficile*), and food poisoning. Noninfectious causes include overfeeding (particularly of fruit juices), irritable bowel syndrome, celiac disease, milk protein intolerance, lactose intolerance after infectious diarrhea, cystic fibrosis, and inflammatory bowel.

B. **Evaluation.**

1. **History.** Acute versus chronic. Volume, frequency, character of stools, presence of blood or mucus. Associated symptoms (vomiting, fever, malaise, etc.). Epidemiologic data (travel, day care, family history).

2. **Exam.** Estimate dehydration (see section on dehydration below). Examine for other infectious process or source. Determine if nutritional status is compromised. Neurologic symptoms, mental status changes or seizures suggest *Shigella* or *Rotavirus*.

3. **Lab tests.** Culture is indicated for acute bloody or guaiac positive diarrhea. **Fecal leukocytes and RBCs are not sensitive or specific**

enough to be useful in the diagnosis of infectious diarrhea; there is a high degree of false negative tests. O&P for prolonged diarrhea or as indicated. Studies for chronic disease as appropriate. An ELISA test is available for *Rotavirus* (Rotazyme). See Chapter 5.

C. **Treatment.**

1. Acute diarrhea with dehydration in the absence of vomiting is treated with large amounts of osmotically balanced clear liquids such as Pedialyte, Ricelyte, or the WHO rehydration formula until rehydration is complete. See dehydration and oral rehydration section.

2. There is abundant evidence that early reinstitution of a lactose-free general diet will decrease the duration and severity of diarrhea. Foods provided should be the same as those in the child's normal diet with the exclusion of high-sugar foods such as apple juice, which may cause an osmotic diarrhea, and milk products with lactose. Breast-fed infants should continue to nurse without restrictions; lactose-free soybean formulas may be used in those who are bottle fed.

3. Avoid the use of antiperistaltic agents in infants and children.

4. Most episodes of diarrhea do not benefit from antimicrobial therapy. Bacterial diarrhea should be treated appropriately after culture results are available, although many would treat heme positive diarrhea presumptively once cultures have been obtained. Caution should be used in the treatment of diarrhea caused by *Salmonella* species because this may prolong the carrier state. However, antibiotics should be used for *Salmonella* in infants <3 months old, patients with symptoms of toxicity, patients with metastatic foci, or with *Salmonella typhi*. See Chapter 5. Avoid treating enterohemorrhagic *E. coli* (O157:H7) with antibiotics, since it increases the risk of hemolytic uremic syndrome (*NEJM* 342:2000.)

5. Diarrhea with vomiting is treated as for vomiting until patient is able to tolerate oral feedings.

6. Racecadotril (acetorphan) has been used successfully in children as young as 3 mon with **watery,** heme-negative diarrhea (*NEJM* 343:463, 2000.)

III. **Dehydration.**

A. **Clinical assessment**

1. **Clinical observation.** See Table 12-6. **Clinical signs and symptoms are neither sensitive nor specific** (only about 75% sensitive) and have a high index of suspicion for dehydration given the proper history.

2. **Laboratory diagnosis.** BUN/Creatinine ratio of >20 is 92% sensitive but only 33% specific for dehydration. Serum bicarbonate, urine specific gravity, etc. are all poor predictors of dehydration.

3. **Degree of dehydration.** Because is it clinically very difficult to determine the percent dehydration, the World Health Organization has suggested categorizing patients as having **"none," "some," or "severe,"** rather than trying to predict a percentage.

4. **In hypotonic dehydration** (Na^+ <130 mEq/L) all manifestations appear with less fluid deficit, whereas in hypertonic dehydration (Na^-

TABLE 12-6

CLINICAL SIGNS ASSOCIATED WITH VARIOUS DEGREES OF DEHYDRATION

Dehydration (%)	Clinical Observation
5-6	Heart rate (10% to 15% above baseline value)
	Slightly dry mucous membranes
	Concentration of the urine
	Poor tear production*
7-8	Increased severity of above
	Decreased skin turgor
	Oliguria
	Sunken eyeballs*
	Sunken anterior fontanelle*
>9	Pronounced severity of above signs
	Decreased blood pressure
	Delayed capillary refill (>2 seconds)
	Acidosis (large base deficit)

*These signs may be less sensitive indicators of dehydration than the others.

TABLE 12-7

INTRACELLULAR AND EXTRACELLULAR FLUID COMPOSITION

Ion	Intracellular (mEq/L)	Extracellular (mEq/L)
Na^+	20	145
K^+	150	3-5
Cl^-	—	110
HCO_3^-	10	20-25
PO_4^-	110-115	5
Protein	75	10

Dehydration for <3 days: 80% extracellular fluid and 20% intracellular fluid losses. Dehydration for >3 days: 60% ECF and 40% ICF losses.

>150 mEq/L) the circulating volume is relatively preserved, and so circulatory disturbances are seen later.

5. **Calculation of electrolyte deficits.** See section V and Table 12-7.

B. **Oral rehydration. There is no role for weak tea, flat soda, Jell-O (gelatin) water, etc.**

1. Concept of "gut rest," that is, stopping oral intake for several hours before refeeding, has been found to have several negative effects, such as increased intestinal permeability and worsening of starvation and dehydration. Studies have shown that stool production is actually less with early refeeding.

2. Oral rehydration is appropriate in most cases of mild to moderate dehydration.

3. Currently only two fluids meet the recommendations of the World Health Organization (WHO) and the American Academy of Pediatrics

for the rehydration phase of the treatment of diarrhea—Rehydralyte. (Ross) and the WHO-ORS product (oral rehydration solution). These are the only two products that contain the 75 to 90 mEq/L of sodium recommended for rehydration. A simple alternative for making a rehydration solution is to mix half a teaspoon of table salt and 8 teaspoons of sugar in 1 liter of water. However, this solution neither replaces potassium nor contains bicarbonate to hasten the resolution of acidosis. One also needs to be sure that the parent is able to mix the solution properly. One can make a more complicated but more complete solution by adding 8 teaspoons of table sugar, half a teaspoon of salt, half a teaspoon of sodium bicarbonate (baking soda), and a third of a teaspoon of potassium chloride (e.g., "light salt products") to 1 liter of water.

4. Oral rehydration should be accomplished over 4 hours. The dose for mild dehydration is 50 ml/kg, or 100 ml/kg for moderate dehydration. If vomiting is occurring, the child may be given frequent small doses of the rehydration fluid and then subsequent maintenance fluids by using a teaspoon or a small oral syringe to provide a rate of approximately 5 ml/min.

5. For replacement of ongoing losses, it is recommended that a fluid with a lower sodium content than the rehydration fluid be used. Pedialyte (Ross) or Ricelyte (Mead Johnson) are examples of appropriate maintenance fluids. **Other solutions, such as weak tea, dilute or full-strength soft drinks, Jell-O (gelatin) water, tap water, apple juice, etc., are contraindicated and may lead to hyponatremia.** Alternatively, the rehydration fluid may be given along with other low-sodium fluids, such as breast milk or formula. Replacement of ongoing losses is advised at a rate of 10 ml/kg or 1/2 to 1 cup of ORS for each diarrheal stool.

C. Intravenous rehydration.
1. **Formulas for calculating electrolyte deficits.**
   a. Sodium deficit (mEq total) = (125 [or Desired serum sodium] − Current serum sodium) × 0.6 × Weight (kg).
   b. Potassium deficit (mEq total) = (Desired serum K [mEq/L] − Measured serum K) × 0.25 × Weight (kg).
   c. Chloride deficit (mEq total) = (Desired serum chloride [mEq/L] − Measured serum Cl) × 0.45 × Weight (kg).
2. **Correction of free-water deficit in hypernatremic dehydration.** Free-water deficit = 4 ml/kg for every mEq that the serum Na exceeds 145 mEq/L.
3. **Maintenance requirements for fluids and electrolytes.**
   a. Fluid maintenance.
      (1) **Weight <10 kg:** 100 ml/kg/day
      (2) **Weight 11 to 20 kg:** 1000 ml + 50 ml/kg/day for every kg over 10 kg

(3) **Weight >20 kg:** 1500 ml + 20 ml/kg/day for every kg over 20 kg
(4) **Adult:** 2000 to 2400 ml/day
4. **Total body water.** 60% of body weight.
5. **Maintenance electrolyte requirements.**
   a. Na^+: 3 mEq/kg/day, or 3 mEq/100 ml of H_2O
   b. K^+: 2 mEq/kg/day or 2 mEq/100 ml of H_2O (adult: 50 mEq/day)
   c. Cl^-: 3 mEq/100 ml of H_2O
   d. Glucose: 5 g/100 ml of H_2O
6. **Replacement of ongoing losses.**
   a. See Table 12-8 for composition of various body fluids.
   b. NG losses usually replaced with D_5 1/2NS with 20 mEq/L of KCl.
   c. Diarrhea usually replaced with D_5 1/4NS with 40 mEq/L of KCl.
D. **General principles in treating dehydration.**
   1. Weigh the child.
   2. Be sure to add ongoing losses to maintenance + deficit fluids and electrolytes.
   3. If moderately or severely dehydrated, give an initial fluid bolus of 20 ml/kg LR or NS over 20 minutes. Repeat bolus if response is inadequate. If poor response after three fluid boluses, that is, poor perfusion, no urine output, abnormal vital signs, may need CVP or PCWP to guide fluid resuscitation.
   4. In hypotonic or isotonic dehydration, calculate the total fluids and electrolytes (maintenance + deficit replacement) for the first 24 hours, give half over the first 8 hours and the other half over the next 16 hours. In hypertonic dehydration, correct the fluid and electrolyte deficits slowly over about 48 hours.
   5. Do not add potassium to IV until urine output is established. Diabetic ketoacidosis may be an exception, where correction of hyperglycemia and acidosis may lead to rapid development of hypokalemia.
   6. Increase maintenance fluids by 12% for each Celsius degree of fever.
E. **Hypotonic dehydration (Na <125 mEq/L).**

12

PEDIATRICS

TABLE 12-8				
ELECTROLYTE COMPOSITION OF VARIOUS BODY FLUIDS				
Fluid	Na (mEq/L)	K (mEq/L)	Cl (mEq/L)	Protein (g/dl)
Gastric	20-80	5-20	100-150	—
Pancreatic	120-140	5-15	40-80	—
Small bowel	100-140	5-15	90-130	—
Bile	120-140	5-15	80-120	—
Ileostomy	45-135	3-15	20-115	—
Diarrhea	10-90	10-80	10-110	—
Burns	140	5	110	3-5

1. Symptomatic earlier than in isotonic or hypertonic dehydration. Therefore use weight loss of 3% = mild, 6% = moderate, and 9% = severe dehydration as a guide.
2. Hypotonic dehydration usually results from replacing losses (vomiting and diarrhea) with low-solute fluids, such as dilute juice, cola, weak tea.
3. Lethargy and irritability are common, and vascular collapse can occur early.
4. **Therapy.** Calculate total fluid and electrolyte needs according to the maintenance and deficit replacement formulas in section C.
   a. Do not try to raise serum Na more than 10 mEq/L (that is, if the current serum sodium is 125, use 135 as the desired serum Na level in the calculation) in first 24 hours.
   b. To calculate the milliequivalents of Na needed in each liter during the first 24 hours of therapy: mEq of Na per liter of IV fluid = total sodium needed in the first 24 hours divided by total volume of fluid needed. (Normal saline = 154 mEq of Na/liter).
   c. Usually D_5 1/2 NS or D_5 NS is used. Potassium can be added after urine output is established. Give half of the calculated total fluid and electrolyte requirements for the first 24 hours over the first 8 hours and the other half over the subsequent 16 hours.
F. **Severe, symptomatic hyponatremia.** See Chapter 6.
G. **Isotonic dehydration (Na = 130 to 150 mEq/L).**
   1. Symptoms are less dramatic than in hypotonic dehydration.
   2. Use estimate (loss of weight) 5% = mild, 10% = moderate, 15% = severe dehydration.
   3. Calculate total maintenance + deficit replacement fluids and electrolytes for first 24 hours.
   4. Treatment is similar to treatment for hypotonic dehydration: give half of first 24 hours needs in first 8 hours, and give the remaining half over the next 16 hours.
   5. Usually can use D_5 1/4 NS or D_5 1/2 NS; may add potassium after urine output established.
   6. Remember to estimate and replace ongoing losses.
H. **Hypertonic dehydration.**
   1. Usually occurs as a result of using inappropriately high solute load as replacement, renal concentrating defect with large free-water losses, heat exposure with large insensible losses, etc.
   2. Typical symptoms include thick, doughy texture to skin (tenting is uncommon), shrill cry, weakness, tachypnea, intense thirst.
   3. Shock is a very late manifestation. If severe dehydration or shock is present, the patient may need an initial fluid bolus of 20 ml/kg NS over the first 20 to 30 minutes.
   4. Free-water deficit (ml) is estimated to be 4 ml/kg × (Actual serum Na (mEq/L) − 145 mEq/L).

5. Replace the free-water deficit **slowly** over 48 hours. Aim to decrease the serum sodium by about 10 mEq/L/day. Reducing serum sodium more rapidly can have severe repercussions, such as cerebral and pulmonary edema.
6. Usual replacement fluid is D_5 1/4 NS or D_5 1/2 NS.
7. If Na >180, may need dialysis.

CONSTIPATION AND ENCOPRESIS

I. **Overview.** Infrequent passage of dry, hard stools. Causes can be organic (Hirschsprung's disease, anal stenosis, anal stricture, drugs, dehydration, neuromuscular disease) or functional (voluntary withholding). Beyond the neonatal period 90% to 95% of constipation is functional.

II. **Causes**

A. **In newborn** must rule out anatomic and congenital causes such as rectal or colonic atresia, myelomeningocele, absent abdominal muscles, cystic fibrosis, Hirschsprung's disease.

B. **In older** children, functional or dietary.
   1. **Dietary.** Lack of dietary bulk, excessive intake of cow's milk, early introduction of cow's milk.
   2. **Stool retention.** Painful defecation caused by fissure, rectal abscess, etc., or conflicts in toilet training. Voluntary withholding results in decreased rectal sensation and rectal distension and subsequent loss of defecation urge. Stooling around impaction with soiling is known as "encopresis" if noted after normal toilet training age of 4 to 5 years.
   3. **Other causes of constipation.** Narcotics, antidepressants and other anticholinergics, overuse of laxatives, hypothyroidism, hypokalemia.

III. **Evaluation**

A. **History.** Age of onset. Parent expectation of stool pattern. Stool consistency, size, frequency, soiling, abdominal pain, anorexia, tenesmus. Infants should pass meconium in first 24 hours.

B. **Exam.** Palpable abdominal mass. Rectal exam reveals hard stool present with dilated ampulla. Anal fissure may be present.

C. **Lab tests.** Abdominal flat plate will show stool filling the colon. Barium enema to demonstrate atresia. Rectal biopsy for Hirschsprung's. Thyroid functions and electrolytes and calcium as indicated.

IV. **Treatment**

A. **Simple constipation in infants** treated with lactulose 2.5 to 10 ml/24 hours, divided TID or QID. Add fruit and fruit juices to diet if older than 4 months. Karo syrup (corn syrup) 15-20ml per 8 oz of formula can be helpful. Previous concerns about the possibility of botulism are unfounded. A glycerin suppository may stimulate the passage of a stool. Changing to Carnation Good Start formula may be helpful with constipation.

B. **In older children,** clear impaction using pediatric enema or cathartic (such as bisacodyl suppositories). Polyethylene glycol (GoLYTELY, MiraLax) may also be used. Give 40 ml/kg over 6 hours. Increase dietary fiber (prunes, figs, raisins, beans, bran, fresh fruits, and vegeta-

12

PEDIATRICS

bles) or use a psyllium supplement. Limit milk if excessive by history. Avoid hypotonic and phosphate enemas, which can cause electrolyte abnormalities and seizures.

C. **Encopresis** (soiling with impaction).

1. Usually starts as a functional voluntary withholding but progresses to decreased urge to defecate because of rectal enlargement and loss of sensation of full rectum.

2. Counseling of patient and parents on cause of soiling. Outline plan to help patient resolve problem.

3. Clear rectum of impaction before starting treatment.

4. Start milk of magnesia (<1 year = 5 ml; >1 year = 7.5 to 30 ml), or mineral oil 5 to 30 ml, and increase until having soft stools. Polyethylene glycol (e.g., Miralax) is also being used for this indication. Start with 1 tsp in 4 ounces of fluid per day and increase to 1 tbsp per day in up to 8 ounces of liquid. Lactulose 5-10 mg PO BID can also be used. Mineral oil should not be used in those <5 years of age. Continue treatment for 2 to 6 months while rectal size and sensation return to normal.

5. When decreasing dose of laxative start toilet-sitting regimen, that is, sitting for 15 minutes after each meal. Consider reward system appropriate to age.

6. Implement dietary changes as above.

GI BLEEDING IN CHILDHOOD

I. **Surgical Causes.**

A. **If less than 1 year of age, think of** anal fissure (43%), intussusception (39%), duodenal-gastric ulcer (15%), gangrenous bowel (9%), Meckel's diverticulum (3.8%).

B. **If more than 1 year, think of** polyps (50%), ulcers (14%), anal fissure (12.5%), esophageal varices (10.5%), intussusception (9%), hemorrhoids (0.8%).

II. **Medical Causes.**

A. **Hematologic abnormalities.** Hemophilia, iron deficiency, thrombocytopenia, vitamin K deficiency.

B. **Systemic causes.** Milk allergy, infectious diarrhea, Henoch-Schönlein purpura, scurvy, uremia, etc.

C. **Drugs.** NSAIDs, iron poisoning.

D. **Swallowed blood.** From nose bleed, maternal blood from breast feeding, etc.

E. **To differentiate swallowed maternal blood (from breast feeding, etc.) from neonatal blood.** Take vomitus, stool, etc., and mix with 5 to 10 parts of water. Centrifuge to remove debris and decant the pink supernatant (if not pink, won't work). Mix 1 ml of 0.25N (1%) sodium hydroxide with 5 ml of supernatant. Read color change in 2 minutes. If remains pink, blood is of fetal origin. If turns brown-yellow, blood is of adult origin. It is helpful to run a control of the infant's blood.

STRIDOR AND DYSPNEA

For differential diagnosis of stridor and dyspnea, see Table 12-9.

I. **Epiglottitis.**

A. **Definition.** Infection of the epiglottis and of the aryepiglottic folds and surrounding soft tissues. Becoming less common since use of *H. influenzae* vaccine. Is more common in adults in whom it presents as a severe sore throat with drooling, neck tenderness.

B. **Cause.** Almost always by *H. influenzae* type B. Other causes: beta-hemolytic streptococci, *Staphylococcus aureus,* and *Streptococcus pneumoniae.*

C. **Clinical presentation.** May occur at any age, with a peak incidence at 2 to 7 years. Presents with sudden onset of high fever, respiratory distress, severe dysphagia, drooling, muffled voice, and a toxic appearance. Stridor, if present, may be mild in comparison to croup. Often there is little or no coughing. Child typically prefers being upright in "sniffing" position.

D. **Lab tests.** Invasive procedures and examinations should be avoided until after airway is secured. CBC and blood and epiglottic cultures may then be obtained. Radiographs of lateral area of neck shows characteristic swollen epiglottis (thumb sign). **Never send a child suspected of having epiglottitis to be radiographed unaccompanied by someone who can emergently manage airway.**

E. **Treatment.**

1. **Do not move, upset, or lay child down unless prepared to manage obstructed airway.**

2. **Airway.** In an emergency, a bag-valve-mask can buy time. **Consider a needle cricothyrotomy.** Controlled intubation by an experienced operator is preferred. Tracheostomy is acceptable if unable to intubate. Usually safely extubated in 48 to 72 hours after appropriate antibiotics are started. **Airway must be secure. Top of size 3 ET tube fits on Luer-lok needle, allowing for easy bagging.**

3. **Antibiotics.** Initiated once artificial airway secure. Cefotaxime 50 to 200 mg/kg/24 hours divided Q6h or ceftriaxone 75 mg/kg Q24h are the first-line drugs with TMP/SMX as a second-line agent.

4. **Admission to ICU.** Use proper sedation and restraints during period of intubation. Antibiotics continue for 7 to 10 days after extubation.

II. **Croup (Laryngotracheobronchitis).**

A. **Definition.** A syndrome of airway swelling in the glottic and subglottic area of viral origin.

B. **Causes.** Parainfluenza virus types 1 and 3 responsible for majority of cases; remainder respiratory syncytial virus, influenza virus, and adenovirus.

C. **Clinical presentation.** Age usually 6 months to 6 years. Symptoms of the common cold usually precede onset. Brassy cough (seal bark), hoarseness, and inspiratory stridor are characteristic. If severe may include retractions, decreased air entry, and cyanosis. Usually benign course but can progress to obstruction.

12

PEDIATRICS

TABLE 12-9

DIFFERENTIAL DIAGNOSIS OF STRIDOR AND DYSPNEA

	Viral Laryngotracheitis	Bacterial Tracheitis	Retropharyngeal Abscess	Epiglottitis
CAUSE	Parainfluenza Influenza RSV	Viral prodrome + Staphylococci Streptococci *Haemophilus influenzae* Enteric pathogens	Beta-hemolytic streptococci anaerobes	*H. influenzae* Staphylococci Streptococci
AGE	3 months to 3 years	3 months to 3 years	6 months to 3 years	2 to 7 years
CLINICAL CHARACTERISTICS	Low-grade fever Coryza Barking cough Hoarse voice Winter/spring peak	Improving croup then sudden increase: temperature, work of breathing, stridor No drooling Fall/winter peak	Initial URI Dysphagia, refusal to feed Drooling, toxic appearance, stridor	Sudden onset of high fever, dysphagia, stridor, drooling. No cough
RADIOGRAPH	Unnecessary (steeple sign unreliable)	Detached pseudomembrane may give soft-tissue shadow	Radiograph shows retropharyngeal soft-tissue density and air-fluid level	Unnecessary (thumb sign)
TREATMENT	Cool mist, epinephrine, steroids	Intubation, antibiotics	Surgical drainage, antibiotics	Intubation, antibiotics

D. May be resolved by presentation to office or ED from exposure to cool air.

E. Must differentiate from epiglottitis and bacterial tracheitis, which require emergent management. See Table 12-9.

F. **Classification.**

1. **Very mild.** Intermittent stridor, present when awake or excited, goes away when sleeping.

2. **Mild.** Continuous stridor when awake or asleep not audible without stethoscope.

3. **Moderate.** Continuous stridor audible without stethoscope and may be accompanied be sternal retractions.

4. **Severe.** Continuous stridor with evidence of respiratory failure, that is, cyanosis, altered mental status.

G. **Lab tests.** Usually not indicated and may induce further agitation with respiratory compromise. If in doubt and no need for emergent airway management, AP radiograph of neck may show subglottic narrowing (steeple sign).

H. **Management.**

1. Calm the child on the parent's lap and provide cool, humidified air.

2. Oxygen if saturation <95%.

3. Reassess status after 15 to 30 minutes.

4. If mild classification, consider discharge with instructions for cool mist humidifier.

5. **If moderate classification.**

a. The traditional treatment has been nebulized racemic epinephrine, 2.25% solution, 0.5 ml diluted in 3 ml of saline.

b. **Nebulized epinephrine,** 5 ml of 1:1000, has been shown to be as safe as, at least as good as, and perhaps superior to racemic epinephrine. May repeat PRN.

c. There is no "rebound effect" from epinephrine, but patients may return to their pretreatment state.

d. **Steroids.** Generally those who need nebulized epinephrine should also be treated with dexamethasone 0.6 mg/kg/dose IM or PO up to 10 mg. Although not standard of care, nebulized budesonide 1 mg given twice at 30-minute intervals is effective in mild-to-moderate croup and may prevent the need for systemic steroids. However, up to now, it has not been compared to dexamethasone in any trial.

e. Continuation of cool, humidified air may also be helpful.

f. **Disposition.** Patients may be discharged with instructions for cool mist humidifier if, after 3 to 6 hours of observation, they require no further treatment with epinephrine and their croup is mild. If patient remains in the moderate classification, hospitalization with epinephrine or racemic epinephrine PRN and dexamethasone 0.25 to 0.5 mg/kg/dose Q6h for 2-4 doses.

12

PEDIATRICS

   6. **If in severe classification,** the decision to intubate should be left to experienced personnel and, when feasible, be performed in the operating room. Management is as above while awaiting trained personnel for sedation and intubation.

III. **Foreign-Body Aspiration.**

A. **Clinical presentation.** Majority 3 months to 6 years. Have triphasic history:
   1. Initial cough, choking, gagging, stridor, wheeze.
   2. FB then passes into smaller airways and have silent phase.
   3. Then have recurrent pneumonia, wheezing, abscess, bronchiectasis.
   4. A third not witnessed or not remembered by caregiver.

B. **Radiographs.** Can show air trapping on exhalation but one fourth have normal radiograph. Radiography is only 50% specific. Do CXR with patient lying on affected side. Dependent lung will not deflate normally if there is foreign body obstruction.

C. **Bronchoscopy.** Diagnostic procedure of choice if there is any question.

D. **Treatment.**
   1. **Without respiratory distress.** Refer for removal by bronchoscopy.
   2. **Respiratory distress present.**
      a. **If the patient is breathing,** do not interfere; allow the child's efforts to attempt to clear the foreign body.
      b. **If not moving air,** American Heart Association obstructed airway maneuvers should be employed. For infants, 5 interscapular back blows with the child's head lower than the chest, alternating with 5 chest compressions. In older children, Heimlich maneuver. Advanced cardiac life support protocol should be initiated if necessary.
      c. Bag-valve-mask ventilations can convert a total obstruction to a partial one by pushing foreign body into a main bronchus.
      d. Immediate direct laryngoscopy and removal with Magill forceps should be performed.
      e. If unsuccessful, cricothyrotomy or intubation if needed.

E. **Prevention.** Infants and young children should not eat nuts, popcorn, hot dogs, uncooked carrots, whole grapes, or hard candies. **Balloons and surgical gloves are especially dangerous for young children.** Dice food. Avoid small toys. Educate parents.

IV. **Bronchiolitis.**

A. **Epidemiology.** Illness of young children and infants. Most serious in first 2 years of life. Respiratory syncytial virus (RSV) principal agent. Also associated with parainfluenza, adenovirus, Influenza virus, rhinovirus. The majority occur during winter but can occur any season.

B. **Clinical presentation.** Rhinorrhea, sneezing, coughing, low-grade fever. Onset of rapid breathing and wheezing. Signs of respiratory distress in severe cases: nasal flaring, tachypnea, prolonged expiratory phase, retractions.

C. **Lab tests.** CBC usually within normal limits. Blood gas, O_2 saturation levels, as appropriate. Nasal wash for RSV culture and antigen assay. CXR can be normal but occasionally shows air trapping and peri-bronchial thickening.

D. **Treatment.**

1. **Indications for hospitalization.** Use clinical judgment. Some suggested criteria include <6 months old, resting respirations >50 to 60, pO_2, <60 mm Hg, pulse oximetry 95%, apnea, unable to tolerate oral feedings.

2. **Supportive measures.** Antipyretics, IV fluids, humidified O_2, nebulized bronchodilators, such as albuterol 2.5 mg in 3 ml of NS; this can be repeated PRN. Oral albuterol can be used (0.1 mg/kg Q8h up to 12 mg) but is much less effective. **Epinephrine, 5 ml of 1:1000 by nebulizer is safe and effective and is an alternative.** Steroids are ineffective. However, they continue to be widely used in doses similar to those for asthma.

3. **Ribavirin aerosol.** The efficacy of ribavirin has recently been called into question. The use of ribavirin even in severely ill patients is at the discretion of the physician. If croup or bronchiolitis secondary to RSV, consider use of ribavirin in high-risk groups.
   - Congenital heart disease
   - Chronic lung disease (such as bronchopulmonary dysplasia)
   - Infants <6 weeks of age
   - Neurologic disorders
   - Immunosuppressed
   - Severely ill infants.
   - PaO_2 <65 mm Hg or SaO_2 <90%
   - Increasing pCO_2

4. Intubation and mechanical ventilation as indicated.

5. **Respiratory syncytial virus immunoglobulin** (RSV-IVIG) 750 mg/kg IV Q30 days can prevent RSV infection and hospitalization in those children with severe underlying illness such as bronchopulmonary dysplasia or prematurity. An alternative is Synagis (Palviziumab), an RSM immunoglobulin that can be given IM (15mg/kg/dose IM Q month). Use with caution in those with thrombocytopenia or coagulation defects because of intramuscular bleeding.

12

PEDIATRICS

LIMP AND JOINT PAIN

I. **Joint Pain.**

A. Will have pain on weight bearing or refusal to bear weight. Pain on passive motion of joints involved with arthritis.

B. Determine if true arthritis by exam, presence of fever, number of joints involved.

II. **Limp.**

A. Pain from hip often felt as knee pain in children.

B. Examine shoes and feet (look for tiny pebble in shoe bottom, etc.).
C. **General approach to the child with a limp.**
   1. A conservative approach indicated, since very few children without systemic symptoms or true arthritis have any significant disorder. If pain persists or you suspect an acute arthritis, diagnostic evaluations can include a CBC with differential, ESR, anti-streptolysin O titer, rheumatoid factor, throat and urine cultures, ultrasonography for joint effusion, and radiographic studies of the hips. A joint tap should be done when there is clinical suspicion of a septic joint and an effusion by U/S.
D. **Differential Diagnosis and Approach**
   1. **Transient tenosynovitis (irritable hip).**
      a. Most common cause of limp (well over 90% in some series).
      b. Frequently follows URI or streptococcal infection.
      c. May have joint effusion but not true arthritis.
      d. ESR—normal or mildly elevated.
      e. Generally resolves within 24 to 48 hours with rest and ibuprofen-acetaminophen. Close follow-up is indicated.
   2. **Septic hip joint. A true emergency** (see also Chapter 7).
      a. Generally febrile with elevated ESR, WBC >18,000/mm^3, but lab values may be normal and may overlap with those of other illnesses.
      b. Will generally look sick and hold hip in flexion and external rotation.
      c. Effusion present on ultrasonography but may also have effusion with transient tenosynovitis (71%). Tap is diagnostic.
      d. Relatively sudden onset and rapid course.
      e. Treat with antistaphylococcal antibiotics. Requires orthopedic consultation and surgical intervention.
   3. **Legg-Calvé-Perthes disease (aseptic necrosis of the femoral head).**
      a. Most common between 5 and 10 years of age.
      b. Slow insidious onset of limp and hip pain, which is progressive. Have limitation of motion of the hip.
      c. Diagnosis by radiography of affected hip (see lucency of femoral head and eventually sclerosis and destruction of femoral head). Bone scan may reveal abnormalities earlier than a plain radiograph.
      d. Treatment requires consultation with orthopedics and includes rest, anti-inflammatories, and casting for more severe cases.
   4. **Slipped capital femoral epiphysis.**
      a. Generally seen in overweight teenagers, especially boys who are prepubertal.
      b. May have insidious onset of pain but can also follow acute trauma.
      c. May be pain with passive motion. Patient will hold hip in external rotation.
      d. Diagnosis by frog-legged radiographs of both hips.
      e. Treatment is by orthopedic referral and surgical fixation.
   5. **Osgood-Schlatter disease.**

a. Characterized by pain over the tibial tubercle, which is usually unilateral. May have swelling over the area of pain.

b. Usually occurs in active children between 10 and 15 years of age.

c. Treatment is rest and NSAIDs and local heat.

6. **Diskitis.**

a. An inflammatory process of the disk or disks (usually L3 to L5), which may be infectious in cause (staphylococcal primarily).

b. Presents with refusal to walk or limp, low-grade fever, and "tripod posturing" - leaning back with back extended onto outstretched arms when sitting.

c. Generally have pain over involved disk area but may also have pain on straight-leg raising, hip motion.

d. Sedimentation rate almost always elevated, but CBC may be normal. Disk space may be narrowed on radiograph. Bone scan will show inflammatory focus.

e. Treatment is generally supportive with anti-inflammatories but may need antibiotics. Orthopedic consultation recommended.

7. **Juvenile rheumatoid arthritis.**

a. Defined as presentation of rheumatoid arthritis before 16 years of age.

b. See chapter 7, rheumatology as well.

c. 20% have "Still's disease," which is JRA plus fever, thrombocytopenia, splenomegaly, generalized adenopathy.

d. 40% have onset in one or a few joints.

e. 40% have polyarticular onset similar to adult onset.

f. 75% have complete remissions.

8. **Rheumatic fever.** See Chapter 7 for details.

9. **Sickle cell** crisis in appropriate populations (see Chapter 6).

10. **Other arthritides** including manifestation of ulcerative colitis, Crohn's disease, etc. Diagnosis by looking for and finding symptom complex.

NOCTURNAL ENURESIS

I. **Definition.** Involuntary loss of urine during sleep. Nocturnal enuresis is a disorder of delayed maturation and generally cannot be officially diagnosed until the child is at least 5 years old.

II. **Primary Enuresis.** Wetting that proceeds more or less continuously for at least 1 year without prior dry spells.

III. **Secondary Enuresis.** The child has been dry at least for 1 year before wetting the bed.

IV. **Epidemiology.** Most often primary, affects 10% to 20% of children 5 to 6 years of age. 1% of adults are affected. Tends to be familial; affects the child's self-esteem. Only 1% to 4% are attributable to uropathies. **Etiology theories:** "Organic" (deficiency in the nocturnal production of ADH, obstructive sleep apnea, need to rule out other organic causes),

12

PEDIATRICS

"psychologic," "sleep stage," and "failure to learn control." The definite cause is yet undetermined.

V. **Evaluation.** History: developmental milestones (assess delay in neurologic development), voiding history, toilet training, social history, child rearing, family milestones. Obtain history of UTI, medical and surgical problems, medications, diet. Gait, posture, spine exam may be important in diagnosing neurologic abnormalities. Abdominal mass, bladder size, UA, and culture to look for urinary tract infection, obstruction with overflow. If child is diurnal and nocturnal wetter, a renal and bladder ultrasonogram should be done. If there is history of UTI should do VCUG.

VI. **Management.**

A. Motivate the child to establish control!

B. **Pharmacotherapy.** DDAVP 1 or 2 sniffs QHS. Oxybutynin 1 to 5 mg QHS (used in daytime also for day wetting); imipramine less effective (25 to 50 mg QHS 6 to 12 years, 50 to 75 mg QHS >12 years). Also must be aware of the risks of overdose of imipramine. Enuresis often recurs when the medication is discontinued.

C. **Behavioral** (most successful). Self-monitoring, motivation and responsibility training, charting of success and failure nights, bladder training, enuresis alarms, nocturnal awakenings, avoid diapers. The enuresis alarms or pagers have been found to be the most effective form of therapy for enuresis.

D. **Diet.** Avoid caffeine, liquids before bedtime. May use DDAVP on sleepovers, travel.

BIBLIOGRAPHY

Adcock PM et al: Effect of urine latex agglutination tests on the treatment of children at risk for invasive bacterial infection, *Pediatrics* 96(5):951, 1995.

Allen UD: Cow's milk versus soy-based formula in mild and moderate diarrhea: a randomized, controlled trial, *Acta Paediatr* 83(2):183, 1994.

Baraff LJ et al: Practice guideline for the management of infants and children 0 to 36 months of age with fever without source, *Ann Emerg Med* 22(7):1198, 1993.

Baskin MN et al: Outpatient treatment of febrile infants 28 to 89 days of age with intramuscular administration of ceftriaxone, *J Pediatr* 120(1):22, 1992.

Bickerstaff DR et al: An investigation into the etiology of irritable hip, *Clin Pediatr* 30(6):353, 1991.

Blumberg DA et al: Severe reactions associated with diphtheria-tetanus-pertussis vaccine: detailed study of children with seizures, hypotonic-hyporesponsive episodes, high fevers, and persistent crying, *Pediatrics* 91(6):1158, 1993.

Bond T, Welch V, Mikula P: Overview and management of sleep enuresis in children, *AUA Update Series,* Lesson 16, vol XV, Baltimore, 1996, American Urological Association.

Bramson RT et al: The futility of the chest radiograph in the febrile infant without respiratory symptoms, *Pediatrics* 92(4):524, 1993.

Chouela EN et al: Equivalent therapeutic efficacy and safety of ivermectin and lindane in the treatment of human scabies, *Arch Dermatol* 135:651-655, 1999.

Committee on Infectious Disease: Therapy for children with invasive pneumococcal infections, *Pediatrics* 99(2), 1997.

Klassen TP et al: Nebulized budesonide for children with mild-to-moderate croup, *N Engl J Med* 331(5):285, 1994.

Larsen PB et al: Aminophylline versus caffeine citrate for apnea and bradycardia prophylaxis in premature neonates, *Acta Paediatr* 84(4):360-364, 1995.

Lucassen PLBJ et al: Effectiveness of treatments for infantile colic: systematic review, *Br Med J* 316(7144):1563, May 23, 1998.

Markestad T: Use of sucrose as a treatment for infant colic, *Arch Dis Child* 76(4):356, April 1997.

McMillin JA et al: *The whole pediatrician catalog,* Philadelphia, 1977, Saunders.

Menon K et al: A randomized trial comparing the efficacy of epinephrine with salbutamol in the treatment of acute bronchiolitis, *J Pediatr* 126(6):1004, 1995.

Metcalf TJ et al: Simethicone in the treatment of infant colic: a randomized, placebo-controlled, multicenter trial, *Pediatrics* 94(1)29-34, 1994.

Muñoz M et al: Appearance of resistance to beta-lactam antibiotics during therapy for Streptococcus pneumoniae meningitis, *J Pediatr* 127(1):98-99, 1995.

Nanulescu M et al: Early re-feeding in the management of acute diarrhoea in infants of 0-1 year of age, *Acta Paediatr* 84(9):1002, 1995.

Nigro G et al: Ganciclovir therapy for symptomatic congenital cytomegalovirus infection in infants: a two-regimen experience, *J Pediatr* 124(2):318-322, 1994.

Nutman J et al: Racemic versus l-epinephrine aerosol in the treatment of postextubation laryngeal edema: results from a prospective, randomized, double-blind study, *Crit Care Med* 22(10):1591, 1994.

Oggero R et al: Dietary modifications versus dicyclomine hydrochloride in the treatment of severe infantile colics, *Acta Paediatr* 83(2):222-225, 1994.

Prasad K et al: Dexamethasone treatment for acute bacterial meningitis: how strong is the evidence for routine use? *J Neurol Neurosurg Psychiatr* 59(1):31, 1995.

Ratnam S et al: Measles and rubella antibody response after measles-mumps-rubella vaccination in children with afebrile upper respiratory tract infection, *J Pediatr* 127(3):432, 1995.

Rimell FL et al: Characteristics of objects that cause choking in children, *JAMA* 274(22):1763, 1995.

Roizen N et al: Neurologic and developmental outcome in treated congenital toxoplasmosis, *Pediatrics* 95(1):11-20, 1995.

Sanford JP: *Guide to antimicrobial therapy,* 1999, Dallas, Antimicrobial Therapy.

Waisman Y et al: Prospective randomized double-blind study comparing l-epinephrine and racemic epinephrine aerosols in the treatment of laryngo-tracheitis (croup), *Pediatrics* 89(2):302, 1992.

Wald ER et al: Cautionary note on the use of empiric ceftriaxone for suspected bacteremia, *Am J Dis Child* 145(12):1359, 1991.

Wald ER et al: Dexamethasone therapy for children with bacterial meningitis, *Pediatrics* 95(1):21, 1995.

Wolke D et al: Excessive infant crying: a controlled study of mothers helping mothers, *Pediatrics* 94(3):322-332, 1994.

12

PEDIATRICS

GYNECOLOGY

Alicia M. Weissman

CONTRACEPTIVES

Table 13-1 lists the percentage of women experiencing an unintended pregnancy during the first year of typical use and the first year of perfect use of contraception.

I. **Combined Oral Contraceptive Pill (OCP).**

A. **Mechanism of action.** Suppresses ovulation through inhibition of the hypothalamic-pituitary-ovarian axis; alters the cervical mucus, retards sperm entry and discourages implantation into an unfavorable endometrium.

B. **Risks and adverse effects.** Hypertension, thromboembolism, stroke, myocardial infarction (especially in smokers), gallstone formation, hepatocellular adenomas or cancer, growth of fibroids. Minimally increases rate of breast cancer, may increase rate of cervical cancer. Possible higher rate of HIV due to intercourse without condoms.

C. **Side effects.** Nausea, breast tenderness, weight gain, decreased libido, leg cramping, headache, bloating, acne, spotting. Depression and migraines can worsen or improve.

D. **Absolute contraindications.** Pregnancy, history of thromboembolic disease, stroke or TIA, focal or severe migraine, ischemic heart disease, severe hypertension, history of breast cancer or estrogen-dependent neoplasms, hepatic dysfunction or tumor, porphyria, current prolonged immobilization or recent surgery on legs, diabetes with end-organ damage, smoker (>20 cigarettes/day) over 35. Ask about family history of venous thromboembolism; if positive, consider screening for Factor V Leiden, etc. (see Chapter 4).

E. **Relative contraindications.** Postpartum less than 3 weeks, lactation, active gallbladder disease, active mononucleosis, undiagnosed abnormal vaginal bleeding, light smoker over 35, long-term use of drugs decreasing the efficacy of the pill (rifampin, rifabutin, griseofulvin, phenytoin, phenobarbital, topiramate, carbamazepine, ampicillin, doxycycline, tetracycline). See below for pill management with antibiotics, etc.

F. **Noncontraceptive benefits of oral contraceptives.** More regular menses, decreased menorrhagia, decreased dysmenorrhea, increased iron stores, treatment of irregular menses secondary to anovulation; improvement in hirsutism; protection from benign breast disease, functional ovarian cysts, PID, ectopic pregnancy, epithelial ovarian cancer and endometrial carcinoma. Also increases bone mineral density.

G. **Benefits in special situations.** Patients with polycystic ovarian disease (PCO), severe dysmenorrhea, premenstrual syndrome (PMS) or amenorrhea can prolong their cycle by taking 2-3 consecutive packages of active pills (63 days, skipping inactive pills), followed by 7 days of inactive pills to allow withdrawal bleeding (and minimize the risk of endometrial

TABLE 13-1

CONTRACEPTIVE FAILURE RATE

Method	Typical Use (%)	Perfect Use (%)
No method	85	85
Oral contraceptives		
Combination	5	0.1
Progestin-only	5	0.5
Depo-Provera	0.3	0.3
Norplant and Norplant-II	0.05	0.05
Intrauterine device		
Copper-T 380A (Paraguard)	0.8	0.6
Progesterone-T IUD (Progestasert)	2.0	1.5
LNg 20-T (Mirena)	0.1	0.1
Condom	9.8	18.5
Female condom (Reality)	21	5
Male	14	3
Spermicide alone	26	6
Diaphragm	20	6
Cervical cap		
Parous women	40	26
Nulliparas	20	9
Sponge		
Parous women	40	20
Nulliparas	20	9
Lactational amenorrhea	2	—
Periodic abstinence	25	—
Calendar	—	9
Ovulation method	—	3
Sympto-thermal	—	2
Postovulation	—	1
Withdrawal	19	4
Female sterilization	0.5	0.5
Male sterilization	0.15	0.10

Adapted from Hatcher et al: *Contraceptive Technology*, 1998.

cancer). However, the long-term effects of this regimen have not been well studied.

H. **Perimenopausal use of oral contraceptives.** Perimenopausal women who still have menses can safely use oral contraceptives if they are non-smokers without other contraindications such as hypertension. Well-controlled hypertension not exacerbated by contraceptives may be acceptable. Use caution in any smoker. To determine menopausal status, ask about hot flashes during the placebo week and check the FSH on the sixth or seventh day of the placebo week. When menopausal, discuss changing directly to HRT.

I. **Managing the patient taking the pill**

1. **When starting OCPs** exclude pregnancy and supplement with alternative contraception during the first month. Recommend the use of condoms with OCPs to reduce risk of STDs and HIV.
2. **Starting regimens.** Start active pills day 1 after the start of menses. Many women choose to start on the Sunday after the start of their menses for convenience. For the post-partum, non-breast-feeding women, start OCP during week 4 after delivery. OCPs can be started the day after an induced or spontaneous abortion. For those who have had major surgery or leg surgery, do not start OCPs until they have been ambulatory for 2 weeks.
3. **Missed pill.** If a pill is missed, it should be taken as soon as possible and the next dose should be taken as usual. If two pills are missed, take two pills together on two consecutive days to catch up. Alternative contraception should be used for 7 days.
4. **If taking antibiotics or other interacting medication for a short time** (United Kingdom National Guidelines): use another form of birth control for the duration of the (antibiotic) treatment and for 7 days afterwards. If this 7 days extends into the next month, the patient should start the active pills without taking the placebo (i.e. skip menses).
5. **For breakthrough bleeding.** Breakthrough bleeding is not uncommon during the first 3 months of OCP use. Generally, breakthrough bleeding in the first 10 days of the cycle is due to inadequate estrogen while breakthrough at other times in the cycle is due to inadequate progesterone. For heavy bleeding in the first 7 days of the cycle, treat with conjugated oral estrogen 1.25 mg or estradiol 2.0 mg PO QD for the first 7 days of the cycle while continuing the contraceptive medication. If breakthrough bleeding continues, consider changing oral contraceptives with additional progesterone or estrogen depending on when in the cycle the problem occurs.
6. **Amenorrhea** is usually due to excess progestin effects. Consider adding conjugated estrogen for the first 7 days of the cycle or change to a higher estrogen or lower progesterone OCP.
7. **Third-generation progestins** Three progestogens, desogestrel, norgestimate, and gestodene with low androgenicity, minimal metabolic effects and good cycle control are available. They are useful for acne and hirsutism. However, they are more expensive, and there is some evidence that the risk of thromboembolic disease may be slightly increased with desogestrel and gestodene (Orthocept and Desogen).

II. **Progestin Only Contraceptives.**
A. **Types of Progestin only Contraceptives.**
   1. **Progestin-Only OCP (Minipill)** Minipills are somewhat less effective than combination pills unless used in women who are breast-feeding full-time. And, they must be taken at the same time every day to be effective making them less suitable for patients who might have irregular work schedules or are prone to missing doses (e.g., adolescents,

etc.). They have no adverse effect on lactation. Adverse effects, advantages, and contraindications as for progestin implants below.

2. **Injectable medroxyprogesterone acetate** (Depo-Provera) is given 150 mg IM every 3 months. Some women (especially if obese) may require higher doses because of higher levels of circulating estrogens. Most women have irregular bleeding for up to a year and then become amenorrheic. Medroxyprogesterone may accelerate the development of breast cancer (acts as a promoter) and decrease bone density. Return to fertility may be delayed up to 10 months due to persistence of the depot medication. Advantages and contraindications as for progestin implants below.

3. **Progestin implants** (Norplant). Subcutaneous insertion of six Silastic capsules containing levonorgestrel for slow release, providing contraception for 5 years. Removal is possible at any time. Long-term safety is unclear. Norplant-II contains two levonorgestrel implantable rods, is effective for 3 years, and has been cleared by the FDA.

B. **Advantages.** Because of their reduced potential to cause clotting abnormalities, progestin-only methods (minipill, Depo-Provera, Norplant) are useful in women with risk factors for cardiovascular disease, such as smokers, women >35 years, and diabetics.

C. **Absolute contraindications.** Pregnancy, undiagnosed abnormal vaginal bleeding, progestin-sensitive breast cancer.

D. **Relative contraindications.** Manufacturers of progestin-only methods continue to list estrogen-related contraindications despite the absence of estrogen in the contraceptives. See combined OCP above for list. Exercise caution when using phenytoin, carbamazepine, primidone, phenylbutazone, rifampin, or rifampicin.

E. **Side effects**: breast tenderness, weight gain, and possible depression.

F. **Fertility.** Usually returns within 2 months after removal.

III. **Intrauterine Devices (IUD).**

A. **Mechanism of action.** Primarily through inhibition of sperm migration, ovum transport and fertilization. No longer thought to be a significant abortifacient, although occasionally failure of implantation may occur.

B. **Safety.** Currently available IUDs are considered safe, with very low complication rates in properly selected patients. Patient selection is extremely important to avoid increasing the risk of infection and infertility. The ideal candidate is a parous woman in a mutually monogamous relationship with no history of PID.

C. **Duration.** Copper-T 380A (Paraguard) is replaced after 10 years. Progesterone-T IUD (Progestasert) is replaced annually. LNg 20-T (Mirena) lasts 5 years.

D. **Other uses.** Progestasert and Mirena offer effective treatment for severe menorrhagia.

E. **Absolute contraindications.** Current, recent (within 3 months) or recurrent endometritis, PID, or STD, pregnancy, anatomically distorted uterine cavity, known or suspected HIV infection. For Progestasert and Mirena, progestin-sensitive neoplasm.

F. **Relative contraindications.** Any history of gonorrhea or chlamydia, multiple sexual partners or a partner with multiple other partners, undiagnosed abnormal vaginal bleeding, known or suspected uterine or cervical malignancy, previous problems with an IUD (pregnancy, expulsion, perforation, pain, heavy bleeding). Use of an IUD in nulliparas is controversial.

G. **Adverse effects.** Include PID after insertion, uterine perforation during insertion. For Paraguard, spotting, heavy menstrual flow, and dysmenorrhea. For Progestasert and Mirena, spotting and amenorrhea.

H. **Special Notes.**
1. **Expulsions.** The patient should check that the string is palpable each month after her menses. Between 2% and 10% of women expel their IUD within the first year.
2. **Ectopics.** The absolute rate of ectopic pregnancy is reduced with the IUD because of its high contraceptive efficacy. However, when accidental pregnancy does occur, there is an increased proportion of ectopics, highest with the Progesterone-T.

IV. **Spermicides** containing nonoxynol-9 destroy sperm cell walls and provide some protection against STDs but may increase the risk of HIV transmission. When used alone, the failure rate is relatively high. When spermicides are used with a condom, the failure rate is comparable to that of oral contraceptives, and much better than for either spermicides or condoms alone. May cause vaginal irritation.

V. **Barrier Devices** (condom, female condom, diaphragm, cervical cap, intravaginal sponge). These methods (especially male condoms) decrease the risk of STDs when used properly. Adverse effects include latex allergy, increased risk of UTI with diaphragm.

A. **Condoms.** Efficacy of condoms is improved when used with vaginal spermicide. Patient education is important to promote proper use.

B. **Diaphragm and cervical cap.** Proper fitting is important. Carefully review product instructions with the patient: comfort with touching oneself, proper insertion technique and correct use of contraceptive cream/jelly is required for maximum efficacy. Have the patient demonstrate insertion and removal in the office before prescribing. The cervical cap is not recommended for use in parous women. The diaphragm is a risk factor for UTIs.

C. **Contraceptive sponge.** Available without a prescription. Not recommended for parous women.

VI. **Lactational Amenorrhea.** Full or nearly full breast feeding (supplements given for less than 5-15% of feeding episodes) is 98% effective for contraception during the first 6 months postpartum but is not reliable after 6 months. Women who do not wish to become pregnant should use an additional contraceptive method during the entire post-partum period but especially if bottle-feeding is increased.

VII. **Periodic Abstinence** during presumed fertile times requires long periods of abstinence. Highest failure rates in women with irregular cycles.

VIII. **Sterilization.**

13

A. **Female sterilization** is a very effective, permanent method of birth control. It has a high initial cost and is associated with an increased risk of ectopic pregnancy should pregnancy occur. When performed immediately postpartum or post-abortion, the health risks are minimized. The procedure can be performed under local or general anesthesia. Failure can occur due to pregnancy at the time of sterilization, tube re-anastomosis, fistula formation, equipment failure or surgical error. **Overall failure rate in 10 years is up to 3.2% with laparoscopic procedures.** Surgical reversibility is limited and expensive, so sterilization should be considered permanent. Careful patient counseling beforehand is essential.

B. **Male sterilization** is also very effective, permanent, costs less than half as much as female sterilization and is less invasive. A waiting period after vasectomy is required to clear the reproductive tract of sperm. The procedure is performed under local anesthesia.

XI. **Emergency Contraception (morning-after pill).** All female patients of reproductive age should be made aware of postcoital contraception (Table 13-2). This knowledge does not increase the likelihood of high-risk behavior. High doses of oral contraceptives, begun within 72 hours of unprotected intercourse decreases the risk of pregnancy by 74%. Only RU-486 (mifepristone) has been shown to be effective after 72 hours; other regimens are unstudied but may be effective. Consider prescribing an antiemetic (e.g., prochlorperazine, metoclopramide), since nausea and vomiting are common side effects.

A. **Regimens:** Effective and well-tolerated regimen is levonorgestrel (marketed as **Plan B**) 0.75 mg PO × 2, 12 hours apart. **Preven,** a convenient emergency contraception kit, includes two doses of medication and pregnancy test. **Mifepristone** (RU 486) 600 mg in one dose is the most effective with the fewest side effects. Doses as low as 10 mg **mifepristone** have been effective up to 5 days after unprotected intercourse.

B. For the drugs in Table 13-2, women should be instructed to take one dose as soon as possible after unprotected intercourse with a second dose 12 hours later. If prescribed, the antiemetic should be taken 1 hour before each dose. If a dose is vomited, the patient should contact the

TABLE 13-2

OPTIONS FOR POSTCOITAL CONTRACEPTION

Brand	Pills Per Dose	Brand	Pills Per Dose*
Plan B (most effective, best tolerated)	1 pill	Tri-Levlen	4 yellow pills
Levlen	4 light-orange pills	Ovral	2 white pills
Lo/Ovral	4 white pills	Alesse	5 pink pills
Triphasil	4 yellow pills	Ovrette	20 yellow pills
Preven	2 pills	Nordette	4 light-orange pills

Adapted from Hatcher et al: *Contraceptive Technology* 1998.
*All regimens are 2 doses, 12 hours apart.

health care practitioner to obtain an additional dose. Patients should avoid unprotected intercourse and if there is no menses within 3 weeks, return for a pregnancy test.

VAGINAL, VULVAR, AND RELATED CONDITIONS

I. **Vestibulitis.** Inflammation, pain and tenderness probably due to up-regulated nerve supply in the vestibular area.

A. **Etiology.** Although the true etiology is unknown, vulvar vestibulitis syndrome is strongly associated with candidal infection.

B. **Clinically.** There is entry dyspareunia, erythema and point tenderness of the vestibule, primarily at the base of the hymenal remnant.

C. **Treatment** may include long-term oral antifungal therapy, topical steroids, or surgery. Mycolog-II (nystatin + triamcinolone) is frequently very effective.

II. **Vulvovaginitis.** All types of vaginitis may produce vulvar itch, irritation, dyspareunia, or dysuria. Evaluation includes history, exam, microscopic exam of secretions with saline and KOH (wet prep obtained from vaginal vault) and vaginal pH with Nitrazine. Consider a UA to rule out UTI, and cervical cultures for infection with gonorrhea and chlamydia if indicated. Obtain a Pap if not done recently, since HPV is also sexually transmitted.

A. **Candidal vaginitis.**
   1. **Etiology.** *Candida albicans,* other *Candida* species (such as *glabrata*), *Torulopsis* species, other yeasts. Not generally sexually transmitted, although in refractory cases treatment of the partner may be needed. Precipitating factors include systemic antibiotic therapy, pregnancy, high-dose estrogen oral contraceptives and tight-fitting undergarments. Recurrent infections may occur in uncontrolled diabetes mellitus, immunosuppression (HIV, corticosteroid use). Asymptomatic colonization does not require treatment.
   2. **Discharge.** Discharge is nonmalodorous, thick, white cottage cheese-like and adheres to vaginal walls.
   3. **Diagnostic tests.** Wet mount: pseudohyphae or budding yeast cells. Wet mount is insensitive (65%-80%); if wet mount is negative, consider empiric treatment for typical pruritus without a watery discharge. Vaginal pH is normal (<4.5). Reserve fungal cultures for recurrent/resistant cases.
   4. **Treatment.**
      a. **Vaginal suppositories** can be used at bedtime for 3 days: clotrimazole 200 mg (100 mg × 2), miconazole 200 mg, or terconazole 80 mg. Single dose treatments are also available (e.g., 1200 mg of miconazole)
      b. **Vaginal creams** are used at bedtime for 7 days: clotrimazole 1% 5 g, miconazole 2% 5 g, or terconazole 0.4% 5 g.
      c. **Oral:** One dose of fluconazole 150 mg PO is effective. Itraconazole 200 mg PO QD for 3 days may also be used.

13

GYNECOLOGY

    d. **Recurrent or resistant cases** may require 10-14 days of topical or oral therapy, followed by suppressive therapy with clotrimazole 500 mg vaginal suppository or fluconazole 100 mg PO once weekly. Clotrimazole and miconazole are available OTC; **terconazole** is prescription and should be reserved for resistant disease. Encourage cotton underwear.

    e. **In pregnancy,** use creams for 7 days and avoid oral therapy.

B. **Bacterial vaginosis (BV).**

  1. **Etiology.** Polymicrobial (*Gardnerella vaginalis, Mycoplasma hominis, Prevotella, Mobiluncus, Bacteroides,* etc.). Not generally considered sexually transmitted but rare in those not sexually active. BV suggests (but does not prove) sexual abuse in the proper population. BV can lead to premature delivery, chorioamnionitis and postpartum endometritis; however, it is not clear that treatment prevents these complications.

  2. **Discharge.** Thin, white, or dull gray, homogeneous malodorous discharge that adheres to the vaginal walls.

  3. **Diagnostic tests.** 3 of 4 criteria: (1) Elevated pH (>4.5), (2) positive whiff or amine test when KOH applied to vaginal secretions, (3) clue cells seen on saline wet mount, (4) homogenous discharge noted.

  4. **Treatment.**

    a. **Oral:** Metronidazole 500 mg PO BID for 7 days or 2 g PO as single dose; clindamycin 300 mg PO BID for 7 days.

    b. **Vaginal:** metronidazole 0.75% gel 5 g per vagina BID for 5 days or clindamycin 2% cream per vagina QHS for 7 days.

    c. **Pregnancy.** During the first trimester avoid oral therapy; use vaginal metronidazole (avoid vaginal clindamycin—higher rate of preterm delivery), but treatment probably does not prevent preterm labor. After the first trimester, use metronidazole 250 mg PO BID for 7 days or 2 g PO as single dose; or clindamycin PO as above.

    d. **Treatment of male partner(s)** does not reduce the rate of recurrence (although condom use will).

C. **Trichomonas vaginitis.**

  1. **Etiology.** Trichomonas vaginalis, a protozoan that is sexually transmitted.

  2. **Discharge.** Copious, yellow gray or green, foamy, malodorous discharge.

  3. **Diagnostic tests.** Elevated pH (>4.5). Presence of mobile, flagellated organisms and leukocytes on wet mount.

  4. **Treatment.**

    a. Metronidazole 2 g PO as a single dose, or 500 mg PO BID for 7 days. Treat partner as well. Vaginal metronidazole is **not** effective. For multiple treatment failures (reinfection excluded) use metronidazole 2 g PO QD for 3-5 days.

    b. **Pregnancy.** During the first trimester, use clotrimazole 100 mg vaginal tabs QHS × 2 weeks. Then retreat in the second trimester with 7 day metronidazole regimen.

D. **Contact irritant/allergic vaginitis.** Itching, burning, soreness, variable discharge, with or without erythema. By definition, an evaluation for other etiologies is negative.
 1. **Etiology.** Obtain a careful history to identify the offending agent, such as menstrual pads, chemicals (soaps, laundry detergent, spermicides, perfumes, feminine hygiene products, etc), latex condoms, antifungal creams.
 2. **Treatment:** avoid the irritant, use bicarbonate sitz baths, topical vegetable oil. Avoid corticosteroids, which cause burning and atrophy.
E. **Atrophic vaginitis.** Predominantly in postmenopausal women, may also occur during lactation or with progesterone-only contraceptives.
 1. **Clinically.** Epithelium has few rugae and is inflamed and dry, producing itching, dyspareunia, spotting and urinary symptoms. May have significant vaginal hemorrhage especially in the elderly. Vaginal pH>6.0. Wet mount may show increased cocci and coliforms, small round parabasal cells, PMNs.
 2. **Treatment** is estrogen, either oral estrogen replacement therapy or topical estradiol 0.01% cream 2-4 g daily for 1-2 weeks, then half the dose for 1-2 weeks, maintenance dose is 1 g 1-3 times per week. Another option is conjugated estrogen cream 2-4 g daily (3 weeks on, 1 week off) for 3-6 months. If estrogen is contraindicated may use glycerin/mineral oil preparations (Replens) symptomatically. If symptoms do not resolve with hormone or antifungal therapy, biopsy is indicated.
F. **Chronic purulent vaginitis** has been reported which is an exudative vaginitis, with purulent discharge and an elevated vaginal pH due to replacement of normal flora with gram-positive cocci and occasional vaginal spotted rash. Responds to clindamycin cream.
III. **Cervical Infections.** Most commonly *Neisseria gonorrhoeae* and *Chlamydia trachomatis*.
A. **Range of symptoms.** From asymptomatic to mucopurulent cervicitis; may have associated urethritis or infection of Bartholin's glands.
B. **Evaluation.** Pelvic exam; look for purulent, yellow or green cervical discharge, >10 WBC/oil field on cervical smear, and check gram stain for gram-negative intracellular diplococci (GC). Cervical cultures for GC/*Chlamydia* should be done. Consider a Pap smear if none recently.
C. **Collecting specimens.** Collect cervical culture for gonococcus culture first, since this organism will be found in the mucus. Endocervical cells are needed for *Chlamydia*, which is intracellular. For both specimens use an endocervical swab held in the cervix for 30 seconds. Twirling the *Chlamydia* swab will increase yield. See Chapter 8 for treatment.
D. **Routine screening** is recommended in high-risk groups such as sexually active teens and women <25 or with new or multiple sexual partners. DNA-based screening tests of vaginal secretions or urine specimens are also available.
IV. **Urethritis.** Causes for urethritis with negative UA include low colony-count UTI (up to 30% of culture proven UTIs have a negative UA),

13

GYNECOLOGY

N. gonorrhea, C. trachomatis, Mycoplasma species, Ureaplasma urealyticum, Trichomonas vaginalis, herpes simplex, Candida, interstitial cystitis, contact sensitivity (to soaps, feminine hygiene products, latex condoms, spermicides, etc). PCR of voided urine can detect Chlamydia. See Chapter 8 for more information.

V. **Proctitis and Proctocolitis** can also be due to sexually transmitted infections such as N. gonorrhoeae, C. trachomatis, and herpes simplex virus when receptive anal intercourse or oral-anal contact is practiced.

VI. **Syphilis, Genital Herpes Simplex, and Other STDs.** See Chapter 8.

PELVIC INFLAMMATORY DISEASE (PID)

I. **General.** PID is an infection that may involve the uterus, fallopian tubes, ovaries, and pelvic cavity, and may produce tubo-ovarian abscesses.

II. **Pathogenesis.** Usually sexually transmitted but may occur after uterine instrumentation. Often polymicrobial, with ascending infection initiated by N. gonorrhoeae or Chlamydia trachomatis, and secondary infection by other organisms including Mycoplasma species, Ureaplasma urealyticum, Bacteroides, Enterobacteriaceae, Streptococci, gram-negative enterics, other anaerobes.

III. **Predisposing Factors.** Multiple sexual partners, non-barrier contraceptive use (especially IUD), transvaginal instrumentation of cervix and uterus, recent menstrual period, current STD infection, history of PID or douching.

IV. **Diagnosis.**

A. **Differential diagnosis.** Appendicitis, ectopic pregnancy, septic abortion, endometriosis, hemorrhagic corpus luteum, ovarian cyst, adnexal torsion, inflammatory bowel disease, mesenteric lymphadenitis, pyelonephritis, or other intra-abdominal processes. See acute abdomen in Chapter 15, surgery, for a more complete discussion of abdominal/pelvic pain.

B. **Evaluation.** Abdominal and complete pelvic exam. Obtain UA, CBC, pregnancy test, Gram stain of cervical discharge, and appropriate cultures: endocervix, rectum, urethra, blood, and peritoneal fluid as indicated. Obtain Pap if none recently.

C. **Criteria for diagnosis.**

1. **Primary criteria:** must have all three. (1) lower abdominal tenderness with or without rebound, (2) cervical motion tenderness, (3) adnexal tenderness. Additionally, there should be no other pathology that explains the symptoms. **The primary criteria alone are sufficient to treat for PID!!**

2. **Secondary criteria** used to confirm the diagnosis: (1) temperature >38.3° C, (2) abnormal vaginal discharge; (3) adnexal mass on bimanual exam or ultrasonography, (4) WBC >10,500/mm^3; (5) elevated ESR or CRP; (6) endocervical Gram stain with gram-negative intracellular diplococci, positive rapid assay for Chlamydia, or other documentation of GC or Chlamydia infection; (7) diagnostic laparoscopy or endometrial histology; (8) culdocentesis with WBCs and bacteria

V. **Treatment.** Because of the risk of infertility, treat all patients meeting the primary criteria presumptively while awaiting cultures even if no secondary criteria are met.

A. **Outpatient therapy** if temperature is less than 38° C, WBC<11,000/mm^3, minimal signs of peritonitis, active bowel sounds, able to tolerate PO, good compliance likely.

1. Ofloxacin 400 mg PO BID × 14 days plus metronidazole 500 mg PO BID × 14 days. **Alternative:** Ofloxacin as above plus clindamycin 450 mg PO QID × 14 days **or** Ceftriaxone 250 mg IM × 1 dose plus doxycycline 100 mg PO BID × 14 days. Reevaluate in 48-72 hours. May also elect IV therapy.

2. Single-dose azithromycin is not adequate therapy for *Chlamydia* in the setting of PID.

B. **Inpatient therapy** if suspected abscess, pregnancy, temperature greater than 38° C, WBC >11,000/mm^3, unable to take PO medication, peritonitis, no response to oral antibiotics within 48 hours, unclear diagnosis, inability to comply with outpatient treatment and follow-up. Some authorities admit all adolescents with PID.

1. Cefotetan 2 g IV Q12h plus doxycycline 100 mg IV/PO Q12h **or** cefoxitin 2 g IV Q6h plus doxycycline 100 mg IV/PO Q12h until improvement. Follow with doxycycline 100 mg PO BID to complete 14 days.

2. In IUD-related infection, suspected abscess, or procedure-related infection: clindamycin 900 mg IV Q8h plus gentamicin loading dose 2 mg/kg IV followed by gentamicin 1.5 mg/kg Q8h until improvement. (Adjust gentamicin dose in renal insufficiency. Can also use single daily gentamicin dosing.) Adding ampicillin 1 g IV Q6h to clindamycin and gentamicin appears to improve efficacy in the setting of abscess. **Alternative:** ofloxacin 400 mg IV Q12h plus metronidazole 500 mg IV q8h. Follow as outpatient with doxycycline 100 mg PO BID or clindamycin 450 mg PO QID to complete 14 days, follow-up in 7 days.

VI. **Complications.** Infection rarely remains confined to fallopian tubes, and peritonitis is common. **Acute complications** include rupture of tubo-ovarian abscess, adnexal torsion, Fitz-Hugh-Curtis syndrome (perihepatic GC) and septicemia. **Long-term** complications include an increased risk of ectopic pregnancy (6-10 times), infertility (20%), and bowel obstruction secondary to adhesions.

BARTHOLIN'S GLANDS

I. **General.** The Bartholin's glands are pea-sized organs situated at the 5 and 7 o'clock positions of the vaginal introitus. When normal they are nonpalpable. A Bartholin's gland may become enlarged from cystic dilatation, abscess, or adenocarcinoma (generally in women >40 years).

II. **Cystic Dilatation** of the Bartholin's duct can result from trauma or inflammation. These cysts are usually asymptomatic, and in women under 40

13

GYNECOLOGY

40, they generally do not require treatment. Symptomatic cysts can be treated with placement of a Word catheter for 4 weeks or marsupialization. In women >40 there is a small incidence of adenocarcinoma in Bartholin's which can be evaluated with drainage and selective biopsy. Try to avoid surgical treatment during pregnancy for uninfected cysts.

III. **Bartholin's Gland Abscess** is a polymicrobial infection accompanied by severe dyspareunia, vulvar pain, difficulty walking or sitting, erythema, edema, and possibly cellulitis of the surrounding tissue.

A. **Etiology:** *B. fragilis, N. gonorrhoeae, Bacteroides* species, Peptostreptococcus, *E. coli,* Proteus, and Klebsiella.

B. **Treatment:** Hot soaks, pain medication, and antibiotics if surrounding cellulitis is present. Abscesses may spontaneously rupture and drain after 4-5 days or may require surgical drainage. A GC culture should be obtained (present in 20%). Antibiotics should be directed against gram negatives and anaerobes (e.g., amoxicillin/clavulanate or metronidazole + TMP/SMX, etc.). IV combinations include metronidazole + gentamicin, Unasyn, etc.

C. **Further management:** Abscesses tend to recur after simple incision and drainage, so placement of a Word catheter for 4 to 6 weeks or marsupialization is recommended. The gland should be excised if the abscess reforms on multiple occasions.

ABNORMAL VAGINAL BLEEDING, MENSTRUAL PROBLEMS, AND SECONDARY AMENORRHEA

See also endometrial abnormalities section below.

I. **Terminology.**

A. **Menorrhagia:** Heavy or prolonged bleeding. **Metrorrhagia:** Intermenstrual bleeding, spotting, or breakthrough bleeding. **Menometrorrhagia:** Heavy irregular bleeding. **Polymenorrhea:** Menstrual interval <21 days. **Oligomenorrhea:** Menstrual interval >35 days. **Amenorrhea:** Absence of menstrual bleeding.

II. **Evaluation.**

A. **History.** Describe bleeding (timing, duration, flow, presence of clots, number of pads used). Obtain menstrual and obstetric history, sexual history, drug and medication use, familial bleeding disorders and bleeding tendencies, contraceptive use, postcoital bleeding (may indicate cervicitis, cervical polyp), galactorrhea, headaches (e.g., from prolactinoma), visual disturbances, menopausal symptoms, change in weight, diet, exercise, stressors.

B. **Physical exam.** Look for obesity or low body weight, acne, hirsutism, Cushingoid habitus. Thyroid exam, check skin for petechiae, ecchymoses. Breast exam, pelvic exam noting vaginal or cervical lesions, uterine size and shape, adnexal masses. Exclude rectal source of bleeding. Obtain Pap if none recently.

C. **Initial lab tests.** Pregnancy test, CBC (for anemia, platelet count), free T4/TSH, GC and *Chlamydia* cultures if sexually active. **As indicated:**

PT, PTT, FSH and LH (elevated ratio of FSH/LH:3:1 in PCOS, see PCOS below), prolactin, UA (for microscopic hematuria) and androgens (testosterone, DHEA-S), 24-hour urinary free cortisol, liver/kidney function tests. Pelvic ultrasound if palpable mass. Consider endometrial biopsy especially if >35 or if obese with >12 months anovulatory bleeding.

III. **Causes of Abnormal Vaginal Bleeding**

A. **Dysfunctional uterine bleeding.** Usually associated with anovulatory cycles and patchy asynchronous sloughing of estrogen-stimulated endometrium due to tonic hormone levels rather than cyclically fluctuating gonadotropins and sex hormones. Common causes include puberty, perimenopause, stress, weight loss (anorexia, athletes), PCOS, and simple obesity. In obesity and PCOS, chronic anovulation results in long-term unopposed estrogen exposure, increasing the risk of endometrial hyperplasia or carcinoma. Failure to establish regular menses at puberty or prolonged absence of regular cycles from weight loss can lead to loss of bone mass. (Female athlete's triad: anorexia nervosa, anovulation, osteoporosis.)

B. **Other endocrinopathies.** Hypothyroidism or hyperthyroidism, hyperprolactinemia, androgen-producing adrenal disorders.

　　1. **Hyperprolactinemia.** Most common lesion is microadenoma of pituitary, but may also be due to hypothyroidism, antipsychotics or other medication. May have headaches or visual symptoms. Check TSH/FREE T4. High-resolution CT of the sella turcica or MRI are the imaging studies of choice. Refer appropriately if imaging is abnormal or, if normal, follow prolactin Q6 months and CT or MRI Q1-2 years. Can treat with bromocriptine to suppress prolactin and shrink adenomas.

C. **Structural lesions.** Cervical polyps, endometrial polyps, leiomyomas. Submucosal fibroids are present in a significant proportion of women with postmenopausal bleeding.

D. **Malignant lesions.** Vaginal, cervical neoplasm; endometrial hyperplasia or carcinoma; estrogen-producing ovarian neoplasms.

E. **Coagulopathies.** Most common is von Willebrand's disease. Also consider leukemias, thrombocytopenias (see Chapter 6).

F. **Pregnancy-related bleeding.** Ectopic pregnancy, threatened abortion, molar pregnancy, placental abruption, placenta previa, implantation of blastocyst.

G. **Infections.** Chlamydia, chronic cervicitis, chronic endometritis.

H. **Miscellaneous.** Atrophic vaginitis, bleeding during ovulation, hormone contraceptive-related breakthrough bleeding, IUD use, some herbal drugs (ginseng), foreign object, trauma, severe organ dysfunction (renal, liver)

IV. **Treatment of Abnormal Vaginal Bleeding**

A. **Ovulatory menorrhagia (heavy menstrual bleeding):** NSAIDS will decrease menstrual bleeding. Treat with maximal doses of NSAID (ibuprofen, naproxen, etc.) beginning 1-2 days before menses. Combination

13

GYNECOLOGY

oral contraceptives are another option to decrease menstrual bleeding. In refractory cases, consider progestin IUD (Progestasert, Mirena).

B. **Acute management of dysfunctional uterine bleeding.**

1. **Severe bleeding requiring inpatient therapy.** (Symptomatic Hb less than 10, hypotension, etc.) may require IV fluid resuscitation and blood transfusion. Use conjugated estrogen 25 mg IV Q4h until bleeding abates or for 12 hours followed by conjugated estrogen 1.25 mg PO QD × 7 days. Antiemetics will help with nausea. After 7 days of estrogen, induce withdrawal bleed with medroxyprogesterone acetate 10 mg PO QD × 7 to 10 days. On day 5 of withdrawal bleeding begin low-dose OCP. Options for refractory hemorrhage include intrauterine tamponade with inflatable catheter, D&C, endometrial ablation, hypogastric artery ligation or embolization, hysterectomy.

2. **Major bleeding not requiring inpatient therapy.** May use conjugated estrogen 1.25 mg or estradiol 2.0 mg PO QD for 7-10 days (for severe bleeding, dose Q4 hours initially for 24 hours). Prescribe antiemetics. Follow with medroxyprogesterone acetate 10 mg PO QD × 7 to 10 days, then low-dose OCPs.

3. **Moderate bleeding.** Use any combined progestin-estrogen OCP, 1 active pill **QID** for 7 days (1.5 packs, avoid placebo pills). Prescribe antiemetics. Expect cessation of flow in 12 to 24 hours. Heavy withdrawal flow with cramping will start 2 to 4 days after regimen completed. On day 5 of withdrawal flow, begin daily low-dose combination OCP or use medroxyprogesterone acetate 10 mg QD × 10 days each month for at least 3 months.

4. **Mild bleeding.** Use medroxyprogesterone acetate 5-10 mg PO QD × 10-14 days to induce a coordinated withdrawal bleed ("medical curettage"). Expect heavy but limited bleed to begin within 5 days afterward. If withdrawal bleed does not occur, further work-up is indicated. After the induced withdrawal bleed, if spontaneous cycles do not resume treat as below under "long-term management". Persistent abnormal bleeding requires reevaluation.

5. **Long-term management of dysfunctional uterine bleeding.** If regular cycles do not resume, induce cycles with combined OCPs especially if contraception is needed. Alternatively, use medroxyprogesterone acetate 5-10 mg QD × 10 days, monthly (or at least every 3 months). Either treatment prevents endometrial hyperplasia.

6. **Management of perimenopausal bleeding.** Work-up usually not needed for a single anovulatory cycle. Determine menopausal status by checking an FSH and treat as per dysfunctional uterine bleeding above. Avoid long-term OCP use in smokers >35 but they may be used in non-smoking, healthy patients premenopausally to prevent dysfunctional uterine bleeding (see section on contraception above for contraindications). Recurrent irregular bleeding should be evaluated with an endometrial biopsy or D & C to exclude endometrial hy-

perplasia or carcinoma. This can be followed by hysteroscopy looking for other organic lesions (polyps, submucosal fibroids) if bleeding continues.

7. **Management of postmenopausal bleeding.** Mild spotting may be observed on initiation of HRT. Otherwise, postmenopausal bleeding always requires complete evaluation for endometrial hyperplasia or carcinoma, with endometrial biopsy or D&C followed by hysteroscopy if bleeding continues. Alternatively, an endovaginal ultrasound showing an endometrial stripe of less than 5 mm excludes endometrial carcinoma with sensitivity close to 100%, specificity 75%. Biopsy is required if stripe is 5mm or greater. The specificity is markedly reduced in women on HRT because of the resulting increase in endometrium. The same contraindications for OCPs should be considered. **For bleeding due to atrophic endometrium,** start HRT, or if already on HRT increase the estrogen component by 50% to 100% for 3 months. **For bleeding due to proliferative endometrium,** start HRT, or if already on HRT increase the progestin component by 50% to 100%.

8. **Less-common therapies.** Persistent bleeding may require prolonged therapy. Depending on the underlying problem, some possible treatments include progestin IUD (chronic illness, renal failure), desmopressin (coagulopathies, renal failure), GnRH agonists (blood dyscrasias, renal failure, transplant patients).

V. **Secondary Amenorrhea.** Absence of menses for at least 3-6 months in a previously menstruating woman. Primary amenorrhea (never menstruated) has a different differential and work-up.

A. **Causes.** Pregnancy, hypothalamic anovulation (hypogonadotropism/hypothalamic related amenorrhea presents with a low LH (<0.5 IU/ml), which can be the result of weight loss, anorexia, or stress), recent discontinuation of hormonal contraceptives, physiologic menopause, premature ovarian failure, hyper- or hypothyroidism, hyperprolactinemia, PCOS, ovarian or adrenal tumor, uterine outflow tract abnormality. Failure to maintain an adequate weight (e.g., in anorexia or the female athlete) is an important cause of secondary amenorrhea.

B. **History and exam** as above for abnormal vaginal bleeding. Consider endometrial biopsy if amenorrheic >12 months.

C. **Initial lab tests. Pregnancy test in all reproductive-age women** with amenorrhea, regardless of reported sexual history. Serum prolactin, TSH/free T4. (May elect to draw FSH, LH as well with initial labs.) If serum prolactin is high, see III B1 above.

D. **Evaluation begins with a progestin challenge test** (if pregnancy test is negative). Give medroxyprogesterone acetate 10 mg QD × 5 days. Withdrawal bleeding within 7 days indicates ovaries are secreting estrogen and rules out premature ovarian failure.

E. **Diagnosis and further evaluation depending on above results.**

1. **Positive progestin challenge.** If expected withdrawal bleed occurs, it indicates sufficient endogenous estrogen is present. If patient has a

13

GYNECOLOGY

normal prolactin level and no galactorrhea, pituitary tumor is effectively ruled out.

 a. **Differential** includes hypothalamic (idiopathic, e.g., stress, weight loss, etc.) anovulation, POCS, ovarian or adrenal tumors if hirsute.

 b. **Treatment in those with idiopathic anovulation and PCOS.** Induce cycles with combined OCPs especially if contraception is needed. Alternatively, use medroxyprogesterone acetate 10 mg QD × 10 days, monthly or at least every 3 months to prevent endometrial hyperplasia. If fertility is desired, treat with clomiphene citrate. See also section on POCS.

 2. **Negative progestin challenge.** No withdrawal bleeding; normal prolactin level. Indicates either insufficient estrogen or outflow tract abnormality.

 a. Next step is **estrogen/progestin challenge test:** give conjugated estrogen 1.25 mg PO QD × 21 days, with medroxyprogesterone acetate 10 mg QD during the last 5 days.

 b. **Positive estrogen/progestin challenge test:** expected withdrawal bleed occurs. Check FSH and LH >2 weeks after challenge test.

 (1) **FSH and LH high:** premature ovarian failure. Evaluate for systemic causes and start hormone replacement. (see section on menopause)

 (2) **FSH and LH normal or low:** indicates pituitary or hypothalamic dysfunction. Evaluate for pituitary tumor and start hormone replacement. See section on menopause.

 c. **Negative estrogen/progestin challenge test:** no withdrawal bleed occurs. May repeat once to confirm result. Differential includes Asherman's syndrome (uterine synechiae) if history of D&C; other outflow tract abnormalities.

ENDOMETRIAL ABNORMALITIES

See previous section on abnormal uterine bleeding.

I. **Endometritis**

A. **Puerperal endometritis** (see Chapter 14).

B. **Acute endometritis** is a component of PID (see section on PID).

C. **Chronic endometritis** is often asymptomatic except for intermenstrual bleeding, menorrhagia, or postcoital bleeding. Patients may complain of a dull heavy discomfort.

 1. **Diagnosis.** Made by endometrial biopsy showing inflammation with plasma cells. Culture endometrial and cervical specimens for *Chlamydia* and gonorrhea. Check wet mount for bacterial vaginosis.

 2. **Treatment.** Doxycycline 100 mg PO BID for 10 days. If bacterial vaginosis is also present, include anaerobic coverage as well.

 3. **IUD-associated** chronic actinomyces infection may occur or *Actinomyces* may be noted on routine Pap smear. Remove IUD.

 4. **Tuberculous** endometritis is rare today.

II. **Endometrial polyps**

A. Bleeding due to polyps may respond to hormonal therapy or NSAIDs.

B. Malignant transformation is rare but can occur.

C. Polypectomy can be done at the time of diagnostic hysteroscopy.

III. **Endometrial Hyperplasia and Adenocarcinoma**

A. **Spectrum.** Hyperplasia may be simple (including cystic hyperplasia), complex (adenomatous without atypia), or atypical (atypical adenomatous). Atypical hyperplasia progresses to adenocarcinoma in about 25% of cases.

B. **Signs and symptoms of endometrial hyperplasia and adenocarcinoma.** Most women present with prolonged, heavy or intermenstrual bleeding and are over age 40 or postmenopausal. The probability that postmenopausal bleeding is caused by an endometrial carcinoma increases with the patient's age. Women receiving hormone replacement therapy who have regular withdrawal bleeding in response to exogenous progestins do not require scheduled monitoring with endometrial biopsy. The presence of atypical glandular cells (AGUS) on a Pap smear also suggests an endometrial problem.

C. **Risk factors.** Chronic anovulation (as in POCS), obesity (increased conversion of androstenedione to estrone by adipose tissue aromatase), unopposed exogenous estrogen use, diabetes mellitus, nulliparity, late menopause, and hypertension.

D. **Diagnosis.** Diagnose with office endometrial biopsy, dilatation and curettage or hysteroscopy. In postmenopausal women, a transvaginal pelvic ultrasound can effectively exclude hyperplasia or cancer if the endometrial stripe measures <5 mm, however many women will have a thicker endometrial stripe and require biopsy.

E. **Treatment.**

1. **Simple hyperplasia:** The risk of malignancy is low. Treatment is with progesterone, induction of regular endometrial shedding, D&C, or observation.

2. **Complex hyperplasia:** Risk of malignancy is slightly higher. Treatment is with intermittent or continuous progestin.

3. **Atypical hyperplasia:** Often total abdominal hysterectomy and bilateral salpingo-oophorectomy is performed. High-dose progestin therapy is an alternative in poor surgical candidates or if fertility is desired, but endometrial surveillance is necessary to watch for progression to cancer.

4. **Endometrial carcinoma:** Total abdominal hysterectomy and bilateral salpingo-oophorectomy plus adjuvant radiation.

13

GYNECOLOGY

DYSMENORRHEA

I. **Characteristics and Etiology**

A. **Primary dysmenorrhea** is defined as menstrual pain in the absence of pelvic pathology, resulting from excessive prostaglandin production with the onset usually before age 20. Pain is crampy and spasmodic in the lower abdomen or back and begins within a day of onset of flow, lasts

24 to 72 hours, and may be associated with headache, fatigue, nausea, vomiting, diarrhea, thigh pain, dizziness. Primary dysmenorrhea usually improves after childbirth.

B. **Secondary dysmenorrhea** is defined as menstrual pain associated with pelvic pathology. Secondary dysmenorrhea usually has an onset after age 20, progresses with age, and is less characteristically timed with menses. Causes include endometriosis, leiomyomas, endometrial cancer, IUD use, polyps, PID, cervical stenosis, ovarian cysts, imperforate hymen or other obstructive malformation, uterine synechiae.

II. **Evaluation**

A. **History.** Past menstrual history, need for contraceptives, family history, review of systems, effect on daily activities or work, and psychologic effect.

B. **Exam.** Pelvic, rectovaginal exam for uterosacral nodules.

C. **Lab tests.** Not usually necessary. If indicated by H&P, consider Pap smear, cultures, wet mount. Endometrial biopsy, ultrasonography or laparoscopy may be useful, especially in diagnosing secondary dysmenorrhea.

III. **Treatment**

A. **Primary.**
   1. **Reassurance**
   2. **NSAIDs** Ibuprofen 400 to 800 mg PO TID; naproxen 500 mg PO BID. Mefenamic acid 500 mg initially and then 250 mg PO TID may be especially effective. Start 3 days before expected menses and continue until flow stops. Reassess the need for medications in 1 year.
   3. **Combination** OCPs, 3 month trial, continue if effective.
   4. If no response, look for organic cause, consider laparoscopy.

B. **Secondary.** Treat underlying cause.

PREMENSTRUAL SYNDROME (PMS)

I. **General.** Constellation of physical, emotional, or behavioral symptoms occurring during the second half of the menstrual cycle (luteal phase, 7 to 10 days before menses), with resolution of symptoms soon after flow begins. There must be a symptom-free interval of at least one week during the first half (follicular phase) of the menstrual cycle. PMS affects 90% of women minimally and 10% severely. It affects primarily those in late 20s to early 30s without racial, socioeconomic, or other demographic predilection. **Hysterectomized patients** can still experience PMS if at least one ovary is present.

II. **Diagnosis is clinical.** See Box 13-1.

III. **Variability** in symptoms can be wide. PMS may be diagnosed even if all criteria for Premenstrual Dysphoric Disorder are not met. Additional symptoms such as flatulence, constipation, diarrhea, sore throat, palpitations, urinary symptoms, dizziness, and others may be present.

IV. **Symptom calendar** is helpful in documenting cyclicity and in monitoring response to therapy.

V. **Causes**

BOX 13-1

DSM IV CRITERIA FOR PMS (PREMENSTRUAL DYSPHORIC DISORDER)

Patients must have 5 or more of the following and at least one of the symptoms in column 1

COLUMN 1

- Feeling sad, hopeless, or self-deprecating
- Feeling tense, anxious or "on edge"
- Marked lability of mood interspersed with frequent fearfulness
- Persistent irritability, anger, and increased interpersonal conflicts

COLUMN 2

- Decreased interest in usual activities, which may be associated with withdrawal from social relationships
- Difficulty concentrating
- Feeling fatigued, lethargic, or lacking in energy
- Marked changes in appetite, which may be associated with binge eating or craving certain foods
- Hypersomnia or insomnia
- A subjective feeling of being overwhelmed or out of control
- Physical symptoms such as breast tenderness or swelling, headaches, joint or muscle pain, sensations of bloating or weight gain with tightness of fit of clothing, shoes, or rings.
- Symptoms interfere with work or usual activities or relationships.

Symptoms cannot be an exacerbation of another disorder like major depression, panic, dysthymia, personality disorder; although it may be superimposed on any of these.

13

GYNECOLOGY

A. **Hormonal and chemical.** Theories abound. Probably a neurotransmitter imbalance induced by the normal hormonal cycle.

B. **Biopsychosocial.** Expectations, beliefs, personality, coping style, sexual experiences, partner responses, social supports, etc. all play a role.

VI. **Treatment**

A. **Validation.** The symptoms are not "all in her head." Consider support groups.

B. **Regular aerobic exercise** helps both mood and somatic symptoms.

C. **Psychological therapy.** Stress management, relaxation therapy, and supportive psychotherapy.

D. **Diet.** Limit salt (fluid retention), caffeine (breast tenderness), alcohol and fat. Increase complex carbohydrates and fiber. Consider vitamin B_6 50 mg PO TID, keeping in mind risk of peripheral neuropathy.

E. **Medications.**

1. **Breast symptoms** may respond to bromocriptine 2.5mg QHS or danazol 200mg/day or BID.

2. **Antidepressants.** SSRIs (fluoxetine, sertraline, etc.) may be titrated to effect. Clomipramine is also effective, 25-75 mg QD. Use only during the luteal phase if possible, all month if necessary. Has been shown to be effective in controlling symptom severity in multiple placebo-controlled clinical trials.

3. **Anti-anxiety medication** such as buspirone 5-10 mg PO TID is useful where anxiety predominates. Benzodiazepines have also been used but are addictive and should be used very cautiously.

4. **Calcium.** 1000-1200 mg daily (divide BID) or magnesium 400 IU PO QD during the luteal phase have both been shown to be effective in placebo-controlled trials.

5. **Diuretics.** Spironolactone 25 mg TID-QID during luteal phase (12 days before menses). Best for those with weight gain, bloating, and edema.

6. **Prostaglandin inhibitors.** Ibuprofen 400 to 800 mg TID, naproxen 500 mg PO BID, or mefenamic acid 500 mg TID 10 days before period through day 2 of menses. Have been shown to reduce the intensity of both the physical and emotional symptoms.

7. **Cycle suppression** with oral contraceptives or Depo-Provera. Rarely, GnRH agonists are used.

8. **Progesterone.** Oral 100-400 mg PO BID. Vaginal or rectal suppository 200 to 400 mg/day during luteal phase. Medroxyprogesterone acetate 10-20 mg PO QD is another possibility.

CHRONIC PELVIC PAIN

See Chapter 15 for acute abdominal and pelvic pain.

I. **Characteristics.** Unpleasant sensation or discomfort in the lower abdomen or pelvis with a duration of greater than 6 months, causing enough physical or psychological suffering to impair the quality of life. Patients usually report incomplete relief by most previous treatments, significantly impaired function at home or at work, signs of depression, pain out of proportion to pathologic condition, altered family roles. **Many have a history of past sexual abuse.**

II. **Etiology.** The biopsychosocial model proposes that precipitating organic symptoms combine with psychosocial variables to produce chronic debilitating pain. In 5% of cases no identifiable somatic source of pain can be found.

III. **Sources of noncyclic pain.**

A. **Gynecologic disorders.** Pelvic inflammatory disease, pelvic adhesions, and cervical stenosis.

B. **Musculoskeletal disorders.** Poor posture, scoliosis, unilateral standing habits, lumbar lordosis, leg-length discrepancy, abnormal gait, abdominal wall trigger points, history of low back trauma, levator syndrome of pain/pressure in the perirectal area.

C. **Gastrointestinal tract disorders.** Irritable bowel syndrome, chronic constipation, and diverticulitis.

D. **Urinary tract disorders.** Chronic urethritis, detrusor instability, recurrent cystitis, interstitial cystitis. Other unusual diagnoses may also provide a source of pain.

IV. **Sources of cyclic pain.** Mittelschmerz, primary and secondary dysmenorrhea, endometriosis, adenomyosis, cervical stenosis, intrauterine device, leiomyomas, PMS, obstructive uterine/vaginal malformation in adolescents.

V. **Psychosocial factors.** Major depression or anxiety disorders, somatoform disorders, sexual or physical abuse, dissociation disorders, post-traumatic stress disorder, marital stress, spouse response to patient's pain, familial model of handling pain.

VI. History. **A comprehensive history** of the pain including cyclicity, association with sexual activity, pinpoint pain (trigger point), associated GI (e.g., such as irritable bowel) or urologic symptoms including bowel and urinary habits. A pain diary may be helpful. 2) **Detailed sexual history** including physical or sexual abuse. 3) Screen for depression (Beck Depression Inventory, see Chapter 19, psychiatry), 4) Psychologic response to pain and its effect on lifestyle, family, and friends, 5) Previous abdominopelvic surgical procedures or episodes of PID.

VII. **Evaluation.**

A. **Physical examination** focusing on the abdomen and pelvis. The examiner should probe for abdominal wall trigger points and evaluate for musculoskeletal disorders and tenderness of the bladder, urethra, and other pelvic organs.

B. **Lab tests.** UA and urine culture, stool guaiac, Pap smear, cervical cultures. Laparoscopy, endoscopy, colonoscopy, barium enema if indicated. Patient-assisted laparoscopy under local anesthesia can provide "pain mapping."

VIII. **Management:** Once a pathologic cause of chronic pelvic pain is ruled out, provide symptomatic relief. Focus on breaking the biopsychosocial cycle of pain and disability. Try to manage rather than eliminate the pain (which is usually unlikely).

A. **Analgesics.** Scheduled dosing of an NSAID (ibuprofen, naproxen). PRN dosing increases attention to pain. Avoid narcotics, which exacerbate dysmotility syndromes and are addictive.

B. **Trigger points** can be injected with 5 to 10 ml of 0.25%-0.5% bupivacaine (may mix with 40 mg of triamcinolone). Repeat this Q2-4 weeks at first, followed by successively longer intervals until the nidus of pain resolves. Alternatives include TENS, acupuncture, and physical therapy.

C. **Antidepressants.** Low doses of tricyclic antidepressants (imipramine, amitriptyline, doxepin 10-25 mg, titrate to 75 mg if needed) taken at bedtime will decrease pain intensity, promote sleep and reduce depressive symptoms. May exacerbate constipation. For treatment of major depression, consider using an SSRI in addition, or increasing the tricyclic. See Chapter 19 for further information.

13

GYNECOLOGY

D. **Functional bowel disorders.** Use daily psyllium supplements (6 g daily or more) with increased dietary fiber to reestablish normal bowel motility. Psychotherapy may be helpful. Use antispasmodics (dicyclomine) only after thorough GI evaluation.

E. **Psychologic therapies.** Cognitive-behavioral therapy to control pain: relaxation techniques, stress management, and pain-coping strategies. Psychotherapy for mood disorders, eating disorders, abuse survivors, etc. Marital/family counseling, sex therapy, substance abuse treatment as indicated.

F. **Ovarian cycle suppression** for cyclic pain. Monophasic oral contraceptives, medroxyprogesterone acetate either injectable (Depo-Provera 150-300 mg Q3 months) or oral (10-30 mg QD).

G. **Antibiotics** if evidence of chronic endometritis, (positive cultures or endometrial biopsy), or for urethritis with pyuria. See appropriate section for management.

H. **Surgical management.** Diagnostic laparoscopy, lysis of adhesions, uterine suspension, uterosacral nerve ablation, presacral neurectomy, hysterectomy (high recurrence rate of pain).

POLYCYSTIC OVARIAN SYNDROME (PCOS)

I. **General.** Persistent anovulation produces polycystic ovaries and a hyperandrogenic state, associated with hyperinsulinemia and obesity. PCOS is also known as Stein-Leventhal syndrome and hyperandrogenemia with chronic anovulation.

II. **History.** Menstrual irregularities usually of teenage onset (patients often state that they never have had regular menses), hirsutism, acne, family history of PCOS (50% chance of first-degree female relatives being affected), or type II diabetes.

III. **Physical.** The traditional description of the patient with PCOS is an obese female with acne and excess body hair. However, not all women with PCOS have these manifestations and those with PCOS may be thin with a fair complexion. Patients may have palpably enlarged ovaries. Virilization is uncommon (deepened voice, etc.)

IV. **Laboratory evaluation.** Work-up of menstrual irregularities (as described under abnormal vaginal bleeding and secondary amenorrhea). LH:FSH ratio >2 or 3 suggests PCOS. Testosterone and DHEA-S levels may be mildly elevated. Consider endometrial biopsy at any age if prolonged amenorrhea or oligomenorrhea, and especially if >35.

V. **Differential diagnoses.** For hirsutism: late-onset adrenal hyperplasia, androgen-producing ovarian or adrenal tumors, Cushing's syndrome, drug-induced, idiopathic hirsutism. For menstrual irregularities, see abnormal vaginal bleeding and secondary amenorrhea sections.

VI. **Sequelae**

A. **Gynecologic.** Infertility, amenorrhea, dysfunctional uterine bleeding, increased risk of endometrial cancer, possible increased risk of breast cancer.

B. **Dermatologic.** Hirsutism, alopecia, acne.
C. **Cardiovascular.** Lipid changes, increased risk of cardiovascular disease.
D. **Endocrine.** Increased risk of insulin resistance, leading to diabetes mellitus.
VII. **Treatment. It is important that women with PCOS have menstrual periods at least every 3-4 months to reduce the risk of endometrial carcinoma.**
A. **Weight loss** if achieved may reduce hirsutism and reverse menstrual irregularities and infertility.
B. **Hormonal therapy.** Weight loss may permit ovulation to resume. Treat menstrual irregularity with medroxyprogesterone or oral contraceptives as described in previous sections. Can induce fertility with clomiphene.
C. **Hirsutism.** Weight loss, depilation, and electrolysis. Oral contraceptives may improve hirsutism (especially those with norgestimate). An alternative is Depo-Provera up to 400 mg IM Q3 months or medroxyprogesterone acetate 30-40 mg PO QD. Spironolactone is an anti-aldosterone diuretic and an antiandrogen, which can be used alone or with hormones. Give up to 100-200 mg PO QD (or in 2 divided doses) initially, reduce to maintenance dosage of 25-50 mg QD after results obtained. Monitor for hyperkalemia and use with effective contraception: spironolactone could feminize a male fetus. Second-line agents have more adverse effects: flutamide, finasteride.
D. **Lipids.** Consider screening for dyslipidemia with a fasting lipid panel.
E. **Insulin resistance.** Consider screening with a 75 g glucose tolerance test. If positive, metformin is useful to reduce insulin resistance, promote weight loss and prevent long-term complications.

13

GYNECOLOGY

ABNORMAL PAP SMEARS

I. **Abbreviations in common usage.**
A. **ASCUS:** Atypical squamous cells of undetermined significance.
B. **AGUS:** Atypical glandular cells of undetermined significance.
C. **LSIL:** Low-grade squamous intraepithelial lesion (encompasses **HPV** and **CIN I**)
D. **HSIL:** High-grade squamous intraepithelial lesion (encompasses **CIN II, CIN III, CIS**)
II. **Who needs a pap smear?** Women who are sexually active (with men or women), women over age 18.
III. **Who does not need a pap smear?** Women who are status posthysterectomy **if the hysterectomy was not for malignancy or cellular abnormality,** women over age 65 who have had 2 negative pap smears.
IV. **Rectal exam** does not add information to the **routine** Pap smear and need not be done.
V. **Approach Based on Pap Smear.** Patients should be aware that Pap smears are not 100% accurate, yet they provide the best way to screen for cervical cancer and precancerous lesions.

A. **If Pap smear is normal.** Repeat every year from onset of coitus or age 18-20. If low risk (mutually monogamous, no prior abnormal Paps, no history of HPV or STDs, nonsmoker, no DES exposure), may change to every 2-3 years after 2 consecutive normals.
B. **If pap reads "no endocervical cells present".** Pap test is considered inadequate and should be repeated.
C. **If pap reads "unsatisfactory for evaluation".** Repeat the Pap.
D. **If pap reads "ASCUS."**
   1. **ASCUS, reactive/reparative changes noted.** Look for causative agent on wet mount or cultures and treat only if a specific organism is identified. Follow-up Paps as detailed below.
   2. **ASCUS (unqualified).** Repeat Pap test every 4-6 months for 2 years, until 3 consecutive negative Pap results are obtained, then return to yearly Paps. If another abnormal within 2 years, proceed to colposcopy. Immediate colposcopy is indicated if the patient is not able to comply with follow-up Pap smears.
   3. **ASCUS, neoplasm favored.** Colposcopy indicated after the first abnormal Pap smear.
   4. **ASCUS in a postmenopausal patient.** Atrophic cells may look like dysplastic cells. Use topical estrogen cream for 4-6 weeks and repeat the Pap smear. If still abnormal, proceed to colposcopy.
E. **LSIL or HSIL:** Proceed to colposcopy.
F. **AGUS.** Colposcopy with endocervical curettage.
G. **Other indications for colposcopy.** Visible lesion (even if Pap normal), squamous cell carcinoma, adenocarcinoma, human papillomavirus infection (cervical or external genitalia), persistent inflammation.
VI. **Colposcopy.** A discussion of colposcopy and the treatment of cervical dysplasia is beyond the scope of this manual.

INFERTILITY

I. **General.** Involuntary infertility is defined as the inability to conceive after one year of unprotected intercourse. Affects 10%-15% of couples. The incidence is increasing because of delayed childbearing and an increased incidence of STDs and PID
A. **Average time to conception.** 3 months: 25% of normal couples conceive in the first cycle, 85% within one year.
B. Acknowledge the emotional nature of problem and define infertility as a couple's shared concern. Inquire about partner responses.
II. **Common major problems.** Anovulation (15%), male factors (35%), tubal and pelvic disease (35%), or a combination of these factors. Less common problems include cervical problems or immune infertility. Smoking decreases female fertility.
III. **Diagnostic Evaluation and Treatment**
A. **Thorough history and physical examination** of both male and female. Ask about menstrual history, obstetric history, previous children fathered, prior contraceptives used, history of STDs or PID, pelvic surgery, cervical

treatments, medications or herbs used. Determine coital frequency, sexual practices, impotence, dyspareunia, use of postcoital douches, lubricants (even K-Y or petroleum jelly can be spermicidal: recommend vegetable oil).

B. **Preconception evaluation to address risk factors before conception (e.g., folate).** See Chapter 14.

C. **Semen analysis. Since 35% of couples have some component of male factor infertility, a semen analysis should be one of the initial tests done.** Collected after a 2 or 3-day period of abstinence in glass container. **Male causes for infertility** include testicular disorders, varicocele, hypospadias, ductal obstruction, endocrine abnormalities, retrograde ejaculation, and genetic disorders (Klinefelter's syndrome).

1. **Normal semen analysis.** (WHO criteria). Volume >2 ml, sperm count >20 million/ml, motility >50% with forward progression, morphology >30% normal forms, WBC <1 million/ml.

2. **If normal,** look for female factors causing infertility.

3. **If pyospermia present** (>1 million WBC/ml), search for and treat infections of urethra, epididymis, or prostate.

4. **If otherwise abnormal, repeat in 2 months.** If abnormalities persist, refer to urologist for further evaluation.

D. **Ovulation assessment.**

1. Symptoms of ovulation (such as Mittelschmerz, PMS), length and regularity of menstrual cycle.

2. Basal body temperature charting. Should see a 0.4-0.6° F rise the day after ovulation that is sustained 11-16 days until menstruation. To maximize the chances of conception, advise coitus every 36-48 hours from 4 days before ovulation until 2 days after (some patients find this schedule difficult psychologically)

3. Evaluate and treat menstrual abnormalities.

   a. **Amenorrhea.** Rule out premature ovarian failure, confirmed by FSH >40 mg/ml and estradiol <40 picograms/ml in same sample.

   b. **Oligomenorrhea with hirsutism or galactorrhea.** Suspect POCS. Assess for hyperprolactinemia, and, if present, work up to exclude pituitary cause. If idiopathic hyperprolactinemia, treat with bromocriptine 2.5 mg QHS until BBT demonstrates ovulation. Dose can be increased by 2.5 mg every 3 days until prolactin normal with maximum daily dose 15 mg divided BID. If no ovulation in 2-3 months, add clomiphene. Hypothyroidism can be associated with hyperprolactinemia and should be evaluated and treated.

   c. **Ovulation induction if documented defect found.**

      (1) **Clomiphene citrate** 50 mg QD for days 5 to 9 after either induced or spontaneous menses. Monitor for ovulation with BBT or ovulation kits that detect LH surge about 12 to 24 hours before ovulation to allow timing of intercourse. If ovulation fails to happen, in the next cycle the dose can be in-

creased to 100 mg QD, up to 200 mg QD in a stepwise fashion each cycle to achieve ovulation. Side effects include ovarian enlargement (pain, bloating) and hot flashes. 5% to 10% of patients have multiple gestation. Advise coitus for 1 week beginning 5 days after the final dose of clomiphene

(2) If ovulation does not occur on maximal doses of clomiphene, or if a short luteal phase is noted, a single dose of HCG 10,000 IU IM can be given 7 days after the final dose of clomiphene. Advise coitus that day and for the following 2 days.

(3) Human menopausal gonadotropin (Pergonal) is used for hypothalamic-pituitary insufficiency. Multiple gestations occur at rates higher than those with other ovulation regimens, and close monitoring of follicle production is required. Consultation is recommended.

d. **Luteal phase defect** is controversial and diagnosis by endometrial biopsy or serum progesterone levels is inexact. Luteal phase defect is suspected when a short interval between ovulation and menses is noted on BBT charting. Clomiphene citrate can be used empirically if no other factors identified.

(1) Low serum progesterone level (<10 mg/ml) on day 21 of cycle is suggestive of luteal phase defect.

(2) Endometrial biopsy between days 22-24 that is out of phase >2 days relative to ovulation estimated by BBT also suggests luteal phase defect.

(3) If these tests are abnormal, treat with supplemental vaginal progesterone suppositories 25 mg BID starting 3 days after ovulation. Continue until menses or if pregnancy occurs, continue until week 10 when placental progesterone is sufficient to support pregnancy.

E. **Tubal functioning** related to prior PID, ectopic, abdominopelvic surgery, IUD use. Hysterosalpingogram should be done to assess tubal patency and identify uterine anomalies, fibroids, and synechiae. Perform 2-6 days after end of menses to minimize possibility of disrupting a pregnancy.

F. **Endometriosis.** Diagnosed by laparoscopy if no cause found after workup as outlined above.

G. **Infections** of the cervix with Ureaplasma and Mycoplasma have been implicated in infertility. Culture cervical mucus; some authorities presumptively treat both partners with doxycycline 100 mg PO BID × 7 days.

H. Cervical factors, postcoital testing, and the role of sperm antibodies are controversial.

IV. **Other Options. Unexplained infertility** and male factor infertility can be treated in specialized centers with intrauterine insemination of washed sperm or in vitro fertilization (IVF) which encompasses gamete intrafallopian transfer (GIFT), intracytoplasmic sperm injection (ICSI) and other techniques. Success rates are generally around 50% after up to 6 cycles in women under 35.

ENDOMETRIOSIS

I. **Definition.** Endometriosis is the presence of functioning endometrial tissue outside its normal location, most frequently on the ovaries, uterosacral ligaments, cul-de-sac, and occasionally uterovesical peritoneum. However, it may occur elsewhere including nasal mucosa, lung or even brain. It is estrogen-dependent and generally regresses after menopause or oophorectomy.

II. **Pathogenesis.** Several factors may play a role including retrograde transport and implantation, metaplastic transformation of "coelomic" peritoneum, lymphatic or hematogenous dissemination, immunological defects, genetic predisposition.

III. **Evaluation**

A. **History.**

1. The most common symptoms associated with pelvic endometriosis are dysmenorrhea (66%), deep dyspareunia (33%), infertility (60%), and low back pain or chronic pelvic pain that worsens with menses. May have premenstrual spotting and menorrhagia. Dysmenorrhea often precedes menses and lasts throughout the period.

2. Less common symptoms include dyschezia (painful defecation), diarrhea, intermittent constipation, cyclic abdominal pain, dysuria, urinary frequency and hematuria.

3. One-third of women with endometriosis are asymptomatic and even extensive disease may be asymptomatic.

B. **Physical examination.**

1. Fifty percent of women have a normal clinical examination.

2. Findings will be accentuated in early menses and may include a fixed, tender, retroverted uterus; tender nodules along the uterosacral ligaments (with obliteration of the cul-de-sac); nodules on the back of the uterus and cervix; unilateral or bilateral fixed asymmetric adnexal masses. Rectovaginal exam is important to assess the posterior uterus and cul-de-sac.

3. Up to 10% of teens with endometriosis have congenital outflow tract obstruction.

C. **Diagnostic aids:**

1. **Laparoscopy** should be done to confirm the diagnosis **if treatment will be more extensive than under "mild disease" below** since the clinical diagnosis may be wrong 30% to 40% of the time. Laparoscopy will help assess the extent and stage of the disease as well as tubal patency. Patient-assisted laparoscopy can improve the diagnostic yield.

2. **Ultrasound** may be helpful with a large pelvic mass, but cannot visualize small implants or differentiate types of cystic lesions.

IV. **Management:** Medical treatment of endometriosis cannot restore fertility (see section on Infertility), but may help with pain or dyspareunia. Pain recurs after treatment in 53%.

13

GYNECOLOGY

A. **Mild disease.** Usually the diagnosis will be suspected but not confirmed, since laparoscopy is usually not indicated. Treatment can include observation and NSAIDS. Additional treatment includes:
   1. Combination oral contraceptives, given for at least 6 months. Response rate is 75%.
   2. Depo-Provera 150 mg IM Q3 months. Return to fertility may be delayed after discontinuation.
B. **Treatment options in moderate disease.** Diagnosis should be confirmed by laparoscopy prior to initiating therapy.
   1. **"Pseudomenopause."** Danazol is a synthetic androgen that suppresses gonadotropins and causes amenorrhea. Side effects include vasomotor symptoms such as atrophic vaginitis, weight gain, fluid retention, migraines, dizziness, fatigue, depression, decreased HDL, acne, hirsutism, and potentially irreversible voice changes. Danazol 200 or 400 mg PO BID for up to 6 months. Begin on the first day of menstruation. Use a barrier contraceptive the first month: female fetuses may be adversely affected. Response rate is 84%-92%.
   2. **"Pseudopregnancy."** Continuous oral contraceptives: use a standard monophasic formulation. Side effects as per OCP. Have the patient take one active pill every day continuously, beginning on the third day of menstruation. When breakthrough bleeding occurs, increase to two pills daily for 5 days, then return to a single pill daily. If necessary, may use up to 3-4 pills daily, although nausea may limit therapy. Maintain amenorrhea for 6-9 months: 80% of patients will experience improvement of symptoms.
   3. **Progestin therapy** is useful if pseudopregnancy is not tolerated or is contraindicated. Side effects include breakthrough bleeding, depression, irritability, lipid changes. Initiate therapy during menses. Progestins appear to be as effective as other treatments.
      a. Depo-Provera 150 mg IM Q3 months, may increase to 200 mg IM Q month $\times$ 4 months if needed to produce prolonged amenorrhea. Return to fertility may be delayed after discontinuation.
      b. Medroxyprogesterone 10-30 mg PO QD is an alternative.
   4. **Conservative surgery** to laparoscopically remove extrauterine endometrial tissue is often performed at the time of laparoscopic diagnosis. May also use pharmacotherapy from 6 weeks before to 3-6 months after surgery. Recurrence rate is 19% over 5 years.
C. **Severe disease.**
   1. **Definitive surgery.** Hysterectomy and bilateral oophorectomy. Recurrence rate is 10% over 10 years.
   2. **GnRH agonists** such as leuprolide acetate (IM), goserelin (SQ implant) or nafarelin (nasal spray) induce an artificial menopausal state. Side effects are similar to menopause, including decreased bone mineral density. Response rate is 90%.

ADNEXAL MASSES

I. **Overview.** Ovaries usually 3 to 5 cm in length but influenced by hormones. Fallopian tubes normally cannot be felt. Ninety percent of adnexal masses involve the fallopian tube or ovary.

II. **Differential Diagnosis** will include ectopic pregnancy and masses arising from nearby structures including bladder, bowel, lymph nodes, or a pelvic kidney. Lateral uterine fibroids may be difficult to distinguish from adnexal masses. Benign parovarian cysts may be difficult to differentiate from ovarian cysts, even on ultrasound.

III. **Evaluation.**

A. **History.**

1. Ovarian neoplasms are often clinically silent, except for nonspecific "pressure" symptoms including urinary frequency, constipation, and pelvic heaviness.

2. Gynecological history including menses and STDs, sexual history including contraceptives, obstetric history, surgical history. Review of systems including bowel and bladder function, endocrine symptoms.

3. Family history of reproductive cancers (breast, uterine, ovarian) from both sides of family is critical because some ovarian tumors are familial (e.g., BRCA gene).

4. Multiparity, late menarche, early menopause, and the use of OPCs have all been shown to be protective against ovarian surface epithelial cell tumors.

5. Large tumors may cause increased abdominal girth and may be confused with pregnancy.

6. Pain may result from stretching of the ovarian capsule, torsion, rupture, or intracystic hemorrhage.

7. Functional cysts may cause menstrual abnormalities.

B. **Physical exam.** (1) **Look for virilization,** adenopathy, check breast, abdominal and pelvic exams including rectovaginal exam; (2) **Benign tumors are characteristically unilateral,** cystic, and mobile and do not cause ascites; (3) **Malignancies are usually solid, fixed,** and nodular and may cause ascites.

C. **Diagnostic evaluation.** Ultrasonography will help characterize the mass. **Large cysts** greater than 10 cm in diameter are more likely to be malignant and require immediate evaluation and probable excision. **Solid ovarian tumors** (by ultrasonography) are almost always malignant and demand immediate and aggressive evaluation and treatment. An exception to this is the rare luteoma of pregnancy. Check pregnancy test. Obtain CBC if there is bleeding, FSH and LH, if virilization present, and additional tests as indicated by the history and physical exam.

IV. **Treatment of Ovarian Masses.** Evaluation and treatment is based on the patient's age and reproductive status.

A. **Premenarchial** ovarian masses are at high risk for malignancy (germ cell tumors)

13

GYNECOLOGY

B. **Premenopausal (benign functional ovarian cysts)**
   1. Women of childbearing age with an easily palpable, smooth, mobile ovarian mass **less than 6 cm diameter** may be observed with repeat pelvic exam in 6 weeks if the clinical picture is most consistent with a benign functional cyst: however, compliance with follow-up must be assured. **Any mass 6 cm or greater should be evaluated by ultrasound.**
   2. **If ultrasound demonstrates a simple ovarian cyst under 6 cm** in diameter, this may be observed with repeat clinical exam and ultrasound in 6-8 weeks. If the cyst persists but decreases in size, it may be observed through another cycle. Oral contraceptives are sometimes used for 1-2 months to suppress ovarian function and prevent further cyst formation.
   3. **If an ovarian mass persists, is greater than 6 cm, or increases in size during an observation period of 2 months, surgical excision is indicated to exclude neoplasm.**
C. **Postmenopausal** ovarian masses are at high risk for malignancy (surface epithelial or stromal tumors) and one should proceed to full evaluation without a period of observation. Early diagnosis is essential and usually necessitates surgical excision. Occasionally a postmenopausal woman will have a simple ovarian cyst less than 5 cm diameter on ultrasound. These cysts can be observed with repeat ultrasound in 2 months, and followed if unchanged or smaller.

PEDIATRIC GYNECOLOGY

I. **General.** Gynecology of infancy and childhood is often neglected, primarily because problems are uncommon before the onset of puberty; however, when such problems arise, they must be appropriately evaluated. If child abuse is suspected, document the exam carefully and report to the appropriate authorities. Consultation with a specialist in pediatric gynecology may be helpful in cases with legal ramifications.
II. **Common Disorders of Infancy and Childhood.**
A. **Vulvovaginitis.** Most common complaint.
   1. **Symptoms.** Soreness, pruritus, discharge, and burning.
   2. **Exam.** Microscopic exam of vaginal secretions, UA, and possible vaginal cultures. Recurrent or refractory infections of foul-smelling, bloody discharge require vaginoscopy to exclude foreign body or tumor.
   3. **Causes** include nonspecific polymicrobial infection secondary to poor hygiene or foreign body, contact irritation from soaps, etc. Primary infections (*Candida, Gardnerella, Trichomonas,* gonorrhea, syphilis, herpes, etc.), pinworms, lichen sclerosus et atrophicus may also occur. Neoplasms are rare.
   4. **Treatment.**
      a. Remove foreign body with warm saline irrigation or bayonet forceps. Obtain vaginal and urine cultures and treat concurrent infection.

   b. Treat specific infections. *Candidiasis:* see previous section in this chapter. **Bacterial vaginosis and *Trichomonas vulvovaginitis:*** metronidazole 35 to 50 mg/kg/day up to 750 mg divided TID for 7 days. **Gonorrhea:** ceftriaxone 125 mg IM $\times$ 1 azithromycin 10 mg/kg PO $\times$ 1 (max 1 g). **UTI:** TMP/SMX. **Scabies and pediculosis pubis:** see Chapter 10. Suspect sexual abuse if BV, trichomonas, gonorrhea, or chlamydia is present.
   c. Educate about perineal hygiene.
B. **Pinworms** *(Enterobias vermicularis).* May cause vulvovaginitis; rectal itching common; frequently have vaginal pain. See Chapter 10 for diagnosis and treatment.
C. **Diaper dermatitis** (primary contact irritant dermatitis).
   1. Caused by irritants in urine, producing red, papulovesicular, shiny rash sparing skin folds; may fissure.
   2. Treat with good hygiene and protection with zinc oxide or white petroleum jelly as well as frequent diaper changes allowing skin to dry fully. Treat secondary infections caused by *Streptococcus, Staphylococcus,* or *Candida* organisms.
D. **Labial adhesions.**
   1. Related to low estrogen levels, poor hygiene and vulvar irritation. Usually asymptomatic but may interfere with urination leading to dysuria and recurrent vulvar and vaginal infections.
   2. Treat with topical estrogen cream BID for 7 to 10 days, which will lyse adhesions. Use surgical intervention only as a last resort.
E. **Neonatal vaginal bleeding.** May occur at 3 to 5 days, representing withdrawal of transplacental estrogens. No treatment except reassurance of parents.
F. **Urethral prolapse.**
   1. Prolapse of estrogen-dependent distal urethral mucosa forming painful, friable mass at vaginal orifice. Catheter passed through center enters bladder.
   2. Treat initially with topical estrogens and antibiotic creams. If urinary retention is present or lesion is large and necrotic, surgical excision may be required.
G. **Rare but serious disorders of infancy and childhood**
   1. **Sarcoma botryoides** (embryonal carcinoma of vagina).
      a. Presents as bloody vaginal discharge most commonly in very young girls (<3 years) with polypoid growth, which may look like a cluster of grapes.
      b. Survival rare but improving with use of combination chemotherapy and radical surgery.
   2. **Ovarian tumors.**
      a. Symptoms include pain, mass, pressure; may cause vaginal bleeding or the precocious development of secondary sex characteristics if hormonally active. Requires complete evaluation by experienced gynecologist.

13

GYNECOLOGY

MENOPAUSE

Menopause is the physiologic cessation of menses due to diminished ovarian function. By definition, the diagnosis is made after 6 months of amenorrhea. Hormone replacement may abolish many of the symptoms and may prevent further health risks including osteoporosis and possibly cardiovascular disease.

I. **Clinical Features. Average age 51 years:** Symptoms begin in premenopausal years and progress as estrogen and progesterone levels decrease. **Vasomotor symptoms:** Hot flashes, night sweats. **Atrophic symptoms:** Vaginal dryness, pruritus, irritation, and dyspareunia; urinary frequency, dysuria, incontinence and increased incidence of cystitis. **Emotional symptoms:** Lability, irritability, depression, and insomnia. **Increased risk of coronary artery disease. Osteoporosis:** 50% of postmenopausal bone loss occurs in the first 7 years; resultant fractures (hip, vertebral) are a major cause of increased morbidity and mortality.

II. **Hormone Replacement Therapy (HRT).**

A. Estrogen.

   1. Benefits.

      a. **Short-term (months):** estrogen effectively controls perimenopausal vasomotor and psychologic symptoms. There are few risks for short-term use beyond venous thromboembolism and endometrial stimulation.

      b. **Long-term (years):** estrogen prevents osteoporosis, decreases osteoporotic fractures, controls atrophic symptoms.

      c. **Cardiac effects:** The overall effect of estrogen/progesterone replacement on the development of cardiac disease is unclear. The HERS trial (a large randomized controlled trial of estrogen/progesterone HRT versus placebo in women with established coronary artery disease) showed that estrogen is ineffective in **secondary** prevention. In fact, there was an **increase** in cardiac events in the first year on hormones but a **decrease** in cardiac events in years 4 and 5 yielding no overall benefit. Patients already on estrogen for cardiac protection may elect to continue it, but new patients should not be counseled to start estrogen specifically for cardio-protection pending further data.

   2. Risks.

      a. **Endometrial hyperplasia** or neoplasia risk doubles if estrogen is used alone; however, when progestin is added, there is less risk of these cancers than in non-hormonally treated patients.

      b. **Breast cancer:** Most recent data indicate that relative risk of invasive breast cancer is about 1.46 in those taking estrogen and progesterone for 5 years or greater, but the excess cancers tend to be less aggressive and are caught earlier, so mortality appears unchanged or decreased. Adding progesterone does not reduce the risk of breast cancer and may increase it.

   c. **Thromboembolic disease:** relative risk is about 2.9 in the first
      year of therapy.
   d. **Gallbladder disease** risk may be doubled with estrogen.
   e. **Contraindications** include unexplained vaginal bleeding, active
      liver disease or chronically impaired liver function, carcinoma of
      the breast, endometrial carcinoma, recent vascular thrombosis, or
      past history of thromboembolic disease with previous hormone
      therapy.
   f. **Relative contraindications** include hypertension, uterine leiomy-
      omas, migraine headaches, familial hyperlipidemia, hypertriglyc-
      eridemia, endometriosis, and gallbladder disease, close family his-
      tory of venous thromboembolism (consider work-up before
      starting estrogen).

III. **Initial assessment.**
A. **History** including family history, focusing on areas of risk and benefit
   from HRT.
B. **Physical exam** highlighting breast and pelvic exam.
C. **Pap smear** at baseline and annually thereafter.
D. **Mammogram** at baseline and annually.
E. **FSH measurement:** if the patient is clearly menopausal, with amenorrhea × 6 months and/or compatible vasomotor symptoms, confirmation
   with serum FSH is not necessary. If the clinical picture is unclear, check
   FSH and start HRT if FSH >30. For women on oral contraceptives, look
   for hot flashes during the placebo week or check FSH on the 6th or 7th
   placebo day.
F. **Endometrial biopsy** is not necessary prior to initiation of HRT unless
   there are risk factors such as abnormal vaginal bleeding, history of
   prolonged anovulation, history of unopposed estrogen use, obesity,
   diabetes.

IV. **Regimens.**
A. **Continuous combined estrogen/progesterone.** Prempro provides continuous combined therapy in one tablet daily. Available with differing progestin dosages.
   1. **Estrogen component:** Premarin 0.625 mg PO QD or estradiol 1 mg
      PO QD or estradiol patch 0.05 mg/day or estropipate 1.25 mg PO
      QD. Dose may be increased to up to double the initial dose if vaso-
      motor symptoms persist. If hot flashes do not resolve on the higher
      dose, obtain an estradiol level and consider psychological causes
      such as stress.
   2. **Progestin component:** medroxyprogesterone acetate 2.5 mg PO QD
      or micronized progesterone 100 mg PO QD or norethindrone 0.35
      mg PO QD. Micronized progesterone and norethindrone may have
      fewer side effects.
B. **Cyclic combined.** Premphase comes in a monthly package similar to
   OCPs to help improve compliance.

13

GYNECOLOGY

1. **Estrogen component:** Daily dose same as above (A1). Older cyclic regimens using only 25 days of estrogen each month produced vasomotor symptoms.
2. **Progestin component:** medroxyprogesterone acetate 5 mg PO QD or micronized progesterone 200 mg PO QD or norethindrone 0.7 mg (2 tabs of 0.35) PO QD for 10-14 days each month. Micronized progesterone and norethindrone may have fewer side effects.

C. **Unopposed estrogen.** Primarily for hysterectomized patients. Daily estrogen dose same as above (section A 1). Very occasionally a patient with a uterus will elect unopposed estrogen due to intolerance of progesterone: if so, annual endometrial sampling is imperative and periodic withdrawal/progestin use to induce menses every 3-6 months is recommended.

D. **SERMs (Selective Estrogen Receptor Modulators)**
   1. **Raloxifene** is indicated for the prevention and treatment of osteoporosis but not vasomotor symptoms. Use **Raloxifene:** 60 mg PO QD. Added progestin is not needed.
      a. **Effects:** estrogenic in bone and lipid metabolism, and antiestrogenic in endometrial and breast tissue. Raloxifene preserves bone density and decreases osteoporotic fractures without increasing the risk of endometrial or breast cancer. Raloxifene's effect on lipids and the cardiovascular system is still under investigation, as is the possibility that Raloxifene decreases breast cancer risk (similar to tamoxifen).
      b. **Side effects** include increased hot flashes, leg cramps and increased risk of venous thromboembolism (consider work-up before starting raloxifene if there is a close family history of venous thromboembolism).
   2. Additional SERMs, such as idoxifene are under clinical development.

V. **Managing vaginal bleeding on combined estrogen-progesterone HRT**

A. **Breakthrough bleeding** occurs in 10%-20% of patients on cyclic HRT and 40%-60% on continuous HRT during the first 6 months. Breakthrough bleeding is more common in women who recently had periods.

B. **Evaluation.** Endometrial biopsy if irregular bleeding continues longer than 6 months. Scant tissue will be recovered if the endometrium is atrophic. Another option is transvaginal ultrasound: endometrial stripe ≥ 5 mm requires endometrial sampling (but this occurs in more than half of patients on HRT). With either test, continued abnormal bleeding will warrant further evaluation such as hysteroscopy.

C. **Treatment options.** In a continuous regimen, double the baseline daily progestin dose (i.e., from 2.5 to 5 mg of medroxyprogesterone) or consider changing to a cyclic regimen. Consider endometrial ablation, progestin IUD, or hysterectomy.

D. **Special considerations**
   1. **Elderly women** who have never taken HRT may still benefit from fracture prevention. Consider risks and benefits for each patient indi-

vidually. Start with lower than usual doses and increase after 6 months to minimize side effects.

2. **Libido.** Women with persistently decreased libido despite HRT may benefit from addition of methyltestosterone (e.g., Estratest)
3. **Endometriosis:** women with a history of endometriosis who have had a hysterectomy should probably be given progestin in addition to estrogen, to avoid adenocarcinoma developing from residual pelvic and intra-abdominal endometrial implants.
4. **Bisphosphonates** and HRT have an additive effect in treating established osteoporosis, and can be used together.

E. **Duration of treatment:** long-term HRT should be continued as long as the benefits are desired. Rapid bone loss ensues after discontinuation

F. **Other treatments** are available for most HRT indications. Osteoporosis can be treated with bisphosphonates; cardiovascular risk can be modified with lipid-lowering agents and aspirin; hot flashes can be treated with progesterone, venlafaxine, clonidine, naloxone, or methyldopa; vaginal atrophy can be treated with topical estrogen cream (although high doses may have systemic effects) or hydrating agents (e.g., Replens).

G. **Other notes.**
   1. **Lower than usual doses** (i.e., 0.3 mg of Premarin) of estrogen probably will prevent bone loss if adequate calcium (1500 mg daily) and Vitamin D intake (400-800 IU daily) are ensured through diet or supplements.
   2. **Phytoestrogens** such as those in soy have been popularized for herbal treatment of menopausal symptoms, but have not been extensively studied. Doses large enough to effect symptomatic relief are likely to also produce estrogen-related side effects such as endometrial stimulation.

SEXUAL ASSAULT

Discussion of exam is beyond the scope of this manual.

I. Rape-Trauma Syndrome

A. **Acute phase.** May last for hours to days and is characterized by a distortion or paralysis of the individual's coping mechanism. Generalized body pain, eating and sleeping disturbances, vaginal discharge, itching and rectal pain, depression, anxiety, and mood swings may be present.

B. **Delayed or organizational phase.** Characterized by flashbacks, nightmares, phobias, and a need for reorganization of thought processes, as well as the gynecologic and menstrual complaints noted above. This phase may occur months or years after the event. Mood disorders and posttraumatic stress syndrome may develop.

C. **Counseling.** Should be phase specific.

III. **Prophylactic Therapy** After Rape. Treat presumptively for *Chlamydia* and gonorrhea (for doses, see Chapter 8). The patient should be instructed to return for repeat STD testing in 3 to 4 weeks. The patient should be counseled about possible HIV infection and offered prophylactic therapy (see Chapter 11). HIV serologic analysis should be obtained at the time of assault and repeated in 6 months. If the patient is at risk for pregnancy, a postcoital contraceptive regimen should be offered (see section on contraception), and a pregnancy test should be performed during the return visit. If the patient becomes pregnant, she should be counseled about all available options. Arrange for follow-up medical care and counseling.

II. **Child Sexual Abuse.**

A. Babies, children, handicapped people, and the elderly can be victims of sexual assault. A high index of suspicion is needed for diagnosis.

B. **Symptoms. Behavioral:** anxiety, sleep disturbances, withdrawal, somatic complaints, increased sex play, inappropriate sexual behavior, school problems, acting-out behaviors, self-destructive behaviors, depression, low self-esteem. **Physical:** unexplained vaginal or rectal injuries, unexplained vaginal or rectal bleeding, bruising, bites, scratches, pregnancy, sexually transmitted disease, recurrent vaginal infections, pain in the anal or genital area, recurrent atypical abdominal pain.

C. Physical findings

1. **Colposcopy** allows a detailed magnified inspection of the vulva to search for physical signs of abuse that may have escaped detection by unaided examination. However, most findings are visible to the naked eye. **Take pictures and document any findings well.** Videocolposcopy is the standard of care.

2. **Nonspecific.** Redness of external genitalia, increased vascular pattern of the vestibule and labia, presence of purulent discharge from the vagina, small skin fissures or lacerations in the area of the posterior fourchette, and agglutination of the labia minora after trauma.

3. **Specific findings.** Recent or healed lacerations of the hymen and vaginal mucosa may indicate abuse. An enlarged hymenal opening of 1 cm or more is non-specific. Procto-episiotomy and indentations in the skin indicating teeth marks (bite marks) or laboratory confirmation of a venereal disease may indicate abuse.

4. **Definitive findings.** Any presence of sperm.

OSTEOPOROSIS

I. **Overview.**

A. **Bone mass** peaks at age 30 and gradually declines thereafter. Bone loss accelerates after menopause to 1.5% per year, then slows again after 10-15 years.

B. **Osteoporosis** is decreased bone mass with normal ratio of mineral to matrix. A bone mineral density (BMD) T score below 2.5 standard deviations below the mean for young adults is considered osteoporosis.

C. **Osteopenia** is decreased bone mass with a T score between 1 and 2.5 standard deviations below the mean for young adults.

D. **Risk factors** for osteoporosis include exercise-related amenorrhea, time since menopause, corticosteroid use, thin body habitus, sedentary lifestyle, inadequate calcium or Vitamin D intake, family history of osteoporotic fractures, white or Asian race, high alcohol consumption, smoking, hyperthyroidism, chronic kidney or liver disease, and long-term therapy with corticosteroids, thyroid hormone, anticonvulsants, or heparin.

E. **Protective factors** include obesity, diabetes mellitus, thiazide diuretic use, and possibly statins.

F. **Fractures resulting from osteoporosis include** hip fractures (with 5%-20% mortality rate within 3 months), vertebral compression fractures (causing loss of height, kyphosis, and resulting pulmonary, GI, and bladder problems), Colles' fracture and tooth loss.

II. **Diagnosis.**

A. **Radiographs** will show osteopenia only after there is 20% to 30% bone loss.

B. **DEXA scan** is the most accurate method of measuring bone mineral density (BMD) but is not recommended as a routine screening test. Measuring BMD is useful when it will make a significant difference in management as in the decision of whether to start hormone replacement therapy.

C. **Osteoporotic fractures** are often the first indication of osteoporosis.

D. **Differential diagnosis.** Once osteoporosis is diagnosed, consider whether there is an underlying condition that might be causing osteoporosis: hyperparathyroidism, chronic renal failure, multiple myeloma, leukemia, lymphoma, hyperthyroidism, excessive thyroid replacement, hypercortisolism, metastatic cancer.

III. **Prevention.**

A. **Calcium intake:** Adolescents and reproductive-age women producing endogenous estrogen require 1000 mg of calcium daily through diet or supplements. Postmenopausal women require 1500 mg daily if not taking estrogen or raloxifene. Calcium should be taken with meals in doses up to 500 mg. Calcium carbonate is cheapest, although calcium citrate is better absorbed.

B. **Vitamin D** intake of 400 IU (perhaps 800 IU after age 70) through fortified milk, multivitamin or supplement is required for absorption of calcium. Deficiency is especially common in winter in the higher latitudes, and in institutionalized patients.

C. **Exercise.** Regular weight-bearing exercise such as running, weight training, aerobics, walking and sports excluding swimming.

D. **Quit smoking** and avoid excessive alcohol use.

E. **Minimize corticosteroid and thyroid hormone use** as much as possible. If on chronic steroids, vitamin D and calcium ± alendronate (or risedronate) should be considered.

F. **Alendronate** 5 mg PO QD **or** 35mg PO once a week is used for prevention of osteoporosis in postmenopausal women as is risedronate 5 mg/day.

G. **Modify the home environment** to identify and eliminate factors predisposing to falls.

13

GYNECOLOGY

IV. **Treatment.** All of the following therapies should be accompanied by adequate calcium and Vitamin D intake.
A. **Hormone replacement** therapy with estrogen or raloxifene especially in women with premature or surgical menopause (see previous section)
B. **Bisphosphonates** are effective monotherapy, and have a small additive effect when given with hormone replacement therapy. They are also useful in corticosteroid-related osteoporosis.
   1. **Alendronate** (10 mg PO once a day **or** 70 mg PO once a week, which is just as effective) has been shown to reduce the risk of vertebral fractures by 90% and nonvertebral fractures by 30%-50% in established osteoporosis. To prevent esophageal ulceration, it must be taken in the morning with 8 oz water at least 1/2 hour before any other foods or fluids are taken and the patient must remain upright until after the first meal.
   2. **Etidronate** is an alternative. It is given cyclically, 400 mg PO QD for 2 weeks, followed by 12 weeks without the drug. It is probably as effective as alendronate.
   3. **Risedronate** is the most potent bisphosphonate **and also has the lowest incidence of GI side effects.** It is approved for osteoporosis in a dose of 5.0 mg/day **for both prevention and treatment.**
   4. **Salmon calcitonin**—1 spray in alternating nostrils each day is expensive but effective in increasing BMD. It relives the pain of vertebral compression fractures.
   5. **Thiazides** especially in patients needing an antihypertensive, increase bone mass and have an additive effect with estrogen.
   6. **Fluoride,** although it increases bone density, actually increases hip fracture risk, so it is no longer used.

ECTOPIC PREGNANCY

Ectopic pregnancy is potentially life threatening but often misdiagnosed. It must be suspected in any woman with vaginal bleeding and lower abdominal pain. Ruptured ectopic is a true medical emergency.
I. **General Information.**
A. **Risk factors.** History of ectopic, PID, tubal or pelvic surgery, pelvic surgery, infertility, endometriosis, anatomical anomalies, DES exposure, cigarette use, older age. Although IUDs do not increase the absolute risk of ectopic, accidental pregnancies with an IUD are more likely to be ectopic than intrauterine. **Fertility treatment** leads to a heterotopic pregnancy (intrauterine with coexistent ectopic) in up to 3%.
B. **Differential diagnosis.** Early intrauterine gestation with implantation bleeding, spontaneous abortion ruptured functional ovarian cyst, appendicitis, PID, other gynecological and abdominal conditions causing pain. See Chapter 15 for further information about the acute abdomen.
II. **Evaluation.**

A. **Symptoms.** Abdominal pain (98%), amenorrhea (65%), vaginal bleed-ing/spotting (80%), with or without symptoms of early pregnancy. **Note that not all patients report amenorrhea or vaginal bleeding!** Patients may have nausea, vomiting, dizziness, syncope, hypovolemic shock, referred shoulder pain, tenesmus and low-grade fever. Usually occurs 6-8 weeks after LMP.

B. **Exam.** Check vital signs. Blood pressure and pulse may be normal even with significant intraperitoneal bleeding! **Pelvic exam may be normal;** only 50% have adnexal mass. Uterus may be enlarged secondary to de-ciduation or blood. Cervical motion tenderness may be found as well as doughy cul-de-sac secondary to bleeding. Marked abdominal tenderness with guarding and rebound suggests ruptured or bleeding ectopic. When an acute abdominal emergency or hemorrhagic shock is suspected, im-mediate surgical consultation is indicated.

C. **Lab tests. Pregnancy test:** Urine pregnancy test may miss a very early ectopic (limit 50 mIU/ml). A serum quantitative beta-hCG is sensitive to 5 mIU/ml. If possible, a quantitative serum HCG should be done. Obtain CBC, type and screen, and transvaginal ultrasound.

III. **Correlate ultrasonography with the serum quantitative HCG.**

A. **Beta-hCG <1500 mIU/ml.** Ultrasonography may not show evidence of a gestational sac. If stable and ultrasound is negative, these patients can be followed-up as per section 4 below. **But do not assume a benign course if the beta-hCG is low. These patients can still rupture an ec-topic if one is present.**

B. **HCG >1500.** If the beta-hCG is above 1500 mIU/ml and the sonogra-pher is reasonably skilled, an intrauterine pregnancy should be de-tectable by transvaginal ultrasonography in 95% of cases. **If an in-*trauterine* sac is not visible with a serum beta-hCG >1,500, suspicion of ectopic is markedly increased.**

C. **beta-hCG >3500.** The *adnexal* gestation is often not visible until the Beta HCG is 3500 to 6500 mIU/ml.

D. **beta-hCG >6000 mIU/ml.** If the patient has a beta-hCG of > 6000 mIU/ml and there is no intrauterine gestational sac seen, it is presump-tive evidence of an ectopic pregnancy.

IV. **Follow-up for the patient in whom the diagnosis of ectopic cannot be proven or ruled out on the first visit.**

A. **In a stable, reliable patient,** if ultrasonography is unable to exclude ec-topic pregnancy, obtain serial quantitative beta-hCG every 48 hours and follow clinical exam. The beta-hCG should approximately double in 48 hours. In an unreliable patient, treat as presumed ectopic.

1. **If beta-hCG rises by >66% in 48 hours,** the pregnancy is continu-ing; repeat the ultrasound when the beta-hCG is >1,500 to differen-tiate between ectopic and intrauterine (should see intrauterine at this point). If still indeterminate, follow-up in another 48 hours with re-peat quantitative beta-hCG and ultrasound. If the beta-hCG is not ris-

13

GYNECOLOGY

ing or is falling, the pregnancy is likely non-viable and a D&C should be done to look for chorionic villi.

2. **Culdocentesis** is used rarely since the advent of transvaginal ultrasonography. Hemoperitoneum (>5 ml of non-clotting blood) in combination with a positive pregnancy test is 99% predictive of a ruptured ectopic.

3. **Serum progesterone** levels are not very helpful.

V. Treatment

A. **Primary treatment is surgical.** Tube-sparing surgical techniques such as laparoscopic salpingostomy allow for preservation of fertility with little increase in risk for recurrent ectopic.

B. **Methotrexate injection is a nonsurgical treatment** for ectopics of less than 3.5 cm with no fetal heart motion. The effect of methotrexate treatment on future fertility needs more study: fertility may be preserved but recurrent ectopics may be more common.

C. **Rhogam. If ectopic or spontaneous abortion is confirmed, remember to give Rh prophylaxis to Rh-negative women.**

BIBLIOGRAPHY

An emergency contraceptive kit, *Med Lett Drug Thera* 40:102-3, 1998.

Blake DR, Duggan A, Quinn T, et al: Evaluation of vaginal infections in adolescent women: can it be done without a speculum? *Pediatrics* 102(4 [Pt1]):939-44,1998.

Brotzman GL et al: The minimally abnormal Pap smear, *Am Fam Physician* 53(4):1154-1162, 1995.

Canavan TP. Appropriate use of the intrauterine device, *Am Fam Physician* 58:2077-84, 1998.

CDC: 1998 Guidelines for treatment of sexually transmitted diseases, *MMWR* 47 (No. RR-1): 1998.

Cerel-Suhl SL, Yeager BF: Update on OPCs, *Am Fam Physician* 60:2073-2084, 1999.

Cervical cytology: evaluation and management of abnormalities: *ACOG Technical Bulletin* 183, Washington, 1993, American College of Obstetricians and Gynecologists.

Chronic pelvic pain: *ACOG Technical Bulletin* 223, Washington, 1996, American College of Obstetricians and Gynecologists.

Colditz GA (for the Nurses' Health Study Research Group): Oral contraceptive use and mortality during 12 years of follow-up: the Nurses Health Study, *Ann Intern Med* 120:821-826, 1994.

Collaborative Group on Hormonal Factors in Breast Cancer. Breast cancer and hormonal contraceptives: collaborative reanalysis of individual data on 53,297 women with breast cancer and 100,239 women without breast cancer from 54 epidemiological studies, *Lancet* 347:1713-27, 1996.

Dardano KL, Burkman RT. The intrauterine contraceptive device: an often-forgotten and maligned method of contraception, *Am J Obstet Gynecol* 181: 1-5, 1999.

del Carmen-Cravioto M, Alvarado G, Canto-de-Cetina T, et al: A multicenter comparative study on the efficacy, safety, and acceptability of the contraceptive subdermal implants Norplant and Norplant-II, *Contraception* 55:359-67, 1997.

Genant HK, Lucas J, Weiss S, et al: Low dose esterified estrogen therapy: effects on bone, plasma estradiol concentrations, endometrium, and lipid levels. Estratab/Osteoporosis Study Group, *Arch Intern Med* 157:2609-15, 1997.

Gilbert DN, Moellering RC Jr, Sande MA, eds: *The Sanford guide to antimicrobial therapy,* ed 29, Hyde Park, Vermont, 1999, Antimicrobial Therapy.

Glasier A: Emergency postcoital contraception, *N Engl J Med* 337:1058-1064, 1997.

Hatcher RA et al: *Contraceptive technology,* ed 17, New York, 1998, Ardent Media.

Hulley S, Grady D, Bush T, et al: Randomized trial of estrogen plus progestin for secondary prevention of coronary heart disease in postmenopausal women. Heart and Estrogen/progestin Replacement Study (HERS) Research Group, *JAMA* 280:605-613, 1998.

Jick H, Jick SS, Gurewich V, et al: Risk of idiopathic cardiovascular death and nonfatal venous thromboembolism in women using oral contraceptives with differing progestagen components, *Lancet* 346:1589-93, 1995.

Lahteenmaki P, Haukkamaa M, Puolakka J, et al: Open randomised study of use of levonorgestrel releasing intrauterine system as alternative to hysterectomy, *BMJ* 361:1122-6, 1998.

Maksymowych WP: Managing acute osteoporotic vertebral fractures with calcitonin, *Can Fam Physician* 44:21606, 1998.

Mazur MT, Kurman RJ: *Diagnosis of endometrial biopsies and curettings: a practical approach,* New York, 1995, Springer-Verlag.

McNeeley SG, Hendrix SL, Mazzoni MM, et al: Medically sound, cost-effective treatment for pelvic inflammatory disease and tuboovarian abscess, *Am J Obstet Gynecol* 178:1272-8, 1998.

Medical management of endometriosis, *ACOG Practice Bulletin* 11, Washington, 1998, American College of Obstetricians and Gynecologists.

Medical management of tubal pregnancy: *ACOG Practice Bulletin* 3, Washington, 1999, American College of Obstetricians and Gynecologists.

Menkes DB et al: Fluoxetine treatment of severe premenstrual syndrome, *Br Med J* 305:346, 1992.

Mishell DR Jr, Stenchever MA, Droegemueller W, et al: *Comprehensive gynecology,* ed 3, St. Louis, 1997, Mosby.

Reiter RC: Evidence-based management of chronic pelvic pain, *Clin Obstet Gynecol* 41:422-35, 1998.

Scott JR et al: *Danforth's obstetrics and gynecology,* Philadelphia, 1994, Lippincott.

Speroff L, Glass RH, Kase NG: Clinical gynecologic endocrinology and infertility, ed 6, Baltimore, 1995, Lippincott Williams & Wilkins.

Spitzer WO: Bias versus causality: interpreting recent evidence of oral contraceptive studies, *Am J Obstet Gynecol* 179:S43-50, 1998.

Tenore JL: Ectopic pregnancy, *Am Fam Physician* 61:1080-8, 2000.

The Writing Group for the PEPI Trial: Effects of estrogen or estrogen/progestin regimens on heart disease risk factors in postmenopausal women, *JAMA* 273:199-208, 1995.

The Writing Group of the PEPI Trial: Effects of hormone replacement therapy on endometrial histology in postmenopausal women, *JAMA* 275:370-375, 1996.

Tintinalli JE et al: *Emergency medicine: a comprehensive study guide,* New York, 1995, McGraw-Hill.

Trussell J, Rodriguiz G, Ellertson C: Updated estimates of the effectiveness of the Yuzpe regimen of emergency contraception, *Contraception* 59:147-51, 1999.

Uterine leiomyomata: *ACOG Technical Bulletin* 192, Washington, 1994, American College of Obstetricians and Gynecologists.

Vaginitis: *ACOG Technical Bulletin* 226, Washington, 1996, American College of Obstetricians and Gynecologists.

Van Winter JT, Bernard ME: Oral contraceptive use during the perimenopausal years, *Am Fam Physician* 58:1373-7, 1381-2, 1998.

Weaver K, Glasier A: Interaction between broad-spectrum antibiotics and the combined oral contraceptive pill—a literature review, *Contraception* 59:71-8, 1999.

Wellerby C: Diagnosis and treatment of endometriosis, *Am Fam Physician* 60:1753-68, 1999.

13

GYNECOLOGY

OBSTETRICS

Sara Mackenzie

PRECONCEPTION CARE

Preconception care is intended to prevent congenital anomalies, maximize maternal health and is offered to all women of childbearing age, since more than 50% of pregnancies are unplanned.

I. **Proven benefits.** Prevention of NTDs by folic acid supplementation. Tight glucose control in DM results in lower incidence of congenital abnormalities. Identify and when possible control factors leading to previous poor results in pregnancy (such as preterm labor from bacterial vaginosis, antiphospholipid antibody syndrome, etc.).

II. **Pre-pregnancy advice.** Proper nutrition, exercise, smoking cessation, abstinence from alcohol and drugs, protection from radiation (x-rays) and workplace exposures, information on prescribed and OTC drugs to avoid teratogenicity, infection control (STD protection and treatment, rubella and hepatitis immunity status), and psychosocial counseling for planning a pregnancy. Assess risk for congenital disease (thalassemia, Tay-Sachs, cystic fibrosis, sickle cell, etc.).

PRENATAL CARE

I. History at Initial Evaluation.

A. **Menstrual history.** Cycle length, age of menarche, pain with menses, duration of flow, characteristics of previous two menses, previous methods of contraception. Establish dates carefully based on first day of last menstrual period and uterine size. Obtain ultrasound if in doubt. Ultrasound dating is most accurate early in the pregnancy.

B. **Medical history.** Underlying problems or illnesses, history of sexually transmitted diseases, medications, family history, and genetic history.

C. **Habits.** Tobacco, alcohol, other recreational drugs, diet, activity, caffeine.

D. **Obstetric history.** Dates of all pregnancies including terminations and spontaneous abortions. Outcome and gestational length. Duration and complications of labor. Particular note should be made of previous shoulder dystocia, premature labor, premature rupture of membranes (PROM), placenta previa, and postpartum hemorrhage. The type of previous deliveries is also important: normal spontaneous vaginal delivery (NSVD), forceps, C-section (indication, type of uterine incision). Weight, sex, and Apgar scores of liveborn infants. Neonatal complications. Number of living children.

E. **Social history.** Occupational hazards, support network, whether or not the father of child is involved, wanted or unwanted pregnancy, expectations, potential stresses, need of social or financial services. Domestic violence or sexual assault. See below.

F. **Prenatal Care for Patients at Risk for Preterm Labor.** Frequent visits during weeks 22 to 32, cervical group B streptococci and urine culture at 24 weeks, vaginal exam for pH and cervical exam, monitor uterine activity, education on nutrition and preterm labor, and reinforce what signs and symptoms to watch for (abdominal cramping, pressure, cramps, backache, increased vaginal discharge, fluid leak, regular uterine contractions).

II. **Physical Exam.**

A. **General physical exam.** Particular attention to height, weight, BP, thyroid gland, dentition, heart, breasts, deep tendon reflexes, signs of underlying heart disease.

B. **Pelvic examination.**

1. **External.** Look for evidence of condylomata acuminata. These lesions may progress during pregnancy, and a small percentage of infants born through involved vaginal tissue will develop laryngeal papillomas or anogenital warts. Podophyllin is contraindicated during pregnancy, but cryotherapy, laser, and TCA may be used. Also look for and culture lesions suspicious for herpes simplex.

2. **Vaginal and cervical.** Look for evidence of condylomas and herpes. Examine vaginal discharge and evaluate for *Candida, Trichomonas,* and bacterial vaginosis (BV); culture cervical discharge for GC and *Chlamydia.* Treat any vaginal infection. It is particularly important to screen for and treat BV, since it is associated with an increased risk of preterm labor, premature rupture of membranes, preterm birth, and histologic chorioamnionitis. (See Chapter 13 for treatment.) Rule out cervical anomalies. Pap smear should be obtained if patient has not had one in last 6 months.

3. **Bimanual.** Rule out adnexal abnormalities. Determine uterine size: 8 weeks = 2 × normal; 10 weeks = 3 × normal; 12 weeks = 4 × normal; 16 weeks = halfway to umbilicus; 20 weeks = at umbilicus; fundal height (weeks of gestation = cm from pubic symphysis to fundus).

III. **Laboratory Evaluation at first prenatal visit.**

A. **Routine.** Pap smear, CBC, UA, and culture to screen for bacteriuria, ABO blood type, Rh type, antibody screen (indirect Coombs'), VDRL test, rubella antibody titer, and hepatitis B surface antigen. Treat asymptomatic bacteriuria to prevent pyelonephritis during pregnancy. Urine should also be screened for protein and glucose by dipstick at each visit. Offer HIV testing. (Many states require testing since AZT administered during pregnancy substantially decreases risk of transmission of HIV to infant—see Chapter 11.)

B. **When indicated.** Cervical culture for GC and *Chlamydia,* Toxoplasmosis antibody test, sickle cell preparation, or hemoglobin electrophoresis in all previously unscreened black women, tuberculin skin testing, HIV antibody testing, and CMV titers.

IV. **Labs During Pregnancy.**

A. **Every visit.** Dipstick urine for protein and glucose.

B. **15 to 20 weeks.** Serum triple-screen (alpha-fetoprotein [AFP], beta-HCG, and estradiol). See below.
C. **14 to 20 weeks.** Amniocentesis, when indicated.
D. **24 to 28 weeks.** Blood glucose screen after 50 g of oral glucose and urine culture.
E. **28 to 32 weeks.** Hematocrit
F. **36 weeks.** Rh antibody screening if indicated. Consider GC, *Chlamydia,* and herpes rescreening in high-risk women. Repeat hematocrit if indicated. Consider testing for group B streptococci at 35 to 37 weeks (see recommendations below). Consider starting acyclovir for patients with genital HSV which has been shown to decrease transmission to the infant if given prophylactically.

V. **Expected Weight Gain.**
A. **First trimester.** Should gain 2 to 5 lb total.
B. **After first trimester.** 3/4 to 1 lb per week.
C. **Average total weight gain.** 25 ± 5 lb.

PRENATAL PATIENT EDUCATION

I. **Nutrition in Pregnancy.**
A. **Caloric requirements.** 30 to 35 kcal/kg/day plus 300 kcal/day. Requirements are higher in adolescence and with multiple gestation.
B. **Calcium.**
  1. **Requirements.** 1200 to 1500 mg of elemental calcium per day.
  2. **Calcium supplements.** Milk, 8 oz glass: 300 mg of calcium, yogurt; generic calcium carbonate (260 mg Ca/650 mg tablet); calcium gluconate chewable (45 mg Ca/500 mg tablets; Tums regular strength (200 mg Ca/500 mg chewable tablet).
C. **Iron.**
  1. **Requirements.** 30 mg of elemental iron per day.
  2. **Additional requirements.** If the pregnant woman is iron deficient or has a multiple-gestation pregnancy, she should take 60 to 100 mg of elemental iron per day. If her Hb is <10, she requires 200 mg/day.
  3. **Iron supplements.**
    a. Ferrous sulfate 65 mg of elemental Fe per 324 mg tablet (20% elemental iron).
    b. Ferrous fumarate 106 mg Fe/325 mg tablet (33% elemental iron).
    c. Ferrous gluconate 38 mg Fe/325 mg (11.6% elemental iron).
D. **Folic acid.**
  1. **Requirements.** 0.4 mg to 1 mg/day. Most prescription prenatal vitamins contain 1 mg of folate. OTC prenatal vitamins contain 0.8 mg of folic acid.
  2. **Sources.** Green leafy vegetables, broccoli, mushrooms, and liver.
  3. **Adequate folate before conception has been shown to reduce the risk of NTDs.**
  4. **Prior history of NTD or family history of NTD**—recommend 4 mg /day for 1 month before pregnancy and during first 3 months gestation.

14

OBSTETRICS

II. **Activity.**

A. **Occupation.** Abstinence from physical work may be recommended if the woman has a history of two previous premature deliveries, an incompetent cervix, or fetal loss secondary to uterine anomalies. No controlled clinical trials have demonstrated efficacy of bed rest for any of these conditions. Women with premature rupture of membranes (PROM), CHF, hemoglobinopathies, Marfan's syndrome, or diabetes with multiple end-organ involvement are also at risk for complications and may benefit from reduced activity as can women with multiple gestations at over 28 weeks. Bed rest is indicated if there is a suspicion of IUGR, preeclampsia, or preterm labor.

B. **Exercise.** (Expert opinion not controlled studies) Avoid in supine position after 1st trimester. Avoid exercise with potential for abdominal trauma. Exercise to fatigue not exhaustion. Contraindicated if pregnancy induced hypertension (PIH), PROM, PTL (preterm labor), incompetent cervix, vaginal bleeding, IUGR.

C. **Other.** There are no routine restrictions on sexual relations, other than comfort and position. Caution should be used if any of the conditions listed above apply.

III. **Habits and Miscellaneous.**

A. **Alcohol.** Increases the risk of midtrimester abortion, mental retardation, behavior and learning disorders. 10% to 30% risk of fetal alcohol syndrome in offspring of women who drink 3 to 5 drinks per day. Risks with lesser consumption unknown.

B. **Tobacco.** Increases the risk of low-birth-weight infants, premature labor, spontaneous abortions, stillbirth, and birth defects.

C. **Crack cocaine or other illicit drug use.** Associated with perinatal addiction, preterm labor, and cognitive and psychologic difficulties in the infant. Cocaine abuse during pregnancy is associated with a significant increase in the incidence of placental abruption.

D. **Caffeine.** 100 mg/day or 1 cup of coffee (approximately 1 cup of coffee per day) does not increase the risk of spontaneous abortions or IUGR.

E. **Seatbelts.** A seatbelt should be worn such that the belts do not directly cross the gravid uterus; lap belt low over hips/ shoulder belt above uterus.

F. **Medications.** In general, no medications should be used without checking with a physician.

   1. **FDA classification of medication with regard to adverse fetal effects. Category A:** proved safe for fetus in human studies (such as prenatal vitamins); **Category B:** adverse effect not demonstrated in animal studies with no human studies, or adverse effects shown in animal studies have not been reproduced in human studies (as with penicillin); **Category C:** no adequate animal or human studies are available, or animal studies show adverse fetal effects with no human data; **Category D:** evidence of fetal risk but benefits believed to outweigh the risks (as with carbamazepine); **Category X:** drugs with proved fetal risks that outweigh any benefits.

2. It is recommended that you confirm the category of all medications in pregnancy before prescribing or recommending them to your patient.
3. Drugs that are used in pregnancy with no known adverse effect at the usual dose (some are class B). Antihistamines, decongestants (e.g., pseudoephedrine), some antibiotics, (penicillin, ampicillin, cephalosporins, erythromycin), non-quinine antimalarials, general anesthetics, acetaminophen, tuberculostatics (INH, PAS, and rifampin), metronidazole (avoid in first trimester if possible, though one study showed no teratogenicity), steroids. Accidental use of clomiphene, bromocriptine, birth control pills, and vaginal spermicides have shown no adverse effects.

G. **Infections.** Avoid children with viral illnesses, especially if not rubella or CMV immune. Avoid direct contact with cat litter and eating raw meat to minimize contact with *Toxoplasma gondii* (toxoplasmosis).

H. **Domestic Violence** Screen all pregnant women for domestic violence. Violence often escalates with pregnancy. Affects 0.9%-20% of pregnant women in US. Ask direct questions, for example, "Have you been hit, pushed or kicked in the last year?"

I. **Potential problems.** Advise patient to contact physician if she experiences vaginal bleeding, leakage of fluid, fever, persistent nausea or vomiting, burning on urination, severe abdominal pain, severe headache or visual disturbance, persistent RUQ pain, peripheral edema, decrease in fetal movement. (Generally after quickening, one should expect 4 or more fetal movements per hour or at least 10 discrete movements in 2 hours.)

RH SCREENING AND RH$_0$(D) Immunoglobulin

I. **Protocol for Routine Rh Screening and Administration of Rh$_0$(D) Immunoglobulin.**

A. **Initial visit.** Draw blood for ABO group, Rh type, and antibody screening (indirect Coombs').

B. **If patient is Rh negative.** Repeat antibody screen at 26 weeks and, if no antibody is detected, give 300 μg of Rh$_0$(D) immunoglobulin (1 vial 5300 μg) IM. Can give Rh$_0$(D) immunoglobulin before knowing antibody result. If antibody is detected, see "additional Rho(D)" below.

C. **After delivery.** Check fetal ABO/Rh type. If infant is Rh positive, mother receives 300 μg of Rh$_0$(D) immunoglobulin IM within 72 hours of delivery.

D. 1 vial suppresses immunity to approximately 30 ml of whole blood (15 ml of Rh(+) packed RBCs).

II. **Additional Rh$_0$(D) Immunoglobulin Requirements.**

A. If at anytime during pregnancy a fetal-maternal hemorrhage is suspected, a Kleihauer-Betke (acid elution) test should be performed. If positive, the mother should receive 10 μg of Rh$_0$(D) immunoglobulin per milliliter of fetal blood calculated to have entered the maternal circulation. However, the Kleihauer-Betke test is not 100% sensitive, and so if

14

OBSTETRICS

there is trauma and a suggestion of fetal-maternal hemorrhage, presumptive use of Rh_o (D) is indicated.

B. A 50 µg dose of Rh_o (D) immunoglobulin (1 vial microdose = 50 µg) is indicated for an Rh-negative woman after a first trimester terminated or spontaneously aborted pregnancy.

C. A 300 µg dose of $Rh_0(D)$ immunoglobulin is indicated for the Rh-negative woman who undergoes amniocentesis, a spontaneous or induced abortion, or who has an ectopic pregnancy.

D. The Kleihauer-Betke test should be performed after delivery if a larger than usual fetal-maternal hemorrhage may have taken place, as with placental abruption. More than the standard 300 µg dose may be required (which protects only up to 15 ml of Rh-positive red blood cells).

III. **Isoimmunization.** If the patient is Rh negative and the antibody screen is positive **before** $Rh_o(D)$ immunoglobulin administration, obtain an antibody titer and refer to a specialist. These infants are at risk for erythroblastosis fetalis.

PRENATAL DIAGNOSIS OF CONGENITAL DISORDERS

I. **Overview.** Major congenital anomalies occur in 3% live born infants at term and represent the leading cause of infant mortality in the United States. Family history should be obtained to evaluate the risk of congenital disease. All women should be offered serum AFP/triple screen. A patient's attitude toward termination should not influence the screening/counseling. Knowledge of fetal abnormality can facilitate psychological adjustment and in the aid care of the fetus.

II. **Methods of Screening/Diagnosis.**

A. **AFP/Triple screen.** Offer to all pregnant women at 15 to 20 weeks (see below).

B. **Chorionic villus sampling** at 10 to 12 weeks (fetal loss rate of 0.5% to 1.5%). No longer associated with increase in limb defects.

C. **Early amniocentesis** performed between 12 and 15 weeks with 1% to 2% fetal loss rate.

D. **Midtrimester amniocentesis** between 15 and 20 weeks with 0.5% to 1% fetal loss rate.

E. **Fetal ultrasound**

ALPHA-FETOPROTEIN (AFP)/TRIPLE SCREEN

I. **Overview.** The measurement of AFP, estriol, and HCG (triple screen) in maternal serum at 15 to 20 weeks of gestation is used as a screening test for fetal structural abnormalities and chromosomal abnormalities (trisomy 21). All three levels are dependent on maternal weight and gestational age. **Since proper interpretation of AFP/HCG/estriol depends on fetal age, women with abnormal values should be referred for ultrasound to confirm gestational age and to evaluate for neural tube defects (NTD) and other structural abnormalities.** In the United States, the incidence of NTD is roughly 1 per 1000 live births.

II. **If Ultrasound Dating confirms the patient's dates** (i.e., the triple screen is abnormal) but no diagnostic structural abnormalities are seen, the patient should be referred for amniocentesis.

III. **Risks.** Psychologic stress, false positive results, false reassurance, and potential fetal trauma secondary to amniocentesis.

IV. **Causes of an elevated AFP.**
A. Underestimated gestational age.
B. Open NTDs (meningomyelocele, anencephaly).
C. Fetal nephrosis and cystic hygroma.
D. Fetal GI obstruction, omphalocele, gastroschisis.
E. Prematurity, low birth weight, IUGR.
F. Abdominal pregnancy.
G. Multiple fetuses
H. Fetal demise.

V. **Causes of a Low AFP.**
A. Overestimated gestational age.
B. Missed abortions.
C. Molar pregnancies.
D. Chromosomal abnormalities (including Down syndrome).

VI. **Causes of a Low Estriol, Elevated HCG, and Low AFP:** Trisomy 21 (Down syndrome).

ANTENATAL FETAL SURVEILLANCE

I. **Obstetric Ultrasound.**
A. **Indications.** Routine ultrasound is **not** indicated but can be used in the following situations:
   1. To determine the presence or absence of an intrauterine pregnancy.
   2. To determine gestational age.
   3. To measure fetal growth and identify intrauterine growth retardation.
   4. To identify multiple-gestation pregnancies.
   5. To detect fetal anomalies (nearly 100% sensitive for detection of NTD).
   6. To detect oligohydramnios or polyhydramnios (if size greater or less than dates).
   7. To demonstrate placental abnormalities (e.g., abruption, placenta previa).
   8. To identify maternal uterine and pelvic anomalies.
B. **Timing.** Will depend on the indication for ultrasound.
   1. In general, the earlier ultrasound is performed in pregnancy, the more accurate is the EDC (first trimester ultrasound gives EDC +/− 5 days; second trimester EDC + 10 days; third trimester EDC +/− 3 weeks). Fetal anomalies may not become apparent until after 20 weeks.
   2. Amniotic fluid volume and fetal movement, tone, and breathing in conjunction with an NST can be used to calculate scores on biophysical profiles (BPP, see below). This can be helpful in the decision to

14

OBSTETRICS

induce or follow postdated pregnancies, high-risk pregnancies, or diabetic pregnancies.

II. **Nonstress Testing (NST).**

A. **Timing.** An NST should be done at the earliest point at which an intervention would be performed if a clearly abnormal result were obtained (generally 32 to 34 weeks).

B. **Indications.** High-risk pregnancies including hypertension, diabetes mellitus, multiple gestation, suspected oligohydramnios or IUGR, known placental abnormality, maternal heart or renal disease, hemoglobinopathy, postdated pregnancies, previous unexplained fetal demise and maternal perceptions of decreased fetal movement.

C. **Equipment.** External fetal heart rate monitor and uterine contraction monitor.

D. **Interpretation.**

1. **A reassuring NST** demonstrates three or more fetal movements accompanied by a fetal heart rate acceleration of 15 beats per minute or more lasting at least 15 seconds during a 20-minute period.

2. **Lack of fetal movement is non-diagnostic** and a repeat NST should be performed after a meal. Lack of movement for short periods of time may be attributable to fetal sleep. However, absence of movement for prolonged periods of time may be ominous.

3. **The NST is abnormal** when the criteria for a reassuring NST are not met or late or variable decelerations are present. A biophysical profile (BPP, below) is then indicated.

III. **Biophysical Profile (BPP).**

A. **Indications.** Same as for NST. May be used as early as 26 to 28 weeks for the surveillance of a complicated or high-risk pregnancy.

B. **Procedural details.** Real-time ultrasound coupled with external fetal heart rate and uterine contraction monitoring.

C. **Interpretation.** Five parameters are evaluated: Fetal breathing movements; gross body movements, fetal muscular tone, amniotic fluid volume (look for pocket of amniotic fluid that measures 2 cm in two perpendicular planes), reactivity of fetal heart rate.

1. Each component of the BPP is given a score of 0 (parameter absent) or 2 (parameter present). The total score ranges from 0 (ominous) to 10 (reassuring; infant at low risk of asphyxia). Further discussion of this topic is beyond the scope of this chapter.

IV. **Amniocentesis.**

A. **Indications:** Done at 14 to 18 weeks of gestation to identify selected inherited disorders in women at increased risk.

1. **Advanced maternal age** (35 years of age or older).

2. **Previous pregnancy** resulting in the birth of a child with a chromosomal abnormality.

3. **Down syndrome or other chromosome abnormality** in either parent or close family member or if either parent is a carrier of a genetically

transmitted disease (Duchenne's muscular dystrophy, hemophilia, metabolic disease, etc.).

4. **NTD** in either parent or a first-degree relative or previous child born with a NTD.
5. **Abnormal serum AFP/triple screen.**
6. **To detect isoimmunization**
7. **Determine fetal lung maturity.**
   a. **Lecithin-to-sphingomyelin (L/S) ratio.** If L/S is >2.0, there is a low risk of respiratory distress secondary to prematurity.
   b. **Phosphatidylglycerol (PG).** PG first appears at 35 weeks gestation and increases in concentration until 40 weeks. If present, it provides reassurance of fetal lung maturity.

14

OBSTETRICS

GROUP B STREPTOCOCCAL (GBS) INFECTION

I. **Risk factors for Neonatal Sepsis.** Intrapartum chorioamnionitis, maternal group B streptococcal (GBS) colonization in the rectum or vagina, prolonged rupture of membranes, and prolonged monitoring with an internal pressure catheter or fetal scalp lead.

II. **Vertical Transmission of GBS.** GBS is the number one cause of neonatal sepsis and meningitis in the United States. Infection occurs in 2 or 3 neonates per 1000 live births. Maternal colonization can be transient, and 20% to 25% of pregnant females are carriers at any given time. In addition to threatening the life of a neonate, GBS is also an important risk factor for the development of chorioamnionitis in the mother, thereby increasing morbidity and the rate of intrapartum complications.

III. **The CDC Recommends 2 Options for GBS.**

A. **Option 1.**
   1. **Culture all women (rectal and vaginal) at 35-37 weeks.** If the patient's recto-vaginal cultures are positive for GBS, she should be offered **intrapartum** antibiotic prophylaxis.
   2. Treatment. Oral antibiotics are ineffective. The following regimens may be used:
      a. **Penicillin G** 5 million units IV and then 2.5 million units Q4h until delivery. Penicillin G is the preferred antibiotic because of its narrow spectrum, making it less likely to select for antibiotic-resistant bacteria.
      b. **Ampicillin** 2 g IV followed by 1 g Q4h until delivery.
      c. **For penicillin allergy.** Either **clindamycin** 900 mg IV Q8h or **erythromycin** 500 mg IV Q6h may be given until delivery.

B. **Option 2.** Screening cultures are not done, but antibiotic prophylaxis is given if any of the following risk factors are present:
   1. **Previously delivered neonate with GBS infection.**
   2. **GBS bacteriuria** during the current pregnancy.
   3. **Labor and delivery occur at less than 37 weeks** of gestation (attack rates for preterm infants are higher).

4. **Membranes** have been ruptured for >18 hours (12 hours in some institutions).
5. **Intrapartum temperature** greater than or equal to 38.0° C (100.4° F).
6. **If PROM occurs at <37 weeks of gestation and the patient is not yet laboring,** GBS cultures should be collected as above. Either of the following regimens may then be used:
   a. **Give IV antibiotics** until culture results are known, or
   b. **Initiate antibiotic therapy only when culture result confirms presence of GBS.**

IV. **Care of the infant of a mother who has had GBS prophylaxis.**

A. **Any infant with symptoms or signs of GBS and those infants born at less than 35 weeks gestation must have a full work-up** (CBC, blood culture, CXR for pulmonary symptoms, LP if indicated). They should be treated until culture results are negative.

B. **For those >35 weeks without symptoms,** approach is stratified based on duration of labor **after the administration of antibiotics.**
   1. If duration of labor **after antibiotics is <4 hours,** infant should have CBC, blood culture, and 48 hours of observation.
   2. If duration of labor **after antibiotics is >4 hours,** observation for 48 hours is indicated.

NAUSEA AND VOMITING OF PREGNANCY

I. **Cause.** Unknown. Probably not related to serum HCG levels, but other hormones have been implicated (estradiol, thyroxine).

II. **Hyperemesis gravidarum.** The incidence of hyperemesis gravidarum (severe nausea and vomiting causing ketosis and dehydration requiring hospitalization) is increased in multiple gestation and molar pregnancies, and so ultrasound is advisable in cases of hyperemesis gravidarum. Exclude organic causes: disorders of GI tract, gallbladder, pancreas, hepatitis, and urinary infection. Recent data suggests an association with *Helicobacter pylori* but this is not yet proven and treatment for *H. pylori* is not yet standard of care. Elevation of serum transaminase and mild jaundice can be observed, which will return to normal after adequate hydration and nutrition. Hyperemesis gravidarum has a 26% recurrence rate in subsequent pregnancies.

III. **Outpatient Management**

A. **Reassurance** that condition improves with time, usually by end of first trimester.

B. **Avoid medications** whenever possible.

C. **Advise patient** to arise slowly and to keep soda crackers at the bedside and eat before rising.

D. **Omit iron supplementation** until nausea resolves.

E. **Eat frequent small meals** and protein snacks at night.

F. **Antiemetics.**
   1. **Doxylamine succinate** (Unisom) 25 mg 1/2 to 1 tablet PO Q AM and Q PM. This can be used in conjunction with pyridoxine.

2. **Diphenhydramine** (Benadryl) 25 to 50 mg PO Q6-8h.
3. **Phosphorylated carbohydrate** (Naus-A-Way, Emetrol, Nausetrol) 15 to 30 ml PO on arising and Q3h PRN for nausea.
4. **Meclizine** 25 to 100 mg PO BID to QID.
5. **Pyridoxine** (vitamin B_6) 25 mg PO TID.
6. **Bendectin** (10 mg of doxylamine succinate and 10 mg of pyridoxine) was removed from the market, although large studies have not shown evidence of teratogenicity.

IV. **Inpatient Management.** For those with severe symptoms, weight loss, dehydration, ketones in urine, or high urine specific gravity. Correct hypovolemia, ketosis, and electrolyte imbalances with IV fluids. Use oral fluids as tolerated.

A. **Monitor** fluid intake and output.
B. **Antiemetics** as above; also consider phenothiazines: prochlorperazine (Compazine), droperidol (Inapsine) and promethazine (Phenergan).
C. **Parenteral nutrition** for prolonged vomiting.
D. **Psychotherapeutic measures,** stimulus control, biofeedback, and imagery can also be helpful.

DIABETES IN PREGNANCY: GESTATIONAL DIABETES MELLITUS (GDM)

I. **Potential morbidity.**
A. Infants born to diabetic mothers have 5 times the normal risk of respiratory distress syndrome, an increased risk of congenital anomalies (especially with first trimester hyperglycemia), an increased risk of neonatal hypoglycemia, hypocalcemia and jaundice.
B. The mother has an increased incidence of preeclampsia, infection, postpartum bleeding, and cesarean section (secondary to macrosomia). There is also an increased risk of maternal injury during vaginal delivery.

II. **Evaluation.**
A. **Glucose challenge test (GCT).**
1. **Timing.** A GCT is performed as a routine screen for GDM in all pregnancies at 24 to 28 weeks of gestation. It should be performed earlier if symptoms are present or if there is a previous pregnancy with GDM.
2. **If there are risk factors for GDM** (e.g., massive obesity, prior history GDM), consider screening at the first prenatal visit if there are risk factors. Repeat at 24 to 28 weeks if initial test is negative.
3. **Procedure.** A blood glucose level is obtained 1 hour after a 50 g oral glucose load.
4. **Interpretation.** A level of 140 mg/dl or greater is abnormal. However, since there are many false positives, a 3-hour fasting glucose tolerance test should be done if GCT is >130 mg/dl.
B. **Glucose tolerance test (GTT).**
1. **Indication.** Follow-up of an abnormal GCT result.
2. **Procedure.** The patient must eat a diet containing at least 150 g of carbohydrate for 2 days. Draw a serum glucose level after an

overnight fast. The patient then ingests 100 g of glucose solution. Serum glucose levels are then obtained at 1, 2, and 3 hours.

3. **Interpretation** (Table 14-1). If two or more of these readings are abnormal, the patient needs treatment for GDM.

C. **Management of gestational diabetes.**

1. **Dietary adjustment is the mainstay of therapy.**
   a. Caloric intake should be 30 to 35 kcal/kg/day. Intake should be reduced to 24 kcal/kg/day if the patient is obese.
   b. Avoid cakes, candy, and other fast-acting carbohydrates.
   c. Dietary composition should be 50% to 60% carbohydrate, 20% to 25% protein, and 20% fat, with high fiber content.
   d. Exercise has shown added benefit along with dietary therapy.

2. **Obstetric surveillance.**
   a. **Early ultrasound** for accurate gestational dating.
   b. **Follow every 2 weeks** until 36 weeks and then weekly.
   c. **Accucheck** QID before meals and at bedtime.
   d. **Check fasting blood** glucose and review home monitoring at each visit. If fasting glucose levels are >105 mg/dl (or postprandial values are 120 to 130), the patient may be hospitalized to ensure adherence to diet. If fasting glucose remains >110 mg/dl, insulin therapy is indicated. Glyburide has been used safely after the first trimester in patients failing insulin. However, this is **not** the standard of care.
   e. **Check for ketonuria daily** to make sure there has been adequate caloric consumption.
   f. **Obtain an ultrasound** if macrosomia is suspected. If the estimated fetal weight is >4000 g, a cesarean section should be **considered** at term.
   g. **Antepartum NST** is often initiated on a weekly basis at 34 to 35 weeks of gestation but may be started earlier. If euglycemia can be documented, consider delaying monitoring until 38 weeks. Delivery is recommended if any sign of fetal compromise is noted.
   h. **Amniocentesis** is helpful in documenting fetal lung maturity before cesarean section, since infants of diabetic mothers have delayed lung maturity.

3. **Postpartum.**
   a. **Infants should be watched for evidence of hypoglycemia** due to high levels of circulating insulin.

TABLE 14-1

UPPER LIMITS OF NORMAL SERUM GLUCOSE LEVELS (MG/DL) WITH 3-HOUR GTT

Fasting	1 Hour	2 Hours	3 Hours
95	180	155	140

b. Gestational diabetics should have a 75 g oral GTT checked 6 weeks postpartum to rule out persistent carbohydrate intolerance. Counsel the patient that she has an approximate 35% risk of developing diabetes at some point in her life.

TRAUMA AND PREGNANCY

I. **Differential.** Retrospective study in tertiary referral center showed etiology of trauma in pregnancy: 54% motor vehicle accidents (MVA), 22% domestic violence, 21% falls, 1.3% burn, puncture, or assault. Up to 50% of falls cause some degree of abruption.

A. **Physical or Sexual Abuse.** Abused women tend to present late for prenatal care. Generally abuse continues and may worsen during pregnancy. Abused patients have an increased risk for: preterm labor, chorioamnionitis and low birth weight infants. Asking direct questions, such as "has anyone hit, slapped or kicked you, etc," is the best way of screening for abuse.

II. **Management.**

A. **Treatment of pregnant woman.** ABC's of evaluating and stabilizing mom take priority. Deflect uterus away from great vessels by placing wedge under right hip or tilt table laterally. Once the mother has been stabilized, consider fetus. If mom is Rh negative, give RhoGam.

B. **Evaluation of fetus.** Trauma increases the risk of placental abruption and fetomaternal hemorrhage. Fetal monitoring and contraction monitoring is the best way to assess for significant abruptio. Ultrasound is less sensitive and MRI is not generally practical (although very sensitive). Monitoring for 2-6 hours is sufficient if no ominous signs (vaginal bleed, contractions, and uterine tenderness) are noted. Make sure that the fetus has a good heart rate and good beat to beat variability as well. If contractions are not detected or occur less than every 10 minutes **and** monitoring of the fetus is normal, an abruption unlikely. Twenty percent of women with contractions greater than every 10 minutes have associated abruption.

C. **Return.** Women should be instructed to return for abdominal cramps, increasing pain or vaginal bleeding.

HYPERTENSION IN PREGNANCY, PREECLAMPSIA, AND ECLAMPSIA

I. **Pregnancy-Induced Hypertension (PIH).**

A. **Definition.** PIH is present when diastolic BP >90 mm Hg **or** a systolic BP >140 **or** a systolic BP rises at least 30 mm Hg over baseline value **or** diastolic BP rises at least 15 mm Hg over baseline value.

B. **Risk factors for PIH.** First pregnancy, multiple gestation, polyhydramnios, hydatidiform mole, malnutrition, positive family history of PIH, underlying vascular disease. Molar pregnancy should be expected if PIH occurs early in gestation.

C. **Treatment.** See section on preeclampsia and chronic hypertension.

II. **Preeclampsia and Eclampsia.**

A. **Preeclampsia.** Defined as the presence of hypertension or PIH accompanied by proteinuria, edema, or both after 20 weeks gestation. Preeclampsia is divided into mild and severe forms.

B. **Criteria for mild preeclampsia.**
1. **Hypertension** as defined above but not meeting the criteria for severe preeclampsia (below).
2. **Proteinuria** >300 mg/24 hours.
3. **Mild edema,** signaled by weight gain >2 lb/week or >6 lb/month.
4. **Urine output** >500 ml/24 hours.

C. **Criteria for severe preeclampsia.**
1. **BP of greater than 160/110** on 2 occasions at least 6 hours apart with patient on bed rest or a systolic BP rise of greater than 60 mm Hg over baseline value **or** a diastolic BP rise of greater than 30 mm Hg over baseline value.
2. The presence of an elevated blood pressure and any of the systemic symptoms noted below categorizes the patient as having severe preeclampsia regardless of the blood pressure.
   a. **Proteinuria** >5 g/24 hours or 3+ or 4+ on urine dipstick.
   b. **Massive edema.**
   c. **Oliguria** <400 ml/24 hours.
   d. **Systemic symptoms** including pulmonary edema, headaches, visual changes, right upper quadrant pain, elevated liver enzymes, or thrombocytopenia.
   e. **Presence of IUGR.**

D. **Eclampsia:** Occurrence of a seizure that is not attributable to other causes in a preeclamptic patient.

III. **Evaluation of PIH and Preeclampsia.**

A. **History.** Document risk factors and any symptoms outlined above.

B. **Physical.** Look for evidence of edema (particularly of the hands and face), BP changes, retinal changes, hyperreflexia, clonus, and RUQ tenderness.

C. **Initial laboratory studies.**
1. **Blood: CBC** (elevated or normal Hb/HCT, low platelet count), electrolytes, **BUN and creatinine** (creatinine >1.0 ng/ml, BUN >10 mg/dl, uric acid (>5.5 ng/dl), **liver function tests** (elevated AST, ALT, LDH), and **coagulation studies** (elevated PT, PTT, and elevated fibrinogen degradation products). Patients may also have **hypoalbuminemia,** as well as **schistocytes** or **helmet cells** on peripheral smear from microangiopathic hemolysis. If patient is in labor, send a blood type and screen.
2. **Uric acid** (>5.5 ng/dl) may be elevated before there are other signs or symptoms of preeclampsia.
3. **24 hour urine** for creatinine clearance, total protein.

IV. **Complications of Preeclampsia.** Eclamptic seizures; *H*emolysis; *E*levated *L*iver function tests, *L*ow *P*latelet count (HELLP) syndrome, hepatic rupture, DIC, pulmonary edema, acute renal failure, placental abruption, intrauterine fetal demise (IUFD), cerebral hemorrhage, cortical blindness, retinal detachment.

V. **Management of PIH/Preeclampsia.**

A. **Outpatient management.** For pregnancy-induced hypertension without significant proteinuria, home bed rest is recommended. Home blood pressure monitoring, weight, and urine protein checks are helpful. Antepartum surveillance (NST) should begin early. Ultrasound exams should be performed periodically to ensure adequate amniotic fluid and to monitor for intrauterine growth retardation (IUGR).

B. **Hospital management.**

1. **Indications.** No improvement of mild pregnancy-induced-hypertension with home bedrest or pre-eclampsia with 2+ proteinuria, evidence of organ system involvement.

2. **Orders.** Bed rest with bathroom privileges is allowed. The goal of IV fluids in severe cases is to replace urine output and insensible losses.

3. **Laboratory evaluation and weights.** Performed daily to every other day. Antepartum surveillance including daily fetal movement count, daily NSTs, and weekly amniotic fluid determinations by ultrasound is essential. Monitor symptoms such as headache, visual disturbances, and epigastric pain.

4. **Delivery is treatment of choice.** Delivery should be accomplished when the fetus is mature but may be required early if maternal health is in danger or if there is evidence of fetal distress. Delivery is indicated when the patient meets criteria for severe preeclampsia. Betamethasone 12.5 mg IM should be given twice 24 hours apart to stimulate fetal lung maturation and can be repeated weekly if pregnancy is prolonged. Electronic FHR monitoring during labor is indicated. *EFM*

5. **Antihypertensive therapy.** Indicated only if BP persistently >160/110. Aim for a diastolic BP 90 to 100 mm Hg. Avoid overcorrection because normal blood pressures can result in placental hypoperfusion.
   a. Diuretics and ACE inhibitor are contraindicated during pregnancy.
   b. Acute management Hydralazine 5 mg bolus and infusion
   c. Long-term medications (if the fetus is immature) include methyldopa (Aldomet), atenolol, and labetalol.

6. **Anticonvulsant therapy.** Seizure prophylaxis is indicated in all preeclamptic patients during labor and delivery and for a minimum of 24 hours postpartum. Seizures may occur in the absence of hyperreflexia, and increased DTRs may be present in the normal population; therefore hyperreflexia is not a useful predictor of who will have a seizure.
   a. **Drug of choice for seizure prophylaxis:** Magnesium sulfate
   b. **The loading dose is** 4 to 6 g of magnesium sulfate IV over 20 minutes and continued at 2 g/hour.

      c. **To treat active seizures.** Magnesium sulfate 1 g/min IV until seizure controlled up to 4 to 6 g maximum. If this fails, see Chapter 2 for management of status epilepticus.

      d. **Continue magnesium sulfate** therapy at least 24 hours postpartum. In 25% of the patients postpartum eclampsia can occur. Monitor urine output postpartum and stop therapy if urine output is >200 ml/hour for 4 consecutive hours. Watch for postpartum hemorrhage because magnesium sulfate can relax the uterus.

  7. **Managing magnesium therapy.**

      a. **Monitor urine output** (100 ml in 4 hours), deep tendon reflexes and serum levels. Therapeutic level is 4 mEq/L but since it takes 12 to 18 hours to equilibrate, serum levels of magnesium sulfate are of dubious value.

      b. **Magnesium toxicity.** Loss of reflexes and drowsiness will herald magnesium toxicity. At levels of 10 to 12 mEq/L and above, muscle weakness, respiratory paralysis, and cardiac depression can occur.

      c. **To treat magnesium toxicity.** 10 ml of 10% calcium gluconate (or calcium chloride) may be administered IV push in the event of magnesium toxicity, or the magnesium infusion can be turned off for 1 to 2 hours.

VI. **Prevention of Preeclampsia.** Aspirin 81 mg a day and calcium supplementation have been used to prevent preeclampsia. However, they have not been shown to be of any benefit in controlled trials and do not change fetal or maternal outcomes.

VII. **Chronic Hypertension Superimposed on Pregnancy.**

A. **Risks.**

  1. **Maternal.** The risk to the mother is the same as in the non-pregnant state. However, in the presence of superimposed preeclampsia (20%), there is increased maternal mortality, frequently from intracranial hemorrhage.

  2. **Fetal.** There is an increased incidence of perinatal death, IUGR, and fetal distress.

B. **Management.**

  1. **Treatment of chronic hypertension** can decrease maternal and, to some extent, fetal morbidity. Appropriate medications include methyldopa, hydralazine, and beta-blockers.

  2. **During pregnancy, it is not appropriate to use:**

      a. Sympathetic ganglion blockers (orthostatic hypotension)

      b. Diuretics (aggravation of volume depletion)

      c. ACE inhibitors (associated with fetal defects and neonatal renal failure)

  3. **Laboratory evaluation** is performed early in pregnancy.

  4. **Obstetric visits** are scheduled every other week at 24 weeks and weekly after 30 weeks.

5. **Early ultrasound** is obtained for dating, and repeated periodically to look for evidence of IUGR.
6. **Antenatal surveillance (NSTs)** should begin at 34 weeks.
7. **Timing the delivery.** The pregnancy should not be allowed to go beyond 40 weeks. Delivery may be required earlier if there is evidence of IUGR or fetal distress or if hypertension cannot be controlled by bed rest and medication.
8. **Intrapartum monitoring** is required during labor.
9. **If there is evidence of IUGR,** cesarean section is preferable to a prolonged induction.
10. **Complicated cases** or women with superimposed preeclampsia should be handled at an appropriate referral center.

14

OBSTETRICS

EARLY ANTEPARTUM HEMORRHAGE

I. **Definition.** Vaginal bleeding at <20 weeks of gestation.
II. **Differential Diagnosis of early vaginal bleeding.**
A. Spontaneous Abortion
   1. **Incidence** 15% to 25% of clinically recognized pregnancies end in a spontaneous abortion.
   2. **Causes.** Fetal abnormalities incompatible with life (chromosomal and other), defective implantation, maternal infection, uterine and cervical anomalies.
   3. Evaluation
      a. **History.** Suggestive of pregnancy (missed period or periods, nausea, vomiting, breast tenderness) followed by cramping and spotting or bleeding often with passage of tissue. All patients should be evaluated to rule out an ectopic pregnancy. Remember patients must be seen within 48 hours for RhoGAM if indicated (i.e., mother is Rh negative)
      b. **Exam.** Including stability of vital signs, orthostatic vital signs, pelvic exam looking for open or closed cervical os, tissue, other causes of vaginal bleeding (such as cervical eversion, polyp, infection, vaginal lesion, ectopic fetus). Size uterus. Check for fetal heart tones with Doppler scanning if 10 to 12 weeks.
      c. Lab tests
         (1) **Urine pregnancy test** is positive in 75% of cases so a negative pregnancy test does **not** rule out spontaneous abortion.
         (2) **CBC, blood type, and antibody screen** in all patients for Rh status. RhoGAM indicated for all Rh-negative, antibody-negative women.
         (3) **Uterine ultrasound** or pathologic exam of tissue if indicated.
         (4) **Serial quantitative HCG** should increase by at least 60% in 48 hours. If it does not rise or drops, it is likely that the pregnancy is nonviable.

B. **Threatened abortion.** Vaginal bleeding ± cramps but with a cervix that is long and closed with a uterus appropriate for gestational age. Roughly 50% progress to inevitable abortion.

C. **Inevitable abortion.** Persistent cramps and moderate bleeding and a cervical os is open. Do not confuse with an incompetent cervix, which is a painless cervical dilatation not associated with cramping and is potentially treatable.

D. **Incomplete abortion.** The same symptoms as an inevitable abortion but with some retained products of conception in the uterus or cervical canal. There is ongoing cramping and excessive vaginal bleeding. Speculum examination reveals a dilated internal os and tissue present within the endocervical canal or vagina. Bleeding may be heavy and clots may be mistaken for products of conception.

E. **Complete abortion.** The entire conceptus is expelled and cramping and bleeding abate or resolve completely. On examination, the uterus is firm, and smaller than one would expect for gestational age.

F. **Missed abortion.** Products of conception retained 3 or more weeks after fetal death. Signs and symptoms of pregnancy abate; pregnancy test becomes negative. Brownish vaginal discharge (rarely frank bleeding) occurs. Cramping is rare. The uterus is soft and irregular. Ultrasound exam rules out live pregnancy.

G. **Septic abortion.** Any of the above scenarios and a temperature of greater than 38° C without other source of fever. Septic abortion is associated with (but does not require) IUD use or instrumentation during abortion. Abdominal and uterine tenderness are present as well as purulent discharge and possibly shock.

H. **Ectopic Pregnancy.** See Chapter 13.

I. **Molar pregnancy** (hydatidiform mole). Placenta undergoes trophoblastic proliferation and typically resembles a cluster of grapes. Occurs more often in women less than 20 or greater than 40 years of age and almost always causes some degree of vaginal bleeding. Hydatidiform moles are associated with hyperemesis gravidarum and the onset of preeclampsia before the third trimester. The uterus is larger than expected for gestational age in 50% of the cases. Ovarian enlargement may occur secondary to thecal lutein cysts. Ultrasound findings typically show a "snowstorm" pattern. Nearly 20% of hydatidiform moles progress to gestational trophoblastic tumor. **Treatment:** Immediate evacuation of mole, subsequent follow-up for detection of persistent trophoblastic proliferation or malignant change

III. **Treatment.**

A. **Assure adequate circulating volume.** Treat with IV normal saline or lactated Ringer's. Consider transfusion if Hb <8 g or patient is unstable.

B. **Threatened abortion.** Bed rest if possible; use acetaminophen for discomfort, nothing in the vagina (no tampons, douches, intercourse), consider ultrasound for gestational sac, cardiac activity, or to rule out ectopic pregnancy. Positive cardiac activity predictive of continued pregnancy >90%. Consider monitoring quantitative beta-hCG with a rise of less than 66% in 48 hours predictive of abortion or ectopic.

C. **Incomplete or inevitable abortion.** Hospitalize if hypovolemic, anemic, or advanced gestation >12 weeks. Tissue visible in os should be gently removed with ring forceps to allow contraction of uterus; but minimize manipulation to decrease risk of infection. Patients with incomplete abortion (tissue passed with continued bleeding) often require suction curettage or D&C. Consider oxytocin drip as an alternative (20 IU in 1000 ml of crystalloid solution at 50 to 100 ml/hour). If unsuccessful, proceed with D&C.

D. **Complete abortion.** Discharge home if vital signs stable, Hb documented to be stable, and bleeding decreased. Consider methylergonovine (Methergine) 0.2 mg PO TID for 3 days if diagnosis certain or after uterine evacuation.

E. **Missed abortion.** Obtain CBC with differential, platelet count, PT and PTT, and DIC (see Chapter 5) panel if indicated. Outpatient management may be considered if retained for less than 4 weeks, if weekly fibrinogen levels are obtained, and if the patient is monitored closely for DIC. Hospitalize if there are signs of infection, DIC, or if the fetus has been retained longer than 4 weeks. Fibrinogen levels of less than 150 mg/dl call for immediate evacuation of the uterus.

F. **Septic abortion.** Obtain CBC, UA, culture of discharge from uterus, blood cultures, chest radiograph for diagnosis of septic emboli and to rule out free air from perforation and abdominal radiograph to evaluate for uterine foreign body. Electrolytes and ABG. Organisms include both anaerobes and aerobes *(Bacteroides, Streptococcus, Enterobacter, Chlamydia, Clostridium)*. Hospitalize, treat sepsis, D&C, IV antibiotics:
   1. **Doxycycline** plus cefoxitin or imipenem or ticarcillin, or
   2. **Clindamycin** plus third-generation cephalosporin or gentamicin
   3. **Discharge** to home with taking oral doxycycline or clindamycin.

G. **Long-Term Management** Give RhoGAM to Rh-negative women. Provide emotional support. Traditional but not well-founded recommendation is to wait 3 months before attempting conception. Having a single spontaneous abortion does not increase the risk of aborting the next pregnancy. Evaluate couple for habitual abortion if the woman has had two or more successive spontaneous abortions. If the patient is a habitual aborter, obtain antiphospholipid antibody titers. Obtain fetal tissue for karyotyping if possible.

14

OBSTETRICS

LATE ANTEPARTUM HEMORRHAGE

I. **Definition.** Vaginal bleeding that occurs after 20 weeks of gestation.

II. **Differential Diagnosis.**

A. **Placenta previa.**
   1. **Incidence.** Occurs in 1 of 200 deliveries. The diagnosis of placenta previa is very common in the second trimester, but more than 95% of these do not have placenta previa at delivery.

2. **Classification.** Placenta previa may be marginal, partial, or total depending on how much of the placenta is over the cervical os.

3. **Diagnosis.** Vaginal bleeding is typically bright red and painless. The blood loss is not massive but tends to recur and become heavier as the pregnancy progresses. Diagnosis may be made by ultrasound. The advisability of a speculum exam is debatable. Digital examination is contraindicated other than in a double setup situation when delivery is desirable and can be rapidly accomplished by C-section. Maternal risk factors include increasing age, multiparity, and prior uterine scar. Associated with breech and transverse presentations.

B. **Placental abruption.**

1. **Incidence.** Placental abruption occurs in 10% of all deliveries. Severe abruption is rare.

2. **Classification.**

a. **Mild.** Slight vaginal bleeding (<100 ml), no FHR abnormalities are present; there is no evidence of shock or coagulopathy.

b. **Moderate.** Moderate vaginal bleeding (100 to 500 ml) and uterine hypersensitivity with or without elevated tone. Mild shock and fetal distress may be present.

c. **Severe.** Extensive vaginal bleeding (>500 ml), tetanic uterus, and moderate to profound maternal shock are present. Fetal demise and maternal coagulopathy are characteristic.

3. **Diagnosis.** The diagnosis of placental abruption is clinical. Although vaginal bleeding is present in 80% of cases, bleeding may be concealed in the remainder (that is, retroplacental bleeding). Thus, the maternal hemodynamic situation may not be explained by observed blood loss. Pain and increased uterine tone are typically present. Risk factors include prior history of abruption, maternal hypertension, cigarette or cocaine use, increasing maternal age or multiparity. Abruption may be associated with premature rupture of membranes, blunt abdominal trauma, and twin gestation after delivery of first infant.

C. **Uterine rupture.** Very rare. May mimic severe abruption. An abdominal film may show free intraperitoneal air or an abnormal fetal position. Accompanied by persistent fetal bradycardia. Emergent C-section and hysterectomy are required.

D. **Other.** Vasa previa (velamentous insertion of the cord). Delivery should be by scheduled C-section. If pregnancy is allowed to progress to term, spontaneous rupture of membrane or amniotomy should be averted because it could lead to fatal bleeding for fetus and possibly mother. Cervical dilation with loss of mucus plug may be confused with other causes of vaginal bleeding or cervical or vaginal lesions (polyps, condylomas).

III. **Laboratory Evaluation** should include a CBC, type and cross, coagulation studies, urinalysis, and ultrasound.

IV. **Management of Placenta Previa and Placental Abruption.**

A. **Placenta previa.**

1. If pregnancy 37 weeks or greater, or if fetal maturity has been documented, a cesarean section is indicated unless only a minimal degree of placenta previa is present.
2. If bleeding is sufficient to jeopardize the mother or fetus despite transfusion, cesarean section may be indicated regardless of gestation.
3. In the preterm gestation, expectant management is indicated in patients with no observed bleeding, reactive nonstress test and stable hematocrit, who are compliant with instructions. Most patients require inpatient observation. Physical activity is restricted. Nothing is allowed in the vagina, including examining fingers. The hematocrit is maintained at 30% or greater. Preterm labor can be managed with magnesium sulfate. Use of beta-adrenergic agents can cause tachycardia and mask the signs of bleeding. Once 36 to 37 weeks of gestation is reached with fetal maturity demonstrated by amniocentesis, the patient is readied for elective double-setup examination.
4. Check for fetal bleeding: To 5 ml of tap water add 6 drops of 10% KOH in two test tubes. Add 3 drops of maternal blood to one tube and 3 drops of vaginal blood to the other. The maternal blood will turn green yellowish brown after 2 minutes. If fetal red blood cells are present, the solution will turn pink. Immediate delivery is indicated.
5. Remember that placenta accreta may complicate placenta previa in women with history of previous C-section. Hemorrhage can necessitate hysterectomy.

B. **Placental abruption.**
   1. Occasionally a small separation occurs without further problem. These patients have no uterine symptoms. Observation is required with fetal heart rate monitoring, serial labs and ultrasound, but if no fetal distress occurs within the next 48 hours, the patient may be sent home.
   2. If placental abruption is mild and the fetus is immature, expectant management may be indicated, with fetal heart rate monitoring and serial laboratory and ultrasound examination.
   3. In all other cases, delivery is indicated. A vaginal delivery is preferred when fetal distress is not present or when the fetus is no longer viable. A C-section is indicated if fetal distress is present. A C-section is also performed when there is a threat to the mother's life or a failed trial of labor.
   4. Shock must be treated with adequate replacement of fluids and packed red blood cells; NS or LR should be used. Urine output must be maintained at 25 to 30 ml/hour. A central venous pressure line or Swan-Ganz catheter will assist in monitoring hemodynamic status. See section on shock in Chapter 2.
   5. Coagulopathy should be treated with fresh frozen plasma. One unit of FFP increases the fibrinogen concentration by 25 mg/dl. Platelet transfusion is required if the count is less than 50,000. Heparin is not used in DIC secondary to placental abruption. See section on DIC in Chapter 6.

14

OBSTETRICS

INTRAUTERINE GROWTH RETARDATION (IUGR)

I. **Definition.** IUGR is defined as a fetus that weighs less than the tenth percentile for its gestational age.

A. **Symmetric IUGR (intrinsic):** normal head circumference-to-abdominal circumference ratio, caused by genetic disease or fetal infection and has a poor prognosis.

B. **Asymmetric IUGR (extrinsic):** increased head circumference/abdominal circumference ratio, caused by placental insufficiency; good prognosis with appropriate treatment.

II. **Risk Factors.**

A. **Chronic maternal disease** including chronic maternal hypertension, PIH, diabetes, cyanotic heart disease, collagen vascular disease, severe maternal anemia, renal disease, multifetal pregnancy, etc.

B. **Fetal genetic disorders** or fetal malformations.

C. **Intrauterine infections.** Rubella, herpes, toxoplasmosis, syphilis, CMV.

D. **Previous history of small-for-gestational-age baby,** smoking, drug, or alcohol abuse.

E. **Abnormalities of the placenta** or placental blood flow.

III. **Diagnosis.** One should be suspicious when the fundal height does not exhibit the predicted 1 cm/week growth between 20 and 36 weeks of gestation. A lag in fundal height by 4 cm mandates ultrasonographic evaluation; otherwise, consider ultrasound on a clinical basis. Serial ultrasonic scanning may confirm the diagnosis.

IV. **Management.** The development of IUGR makes the pregnancy high risk. Stillbirth, oligohydramnios, and intrapartum fetal acidosis are common antepartum complications. Close antepartum surveillance is required, and the decision about when to deliver the infant is complex. Neonatal complications include persistent fetal circulation, meconium aspiration syndrome, hypoxic ischemic encephalopathy, hypoglycemia, hypocalcemia, hyperviscosity, and defective temperature regulation. A perinatologist should manage these pregnancies.

LABOR

Introduction. This section is organized sequentially as events happen during labor and delivery. It starts with the management of preterm labor and postdate pregnancies. It then discusses the stages and management of labor, as well as the induction of labor. Finally, it discusses the delivery itself.

PRETERM LABOR

I. **Definition.** Onset of regular contractions between 20 and 37 weeks of gestation occurring at least every 10 minutes and lasting 30 seconds with cervical change. Discrimination from "false labor" is difficult. Postponement of treatment until cervical change occurs may lower the chances of success.

II. **Causes.** Frequently unknown. Several factors have been associated with preterm labor.

A. **Maternal factors.** Infections (systemic, vaginal, urinary tract, amnionitis), uterine anomalies, fibroids, retained IUD, cervical incompetence, overdistended uterus (polyhydramnios, multiple gestation), rupture of membranes.

B. **Fetal factors.** Congenital anomalies, intrauterine death.

III. **Management.**

A. **Initial examination.**

1. **Estimate fetal weight and age** by ultrasound if necessary.

2. **Document FHR and uterine activity** with external monitoring.

3. **Pelvic examination.** Attempt to limit to one examiner and use sterile technique. Rule out ruptured membranes by looking for vaginal pooling of amniotic fluid and by nitrazine paper testing (turns blue if amniotic fluid present) and evaluate sample of fluid for ferning via microscope. Obtain cervical cultures for group B streptococci and do rapid group B streptococci antigen testing if available. If membranes are ruptured, one can used pooled amniotic fluid to determine fetal maturity by looking at the L/S ratio and PG levels; otherwise amniocentesis may be necessary.

4. **Obtain cath UA** and culture.

5. **Consider fibronectin** test-swab of posterior vagina.

B. **Tocolysis.**

1. **Contraindications.** Evidence of fetal distress, fetal anomalies, abruptio placentae, placenta previa with heavy bleeding, severe maternal disease.

2. **Risks of treatment.** If membranes are ruptured, there is increased risk of cord prolapse and amnionitis. Fetal mortality is increased if labor is suppressed when there is IUGR. Mother may experience tachycardia, nervousness, or pulmonary edema secondary to medication.

3. **Tocolysis most likely will be ineffective** if labor is well established or if the cervix is dilated to 4 cm or more. Preparation should be made to deliver in the optimal setting. Up to now there have been no large-scale controlled clinical trials demonstrating that tocolytics delay delivery.

4. **Beta-adrenergic receptor agonists** may inhibit uterine contractility but only prolong gestation for about 48 hours. To a large extent, the goal of tocolysis is to arrest labor long enough for exogenous steroids to stimulate fetal surfactant production so as to prevent the pulmonary complications of preterm birth.

a. **Protocol.**

(1) **Bed rest** in left lateral decubitus position. Effective alone in 50% of patients.

(2) **Sedation** (100 mg of **secobarbital** or 50 mg of hydroxyzine).

(3) **Hydration,** but avoid large boluses (should not exceed 500 ml).

(4) **Antibiotics** controversial. Do not use for >2 days, to limit incidence of resistance.

(5) **FHR** and uterine activity monitoring.

      (6) **Steroids** accelerate fetal lung maturation (betamethasone or dexamethasone 12.5 mg IM Q24h for 48 hours).

  b. **Drug therapy (tocolytics)**

     (1) **Terbutaline. Infusion** should be titrated on an individual basis so as to maximize inhibition of uterine activity and minimize maternal side effects. **Alternative to infusion:** 0.25 mg SQ Q20-60 min until contractions have subsided. **Continue** 2.5 mg PO every 2 to 4 hours. Doses up to 5.0 mg can be used.

     (2) **Magnesium sulfate.** MgSO4 also decreases uterine contractility but is not useful long-term. It can be an adjunct to terbutaline.

     (3) **Other.** Prostaglandin synthetase inhibitors (such as indomethacin), calcium-channel blockers, aminophylline, and progesterone are under investigation.

PREMATURE RUPTURE OF MEMBRANES (PROM)

I. **Definitions.**

A. **"Premature"** rupture of membranes occurs if there is a delay of greater than 1 hour until onset of labor.

B. **"Preterm premature"** rupture of membranes occurs before 37 weeks of gestation.

II. **Diagnosis.**

A. **History of fluid gush** per vagina. Urine can sometimes be confused with the rupture of membranes.

B. **Sterile speculum exam.**

  1. **Exam will show** pooling of fluid in vaginal vault.

  2. **pH determination.** Amniotic fluid typically turns nitrazine paper blue. Contamination with vaginal-cervical mucus, blood, or urine may lead to false positives.

  3. **Fern test.** Allow a sample of fluid to air dry on a glass or slide. Examination of amniotic fluid under the microscope reveals a classical "fern" pattern.

  4. **Cervical digital examination increases risk of chorioamnionitis!** Evaluate cervix visually with sterile speculum. Avoid digital exams if possible unless patient is in labor and delivery is inevitable. Check for cord prolapse.

III. **Management.**

A. **PROM at term.** Most sources recommend induction and delivery within a range of 24 to 36 hours after admission.

B. **Preterm PROM.** Fetal maturity must be considered. Manage expectantly until the fetus is mature unless chorioamnionitis (see below), fetal distress develops, or labor cannot be inhibited with tocolysis (see above). Positive cervical cultures should be treated but do not necessitate induction without other signs of chorioamnionitis or fetal distress. Follow maternal and fetal vital signs, including temperature every 8 hours and WBC counts as indicated. Antibiotics have been shown to prolong pregnancy. Randomized double blind placebo controlled study showed decreased infant morbidity with antibiotic therapy (ampicillin and erythromycin).

C. **Deliver if amnionitis.** Signs include maternal or fetal tachycardia, maternal fever, uterine tenderness, foul cervical discharge, uterine contractions, leukocytosis, and the presence of leukocytes or bacteria in amniotic fluid.

POSTDATE PREGNANCY

I. **Definitions.**

A. **Prolonged pregnancy.** Longer than 40 weeks of gestation.

B. **Postdate pregnancy.** Longer than 42 weeks.

C. **Postmature pregnancy.** Longer than 42 weeks with evidence of placental dysfunction.

II. **Etiology.**

A. **Most common.** Error in estimating EDC.

B. **Risk factors.** History of prior prolonged gestation (50% risk), older age, anencephaly, or fetal endocrinopathy.

III. **Potential Morbidity.**

A. **Maternal.**

    1. **Birth trauma** secondary to macrosomic infant because of shoulder dystocia.

    2. **Operative delivery, secondary infection and hemorrhage** are more common with postdate pregnancies.

B. **Neonatal.** Meconium aspiration syndrome, polycythemia, hyperbilirubinemia, hypoglycemia, and anoxic organ damage.

IV. **Management: Delivery Should Be Accomplished by 42 Weeks.**

A. **Antepartum fetal surveillance** with NST and amniotic fluid index assessment should be done at 40 and 41 weeks and twice weekly thereafter.

B. **Indications for immediate delivery.** Cervix is ripe, decreased amniotic fluid, large fetal size (abdominal circumference), nonreactive NST, and presence of meconium in fluid. Pregnancies complicated by hypertension and diabetes should be induced at or near term.

C. **Induction of labor** can be preceded by cervical ripening using PGE_2 gel or insert. PGE_2 gel (1 mg placed intracervically) has been shown to decrease the amount of oxytocin needed to establish labor and rate of cesarean section in patients induced for medical indications before 41 weeks of gestation. Decreased amniotic fluid leading to variable decelerations and meconium staining may be managed with amnioinfusion (see below). Nasopharyngeal aspiration at the perineum and endotracheal aspiration should be performed once the baby is born to prevent meconium aspiration. Anticipate shoulder dystocia.

VAGINAL BIRTH AFTER CESAREAN SECTION (VBAC)

I. **Definition.** Attempted vaginal delivery in a woman who has undergone previous cesarean section.

II. **Decision to Attempt VBAC.**

A. **Advantages include** overall reduced morbidity, mortality and cost compared with elective C-section. Additionally, many women prefer a vaginal delivery.

A. **Disadvantages include** the requirement for closer intrapartum monitoring and a higher risk of infection compared to an elective C-section if a C-section is required.

C. **Contraindications include** a history of previous classical, T-shaped, or unknown uterine incision, multiple gestation, an estimated birth weight >4000 g, a non-vertex presentation or inadequate facilities or personnel for emergency C-section.

D. **Probability of success.** Depends primarily on the indication of the previous C-section. If the primary C-section was for breech position, abruption, placenta previa, cord accident, antepartum hemorrhage, hypertensive disorder, or fetal distress, there is a 74% to 94% rate of success. If the primary C-section was for cephalopelvic disproportion (CPD) or failed induction, there is a 35% to 77% rate of success.

III. **Risks.** In addition to the usual risk of delivery, other risks include:

A. **Uterine rupture.** Very rare. Incidence increased if prior C-section was classical.

B. **Cesarean section.** Increased risk of C-section morbidity relative to elective C-section.

IV. **Management.**

A. **Preparation.**

   1. Type and screen for 2 units of packed cells; intravenous line should be inserted.
   2. The anesthesiologist, surgeon, and physician caring for the newborn infant must be notified in advance and be available.

B. **Labor.**

   1. **Electronic fetal monitoring** is recommended.
   2. **Oxytocin** may be cautiously used to augment labor, and close monitoring of uterine contractions (using intrauterine pressure catheter) is necessary. **Oxytocin must be titrated with great care in a VBAC.**
   3. The same expectations of normal progression during labor should be applied to patients with a prior C-section.
   4. An experienced physician should be in attendance throughout labor and delivery.
   5. **Postpartum.** Manual exploration of the uterus after delivery of the placenta is indicated to assess scar integrity.

EVALUATION OF LABOR (BOX 14-1)

I. **Collect the information in Box 14-1 on admission to labor and delivery.**

II. **Pelvic Exam.**

A. **Inspection.**

   1. Look for herpetic lesions, condylomas, and lacerations.
   2. Speculum examination may reveal pooling of vaginal fluid, consistent with rupture of membranes. A nitrazine paper test or swab of vaginal fluid on a glass slide may be necessary to prove the presence of am-

---

BOX 14-1		
ADMISSION INFORMATION FOR LABOR AND DELIVERY		
Gravida/Para	Blood type	Contraction onset, duration,
Complications?	Rho (D) administered?	frequency
LMP and EDC?	VDRL	Membranes intact or
Length of gestation	Rubella	ruptured
Coexisting medical	Hb/HCT	Fetal movement
problems?		Fetal position
Weight gain during		Fundal height
pregnancy		Auscultate fetal tones

niotic fluid in the vagina. The basic pH of this fluid will turn the nitrazine paper blue. Care must be taken to avoid the cervical mucus, which is also basic and may give a false-positive test. If an air-dried sample of fluid reveals a fern-like pattern, the presence of amniotic fluid is confirmed.

B. **Palpation of the cervix.**
   1. **Dilatation of the cervical os.** Dilatation may range from 0 to 10 cm.
   2. **Effacement.** The degree of thinning of the cervix. The cervix may range from 3 cm long (thick or with no effacement) to paper thin (100% effaced). In nulliparas effacement often precedes dilatation. Simultaneous effacement and dilatation is seen in multiparas.
   3. **Palpation of the presenting part.**
      a. **Identification.** Head, foot, buttock, other.
      b. **Station.** Station is described as the relationship of the fetal presenting part to the level of the ischial spines in the maternal pelvis. Station may range from -3 to $+3$. Zero station (engagement) occurs when the lower most presenting part is palpable at the level of the ischial spines. Always assess station by both abdominal method and pelvic method to avoid errors caused by caput.
      c. **Position.** Position is described as the orientation of the presenting part in regard to the maternal pelvis. Vertex presentation with the occiput positioned either to the right or left anteriorly is the most common.

NORMAL LABOR AND LABOR DYSFUNCTION

I. **Normal Phases of Labor.**
A. **Latent phase.** Slow rate of dilatation, <0.6 cm/hour.
B. **Active labor.**
   1. **Acceleration.** Dilatation rate >0.6 cm/hour.
   2. **Maximum slope of dilatation.** Cervix >5 cm or rate >1.2 cm/hour for nullipara and >1.5 cm/hour for multipara.
   3. **Deceleration.** Cervix >9 cm, not completely effaced.

II. **Problems with the Progression of Labor.**

A. **Prolonged Latent Phase.** Defined as >20 hours in nullipara; >14 hours in multipara. Cause: unripe cervix, false labor, sedation, and uterine inertia. **Management:** observation, need for oxytocin stimulation. Avoid amniotomy. Good prognosis for vaginal delivery.

B. **Protracted Active Phase.** Rate of dilatation: <1.2 cm/hour in nullipara; <1.5 cm/hour in multipara. **Cause:** fetal malpositions (occiput posterior), CPD, hypotonic uterine contractions, and anesthesia. **Management:** oxytocin stimulation. 70% require C-section.

C. **Secondary Arrest of Cervical Dilatation.** Cessation of dilatation for >2 hours. High incidence of CPD: frequently require a cesarean section.

D. **Failure of Descent.** Arrest of descent during second stage. High incidence of CPD: frequently required cesarean section.

E. **Protracted Descent.** Nullipara <1 cm/hour; multipara <2 cm/hour. Causes include CPD, full bladder, and macrosomia. Inadequate pushing because of anesthesia can also cause this disorder.

F. **Precipitous Labor** >5 cm/hour dilatation in nullipara; >10 cm/hour in multipara. **Complications:** trauma to birth canal, fetal distress, and postpartum hemorrhage.

INTRAPARTUM MONITORING AND MANAGEMENT

I. **Fetal Heart Rate.** Electronic fetal heart rate monitoring may be performed by means of external Doppler, or direct scalp lead when membranes are ruptured.

A. **Indications.** Meconium staining, use of oxytocin; delivery of an anticipated premature, postmature, Rh-sensitized, or growth-retarded infant; medical complications associated with uteroplacental insufficiency (hypertension, diabetes, severe anemia, heart disease, renal disease), presence of abnormal FHR by Doppler scanning, VBAC, other intrapartum obstetrical complications (failure to progress, excessive vaginal bleeding).

B. **Fetal heart rate tracing interpretation.**

1. **Baseline fetal heart rate.**
   a. **Normal** 120 to 160 bpm.
   b. **Tachycardia** >160 bpm. **Cause:** fetal hypoxia, maternal fever, maternal hyperthyroidism, parasympatholytic or sympathomimetic drugs.
   c. **Bradycardia** <120 bpm. **Cause:** fetal asphyxia, anesthetics, fetal cardiac conduction defect. Usually benign if good variability is present.

2. **Variability.**
   a. **Short-term variability.** Beat-to-beat variation is normally 5 to 10 bpm (reliably assessed with only a scalp lead).
   b. **Long-term variability.** Waviness of the FHR tracing, which normally has a frequency of 3 to 10 cycles/min and an amplitude of 10 to 25 bpm.
   c. **Decreased variability.** Variability may be decreased by fetal sleep cycles, CNS depression secondary to hypoxia or drugs, parasympatholytic agents, extreme prematurity, or congenital anomalies.

Loss of variability is associated with a high incidence of fetal acidosis and low Apgar scores.

3. **Common periodic patterns.**
   a. **Accelerations.** Reassuring if associated with fetal movement. May be compensatory before or after deceleration.
   b. **Early decelerations.** Occur coincidentally with uterine contractions and are associated with fetal head compression. These are vagally mediated and not ominous when they occur late in labor. These start early in the contraction phase, reach their lowest point at the peak of the contraction, and return to baseline levels as the contraction finishes. The FHR does not fall below 100 bpm.
   c. **Late decelerations.** Transient but repetitive deceleration of the FHR observed to occur late in the contraction phase. Reaches its lowest point after the acme of the contraction and returns to baseline rate once the contraction is over. Late decelerations result from fetal hypoxia, indicate uteroplacental insufficiency, and are always considered ominous.
   d. **Variable decelerations.** Characterized by variable duration, timing in relation to contraction and intensity. This is a reflex pattern, typically secondary to umbilical cord compression. May benefit from amnioinfusion. Poor prognostic signs are the following:
      (1) Association with poor FHR baseline variability.
      (2) Lack of pre-deceleration and post-deceleration accelerations.
      (3) Slow return to baseline or failure to return to baseline.
      (4) Biphasic shape (W = knot in cord).
   e. **Prolonged decelerations.** Isolated decelerations >120 seconds can be seen with maternal hypotension, maternal hypoxia, tetanic contractions, prolapsed umbilical cord, fetal scalp procedures (vagal), and paracervical or epidural anesthesia. A prolonged deceleration after severe variable deceleration may signal impending fetal demise.

4. **Management of abnormal FHR pattern or fetal distress.**
   a. **Turn patient onto left side to** alleviate vena cava compression.
   b. **Discontinue intravenous oxytocin.**
   c. **Apply 100% oxygen** to mother by face-mask.
   d. **Correct maternal hypotension or hypertension.**
   e. **Vaginal examination** to rule out prolapsed cord.
   f. **Consider fetal scalp blood sampling** for pH determination (Table14-2).
   g. **With decreased variability,** consider fetal scalp stimulation. The return of variability is reassuring. If tracing maintains poor variability, consider points a to f above.
   h. **With prolonged bradycardia** unresponsive to other maneuvers or late decelerations with worsening fetal acidosis (pH <7.20), consider delivery by C-section.

14

OBSTETRICS

TABLE 14-2

INTERPRETATION OF FETAL SCALP PH

Fetal Scalp Blood pH	Interpretation	Management
>7.25	Normal	Continue FHR monitoring and re-sample if appropriate.
7.20-7.24	Preacidotic	Consider re-sampling and continue FHR monitoring.
<7.19	Fetal acidosis	Re-sample in 5 to 10 minutes and prepare for immediate delivery if low scalp pH is confirmed.

II. **Uterine Activity.** May be determined by an indirect (external) pressure monitor, or by an intrauterine pressure transducer when more accurate estimations are required.

A. **Contractility.** Effective contractions should have an amplitude of 50 to 75 mm Hg, duration of 45 to 90 seconds, and frequency of every 3 to 5 minutes.

B. **Resting tone.** Spontaneous labor 5 to 10 mm Hg. Induced labor 15 to 20 mm Hg.

C. **Rhythmicity.** Presence of coupling or tripling may represent hyperstimulation.

D. **Configuration.** Typically bell shaped. May become rectangular during pushing. The area under the curve when an internal transducer is used may be calculated to determine the adequacy of uterine contractions.

III. **Fetal Stimulation.** When the scalp is stimulated and there is an acceleration of 15 bpm lasting 15 seconds, it denotes fetal pH value of 7.22 or greater. Reverse is not true. Obtain baseline fetal scalp pH in meconium staining. Draw maternal venous blood simultaneously for comparison. In the case of maternal fever do not rely on fetal scalp pH because fetal compromise can occur with normal values.

AMNIOINFUSION

I. **Definition.** Amnioinfusion is a procedure in which a physiologic solution (such as normal saline) is infused into the uterine cavity to replace the amniotic fluid.

II. **Indications.**

A. **Correcting variable decelerations because of cord compression.**

B. **Reduce fetal distress caused by meconium staining** of fluid (rule out concurrent signs of fetal stress).

C. **Correction of oligohydramnios.**

III. **Technique.**

A. **Catheter.** Double-lumen catheter: expensive but helps monitor uterine contractions.

B. **Infusate.** Normal saline, lactated Ringer's (like amniotic fluid).

TABLE 14-3				
BISHOP SCORING SYSTEM				
Cervix	Score			
	0	1	2	3
Position	Posterior	Midposition	Anterior	—
Consistency	Firm	Medium	Soft	—
Effacement (%)	0-30	40-50	60-70	>80
Dilation (cm)	Closed	1-2	3-4	>5
Station	−3	−2	−1	+1, +2

Bishop score of >9 indicates induction should be successful.

Modified from Romney S et al, editors: *Gynecology and obstetrics: the health care of women,* ed 2, New York, 1981, McGraw-Hill.

C. **Temperature.** Room temperature fluid can cause fetal bradycardia if infused rapidly. Body temperature is more physiologic.
D. **Methods.** Continuous infusion by gravity drainage or by infusion pump 10 to 15 ml/min or intermittent infusion by gravity drainage (1 L over 20 to 30 minutes, repeat Q6h). Small risk of uterine rupture if efflux of infusate blocked.

IV. **Efficacy.**
A. **Oligohydramnios.** Lower rate of C-section for fetal distress and higher umbilical artery pHs at birth compared to those in patients not receiving amnioinfusion.
B. **Moderate to thick meconium.** Decreased rate of operative delivery, increased average 1-minute Apgar scores, less meconium aspirated from below neonate's vocal cords, and a lower incidence of meconium aspiration syndrome compared to that in patients not treated with amnioinfusion.

INDUCTION OF LABOR

I. Indications and Contraindications.
A. **Indications.** Pregnancy-induced hypertension, premature rupture of membranes, chorioamnionitis, postdate pregnancy, IUGR, isoimmunization, other evidence of hostile intrauterine environment, diabetes mellitus, other selected maternal diseases, fetal demise.
B. **Contraindications.** Placenta previa, cord presentation, floating presenting part, abnormal fetal lie, active genital herpes, invasive cervical carcinoma, pelvic structural deformities, prior classical uterine incision. Oxytocin stimulation would be relatively contraindicated in conditions that predispose to uterine rupture (high parity, advanced maternal age, fetopelvic disproportion, uterine overdistension, prior uterine scar).

II. Induction Methods. Assess the inducibility of the cervix using Bishop score (Table 14-3). Determine route of induction.
A. **Amniotomy.**
    1. Cervix should be dilated enough to allow reaching the membranes with the amniotomy hook. The fetus should be vertex (unless breech

delivery is planned) with the presenting part well engaged and well applied to the cervix. The umbilical cord should not be palpable.
2. Membranes are hooked, and a gentle tug should cause release of amnionic fluid. Assess fluid for presence of meconium.
3. **Monitor fetal heart tones** before and after the procedure.
4. **Risks:** cord prolapse, injury to fetal part (unlikely with amnio hook)

B. **Dinoprostone (PGE2)**
1. **Indicated** for cervical ripening if Bishop score <5 (see Table 14-3)
2. **Cervidil** (10 mg dinoprostone). Administer as vaginal insert. 1 dose. Monitor for 120 minutes postinsertion.
3. **Prepidil** (0.5 mg dinoprostone) Administered intracervically. Monitor for 60-120 minutes. May repeat after 6 hours. No more than 3 doses in 24 hours.
4. **Risks.** Hyperstimulation and uterine rupture.
5. **Endpoint.** Bishops score of 8 or higher, strong uterine contractions or change in maternal/fetal status.

C. **Misoprostol (PGE1)**
1. Currently not FDA-labelled for cervical ripening but meta-analysis compared use of intravaginal misoprostol with dinoprostone, oxytocin, and placebo. Lower rate of cesarean section, higher incidence vaginal delivery within 24 hours, and reduced need for oxytocin augmentation.
2. Most common dose 25-50 μg inserted every 4-6 hours up to 6-8 doses. Continuous fetal monitoring recommended for 3 hours after dose.
3. **Risks.** Hyperstimulation, possible increased meconium staining, uterine rupture

D. **Oxytocin administration.**
1. Can use to ripen cervix but often used after one of the above methods of cervical ripening.
2. **Close monitoring** of the parturient and fetus is essential. Most hospitals have written protocols available.
3. **Place 10 units of oxytocin** in 1000 ml of D_5NS or D_5LR. Begin with a low dose of oxytocin: 0.5 to 2 mU per minute. (Each milliliter of the above solution contains 10 mU.).
4. **Advancing dose.** Various protocols exist regarding the rate for increasing the dose and the maximum dose. If little uterine response is observed, the dose can be increased by 1 to 2 mU/min every 30 minutes. Most patients respond to rates of 20 mU/min or less. The faster the increase, the more likely the risk of hyperstimulation. The rate of administration is held steady when a good labor pattern (contractions every 2 to 3 minutes lasting 60 to 90 seconds with an intrauterine pressure of 50 to 60 mm Hg and a resting tone of 10 to 15 mm Hg) is achieved. Ideally you want 150 to 250 Montevideo units. Montevideo units = Number of contractions/10 min × (Average peak of contraction − Average baseline of contraction).

5. If at any point the fetal heart rate indicates distress, the patient should be placed on her left side, oxygen administered, and oxytocin discontinued. Reinstatement of oxytocin drip requires reassessment of the situation.

OBSTETRIC ANESTHESIA AND ANALGESIA

I. **Overview.** Pain during first stage of labor is attributable to uterine contractions and cervical dilatation. During the second stage, pain occurs from distension and stretching of pelvic structures and the perineum. Pain is conducted along the paracervical or inferior hypogastric plexus.

II. **Systemic Narcotics. Meperidine** 25 mg IV or **nalbuphine** (Nubain) 10 mg IV are given early during labor and usually avoided at or near delivery. **Maternal complications:** nausea, vomiting, decreased gastric motility, respiratory depression. **Fetal complications:** respiratory depression, CNS depression, and impaired temperature regulation. Naloxone (0.01 mg/kg) can be administered to depressed newborn as IV bolus for counteracting the effect of narcotics. Naloxone may also be given IM.

III. **Local Anesthesia.**

A. **Pudendal block.** Provides analgesia to vaginal introitus and perineum. Usually used in second stage of labor. Technique is beyond the scope of this manual.

B. **Paracervical block.** Provides analgesia during active phase of labor. Blocks pain caused by uterine contractions. Technique is beyond the scope of this manual.

C. **Lumbar epidural anesthesia.**
   1. **Associated with prolonged labor and an increased risk of chorioamnionitis.**
   2. **Contraindications include** maternal fever, preexisting CNS disease, severe hypertension, hypotension, hypovolemia, and coagulopathy.

IV. **Psychologic Methods of Pain Relief.** Lamaze classes aid in preparation; hypnosis, acupuncture, and biofeedback are also used.

VAGINAL DELIVERY

I. **Normal Spontaneous Vaginal Delivery.**

A. **Cardinal movements (for vertex presentation).**
   1. **Engagement.** Occurs late in pregnancy for primigravida, at the onset of labor for multigravida.
   2. **Flexion.** Of the neck so that the smallest diameter possible presents. If the neck does not flex, it may actually extend during labor, producing a brow or face presentation.
   3. **Descent.** Progressive with thinning of the cervix and lower uterine segment. Depends on the force of contractions and on pelvic and presenting part configuration.
   4. **Internal rotation.** Occurs during descent. Vertex rotates from transverse to either posterior or anterior position to pass the ischial spines.

14

OBSTETRICS

5. **Extension.** Occurs as the head distends the perineum and the occiput passes beneath the symphysis.
6. **External rotation.** Occurs after delivery of the head with the head rotating back to a transverse position as the shoulders internally rotate to an anteroposterior position.

B. **Management of vertex delivery.**
   1. **Preparations for delivery.** Should be made when the presenting part begins to distend the perineum, sooner for multigravida. (Local or pudendal anesthesia can be administered at this time.) Episiotomy (if needed) is not performed until delivery is imminent. Episiotomy likely increases the risk of third- and fourth-degree tears.
   2. **Delivery of the head.**
      a. Controlled so that there is no forceful, sudden expulsion that may produce injury. As the vertex appears beneath the symphysis, the perineum is supported by direct pressure from a draped hand over the coccygeal region (Ritgen's maneuver). This will protect the perineum and assist in extension of the head as the vertex passes the symphysis.
      b. As the head is delivered, it will rotate to a transverse position, at which time the baby should be checked for the presence of umbilical cord about the neck. If present, it should be gently slipped over the infant's head (or double clamped and cut if this cannot be done easily).
      c. The mouth and nose should be cleared of secretions with a bulb syringe or DeLee suction trap.
   3. **Delivery of the shoulders.** Shoulders should be rotated to an AP position in the pelvic outlet as the head externally rotates. Gentle traction downward on the head will assist in bringing the anterior shoulder beneath the symphysis. Gentle elevation of the infant head toward the symphysis will release the posterior shoulder.
   4. **Delivery of the body.** The rest of the body will generally deliver spontaneously and quickly after delivery of the shoulders. Care must be taken to control the delivery of the body to prevent unnecessary injury.
   5. **Immediate care of the infant.** Includes double clamping and cutting of the umbilical cord. Do not milk the cord. The clamp closest to the umbilicus should be just distal to the skin or longer if anticipate a need for an umbilical line. A clear airway must be assured and body temperature maintained by drying and wrapping, placing under a radiant heater, or in skin-to-skin contact with mother's chest.

C. **Forceps delivery:** Forceps are generally used to shorten the second stage of labor when in the best interest of the mother or the fetus. A fully dilated cervix and experienced physician are required. Advantages must be weighed against the increased risk of maternal lacerations.
   1. **Indications.**
      a. **Prolonged second stage.**
         (1) Primigravida with regional anesthesia >3 hours.

(2) Primigravida without regional anesthesia >2 hours.
(3) Multigravida with regional anesthesia >2 hours.
(4) Multigravida without regional anesthesia >1 hour.
   b. **Fetal distress.**
   c. **Maternal exhaustion.**
2. **Requirements.**
   a. Fetal head engaged and in vertex-face presentation.
   b. Position of head known exactly.
   c. Membranes ruptured.
   d. Cervix fully dilated.
   e. No clinical evidence of cephalopelvic disproportion.
3. **Definitions.**
   a. **Outlet forceps.** The fetal scalp is visible at the introitus. The head is at or on the perineum, and the sagittal suture is in the AP plane or rotated up to 45 degrees.
   b. **Low forceps.** The leading point of the skull is at least at +2 station.
   c. **Midforceps.** The leading point of the skull is engaged but is above +2 station. (Midforceps delivery should be attempted only in extreme situations while simultaneously preparing for C-section.)
4. **Selection of forceps.**
   a. **Simpson.** Good for primigravida with prolonged second stage (molded fetal head).
   b. **Elliot.** Better if multigravida and if less molded fetal head.
   c. **Tucker-McLane.** Has sliding lock, good for asynclitic fetal head.
   d. **Kielland.** Has minimal pelvic curve, often used for rotation.
   e. **Piper.** Used in breech extractions.
D. **Vacuum Extraction** A safe, effective alternative to forceps delivery. A term, vertex fetus is required. Delivery should not be one that will require rotation or excessive traction. Prior scalp sampling is a contraindication.
1. **Advantages.**
   a. Simpler to apply with fewer mistakes in application.
   b. Less force applied to fetal head.
   c. Less anesthesia necessary (local anesthetic may suffice).
   d. No increase in diameter of presenting head.
   e. Less maternal soft-tissue injury.
   f. Less fetal injury.
   g. Less parental concern.
2. **Disadvantages.**
   a. Traction applied only during contractions.
   b. Proper traction necessary to avoid losing vacuum.
   c. Possible longer delivery than with forceps.
   d. Small increase in incidence of cephalohematomas.
3. **Technique.**
   a. Ascertain that the cervix is fully dilated and the head is in low or outlet position.

14

OBSTETRICS

b. The head is then wiped clean, the labia are spread, and the cup is compressed and inserted. Pressure is applied inward and downward until contact is made with the fetal scalp. The cup should be placed over the posterior fontanelle.

c. A finger is swept around the cup to make sure no maternal tissue is within the cup. Suction pressure is raised to 100 mm Hg, and the location of the cup is rechecked.

d. With the onset of a contraction, suction pressure is raised to a range of 380 to 580 mm Hg. (Negative pressure should not exceed 600 mm Hg.) Traction is applied perpendicularly to the cup, in line with the maternal axis.

e. Should the cup be dislodged, the fetal scalp is to be checked before the cup is reapplied.

f. When the contraction subsides, the suction pressure is reduced to 100 mm Hg.

g. As the head crowns, an episiotomy may be cut but likely increases the risk of third- and fourth-degree tears. Traction is then changed to a 45-degree angle upward as the vertex clears the symphysis.

h. Suction is released and the cup removed after delivery of the fetal head.

i. The procedure should be discontinued if one fails to achieve extraction after 10 minutes at maximal pressure, extraction is not achieved within 30 minutes of initiation, the cup disengages three times, fetal scalp trauma is sustained, or no progress is made after three pulls.

BREECH DELIVERY

I. **Overview.**

A. **Incidence.** 25% of all pregnancies <28 weeks of gestation, 3% to 4% of all pregnancies at or beyond 34 weeks of gestation.

B. **Cause.** Low birth weight, placenta previa, uterine and fetal anomalies, contracted pelvis, multiple fetuses all contribute to breech presentations.

II. **Types of Breech.**

A. **Frank.** Thighs and hips flexed, knees extended. 65% of cases are frank.

B. **Complete.** Thighs and hips flexed, one or both knees flexed. 10% of cases.

C. **Incomplete or footling.** One or both thighs extended, one or both knees below the buttocks. 25% of cases.

III. **Criteria for Vaginal Delivery of Breech Presentation.** (Technique is beyond the scope of this manual.)

A. **Frank breech presentation.**

B. **Fetal weight** 2500 to 3800 g.

C. Fetal head flexed.

D. Gestational age at or beyond 36 weeks.

E. Adequate maternal pelvis.
F. No other maternal or fetal indicator for C-section.

EPISIOTOMY

I. **Overview.** A deliberate incision in the perineum used to facilitate vaginal delivery. Stretching of the vaginal tissues manually may prevent the need for episiotomy and minimize the risk of tears.
II. **Midline.** Good anatomic results, easy repair, low incidence of postpartum pain or dyspareunia. **However, increases the risk of a third or fourth degree laceration compared to patients without an episiotomy.**
III. **Mediolateral. Less likely to extend through the sphincter** but more likely to cause pain during healing, dyspareunia, or excessive blood loss. Good anatomic results are more difficult to obtain.

SHOULDER DYSTOCIA

I. **Incidence.** Directly related to fetal size: >2500 g 0.15%; >4000 g 1.7%; >4500 g 10.0%.
II. **Diagnosis.** Suspect shoulder dystocia if there is reason to suspect macrosomia (gestational diabetes, history of large infants, large maternal size, prolonged gestation), or if second stage is prolonged. Consider C-section. In vaginal deliveries, suspect dystocia if the head pulls back against the perineum after delivery, and external rotation is difficult.
III. **Management.**
A. Ensure adequate maternal anesthesia and cut a very generous episiotomy.
B. Attempt McRobert's maneuver. The mother's thighs are hyperflexed, bringing her feet "to her ears." Have an assistant apply suprapubic pressure. This causes the shoulder to move under the symphysis pubis. Attempt delivery with gentle downward traction.
C. Attempt the Wood's screw maneuver. Gently rotate the posterior shoulder by pushing on the posterior scapula until the shoulder passes under the symphysis and can be delivered as the anterior shoulder.
D. If this is unsuccessful, try delivering the posterior arm first and then rotating the anterior shoulder into the oblique position for delivery.
E. If all else fails, one may attempt deliberate fracture of the clavicle of the impacted shoulder. The thumb and forefinger are used to push the clavicle outward to avoid a pneumothorax. Although the fracture will heal, damage to cervical nerve roots may occur and cause permanent sequelae.

CESAREAN SECTION

I. Indications.
A. **Maternal and fetal.** Cephalopelvic disproportion, failed induction or progression of labor, abnormal uterine contraction pattern.
B. **Maternal.**
   1. **Maternal diseases.** Eclampsia or preeclampsia with non-inducible cervix, diabetes mellitus (if macrosomic infant precludes vaginal de-

14

OBSTETRICS

livery), cardiac disease, cervical cancer, active herpes genitalis. One double-blind clinical trial showed that acyclovir suppression (400 mg PO TID) given after 36 weeks of gestation significantly reduces the need for cesarean section by preventing a herpetic outbreak at term.

2. **Previous uterine surgery.** Classic cesarean section, previous uterine rupture, full-thickness myomectomy. If there is any question about the type of incision made during a previous cesarean section, the operative report for that delivery must be obtained so that incisional type can be known with certainty.

3. **Obstruction to the birth canal.** Fibroids, ovarian tumors.

C. **Fetal.** Fetal distress, cord prolapse, fetal malpresentations.

D. **Placental.** Placenta previa (unless marginal) and abruptio placentae.

II. **Risks.**

A. **Maternal.** Infection, hemorrhage, injury to urinary tract, adverse reactions to anesthesia, prolonged recovery.

B. **Fetal.** Depends on gestational age and indications for C-section. Less birth trauma, though injury can be sustained during operative delivery. May have increased incidence of respiratory distress syndrome.

III. **Antibiotic Prophylaxis.** Reduced incidence of endometritis, wound infection, urinary tract infection and fever post-op with single dose of antibiotic (e.g., ceftriaxone, cefotetan) prior to caesarean delivery.

POSTPARTUM HEMORRHAGE

I. **Definition.** Postpartum hemorrhage is most often defined as a blood loss greater than 500 ml in the first 24 hours after delivery. However, blood loss after spontaneous vaginal delivery is frequently up to 600 ml and between 1 and 1.5 liters after instrumental or operative delivery. Therefore, clinical experience is necessary to determine when bleeding is occurring too rapidly, at the wrong time or is unresponsive to appropriate treatment. Blood loss will be less well tolerated if the patient has not had the normal expansion of blood volume during pregnancy, as in cases of preeclampsia.

II. **Risk Factors.** Multiparity (>5 babies), previous postpartum hemorrhage, manual removal of the placenta, placental abruption or placenta previa, polyhydramnios, prolonged labor, precipitant labor, difficult forceps delivery, prolonged oxytocin administration, breech extraction.

III. **Etiology.** Uterine atony accounts for most cases. Other causes include retained placenta, cervical or vaginal tear, and coagulopathy.

IV. **Physical Exam.**

A. **Vital signs.** BP and pulse abnormalities are very late signs of bleeding due to hemodynamics of pregnancy and usual young age of patient.

B. **Uterus should be palpated** for evidence of atony, tenderness, or lack of involution.

C. **Vaginal exam** may reveal evidence of laceration (generally bright red blood) or atony (darker blood). Bimanual exam may reveal mass (suggestive of broad ligament or paravaginal hematoma).

D. **Hematocrit** is helpful only in comparison to the value before delivery. It will not adequately reflect acute blood loss.

V. **Management.**

A. **Reliable IV access** must be obtained with 2 large-bore IVs. Monitor vital signs and maintain circulatory status with fluids. If the patient shows evidence of symptomatic hypovolemia, blood should be sent for type and cross. Coagulation profile should also be obtained.

B. **Review clinical course for probable cause** (see predisposing factors listed above).

C. **Perform bimanual examination** in recovery area or delivery room.

D. **Managing specific causes of postpartum hemorrhage.**

  1. **Uterine atony:**

    a. **Uterine massage.**

    b. **Oxytocin** IM (10-20 U)/IV (40 U/L at 250 ml/hr) if no contraindications.

    c. **Methergine** IM (0.2 mg) contraindicated if hypertension, preeclampsia hypersensitivity.

    d. **Prostaglandin F2 (Hemabate)** IM or intramyometrially 0.25 mg Q15 minutes up to 8 doses. Contraindicated if active cardiac, renal, pulmonary, or hepatic disease.

  2. **Retained placenta or invasive placenta.** Manual removal of placenta, identify cleavage plain with intrauterine hand, advance fingertips to separate. If can not identify cleavage- probably invasive placenta and requires surgery.

  3. **Trauma.** Identify laceration or hematoma and repair. Consider uterine inversion and uterine rupture.

  4. **If cause is not identified** or fails to respond to the above measures, notify obstetric physicians, anesthesia, and operating room personnel of potential need for surgical intervention. Inform patient of the problem and what measures are being taken to correct it. Get an appreciation of her desires regarding further childbearing and hysterectomy.

  5. **If uterine bleeding persists,** surgery must be considered. Packing or balloon tamponade (e.g., 24 French Foley with 70-80 cc water) is a temporary measure and is rarely effective. Surgical alternatives include uterine artery and hypogastric artery ligation. Hysterectomy is the treatment of last resort when the patient desires future fertility but may be preferred if sterility is desired.

14

OBSTETRICS

POSTPARTUM CARE

I. **Examples of Orders after Routine Vaginal Delivery.**

A. **Immediately postpartum:**

  1. **Pitocin** 10 units IM.

  2. **Bed rest,** and vitals Q15 min for 1 hour postpartum.

  3. **Ice pack** to perineum immediately postpartum PRN.

B. **Thereafter:**

  1. **Ambulate** as soon as possible.

    2. **Diet.** General or other.
    3. **Vital signs.** Q4h.
    4. **Tucks** to perineum PRN.
    5. **Sitz baths** TID and HS PRN.
    6. **IV (if present).** Discontinue when vital signs are stable and uterine bleeding is normal.
    7. **Bladder catheterization** if unable to void in 6 to 8 hours.
    8. **Breast binder** if not nursing.
    9. **CBC** postpartum day 2.
    10. **Administer $Rh_o(D)$** immunoglobulin if indicated.
    11. **Medications.**
        a. **Vitamins.** Continue prenatal vitamins; additional $FeSO_4$ if anemic.
        b. **Pain.** Acetaminophen 650 mg PO Q4-6h PRN or ibuprofen 400 to 600 mg PO Q4-6h for cramping pain. Narcotics as needed (but be careful if breast feeding).
        c. **Bowels.** Docusate sodium 100 mg PO BID; milk of magnesia 30 ml PO QD PRN; bisacodyl 10 mg PO or PR PRN.

II. **Hospital Care.**
A. **Physical examination.**
    1. **Monitor uterine changes.** The fundus should be firm and at or below the umbilicus. Gradual involution occurs over the next 6 weeks.
    2. **Lochia** (uterine drainage) is initially red or bloody, gradually becoming serosanguineous. By 2 to 3 weeks it should be white. Tampons are contraindicated.
    3. **Breasts** are examined for signs of infection and presence of milk. Colostrum is present initially. Milk production should occur by the third to fifth day in primiparas, sooner in multiparas. Breast feeding should not be allowed for greater than 15 minutes on each side per feeding initially to help prevent soreness.
    4. **Legs** should be examined for evidence of thrombophlebitis.

III. **Parent Education.**
A. **Newborn care.**
B. **Breast feeding** and prevention of lactation or engorgement if applicable.

IV. **Discharge.**
A. **Discharge instructions.**
    1. **Rubella vaccination,** if indicated, before discharge.
    2. **Instruct regarding signs of puerperal infection,** postpartum hemorrhage, and mastitis.
    3. **Counsel on avoidance of intercourse** and tampons for 4 weeks.
    4. **Contraception counseling.** OCPs can be started during week 4, if desired. Low-dose or progestin-only pills and Depo-Provera have less influence on lactation.
    5. **Nutrition.** Especially if breast feeding.
    6. **Medications.** Vitamins, iron, stool softener, when appropriate. Counsel on medications to avoid during breast feeding.

7. **Discuss need for rest,** possible stresses that can occur with new infant at home, possibility of postpartum depression.

V. **Follow-up Exam.**

A. **Postpartum check** at 4 to 6 weeks.

B. **Newborn checkup** typically at 1 to 2 weeks.

PUERPERAL FEVER

I. **Definition.** Temperature >38.4° C in first 24 hours or >38.0° C for 2 consecutive days in the 9 days following delivery.

II. **Differential Diagnosis.**

A. **Endometritis.**

1. **Etiology.** Polymicrobial with a mixture of aerobic and anaerobic organisms. In particular, high fever within the first 25 hours after delivery may be caused by gram-negative sepsis, group B streptococcal disease, clostridial sepsis, or toxic shock syndrome. Those 2 days to 6 weeks postpartum may be secondary to *Chlamydia*.

2. **Risk factors.** C-section (20 times greater than vaginal delivery), chorioamnionitis, prolonged rupture of membranes or premature labor, multiple vaginal exams, retained products, manual exploration of the uterus, low socioeconomic status.

3. **Treatment.**

a. Cultures of the cervix and blood may help identify the causative organism, but treatment is often started empirically. If *Chlamydia* is isolated or suspected based on late presentation, add doxycycline or azithromycin to the regimen.

b. There is no consensus on the safest and most effective antibiotic regimens, only that it must have a broad spectrum. Antibiotics are usually continued for 4 or 5 days and for 24 to 48 hours after defervescence.

c. "Gold standard" = Gentamicin (2 mg/kg IV loading dose, followed by 1.5 mg/kg IV Q8h) + Clindamycin (900 mg IV Q8h).

d. Newer regimens (second- or third-generation cephalosporins, semisynthetic penicillins).

(1) Cefoxitin 1 to 2 g IV Q6-8h.

(2) Ampicillin/sulbactam 1.5-3 g IV Q6h.

e. If no response (maximum temperature not dropping within 48 hours of initiation of therapy), start triple-agent therapy: ampicillin and gentamicin and clindamycin, or ampicillin/sulbactam or cefotoxin + ampicillin.

B. **Pelvic abscess.** Suspect if patient develops a pelvic mass or has persistent fever and pain despite therapy for aerobic bacteria. Frequently develops 5 or more days after delivery. Must add therapy for anaerobic bacteria and consider surgical or percutaneous drainage.

C. **Septic pelvic thrombophlebitis.** Symptoms include spiking fevers with or without pain despite antibiotic therapy. The patient may have a tender

14

OBSTETRICS

palpable mass. May have a diagnostic response with improvement of symptoms after beginning intravenous heparin and antibiotics. CT and MRI have been used to diagnose this illness.

D. **Wound infection.** Presentation includes fever, a tender, erythematous, or fluctuant incision, drainage of pus or blood. Usually occurs after the fifth postoperative day. Risk factors include having an intrapartum cesarean section; emergent abdominal delivery, use of electrocautery, placement of open drains, obesity, and diabetes.

E. **Pulmonary atelectasis.** See Chapter 15 for a discussion of pulmonary atelectasis and fever.

F. **Deep vein thrombosis.** Symptoms include fever and lower extremity pain, swelling, and pallor. Traumatic delivery, cesarean section, delay in the resumption of ambulation, and varicose veins all increase likelihood for DVT formation. See Chapter 4.

G. **Pyelonephritis.** Often accompanied by fever, malaise, flank pain, costovertebral angle tenderness, and pyuria. Risk factors include occult bacteriuria, bladder trauma, and Foley catheterization.

H. **Mastitis.** Suggested by fever and swollen, tender breast. Typically occurs 3 to 4 weeks after delivery. Breast feeding and contact with a carrier of *Staphylococcus aureus* are the two prime risk factors.

BIBLIOGRAPHY

ALSO course syllabus, ed 3, American Academy of Family Practice.

Antepartum fetal surveillance: ACOG Technical Bulletin 107, Washington, 1987, American College of Obstetricians and Gynecologists.

Centers for Disease Control and Prevention: Prevention of perinatal group B streptococcal disease: a public health perspective, *MMWR* 45(RR-7):16, 1996.

Connoly Am et al: Trauma and pregnancy, *Am J Perinatol* 14(6):331-6, 1997.

Darroca RJ et al: Prostaglandin E₂ gel for cervical ripening in patients with an indication for delivery, *Obstet Gynecol* 87:228, 1996.

Harman JH et al: Current trends in cervical ripening and labor induction, *Am Fam Physician* 60(2): 477, 1999

Harris BA Jr: Shoulder dystocia, *Clin Obstet Gynecol* 27(1):106, 1984.

Hauth JC et al: Reduced incidence of preterm delivery with metronidazole and erythromycin in women with bacterial vaginosis, *N Engl J Med* 333:1732, 1995.

Hofmeyr S: Antibiotic prophylaxis for Cesarean section, *Cochrane Review* February 25, 1999.

Induction and augmentation of labor, *ACOG Technical Bulletin* 110, Washington, 1987, American College of Obstetricians and Gynecologists

Marcovici I et al: Postpartum hemorrhage and intrauterine balloon tamponade: a report of three cases, *J Reprod Med* 44(2):122, 1999.

McDonald HM et al: Bacterial vaginosis in pregnancy and efficacy of short-course oral metronidazole treatment: a randomized controlled trial, *Obstet Gynecol* 84:343, 1994.

Mills JL et al: Moderate caffeine use and the risk of spontaneous abortion and intrauterine growth retardation, *JAMA* 269:593, 1993.

Petersen R et al: Violence and adverse pregnancy outcomes: a review of the literature and directions for future research, *Am J Prevent Med* 13(5):366-73, 1997.

Prevention of perinatal group B streptococcal disease: A public health perspective, *MMWR* 45(RR-7): 1-24, 1996.

Ramin SM et al: Randomized trial of epidural versus intravenous analgesia during labor, *Obstet Gynecol* 86(5):783, 1995.

Rouse DJ et al: Screening and treatment of asymptomatic bacteriuria of pregnancy to prevent pyelonephritis: a cost-effectiveness and cost benefit analysis, *Obstet Gynecol* 86:119, 1995.

Scott LL et al: Acyclovir suppression to prevent cesarean delivery after first-episode genital herpes, *Obstet Gynecol* 87:69, 1996.

Usta IM et al: The impact of a policy of amnioinfusion for meconium-stained amniotic fluid, *Obstet Gynecol* 85:237, 1995.

Wenstrom K et al: Amnioinfusion survey: prevalence, protocols, and complications, *Obstet Gynecol* 86:572-576, 1995.

Yancey MK et al: Peripartum infection associated with vaginal group B streptococcal colonization, *Obstet Gynecol* 84:816, 1994.

Yancey MK et al: Risk factors for neonatal sepsis, *Obstet Gynecol* 87:188, 1996.

14

OBSTETRICS

GENERAL SURGERY

Mark A. Graber

15

WOUND MANAGEMENT

I. **General Principles.**
A. The goal of wound management is primarily restoration of function, which requires minimizing risk of infection and repair of injured tissue with a minimum of cosmetic deformity. **Be sure to maintain standard precautions.**

II. **Significant History.**
A. **Mechanism of injury**
   1. **Blunt trauma.** Split or crush type of injuries will swell more and tend to have more devitalized tissue and a higher risk of infection.
   2. **Sharp trauma.** Clean edges, low cellular injury, and risk of infection.
   3. **Bite injury.** See Chapter 2.
B. **Contaminants.** Wound contact with manure, rust, dirt, etc. will increase risk of infection. Wounds sustained in barnyards or stables are considered contaminated. *Clostridium tetani* is indigenous in manure.
C. **Time of injury.** After 3 hours, the bacterial count in a wound increases dramatically. Wounds may be closed primarily up to 18 hours out; clean well and use clinical judgment when choosing which wounds to close. Wounds up to 24 hours old on the face may be closed after good cleaning. The blood supply in this area is much better and the risk of infection therefore much less. The risk of infection may be reduced in wounds by use of tape closures (such as Steri-Strip tape).
D. **Tetanus status** (Table 15-1).
E. **Other medical illnesses.** Diabetes, chemotherapy, steroids, peripheral vascular disease, and malnutrition may delay wound healing and increase the risk of infection.

III. **Physical Exam.**
A. **Vascular injury.** Direct pressure is the first choice for controlling bleeding. If a fracture is involved, immobilization will help control bleeding. Do not clamp vascular structures until it is determined if it is a significant vessel needing repair. If the anatomy is suspicious for injury to major vascular structures, obtain angiogram and consider surgical consult. Capillary refill should be checked distally. Bleeding on the scalp is best controlled by suturing the wound. For extremities, inflating a blood pressure cuff above systolic pressure assists in wound inspection and repair. **However, be careful not to cause ischemic injury to the extremity.**
B. **Neurologic injury.** Check distal muscle strength and sensation. Always check sensation before administering anesthesia. For hand and finger lacerations check 2-point discrimination, which should be less than 5 mm at the fingertips. A crush injury may also decrease 2-point discrimination. This may take several months to recover. A lacerated nerve may be repaired immediately or have repair delayed. Loss of sensation

TABLE 15-1

TETANUS STATUS

Last Tetanus Booster	Clean Wound	Dirty Wound
Unknown or never immunized	0.5 ml of tetanus toxoid. Repeat immunization at 6 weeks and 6 month to 1 year	0.5 ml of tetanus toxoid. Repeat immunization at 6 weeks and 6 month to 1 year 250 U of human tetanus immune globulin
>5 yrs to <10 yrs	None (consider 0.5 ml of tetanus toxoid	0.5 ml of tetanus toxoid
10 yrs	0.5 ml of tetanus toxoid	0.5 ml of tetanus toxoid

may be the first sign of a developing compartment syndrome. See Chapter 2 for a full discussion of compartment syndrome.

C. **Tendons.** Can be evaluated by inspection, but individual muscles must also be tested for full range of motion and full strength. Patients with a lacerated tendon may still have digit motion secondary to intrinsic muscles so always compare strength to the uninvolved side.

D. **Bones.** Check for open fracture or associated fractures. X-ray if any question. An open fracture is an indication for surgical débridement and repair except in the case of a distal phalanx fracture where copious irrigation and oral antibiotics are acceptable treatment if the injury can be watched carefully for infection.

E. **Foreign bodies.** Inspect and x-ray the area. Remember that wood or low-lead glass may not show on radiograph. Wound markers can be used during radiography, and views obtained in two planes can help localize the object for recovery. Glass may penetrate at an angle and be buried deeper than it appears to be. Ultrasonography is very sensitive at picking up foreign bodies if radiograph is questionable or there is strong clinical suspicion.

IV. **Repair**

A. **Wound healing.**

1. **Collagen formation.** Peaks at day 7. The wound has 15% to 20% of full strength at 3 weeks and 60% of full strength at 4 months. Epithelialization occurs in 48 hours under optimal conditions. The wound is then completely sealed.

2. **Scar formation.** Requires 6 to 12 months for a mature scar. The smallest scar will be formed when the wound is not under tension. Scars should not be revised until 12 months have passed. Contractures can develop when a scar intersects perpendicularly to a joint crease.

B. **Anesthesia.**

1. **Topical anesthesia.** LAT and TAC can be used alone or can be used to greatly decrease the pain of infiltration.

   a. **LAT.** 4% lidocaine, 1:2000 epinephrine (also known as adrenaline), and 0.5% tetracaine. 5 ml on cotton ball and placed in wound.

(1) Works as well as TAC and does not need to be locked up as controlled substance, takes 10 to 30 minutes to work, and is cheaper than TAC ($3.00 versus $35.00 per dose).

(2) **Precautions.** Avoid use on face or near mucous membranes (absorption through mucous membranes may cause seizures). Avoid LAT in areas where epinephrine would be contraindicated, as on distal digits, tip of nose, ears, and penis.

b. **TAC.** (0.5% tetracaine, 1:2000 epinephrine (also known as adrenaline), 11.8% cocaine); requires approximately 30 minutes for onset of action. Put 5 ml on a cotton ball and then place in wound. Same precautions as with LAT.

2. **Local.** Use 27- or 30-gauge needle and infiltrate slowly and through the open wound edge avoiding the intact skin. This decreases the pain of infiltration. The addition of bicarbonate to lidocaine before infiltration has been shown to significantly decrease the pain of injection (9 ml of lidocaine and 1 ml of bicarbonate).

a. **Lidocaine** (0.5% to 2%) most frequently used with onset 2 to 5 minutes, duration 60 minutes. Can use 3 to 5 mg/kg with not more than 300 mg total (in adults). Avoid using lidocaine with epinephrine on distal extremities such as the ears, fingers, toes, and penis. **However, if lidocaine with epinephrine is accidentally injected into a finger, don't panic. It is *very* rare to get a complication.**

b. **Bupivacaine** (Marcaine) has onset 2 to 5 minutes, duration of hours, and is the longest lasting of the local anesthetics. Intravenous administration may cause serious arrhythmias.

c. **For "caine" allergies,** use diphenhydramine diluted to 1%. Mix 5% diphenhydramine 1:4 ml with normal saline to make a 1% solution. Onset of anesthesia takes longer and does not last as long as with lidocaine. Stronger solutions may cause tissue necrosis.

3. **Regional anesthesia.** Especially good for fingers, hands, feet, toes, mouth, and face. See Chapter 21 for common blocks.

C. **Wound prep.**

1. **Débridement.** Using aseptic technique, devitalized tissue should be removed; avoid taking healthy tissue. High-pressure irrigation is the most effective means of cleansing a wound. Can use a 35 ml syringe with a 19-gauge needle and normal saline. Scrubbing does not cleanse the wound as well and using any disinfectant in the wound damages healthy cells needed for healing.

2. **Skin disinfection.** Can be performed with povidone-iodine solution or chlorhexidine. Avoid getting these solutions in the wound because they impede wound healing. Shaving the area increases the risk of infection. Hair can be clipped in the area if necessary. Never shave eyebrows because they are needed for alignment of the wound and may not grow back.

D. **Wound closure.**
1. Avoid primary closure of infected and inflamed wounds, dirty wounds, human and animal bites (dog bites without crushed tissue is an exception, see Chapter 2, emergency medicine), neglected and severe crush wounds.
2. **Tape closure (with Steri-Strips or others).** Strips carry a lower risk of infection than suturing does and may be a consideration for higher-risk wounds.
3. **Open wound care.** Saline wet to dry dressings with gauze will keep the tissue moist and help débride, Gentle washing of the wound 2 to 3 times per day will remove bacterially contaminated secretions (showers are appropriate for this). Avoid iodine dressings because they damage healthy tissue and will slow granulation. When clean granulation tissue is apparent, secondary closure may be considered or can change to dry, sterile, packing material.
4. **Suturing.** The two types of sutures are: (1) absorbable and (2) non-absorbable. Precision-point cutting needles and small-sized suture (5-0 or 6-0) should be chosen for skin when a cosmetic closure is important as on the face. Conventional cutting needle is used for routine skin closure. 4-0 or 3-0 nylon may be used on extremities. Noncutting needle should be used for subcutaneous tissue. Extensor tendons are slow healing and should have permanent suture of small size chosen (such as polypropylene). Depending on your practice situation, a surgical consultation should be considered. The majority of subcutaneous or dermal suturing may be performed with an intermediate-duration absorbable suture. However, some wounds require permanent sutures (such as stainless steel wires in sternotomy) (Table 15-2).
5. **Staples.** Can be used on the scalp and abdomen with good result. However, avoid use on face, hand, or other areas where structures such as tendons and nerves may become entrapped by the staples.
6. **Glue** (Octylcyanoacrylate, e.g., Dermabond) can be used to close wounds once bleeding has stopped. Avoid use on palms and soles, which are areas of high moisture. Is less effective in high stress areas such as over knee and elbow joints.
7. **Dressings.** Consider antibiotic ointment on face and torso. Antibiotic ointment should be avoided on distal extremities for more than 24 to 48 hours because it may lead to maceration and delayed wound healing. Immobilize if motion of a joint is going to increase skin tension. Keep the wound dry for 24 hours, after which time most wounds do not require a dressing.
8. **Facial wounds** should have crusts soaked off and bacitracin or other ointment applied QID × 5 days to reduce scar formation.
9. **Antibiotics.** There is no medical indication for using prophylactic antibiotics in routine, non-contaminated, skin wounds.

TABLE 15-2
SUTURE MATERIALS AND CHARACTERISTICS

Suture	Strength	Inflammatory Reaction	Ease of Use	Infection Resistance	Notes
NONABSORBABLE SUTURES					
Nylon monofilament	+++	++	+++	+++	Good for skin closure Use two throws on the first knot
Polypropylene (Prolene) monofilament	++++	+	+	++++	Good for skin More difficult to use than nylon
Silk	+	++++	++++	++	Has fallen out of favor Used mostly intraorally
ABSORBABLE SUTURES					
Gut or chromic gut	++	+++	++	+	Rarely used Can almost always be replaced by Dexon or Vicryl
Dexon (polyglycolic acid braided polymer)	++++	+	++++	++++	A good choice for subcutaneous and intraoral sutures
Vicryl (polyglactin 910 braided polymer)	++++	+	++++	+++	Same as above

Adapted from Barkin R, Rosen P, editors: *Emergency pediatrics*, St. Louis, 1986, Mosby.

15

GENERAL SURGERY

a. Consider antibiotic use for patients prone to endocarditis, patients with hip prostheses, lymphedema, contaminated foot wound in diabetics, or others with peripheral vascular disease.

b. See Chapter 2 for antibiotic choices for bite wounds.

V. **Follow-Up Care.**

A. Risk of infection highest 24 to 48 hours, and so all wounds should be rechecked.

B. **General guidelines for suture removal:**

1. **Face,** 3 to 5 days with tape or glue reinforcement after suture removal.

2. **Scalp,** 7 to 10 days; **trunk,** 7 to 10 days; **arms,** 7 to 10 days; **legs,** 10 to 14 days; **joints, dorsal surface,** 14 days.

3. Increase length for diabetics or steroid-dependent patients who may require several weeks to heal.

PREOPERATIVE CARDIAC RISK ASSESSMENT

I. Approximately 8 million surgeries in the United States are performed on patients with known or suspected cardiac disease. Preoperative evaluation can help stratify risk.

A. **The Goldman index.** Useful in predicting cardiac events in an unselected, random group of patients. However, it does not work well when applied to subgroups, such as all those with known heart disease. The type and extent of surgery anticipated needs to be taken into account when one is interpreting the results of the Goldman index. See Table 15-3 for Goldman index, Table 15-4 for risks, and Table 15-5 for preoperative characteristics and testing required. (This approach is suggested by Mangano and Goldman: *N Engl J Med* 333(26):1750, 1995.)

B. **Functional status.** If patient can walk up stairs while carrying a load (functional status class I and II), has a low Goldman index and no known cardiac disease, there is a very low risk of cardiac complications.

C. **Electrocardiography.** Ischemia on a resting ECG is suggestive of a worse outcome. **However,** exercise tolerance appears to be more important than ECG changes in predicting outcomes. So if functional status is good (class I or II), GXT need not be done. Reserve GXT for recent-onset chest pain and unclear functional status.

D. **Echocardiography.** Should be reserved for those who would need an echocardiogram even if they were not having surgery, such as those with murmurs that have not been previously evaluated and those with CHF of unknown cause (diastolic versus systolic versus valvular, etc.). Stress echocardiography can be used as a replacement for the GXT.

E. **Radionuclide ventriculography determined ejection fraction.** Has not been shown to be useful in determining risk for infarction perioperatively. Note, however, that this type of datum is taken into account with clinical measures in the Goldman index (S3 gallop, JVD) and in functional status (class).

TABLE 15-3

GOLDMAN INDEX

Factor	Definition	Number of Points
Ischemic heart disease	MI within 6 months	10
Congestive heart failure	S3 gallop, JVD	11
Cardiac rhythm	Rhythm other than sinus or premature atrial contractions on first preoperative ECG or >5 premature ventricular contractions per minute at any time before surgery	7
Valvular heart disease	Significant aortic stenosis	3
General medical status	pO_2 <60 mm Hg, pCO_2 >50 mm Hg, K <3.0 mmol/L, bicarbonate <20 mmol/L, BUN >50 mg/dl, creatinine >3.0 mg/dl, abnormal AST, signs of chronic liver disease, patient bedridden from noncardiac causes	3
Age	>70	5
Type of surgery	Intraperitoneal, intrathoracic, aortic or emergency operation	3

Class I, 0-5 points; class II, 6-12 points; class III, 13-25 points; class IV, >25.

Modified from Mangano DT, Goldman L: *N Engl J Med* 333(26):1750, 1995.

15

GENERAL SURGERY

TABLE 15-4

RISK OF MAJOR CARDIAC COMPLICATIONS OF DIFFERENT PATIENT GROUPS USING THE GOLDMAN INDEX

Goldman Index Class	Unselected Patients Over 40 Years of Age (%)	Patients With Known Coronary Disease or Other High-Risk Patients (%)	Unselected Patients Undergoing Minor Surgery (All Patients) (%)
I	1.2	3	0.3
II	3.0	11	1
III	12	30	About 2.8
IV	48	75	About 19

Modified from Mangano DT, Goldman L: *N Engl J Med* 333(26):1750, 1995.

TABLE 15-5

PATIENT CHARACTERISTICS AND PREOPERATIVE TESTING REQUIRED

Characteristics of Patient	Preoperative Diagnostic Testing	Special Perioperative Treatment
No known cardiac disease, good functional status, class I or II on the Goldman index	None except routine ECG and CXR if indicated	None
Known stable coronary artery disease and good functional status (function class I or early class II)	None except routine ECG and CXR if indicated	Conservative treatment*
Known coronary artery disease, functional status unclear	Noninvasive testing†	If test is negative, conservative treatment.* If test is positive, aggressive medical therapy‡ or angiography; then retest. If retest is positive, aggressive medical treatment‡ including medication intensification and addressing risk factors (such as smoking) and repeat test. If retest now negative, use conservative treatment.* If retest still positive, consider more aggressive treatment and repeat noninvasive test. If still positive, consider coronary angiography and revascularization (such as PTCA) if indicated.

	None except routine ECG and CXR if indicated	Aggressive medical treatment‡ or angiography if indicated.
Known coronary artery disease, poor cardiac functional status		
Poor noncardiac functional status, no known coronary artery disease or status unclear (below)	Stratified by risk factors (below)	Stratified by risk factors (below)
1. No or few risk factors§	1. If no or few risk factors, none.	1. If no or few risk factors, none.
2. Multiple risk factors§	2. If multiple risk factors, noninvasive testing.†	2. If multiple risk factors and tests is negative, conservative treatment.* If test is positive, aggressive medical‡ treatment or angiography.
Coronary artery disease and either class III or IV on Goldman cardiac risk index	None	Aggressive medical treatment or angiography.

Modified from Mangano DT, Goldman L: *N Engl J Med* 333(26):1750, 1995.

Conservative treatment: Continue cardiac medications, postoperative ECG day 1, after any suspicious perioperative events, and before discharge.

†*Noninvasive testing:* Exercise stress testing if patient can exercise. If patient cannot exercise, use stress echocardiogram, dipyridamole-thallium scan, or ambulatory monitor for ischemia.

‡*Aggressive medical therapy:* Aggressive medical treatment including medication intensification and addressing risk factors (i.e., smoking) followed by repeat noninvasive testing. Modified from Mangano DT, Goldman L: *N Engl J Med* 333(26):1750, 1995.

§Risk factors include age >70 years, diabetes mellitus, CHF, important arrhythmias, known vascular disease, need for aortic, abdominal, or thoracic surgery.

Functional class I or II: Can walk up steps carrying groceries or similar load.

15

GENERAL SURGERY

F. **Thallium scanning.** Thallium scanning seems to be highly sensitive at selecting those who will have postoperative cardiac problems. Specificity is a problem (53% to 80%) unless restricted to a high-risk group. The use of thallium scanning should be restricted to those individuals who cannot exercise (therefore the functional status of these patients cannot be determined) and those whose risk cannot be determined by clinical criteria.

G. **History of MI.** <3 weeks has 25% mortality; urgent procedure only. At 3 months 10% mortality; semiurgent procedures. At 6 months 5% mortality: elective. At 1 year, same risk as asymptomatic patient with cardiac disease.

II. **Beta-blockers reduce perioperative ischemia** in those undergoing non-cardiac surgery who have known coronary artery disease or a high risk of coronary artery disease (2 or more risk factors). Atenolol started preoperatively and continued until discharge from the hospital may decrease overall mortality at 2 years. Most of the lower mortality is attributable to lower cardiac mortality in the 6 to 8 months after surgery. Others have used bisoprolol with similar results. See *N Engl J Med* 335:1713-1720, 1996; *Anesthesiology* 1:7-17, 1998; and *N Engl J Med* 341:1789-94, 1999.

PREOPERATIVE PULMONARY EVALUATION

I. **Postoperative pulmonary complications** are up to 4.3 times more frequent in smokers.

II. **Patients should stop smoking at least 8 weeks before surgery.** Paradoxically, patients who quit less than 8 weeks prior to surgery may have increased risks. For patients with a symptomatic exacerbation of COPD, surgery should be delayed if possible and aggressive management with usual agents prior to surgery is recommended. Additionally, a two week course of corticosteroids may be helpful.

III. **Preoperative spirometry** has a variable predictive value. Clinical findings seem to be a better predictor of outcome.

IV. **See section on postoperative orders** on p. 603 for pulmonary treatment postoperatively.

PREOPERATIVE LABORATORY EVALUATION

I. **A complete history and physical examination** will uncover most abnormalities and preoperative lab testing can be targeted to those in whom it is indicated. One guideline from Mayo Clinic suggests that the minimal preoperative test requirements are (1) an ECG and determination of creatinine and glucose in apparently healthy patients 40 to 59 years of age; (2) an ECG, chest radiograph, and determination of the CBC, creatinine, and glucose in patients 60 years of age or older; and (3) no testing for apparently healthy patients below 40 years. Other literature would suggest the approach in Table 15-6 in the healthy patient who is having an elective procedure.

TABLE 15-6

PREOPERATIVE TESTING

Test	Routine Use Indicated?	Indications
Coagulation studies (PT/INR, PTT).	No	Stigmata liver disease, hx coagulopathy, possible DIC, anticoagulation, alcohol abuse
Bleeding Time	No	Unreliable test. Very subjective.
CBC	No	Possible hematologic or infectious process, significant blood loss predicted
Electrolytes	No	Diuretic use, hx or renal or cardiac disease, possible dehydration by history or physical
Glucose	No	Diabetics, obese patients, undergoing vascular procedures, other reason for increased glucose (e.g., steroids)
BUN/Creatinine	No	Over 60, history renal, cardiac or vascular disease
Urinalysis	No	Symptomatic patients, diabetics, pregnancy
Pregnancy	No	If indicated by history
Liver Enzymes	No	Historical or physical evidence of liver disease
ECG and CXR	No	As indicated by history and physical

15

GENERAL SURGERY

PREOPERATIVE MANAGEMENT OF ANTICOAGULATION

See Table 6-3 for preoperative management of anticoagulation.

PREOPERATIVE CARE AND EVALUATION

I. Admit Orders Note: Supplemental oxygen during and for 3 hours after surgery (80%) can reduce wound infections.

A. Admit to ward or primary physician.

B. Diagnosis and planned procedure.

C. Condition.

D. **Vital signs.** For elective procedure every shift. For emergency procedure as dictated by condition.

E. **Allergies.** Medications (especially antibiotics), foods, dressing materials (such as tape), etc.

F. **Activity.** Bed rest if unstable vital signs or other indication; otherwise encourage activity to avoid DVT, muscle atrophy, pneumonia.

G. **Nursing.** Neurologic checks, monitoring lines (CVP, Swan-Ganz), preoperative teaching, PCA pump, pulmonary toilet, etc.

H. **Diet/NPO.** Determined by rest of medical history and the preparation required for surgery. Period of NPO before surgery dependent on age of patient and anesthesia class. Canadian Anaesthetist Society recommends only 3 hours of NPO in healthy patients (class I and II). Stomach volumes are actually larger in patients who have a prolonged fast. Class III and IV patients should be NPO at least 6 to 8 hours.

I. **Intake and output.** Fluids for rehydration (NS or LR), maintenance and correction of electrolyte imbalance. Blood products if needed. Monitoring of fluids and fluid status (CVP/Swan-Ganz, Foley). Swan-Ganz may increase mortality, however.

J. **Special tests.** As indicated by diagnosis (such as endoscopy before colorectal surgery for cancer).

K. **Special medications.**
1. Patient's routine medications; change medications to IM or IV as needed.
2. Mupirocin to nares preoperatively reduces rate of wound infection.
3. Increased steroids preoperatively if steroid dependent. Stress doses: hydrocortisone succinate-100 mg IV Q6-8 hours
4. Pain medications as needed.
5. Antibiotics as indicated for infection and sepsis or prophylaxis of endocarditis, indwelling hardware or graft placement.
   a. Preoperative antibiotics are most effective when given within 2 hours before surgery. Cefotaxime 1 g IV or cefoxitin 2 g IV have been shown to reduce infection rates for intra-abdominal surgery and should be used.
   b. There is no evidence that continuing "prophylactic" antibiotics postoperatively is helpful. However, antibiotics should be continued if there is active infection or contamination.
   c. For cardiac valvular disease, history of artificial valve, etc, use additional prophylactic antibiotics as recommended by the American Heart Association (see Chapter 3).
6. Prep for surgery. Bowel preps, DVT (see next section for DVT prophylaxis recommendations), and antiseptic shower and hair clipping, if indicated.
7. Premedication by anesthesia to lower anxiety, lower secretions, and interact with narcotics for sedation.

L. Lab tests. See previous section for suggested routine lab tests.

II. **Medical History of Major Importance.**

A. **Neurologic disorders.** Some anticonvulsants are oral only. May need to change medications if patient will be NPO for long period of time.

B. **Hematologic disorders.**
1. **Positive sickle cell screen.** Needs Hb electrophoresis. If majority is Hb S will need partial exchange transfusion before surgical procedure (see Chapter 6).
2. **Clotting disorders.** May need evaluation, treatment (see Chapter 6).
3. **Anemia.** Ideally HCT >30%, with Hb >10 g at surgery. No evidence that anemia contributes to surgical morbidity in the well-hydrated, hemodynamically stable patient with a Hb >7.0 g.

C. **Integument disorders.** If possible, avoid operating when there are active skin infections present. Chronic skin disorders should be optimally controlled for postoperative healing. For those who form keloids, may need to consider different closure techniques.

D. **Nutritional status.**
1. For elective or semielective surgery consider optimizing nutritional status if patient has chronic disease.
2. **Obesity.** Weight loss to improve cardiopulmonary status and decrease problems with healing.
E. **Cardiac.** See preoperative cardiac evaluation above.
F. **Pulmonary.**
1. **COPD.** Optimize pulmonary toilet and use incentive spirometry to encourage lung expansion. See section on pre-operative pulmonary evaluation above.

III. **Operative Note**
A. Preoperative diagnosis.
B. Postoperative diagnosis.
C. Procedure or operation performed.
D. Surgeon, assistants.
E. Anesthesia. General endotracheal, general mask, spinal, epidural, regional block, local, etc., include specific agent used.
F. Findings.
G. Specimen. Frozen section if obtained, pathologic and microscopic characteristics, etc.
H. Estimated blood loss.
I. Intraoperative fluids and blood products administered.
J. Drains and tubes placed.
K. Complications.
L. Patient's condition and disposition.

15

GENERAL SURGERY

POSTOPERATIVE CARE

I. **Orders.**
A. Admit to ward, ICU, or recovery room.
B. **Diagnosis.** Operation.
C. **Vital signs.** Every 30 minutes for first few hours and then reduce as stable.
D. Allergies.
E. **Activity.** Bedrest until fully awake; up walking that night or next morning depending on surgery. Up to chair QID if unable to ambulate.
F. **Diet.** NPO until nausea resolves or resumption of bowel activity as determined by bowel sounds, passing gas, or having bowel movement. Start with clear liquids and advance as tolerated.
G. **Pulmonary.** Deep breathing, and incentive spirometry. Deep breathing has been shown to significantly reduce the rate of respiratory complications such as pneumonia. Intermittent or continuous positive pressure breathing (including nasal bilevel) can also reduce postoperative pulmonary complications but are more expensive and should be used only in those unable or unwilling to take deep breaths or incentive spirometry. **Pain management is critical for good pulmonary function (deep breathing, etc.).**

H. **Intake and output.**
   1. Record intake or output every shift or more frequently if patient's condition is unstable.
   2. **IV fluids.** With surgeries involving third spacing replace with isotonic solutions for first 24 hours. NG losses should be replaced with 0.45 NS, and if in exceptionally large amounts, replace losses milliliter for milliliter. Maintenance fluids should generally be 0.2 NS or D_5 1/2 NS. Potassium is normally included in replacement solutions but is excluded from maintenance solutions until normal renal function is established. Colloids do not provide any survival benefit and are expensive. See below for evaluation of postoperative oliguria.
   3. Instructions for care of all tubes and drains including a Foley catheter and nasogastric tube. NG tube should be connected to low intermittent suction and irrigated frequently to ensure patency. **Remove Foley and other tubes as soon as possible. Prolonged indwelling catheters predispose to infection.**

I. **Nursing.**
   1. Encourage turning, coughing, deep breathing, and incentive spirometry.
   2. Dressing changes.
   3. Parameters to notify doctor such as urine output ($<$0.5 ml/kg/hour), fever, hypertension or hypotension, tachycardia or bradycardia, inability to void within 8 hours of beginning surgery, or unusual drainage on dressings, tachypnea, or bleeding.
   4. Specify neurologic or vascular checks.

J. **Medications.**
   1. **Pain medications.** Oral or IV (by PCA or injection). PCA provides better analgesia, and patients generally require less narcotic than with IM treatment; there is little indication for IM pain medications. Adequate doses of pain medications improve mobility and thus decrease complications such as respiratory and thromboembolic problems. PRN orders provide worse pain management than do standing orders. If cannot use PCA, use scheduled IV doses of morphine (e.g., 2-5 mg IV/hr).
   2. There is no evidence that hydroxyzine or promethazine HCl (Phenergan) have an opiate-sparing effect. In fact, Phenergan may have an antianalgesia effect. They are, however, sedatives.
   3. Tramadol (Ultram) has been shown to be ineffective in postoperative pain.
   4. Propoxyphene-acetaminophen combinations have not been shown to be any better than acetaminophen alone.
   5. Hydrocodone combinations (such as Lortab, Vicodin) are as effective as or more effective than codeine combinations (Tylenol 3 and others) and have fewer GI and CNS side effects. Oxycodone (Percodan and others) are also effective.
   6. **Patient-controlled analgesia. This is the preferred modality but will not work in the patient with dementia.**

a. **Morphine.** Bolus with 2 to 10 mg over 20 to 30 minutes. Use PCA pump that delivers 1.0 mg aliquots with an initial lockout time of about 5 to 15 minutes (therefore 4 to 12 mg/hour). Generally start at 10-minute lockout and adjust from there.

b. **Meperidine.** Bolus 20 to 100 mg over 20 to 30 minutes and then PCA pump that delivers 10 mg aliquots with a lockout time of 5 to 20 minutes. Generally start at 10-minute lockout and adjust from there. Meperidine is metabolized to normeperidine, which can cause agitation and seizures, especially in the elderly.

7. **If using IM.**
   a. **Morphine:** 0.05 to 0.1 mg/kg IM Q3-6h.
   b. **Meperidine:** 0.5 to 1.0 mg/kg IM Q3-6h.

8. **Antiemetics.** First consider if medications may be causing nausea, if NG tube is plugged, or if this is postanesthetic nausea. Some options are:
   a. **Prochlorperazine** (Compazine and others) 5 to 10 mg IV Q6h. May cause hypotension and dystonic reactions.
   b. **Metoclopramide** (Reglan and others) 5 to 10 mg or more (up to 30 mg) IV Q6h. May cause dystonic reactions.
   c. **Droperidol** (Inapsine) 1.25 to 2.5 mg IV. May be sedating.
   d. **Ondansetron** (Zofran) 4 mg IV over 15 minutes (good but expensive). Does not cause dystonia. Alternatives include granisetron, dolasetron.
   e. Watch for dystonic reactions and confusion with a, b and c. Diphenhydramine 25 to 50 mg IV/IM or benztropine 1-4 mg IV/IM can be used to counteract dystonia.

9. Antibiotics. For infection.
10. Routine medications that need to be renewed.
11. PRN medications such as laxatives, sleeping medications, and antacids.

K. **Special tests,** such as follow-up CXRs or serial ECGs. ECG should be performed on postoperative day 1 for high-risk patients.

L. **Laboratory.** Follow-up CBC for possibility of hemorrhage or for large amount of blood loss. If patient continues on IV fluid, check daily electrolytes.

M. See below for postoperative DVT prophylaxis.

II. **Postoperative Fevers by Organ System.**

A. **Respiratory**
   1. Early fever may be secondary to aspiration.
   2. Fever at 24 to 48 hours postoperatively most commonly blamed on atelectasis but recent data has called this association into question. Do not ignore an emerging pneumonia.
   3. After 48 hours most likely is a developing pneumonia.

B. **Wound infections**
   1. Supplemental oxygen (80%) intraoperatively and postoperatively will reduce wound infections.

    2. First 24 hours suggestive of *Clostridium.*

    3. 48 to 72 hours most commonly caused by Streptococci.

    4. 4 days consider enteric aerobes and anaerobes and Staphylococci.

C. **Thrombophlebitis.** Occurs intraoperatively, and fever usually begins after 24 hours.

D. **Urinary tract infections.** Usually related to instrumentation or indwelling Foley catheter and occurs after 24 hours. Remove Foley as soon as possible.

E. **Less common causes of perioperative fever.**

    1. **Transfusion reaction.** Immediate (see Chapter 6).

    2. **Malignant hyperthermia.** Starts intraoperatively and is generally secondary to anesthetic drugs (see Chapter 2, emergency medicine).

    3. Drug reaction.

    4. Endocrine, such as thyroid storm.

    5. Thrombophlebitis from IV site.

    6. Intraabdominal abscess.

III. **Postoperative Oliguria.**

A. **Oliguria** (see also renal failure in Chapter 8) is defined as urine output less than 30 ml/hour or 1ml/kg/hour in children. Postoperative oliguria can be divided into:

    1. **Prerenal azotemia.** Caused by decreased glomerular filtration rate secondary to hypovolemia or hypotension. This can occur with hemorrhage, GI loss, excessive renal loss, and third spacing. BUN/Cr ratio >20.

    2. **Acute tubular necrosis** (renal failure). Often develops postoperatively when there is either preexisting renal disease, long periods of hypotension, use of nephrotoxic agents, septicemia, or hemolysis. (See Chapter 8 for a detailed discussion of diagnosis and management.)

    3. **Other causes.**

        a. Reflex spasm of voluntary sphincter because of pain or anxiety.

        b. Medications such as anticholinergics and narcotics.

        c. Detrusor atony as result of surgery and manipulation (especially after retroperitoneal or pelvic surgery).

        d. Preexisting partial bladder outlet obstruction such as an enlarged prostate.

        e. Mechanical obstruction such as an expanding hematoma or fluid collection, or occluded Foley catheter.

B. **Diagnosis.** Look for signs of hypovolemia such as decreased skin turgor or dry mucous membranes, tachycardia, hypotension. If patient cannot or has no desire to urinate after several hours postoperatively, consider oliguria secondary to hypovolemia. A palpable bladder is a sign of urinary retention.

C. **Treatment.** Relieve pain. If condition permits, perhaps standing or sitting may facilitate voiding.

    1. **Hypovolemia.** Treat hypovolemia if present with a bolus of normal saline (250 ml aliquots) until maintaining urine output at 30 to

60 ml/hour in adults and 0.5 to 1 ml/kg/hour in children. Diuretics will worsen prerenal azotemia.

2. **Mechanical obstruction.** If mechanical obstruction, such as enlarged prostate, consider intermittent catheterization. If the patient already has a Foley catheter, irrigate it to assess for obstruction. There is no need to gradually release urine from the bladder. Drainage of even 1 liter of urine is not associated with hypotension, etc.

IV. **Postoperative Ileus.**

A. Maintain NPO with NG suction; check electrolytes including calcium and potassium. Avoid anticholinergics, narcotics (unless needed for pain) and calcium channel blockers.

B. If prolonged, consider pancreatitis, peritonitis, intra-abdominal abscess, pneumonia, free blood in the peritoneum, etc.

C. For adynamic ileus with colonic distension (cecal diameter 9cm or greater, AKA Ogilvie's syndrome), neostigmine-2mg IV will frequently lead to prompt resolution of the problem. An alternative is colonoscopy with decompression.

POSTOPERATIVE DVT PROPHYLAXIS

I. **General.** 40% to 50% of those with hip surgery will develop a DVT postoperatively; 16% will develop DVT even with the best prophylaxis. If not given prophylaxis, 15% to 30% of those with abdominal surgery will develop a DVT; DVT prophylaxis after surgery is cost effective and reduces the incidence of DVT and PE. Early ambulation is important. Enoxaparin is approved for post-hip surgery prophylaxis; dalteparin is approved for post-abdominal surgery prophylaxis.

II. **Options for DVT Prophylaxis.**

A. **Enoxaparin.** 30 mg SQ BID started within 24 hours following surgery. Alternative is 40mg SQ QD starting 12 hours **before** surgery. Subcutaneous low-molecular-weight heparin is the most effective form of prophylaxis and has fewer complications than unfractionated heparin and may also be cost effective. Continue until patient is ambulatory or up to 14 days. Can also be used for DVT prophylaxis after other surgery, such as abdominal surgery. May have delayed excretion with renal failure.

B. **Dalteparin.** 2500 anti-factor Xa IU SQ QD starting 1 to 2 hours before abdominal surgery and continuing for 5 to 10 days postoperatively. Must be adjusted for renal function. Use with caution in renal and hepatic disease.

C. **Heparin (unfractionated).** 5000 units SQ Q12h.

D. **Graded compression stockings.** Effective and have few side effects.

E. **Warfarin.** Less effective than low-molecular-weight heparin and has greater bleeding complications.

F. **Aspirin.** Not very effective in postsurgical DVT prophylaxis, and other choices, especially enoxaparin, are preferred.

15

GENERAL SURGERY

G. Only low-molecular-weight heparin and graded compression stockings have been shown to reduce the incidence of pulmonary embolism.

ABDOMINAL PAIN

Although classic surgical teaching has been that pain medication may confuse the diagnosis of abdominal pain, this is not supported by the literature. In fact, if anything, the diagnosis may be clarified by judicious pain relief resulting in fewer unnecessary surgeries. Clearly we need to work with our surgical colleagues and should discuss this with them before the need arises.

I. **History.**
A. The area of the pain, including its origin and pattern of radiation, time of onset, nature, and associated symptoms will frequently make the diagnosis (Table 15-7). A menstrual history should be obtained.
B. **Associated symptoms.**
   1. Weight loss, which might indicate malignancy or malabsorption.
   2. Vomiting as with a small bowel obstruction or volvulus (obstruction especially if fecal).
   3. Diarrhea and constipation, which might indicate inflammatory bowel disease, cancer, obstipation, malabsorption.
   4. Melena or blood per rectum: check with Hemoccult. If negative, consider foods (Kool-Aid, beets) or medicines (iron).
C. **Jaundice.** Consider pancreatic cancer (painless), hepatitis, hemolysis (sickle cell, G6PD deficiency, transfusion reaction: see Chapter 6), alcoholic hepatitis, choledocholithiasis, primary biliary cirrhosis, etc.
D. **Urinary symptoms.** Dysuria, frequency, urgency, hematuria. Renal problems often present as a complaint of abdominal pain. Consider urolithiasis, UTI, testicular torsion, etc.
E. **Sexual activity,** last period, birth control, history of venereal disease, vaginal discharge, spotting or bleeding. Consider ectopic pregnancy, PID, ovarian torsion, ruptured ovarian cyst, etc.
F. **Past medical history: Medical problems that can present as abdominal pain include** DKA, hypercalcemia, Addison's disease, pneumonia, cardiac disease and acute angle glaucoma. History should include other major illnesses, prior surgeries, prior studies performed for evaluation of abdominal problems, family history of any similar complaints.
G. **Medications.** Especially digoxin, theophylline, steroids, tetracycline/alendronate (esophageal ulcers), analgesics, antipyretics, antiemetics, barbiturates, and diuretics.
II. **Physical Examination**
A. **Vital signs.** Observe for signs of shock, elevated temperature.
B. **Abdominal exam.**
   1. **Inspection.** Scaphoid appearance or distension, point of most severe pain, hernia, scars.
   2. **Auscultation.** High-pitched bowel sounds are suggestive of an obstructive process. Absent bowel sounds are suggestive of an ileus.

Text continued on p. 613

TABLE 15-7

ABDOMINAL PAIN BY MAIN LOCATION

Diagnosis	Usual Pain Location	Diagnostic Studies	Pain Radiates to and Comments
UPPER QUADRANTS/MIDEPIGASTRIC			
Hepatitis (see Chapter 5), subphrenic abscess, hepatic abscess	RUQ	U/S, CT	Right shoulder; elevated liver enzymes, jaundice
Cholecystitis, cholelithiasis, choledocholithiasis, and cholangitis	RUQ	U/S	Back, right scapula, midepigastric; sudden onset with associated nausea. May be related to food.
Fitz-Hugh-Curtis syndrome	RUQ and signs of PID	Perihepatitis: elevated liver enzymes, associated with Gonorrhea	Right shoulder and back
Pancreatitis (see Chapter 5)	Midepigastric region	Elevated amylase, lipase, WBC. May have normal amylase and lipase if chronic pancreatitis. CT scan or U/S will show edema	Radiates to back; may have peritonitis
Cardiac disease (see Chapters 2 and 3)	May present as epigastric pain	ECG and enzymes to rule out cardiac disease	May be confused with esophageal reflux
Duodenal ulcer or gastric ulcer (see Chapter 5)	Midepigastric/LUQ pain	UGI or endoscopy	Radiation to back if posterior ulcer
		Usually historical (see Chapter 5)	Peritonitis/sudden onset of severe abdominal pain with perforation
Superior mesenteric artery syndrome	Midepigastric pain, especially after eating	Upper GI may show duodenal outlet obstruction	Usually thin individuals with a midepigastric bruit

Continued

15

GENERAL SURGERY

TABLE 15-7

ABDOMINAL PAIN BY MAIN LOCATION—cont'd

Diagnosis	Usual Pain Location	Diagnostic Studies	Pain Radiates to and Comments
UPPER QUADRANTS/MIDEPIGASTRIC—cont'd			
Splenic hematoma or enlargement	LUQ pain	U/S or CT	Hypotension; peritonitis if ruptured
LOWER QUADRANTS			
Aortic aneurysm (see Chapter 2)	Periumbilical especially into back flanks May be colicky	U/S or CT	May present as epigastric or back pain, flank, hip pain Rule out in proper age group if history suggestive of renal stones Hypotension if ruptured
Appendicitis	Early periumbilical Late RLQ	CT or U/S may show abscess, enlarged appendix	May present with peritoneal signs
Cecal volvulus	RLQ pain with sudden onset	Seen on flat plate radiograph as RUQ distended bowel	May be generalized with persistent obstruction Generally elderly patients.
Crohn's disease or ulcerative colitis	RLQ but may be LLQ	Sedimentation rate, ANCA, endoscopy (see Chapter 5)	Diarrhea (bloody in ulcerative colitis), cramps, elevated sedimentation rate
Mesenteric adenitis	RLQ	Diagnosis of exclusion	Pain secondary to enlarged mesenteric nodes from streptococcal pharyngitis
Pneumonia (see Chapter 4)	May mimic appendicitis	CXR	Cough, etc.
Diverticulitis	Generally LLQ, very rarely RLQ	Clinical diagnosis (LLQ pain, diarrhea, vomiting, fever), CT scan most sensitive test	May be generalized

Condition	Clinical features	Diagnosis	Notes
Gynecologic disease (see Chapter 13)	Pain in pelvis, either adnexal area	Pregnancy test, cervical cultures, US	Radiation to groin, may radiate to right shoulder if free of intraperitoneal bleeding
Ovarian torsion, *Mittelschmerz*, ruptured ovarian cyst	Sudden onset colicky lower abdominal pain	Pregnancy test, cervical cultures, US	May have marked cervical motion tenderness
PID (see Chapter 13)	Gradual onset, fever, constant aching pain, vaginal discharge	Pregnancy test, cervical cultures, US	Marked cervical motion tenderness
Urolithiasis or nephrolithiasis (see Chapter 8)	Either flank	Noncontrast CT most sensitive modality.	May radiate to labia or testicles. May mimic AAA
Cystitis (see Chapter 8)	Suprapubic pain	UA	
GENERALIZED (SEE NOTES, SOME MAY LOCALIZE)			
Spontaneous bacterial peritonitis	Generalized with peritoneal signs	Paracentesis	Usually in alcoholics or those with indwelling dialysis catheters
Large bowel ischemia	Acute onset lower abdominal pain followed within 24 hours by bloody diarrhea or blood per rectum	Clinical diagnosis, colonoscopy	Patients generally >60 yrs
Mesenteric thrombosis	Sudden onset of severe generalized abdominal pain without peritoneal signs and out of proportion to physical findings. May have antecedent history of bowel angina (postprandial abdominal pain).	May have elevated serum phosphate, serum lactate, amylase, acidosis. CT scan may show bowel edema. Angiography diagnostic	Patients generally >50 yrs with a history of other vascular disease, low flow states (e.g., CHF, hypovolemia). Must rule out urolithiasis, AAA, perforated ulcer, etc.

Continued

15

GENERAL SURGERY

TABLE 15-7

ABDOMINAL PAIN BY MAIN LOCATION—cont'd

Diagnosis	Usual Pain Location	Diagnostic Studies	Pain Radiates to and Comments
GENERALIZED (SEE NOTES, SOME MAY LOCALIZE)—cont'd			
Intussusception	Cramping abdominal pain with asymptomatic periods Mental status changes common with periods of lethargy Bloody "currant jelly" stools are a late sign Few have palpable sausage-shaped mass in RLQ	Air enema (has replaced barium for this indication) is often curative (see text)	Generally 2 weeks to 2 yrs old
Metabolic disease: DKA, Addison's disease	Diffuse pain, associated nausea, vomiting, may have guarding		
Acute intermittent porphyria	Diffuse and especially into back	24-hour urine for ALA, PGB (porphobilinogen), porphyrins Screening urine for PGB is also available	Colicky abdominal pain that is intermittent may be associated with dark urine Associated psychiatric/neurologic symptoms: sensory changes, paresthesias, psychosis Exacerbated by medications (estrogens, alcohol, sulfonamides), menstruation, weight loss May have photosensitivity
Hemolysis (see Chapter 6)	Back and CVA pain	Reticulocyte count, serum free hemoglobin, LDH	G6PD deficiency; transfusion reactions, paroxysmal nocturnal hemoglobinuria
Meckel's diverticulum	Below or left of umbilicus		May be recurrent with rectal bleeding or intestinal obstruction

3. **Palpation and percussion.** Muscle rigidity (voluntary/involuntary), localized tenderness, masses, pulsation, hernias, peritoneal irritation (rebound: cough or jumping also may elicit "rebound"), involuntary guarding, obturator sign (pain on internal and external rotation of hip), psoas sign (pain on straight leg raising by using obturator muscle, may indicate abscess, etc.), Murphy's sign (RUQ pain when breathing in and pressing over the liver), liver dimension and spleen dimension.
4. **CVA tenderness.**
5. **Pelvic exam in women.**
6. **Rectal exam.** To rule out GI bleeding, prostatitis, etc. The absence of rectal tenderness does not preclude the diagnosis of appendicitis nor does it make the diagnosis of appendicitis. The rectal examination should be used to add to your entire clinical picture.

15

II. **Laboratory**
A. CBC with differential and urinalysis is routinely done on most cases of abdominal pain.
B. Electrolytes, BUN, creatinine with vomiting or diarrhea.
C. Glucose and calcium to rule out DKA and hypercalcemia respectively.
D. Liver function tests and liver enzymes; amylase and lipase for upper abdominal pain.
E. **Other studies as indicated: chest radiograph (upright) for pneumonia or free air (best radiograph for free air).** Abdominal flat plate and upright for bowel obstruction, ileus, free air, abnormal calcification. Ultrasonography or CT to look for peritoneal fluid. ECG for acute MI, ischemia, or arrhythmias. Paracentesis may be important with fluid in the abdomen or in evaluation of abdominal trauma. Culdocentesis has largely been replaced by ultrasonography but can be used to check for intraperitoneal blood (e.g., as in a ruptured ectopic pregnancy).
F. **Pelvic ultrasound or CT.** Useful to distinguish intrauterine from extrauterine pregnancy, also helpful in diagnosing appendicitis, luteal cysts, tubal abscesses, spontaneous abortion. Be sure to check blood flow to both ovaries to rule out ovarian torsion. **Transvaginal ultrasound** can be more helpful as an initial test in the reproductive age female since it is better at detecting GYN disease (e.g., ectopic pregnancy, ovarian torsion). **CT** can be used as a follow-up test in the female patient if the ultrasound (transvaginal) is negative.
G. **Pregnancy test on all reproductive-age females** unless status-post hysterectomy. Sexual history is often unreliable in the emergency setting and **up to 3% of tubal ligations fail!!** Urine pregnancy test may miss very early ectopics. Serum RIA is very sensitive and picks up virtually all pregnancies.
H. **Look for signs of pregnancy** (nausea, breast tenderness, and urinary frequency).
IV. **Special Considerations in the Reproductive-Age Female.**

A. **Pelvic exam.** Complete vulvar and vaginal exam, cervix (dilatation, tissue at os, lesions, motion tenderness), uterine size and tenderness, and adnexa (masses, tenderness, unilateral or bilateral). Obtain cultures for GC and Chlamydia, wet mount.

B. **Culdocentesis.** Less useful with the advent of accurate ultrasound and CT. Culdocentesis will be positive with any intraperitoneal bleeding (such as ectopic pregnancy, bleeding corpus luteum cyst, ruptured liver adenoma, ruptured spleen, peptic ulcer). The absence of fluid is non-diagnostic and does not help in differentiating the cause of pain.

C. **Partial differential diagnosis of pelvic pain.**
   1. Ectopic pregnancy (see Chapter 13), appendicitis, pyelonephritis, ovarian cysts, spontaneous abortion (see Chapter 14), pelvic inflammatory disease (see Chapter 13), ovarian torsion, Mittelschmerz, dysmenorrhea, endometriosis, uterine fibroids, ureteral stone, cystitis, diverticulitis, inflammatory bowel disease, irritable bowel syndrome, bowel obstruction, inguinal hernia, among other causes.
   2. **Sudden onset** is suggestive of ovarian torsion, Mittelschmerz, urolithiasis, ruptured corpus luteum cyst, ruptured ectopic pregnancy. **More gradual onset** is suggestive of appendicitis, PID, abscess, etc.

V. **Initial Treatment**

A. Decide whether to admit and observe, discharge, operate. Serial exams may clarify the diagnosis.

B. Keep NPO until diagnosis is clear.

C. IV fluids: Decide on expected fluid losses and current level of hydration.

D. NG tube for vomiting, bleeding or obstruction.

E. Foley catheter to monitor fluids.

F. The judicious use of pain medications (e.g., morphine 2mg IV) will often help clarify the diagnosis.

G. Serial labs may be helpful, especially CBC, cardiac enzymes.

APPENDICITIS

I. **Overview.** Appendicitis is a common cause of abdominal pain. However, the presentation is not always classic and a high index of suspicion is necessary. Affects any age group but is rare in infants, most common in adolescence and young adult years. Generally occurs from obstruction of the appendiceal lumen by lymphoid hyperplasia or a fecalith.

II. **Clinical Presentation.**

A. **History.** Classic history is that of periumbilical or epigastric pain that migrates to right lower quadrant. **Pain may be felt in flank (retrocecal appendix, pregnancy), testicle (retroileal appendix), or bladder.** Anorexia, nausea, and vomiting may occur after the onset of pain. Anorexia is less likely to be present in children. Presentation is more likely to be atypical in very young, very old, and pregnant patients. Maintain a high index of suspicion in any patient with abdominal pain.

B. **Physical exam. Fever is only found in 15%.** High temperature is not common unless perforation has occurred. Abdominal exam reveals right lower quadrant pain, possibly with rebound or guarding. Psoas sign (pain on active elevation of the legs) may be present, as may be the obturator sign (pain on internal and external rotation of the hip). Rectal exam may reveal localized tenderness but cannot be used to differentiate between those with and those without appendicitis. Pelvic exam should be performed to rule out other illness (such as PID).

C. **Lab tests.** CBC with differential, UA, and pregnancy test (women only) should be obtained on all patients with lower abdominal pain. Obtain cervical or urethral culture if indicated. Mild to moderately elevated WBC with left shift is typical but **WBC is normal in 10%.** UA may show ketonuria or a few RBCs or WBCs, but the presence of significant hematuria or pyuria is suggestive of urinary tract as source of pain.

III. **Management.**

A. **Classical presentation.** Consultation with surgeon for appendectomy. Pain relief may help clarify the situation (small doses of IV morphine). Patient should be kept NPO after arrival at emergency department or clinic and hydrated IV.

B. **If going to the operating room,** the patient should receive IV antibiotics within 2 hours of procedure (such as cefoxitin).

C. **Unclear presentation.** In general, the history and physical exam are more reliable indicators of appendicitis than is the WBC count. Surgeon should be consulted for suspected appendicitis if history and exam suggest the diagnosis. If minimal findings are present on exam, consider observation for several hours with repeated exams (including vital signs and temperature) and CBC Q4h during observation period. CT has largely replaced ultrasonography in questionable cases of appendicitis. CT can reduce unnecessary surgery but need not be done on those with obvious appendicitis.

15

GENERAL SURGERY

GALLBLADDER DISEASE

I. **Overview.** Asymptomatic cholelithiasis, choledocholithiasis, biliary colic, and acute cholecystitis are very common with cholelithiasis being found in 10% of the population. The incidence of cholelithiasis increases with age and is more common in women. Other predisposing factors include obesity, pregnancy, diabetes, and chronic hemolytic states.

II. **Asymptomatic Cholelithiasis.**

A. **Course.** 80% of gallstones are asymptomatic, with a small percentage becoming symptomatic each year (10% at 5 years, 15% at 10 years, 18% at 15 years). Stones are composed of bile salts, cholesterol (80% in the United States are cholesterol stones), phospholipids, or unconjugated bilirubin. Calcification may occur and results in about 15% of the stones becoming radiopaque.

B. **Management.** Asymptomatic patients do not require surgery. Previously, diabetes was considered an indication for cholecystectomy in the asymptomatic patient, but this recommendation has been changed. Consider surgery for those asymptomatic individuals with calcified gallbladder, those with particularly large stones (>3 cm), and those who are at a high risk for gallbladder cancer (Pima Indians and others). See below for medical management.

C. **Percutaneous, ultrasound guided cholecystostomy.** For critically ill patients who are not currently good surgical candidates, this is a less invasive procedure to temporize until the patient has recovered from the acute illness.

III. **Evaluation of the Gallbladder.**

A. **Laboratory tests** including liver function tests, amylase/lipase for evidence of pancreatic involvement. WBC if symptoms acutely present. An elevated alkaline phosphatase is possibly the most sensitive and specific indicator of biliary disease. However, the ALT and AST may become elevated before the alkaline phosphatase.

B. **Plain radiographs** may help, since about 15% of stones are radiopaque, but need not be done if other modalities available.

C. **Ultrasonography** should be the initial exam used to evaluate for cholelithiasis. Can visualize stones, and evaluate biliary ducts and pancreas. Obesity and overlying abdominal gas decrease the quality of the exam. Overall sensitivity is 90%, specificity 85%. CT has a lower sensitivity.

D. **Oral cholecystogram** is performed by having patient ingest 3 g of iopanoic acid about 12 hours before study. Failure of the gallbladder to opacify indicates gallbladder disease. Is not reliable in setting of significant hyperbilirubinemia or acute cholecystitis and has largely been replaced by ultrasonography.

E. **Radionuclide hepatobiliary scan** (e.g., HIDA scan) can be used when there is a consideration of acute cholecystitis or biliary outlet obstruction. Failure of gallbladder to visualize when there is the presence of radioisotope in common bile duct 4 hours after injection indicates dysfunction of the gallbladder such as cholecystitis or outlet obstruction (e.g., tumor, choledocholithiasis).

F. **Endoscopic retrograde cholangiopancreatography (ERCP)** may also be used to define the anatomy of the biliary tree and may be a better choice than radionuclide scanning in many situations. This is especially true if consideration is being given to laparoscopic surgery and a common duct stone needs to be ruled out.

G. **Endoscope-guided ultrasonography.** Not commonly available but sensitive at picking up common duct stones.

III. **Biliary Colic.**

A. **Caused by** intermittent obstruction of the cystic duct by gallstones. History will generally include episodes of epigastric and RUQ pain, which may radiate to back. Pain is usually constant, is abrupt in onset, and subsides slowly. Nausea is commonly associated. Attacks may be precipitated by ingestion of fatty foods. Consider also choledocholithiasis (stone in common duct).

1. **Spasm of the sphincter of Oddi** can cause similar symptoms and is more common after cholecystectomy. This will respond to SL NTG or oral nifedipine.

B. **Physical exam** will reveal absence of fever, possible RUQ or midepigastric tenderness without rebound. Gallbladder may be palpable and the patient may have a positive Murphy's sign (sudden increase in pain with palpation of RUQ during deep inspiration).

C. **Laboratory evaluation.** CBC with differential should be obtained and consider amylase and lipase. WBC should not be significantly elevated. LFTs may be normal or slightly elevated.

D. **Treatment.** Analgesics and antiemetics (prochlorperazine, metoclopramide) should be provided acutely. Morphine may increase biliary pressure and is contraindicated. Ketorolac 30 to 60 mg IM or 15 to 30 mg IV is especially useful in this condition. Meperidine IV in 25 mg aliquots may be used to supplement the ketorolac. If pain resolves, further evaluation may be obtained as convenient in the next few days with the patient instructed to avoid fatty foods. Cholecystectomy should be performed electively.

IV. **Acute Cholecystitis.**

A. 95% of those with cholecystitis will have cholelithiasis.

B. **Presentation** is similar to biliary colic (nausea, vomiting, abdominal pain, RUQ tenderness) with the additional features of fever, leukocytosis, mild elevation of bilirubin, elevated alkaline phosphatase. Murphy's sign may be present.

C. **Ultrasound** only 50% sensitive for cholecystitis. U/S may miss pericholic fluid collections, etc. HIDA scan is diagnostic modality of choice.

D. **Treatment.** Consultation with surgeon is required. Antibiotics are indicated for acute cholecystitis. A third-generation cephalosporin and metronidazole or ampicillin-sulbactam (Unasyn) will cover the most common organisms. There are advantages and disadvantages to early or delayed surgery, though early surgery generally results in lower morbidity and shorter hospitalizations. Surgeon will ultimately need to decide based upon the particular features of the case.

V. **Biliary Sludge**

A. **General.** May be a cause of right upper quadrant pain. Also implicated in 31% of non-alcoholic pancreatitis and 74% of "idiopathic" pancreatitis (e.g., alcohol, gallstones, metabolic problems, drugs have been excluded). Predisposing factors include prolonged CVN, fasting, pregnancy, rapid weight loss, transplant patients and ceftriaxone use.

B. **Diagnosed on ultrasound** but the sensitivity is only about 55% while endoscopic ultrasound has a sensitivity of 98%.

C. **Course is variable.** The majority remain asymptomatic. Of those with symptoms at time 0, 50% become asymptomatic and 20% remain symptomatic over 3 years. Of those asymptomatic at time 0, 10%-15% become symptomatic over 3 years and another 5%-15% develop stones.

15

GENERAL SURGERY

VI. **Medical Management of Cholelithiasis.**

A. **Surgical therapy** is considered the treatment of choice for cholelithiasis. However, in patients in whom this is not practical, other modalities may be used.

B. **Cholesterol stones** may be dissolved using ursodeoxycholic acid. About 70% of cholesterol stones will respond. However, stones tend to recur when ursodeoxycholic acid is discontinued.

C. **Lithotripsy** can be used to fragment stones, which are then passed spontaneously. ERCP may help with stone removal, and use of ursodeoxycholic acid may prevent recurrence.

D. **ERCP** with sphincterotomy may assist in passing stones.

INTESTINAL OBSTRUCTION

I. **Classification.**

A. **Mechanical obstruction.** Complete or partial physical blockage of intestinal lumen (Table 15-8).

B. **Simple obstruction.** Implies one obstruction point.

C. **Closed-loop obstruction.** Blockage at two or more points.

D. **Paralytic (adynamic) ileus.** Impairment of muscle function (such as after abdominal surgery, trauma, peritonitis, spinal injury, pneumonia, hypokalemia, uremia, pancreatitis, etc.), intestinal paracytic infection.

E. **Strangulating obstruction.** When obstructing mechanism occludes mesenteric blood supply on wall of lumen. Necrosis occurs in 3 to 4 hours. Difficult to diagnose preoperatively.

F. Think of GI neoplasm, hypokalemia, intra-abdominal process such as irritation from free blood (as from an ovarian cyst rupture), localized inflammatory process (pancreatitis, pneumonia, PID), toxic megacolon, adhesions, intussusception (see below), peritonitis, etc.

II. **Small Bowel Obstruction.**

TABLE 15-8

CAUSES OF MECHANICAL INTESTINAL OBSTRUCTION IN ADULTS

Site of Obstruction	Cause	Relative Incidence (%)
SMALL INTESTINE (85%)		
	Adhesions	60
	External hernia	15
	Neoplasm	15
	Miscellaneous	10
LARGE INTESTINE (15%)		
	Carcinoma of colon	65
	Diverticulitis	20
	Volvulus	5
	Miscellaneous	10

A. Clinical manifestations.
  1. **Cramping abdominal pain.** Crescendo-decrescendo pattern. Continuous pain is suggestive of strangulation.
  2. **Vomiting.** Earlier in high obstruction. Feculent vomiting, caused by bacterial overgrowth, may be seen especially with distal obstruction.
  3. **Distension.** More in lower obstruction.
  4. **Obstipation.**
  5. **High-pitched bowel sounds.**
  6. **Secondary electrolyte abnormalities.**
B. Work-up.
  1. CBC with differential, electrolytes.
  2. Supine and upright abdominal radiographs with stepladder pattern of air-fluid levels and no colonic gas are suggestive of obstruction.
  3. History and physical examination may point to a particular cause such as adhesions or obstipation.
C. Treatment.
  1. Fluid and electrolyte resuscitation and supportive care.
  2. If partial obstruction with patient passing gas may treat with NG tube. This may relieve vomiting and decompress distension.
  3. Surgical intervention is indicated if obstruction does not resolve with conservative treatment.

III. **Large Bowel Obstruction.**
A. Clinical manifestations.
  1. Cramping pain, little vomiting (less with competent ileocecal valve, vomitus rarely feculent), constipation and obstipation, distension (severe), loud borborygmi and little loss of electrolytes.
B. Work-up.
  1. Electrolytes, glucose, BUN/creatinine, UA and CBC, other labs as indicated.
  2. Colonoscopy or flexible sigmoidoscopy may reveal obstructive lesion.
  3. Radiograph will reveal gas-filled colon with absence of gas beyond obstruction.
C. Treatment.
  1. Nasogastric tube.
  2. IV fluids and appropriate monitoring. Antibiotics only if suspect perforation or abscess formation.
  3. Sigmoidoscopy may reduce a sigmoid volvulus.
  4. Surgical intervention if above measures not successful in relieving obstruction.

IV. **Intussusception.**
A. General.
  1. Intussusception is the most common cause of bowel obstruction in those 3 months to 6 years of age. Rare under 3 months and most commonly occurs between 4 and 12 months.
  2. Less than 10% have a "lead point" but may be secondary to polyp, sarcoma, Henoch-Schönlein purpura, etc.

15

GENERAL SURGERY

3. Ileocecal valve area is the most commonly involved.
4. Male to female ratio is 4:1.

B. **Clinically.**
  1. Main presenting symptom is intermittent, inconsolable crying with asymptomatic periods. **Frequently have mental status changes with lethargy between episodes of abdominal colic.**
  2. Vomiting will develop 6 to 12 hours after onset of colicky pain. Eventually will vomit bilious material.
  3. "Currant jelly" stools are late finding after venous stasis and bowel wall necrosis. Generally pale and shocky by this point.
  4. Abdominal exam may be negative. "Sausage-shaped mass" in only two thirds.
  5. Rule out other causes of pain such as bone injury, hairs around fingers, toes, penis, otitis media.

C. **Diagnosis.**
  1. Ultrasonography has been used successfully.
  2. Plain film may be negative.
  3. Early lab test data are not helpful. Fever and elevated white blood cell count are late findings.
  4. Only about 70% have guaiac-positive stool.
  5. Barium or air enema diagnostic and therapeutic.

D. **Treatment.**
  1. Barium or air enema successful in 75% if caught early but only 25% successful if it has been over 1 or 2 days. Air enema preferred because of risk of barium peritonitis if perforation.
  2. Surgical intervention if this doesn't work
  3. Admit for 24 hours if reduced with enema. About 25% will recur.

BIBLIOGRAPHY

Attard AR et al: Safety of early pain relief for acute abdominal pain, *Br Med J* 305:554, 1992.

Brogan GX et al: Comparison of plain, warmed, and buffered lidocaine for anesthesia of traumatic wounds, *Ann Emerg Med* 26(2):121, 1995.

Classen DC et al: The timing of prophylactic administration of antibiotics and the risk of surgical wound infections, *N Engl J Med* 326(5):281, 1992.

Cummings P et al: Antibiotics to prevent infection of simple wounds: a meta-analysis of randomized studies, *Am J Emerg Med* 13(4):396, 1995.

Daneman A et al: Perforation during attempted intussusception reduction in children—a comparison of perforation with barium and air, *Pediatr Radiol* 25(2):81-88, 1995.

Dixon JM et al: Rectal examination in patients with pain in the right lower quadrant of the abdomen, *Br Med J* 302(6773):386, 1991.

Engoren M: Lack of association between atelectasis and fever, *Chest* 107(1):81, 1995.

Ernst AA et al: LAT (lidocaine-adrenaline-tetracycline) versus TAC (tetracaine-adrenaline-cocaine) for topical anesthesia in face and scalp lacerations, *Am J Emerg Med* 13(2):151, 1995.

Forbes JA et al: Evaluation of two opioid-acetaminophen combinations and placebo in postoperative oral surgery pain, *Pharmacotherapy* 14(2):139-146, 1994.

Glazier HS: Potentiation of pain relief with hydroxyzine: a therapeutic myth? *Ann Pharmacother* 24:484, 1990.

Goswick CB: Ibuprofen versus propoxyphene hydrochloride and placebo in acute musculoskeletal trauma, *Curr Ther Res* 34(4):685, 1983.

Greenfield SM et al: Drinking before sedation: preoperative fasting should be the exception rather than the rule *Br Med J* 314(7075):162, January 18, 1997

Hale DA et al: Appendectomy: a contemporary appraisal, *Ann Surg* 225:252-261, 1997.

Hall JC et al: Prevention of respiratory complications after abdominal surgery: a randomised clinical trial, *Br Med J* 312(7024):148-152, 1996.

Houry S et al: A prospective multicenter evaluation of preoperative hemostatic screening tests, *Am J Surg* 170(1):19, 1995.

Kirks DR: Air intussusception reduction: "the winds of change" [review], *Pediatr Radiol* 25(2):89-91, 1995.

Lovecchio F et al: The use of analgesics in patients with acute abdominal pain, *J Emerg Med* 15(6):775, 1997.

Mangano DT et al: Effect of atenolol on mortality and cardiovascular morbidity after noncardiac surgery, *N Engl J Med* 335:1713-1720, 1996.

Mangano DT, Goldman L: Preoperative assessment of patients with known or suspected coronary disease, *N Engl J Med* 333(26):1750, 1995.

Narr BJ et al: Preoperative laboratory screening in healthy Mayo patients: cost effective elimination of tests and unchanged outcomes, *Mayo Clin Proc* 66(2):155, 1991.

Nyman MA et al: Management of urinary retention: rapid versus gradual decompression and risk of complications, *Mayo Clin Proc* 72:951, October 1997

Pace S, Burke TF: Intravenous morphine for early pain relief in patients with acute abdominal pain, *Acad Emer Med* 3:1086-92, 1996.

Ransohoff DF, Gracie WA: Treatment of gallstones, *Ann Intern Med* 119(Pt 1):606-619, 1993.

Rao PM et al: Introduction of appendiceal count: impact on negative appendectomy and appendiceal perforation rates, *Ann Surg* 229(3):344, 1999

Scholer SJ et al: Use of the rectal examination on children with acute abdominal pain, *Clin Ped* 37:311, May 1998.

Stubhaug A et al: Lack of analgesic effect of 50 and 100 mg oral tramadol after orthopaedic surgery: a randomized, double-blind, placebo and standard active drug comparison, *Pain* 62(1):111, 1995.

Sunshine A et al: Analgesic oral efficacy of tramadol hydrochloride in postoperative pain, *Clin Pharmacol Ther* 51(6):740-746, 1992.

15

GENERAL SURGERY

ORTHOPEDICS

David C. Krupp
Mark A. Graber

LOW BACK PAIN

I. **Overview.** Low back pain is the second most common cause of lost work time. Most cases (90%) resolve within 6 weeks, 40% in 2 weeks; 5% of cases of low back pain become chronic in nature.

II. **Etiology.**

A. **Mechanical causes.** Account for up to 98% of cases of back pain.

1. **Disk injury.** Herniation of the nucleus pulposus usually occurs posteriorly. May impinge on nerve roots, particularly at the L4-L5-S1 levels. Typically pain increases with coughing, sneezing, riding in a car or trunk flexion and includes radicular symptoms and signs. Associated bowel or urinary abnormalities is a surgical emergency (cauda equina syndrome)

2. **Degenerative changes in facet joints.** Result in nerve root impingement at the foramina. Sudden attacks lasting for a few days with symptom-free intervals. Typically pain is worse with trunk extension.

3. **Spondylosis.** Spondylosis is defined as degenerative changes in vertebral bodies and disks. This may cause a nerve root impingement.

4. **Spondylolisthesis.** Slippage of one vertebra anteriorly in relationship to the vertebral body below it. 80% occur at L5-S1.

5. **Spondylolysis.** A defect in the pars interarticularis generally the result of repeated lumbar stress and hyperextension. It generally occurs in the younger patient (18 to mid-twenties) and occurs in 6% of the population. It is much more common in gymnasts. Pain is worse with extension and better with flexion.

6. **Vertebral body fracture.** After trauma or spontaneous "wedge" fractures in elderly with osteoporosis or those using steroids (see Chapter 13 for a discussion of osteoporosis-related fractures).

7. **Spinal canal stenosis.** Irritation during activity results in pain in one or both extremities while walking (similar pain to claudication). Relieved with rest. Exacerbated with back extension, relieved with flexion. Common in the elderly.

8. **Myofascial or soft-tissue injury or disorder.** May have history of trauma, heavy work, or unusual activity.

9. **Arachnoiditis and postoperative scarring.**

10. **Children.** *Under 10 years old:* diskitis (see Chapter 12), tumor, AV malformations, and osteomyelitis. *Over 10 years old:* spondylolisthesis, herniated disks, juvenile kyphosis (Scheuermann's disease—an osteochondritis that leads to wedging of the vertebrae and kyphotic posture), overuse syndrome, tumor, spondylolysis.

11. **Sacroiliitis.** Inflammation of SI joints. Pain exacerbated with pressure on sacroiliac joint (although this is nonspecific for sacroiliitis).

16

B. **Systemic disorders.**
1. **Malignancy**
   a. **Primary tumors.** Multiple myeloma most common.
   b. **Metastatic disease.** 85% are from the breast, prostate, lung, kidney, and thyroid. Most cause lytic lesions with the exception of prostate and thyroid cancer, which cause sclerotic lesions. About 30% bone loss is required before lytic changes will be visible on radiographs.
2. **Miscellaneous.** Osseous, disk, or epidural infection; spondyloarthropathy; metabolic bone disease, including osteoporosis; vascular disorders such as atherosclerosis or vasculitis.

C. **Neurologic causes.**
1. Myelopathy from intrinsic or extrinsic processes
2. Lumbosacral plexopathy, especially in diabetes
3. Neuropathy, including mononeuropathy and inflammatory demyelinating diseases
4. Myopathy, including myositis and metabolic causes

D. **Referred pain,** including GI disorders such as pancreatitis and perforated ulcer; GU disorders, including nephrolithiasis, prostatitis, and pyelonephritis; gynecologic disorders, including ectopic pregnancy and pelvic tumors; abdominal aortic aneurysm; or hip disorder.

III. **Work-up.**

A. **Physical examination.**
1. **Standing.** Examine for obvious defects. Palpate for tenderness or muscle spasm. Test the mobility of the lumbar spine with flexion, extension, and lateral flexion. Observe the patient's gait and have the patient walk on toes (foot plantar flexion test S1) and heels (foot dorsiflexion test L5).
2. **With the patient sitting, do straight-leg raising (SLR) test:** passive extension of the knee. A positive test is radicular pain (e.g., pain, paresthesias down the leg, not back pain or thigh pain from muscle stretching) at less than 60 degrees. However, straight leg raising is neither sensitive nor specific for disk disease. "Crossover" pain with radicular symptoms in the leg **not** lifted is very specific for disk disease.
3. **Reflexes.** Patellar reflex tests the L4 root; Achilles tendon reflex tests the S1 root (L5-S1 disk). **Babinski sign:** if present, indicates disorder above the lumbar region such as cord tumor or CVA.
4. **Sensation.**
   a. **See dermatomal chart (see Figure 23-9)** for a description of radicular sensory findings.
   b. Check hip abduction (L5 motor), perianal sensation (S3-5: also controls anal and urethral sphincter tone), hip extension (L5 motor). Saddle anesthesia and decreased anal sphincter tone indicate a surgical emergency.

B. **Laboratory and imaging studies.**

1. Lumbar spine films are not necessary in most patients. **Plain films should be obtained** if (1) symptoms last more than 6 weeks, (2) there is suspicion or history of malignancy, (3) the patient is using steroids, (4) is over 50 years of age, (5) has a history of trauma, or has neurologic deficits, or (6) is younger than 20 years of age. There is no need to obtain radiographic evaluation for history consistent with muscle strain.

2. Patients suspected of having infectious or neoplastic causes of low back pain should have an imaging study such as a bone scan, CT, or MRI.

3. If severe symptoms persist for several weeks despite conservative therapy and disk herniation or another surgically correctable disorder is suspected, then CT or MRI imaging may be useful. Generally, since surgery is not indicated unless pain is present for at least 6 weeks or there are signs of cauda equina syndrome, there no need for these imaging studies unless there is some indication other than pain. Electromyogram and nerve conduction velocity can be used to evaluate suspected nerve root involvement.

4. **Blood tests.** Differential CBC with ESR, and biochemical screening (calcium, phosphate, alkaline phosphatase) should be performed when a systemic cause for back pain is suspected.

5. **Immunoelectrophoresis of serum and urine samples.** Allows diagnosis of most cases of myeloma (Bence-Jones proteins).

IV. Treatment.

A. **Acute back pain** (no longer than 6 weeks).

1. There is no difference in outcome when patients with acute back pain are treated by a family physician, a chiropractor, or an orthopedic surgeon. Therapy by a family physician is the most cost effective.

2. Regardless of the method of treatment, 40% are better within 1 week, 60% to 85% in 3 weeks, and 90% in 2 months. Negative prognostic factors include more than 3 episodes of back pain, gradual onset of symptoms, and prolonged absence from work.

3. **Bedrest.** Should be kept to a minimum and early mobilization encouraged. This is true in both back strain and radicular disease. If symptoms recur or considerable pain develops in relation to a specific activity or level of activity, the patient should temporarily limit that activity for several days but should not cease all activity.

4. **Analgesia.** NSAIDs provide pain relief and decrease inflammation but have side effects. Acetaminophen provides analgesia but has no anti-inflammatory properties and may be used with or instead of NSAIDs. Narcotics should be used short term as needed. Muscle relaxants such as cyclobenzaprine or diazepam work mostly by sedating patients and preventing activity. However, they probably have little effect on muscle spasm.

5. **Physical therapy.** Although classically several modes have been used to hasten resolution of back pain, most physical therapy modalities

16

ORTHOPEDICS

have no effect when rigorously tested. Traction, local application of heat, cold, and ultrasound, and corsets have been shown to have no effect. Proper lifting, strengthening, and weight loss may prevent recurrence. Transcutaneous electrical nerve stimulation may provide short-term symptomatic relief but has no proven long-term benefit. Acupuncture may also be of help.

6. **Epidural steroid injections.** These have been classically used but a randomized trial shows that there is no benefit.

7. **Rehabilitation exercises.** Trunk extensors, abdominal muscles, aerobic conditioning. The main benefit is that they promote early mobilization, which is critical in treating acute back pain. The specific exercise does not matter as much as the mobilization.

8. Back support belts are ineffective in preventing back pain.

B. **Chronic back pain.** Once back pain has been established for more than 1 year, the prognosis is poor. Mild analgesia should be used. Avoid chronic reliance on narcotics if possible (although addiction rates are low with chronic pain). If depression is encountered, it should be treated. Other modalities for chronic pain include tricyclics, carbamazepine and gabapentin. Physical modalities include transcutaneous electrical nerve stimulation or acupuncture with electrical stimulation. Both are effective but for a limited duration of time.

C. **Indications for admission and referral.** Cauda equina syndrome (urinary retention, sphincter incontinence, saddle anesthesia), severe neurologic deficits (footdrop, areflexia, gastrocnemius-soleus or quadriceps weakness), progressive neurologic deficit, or multiple nerve root involvement.

SHOULDER PAIN

After knee pain, shoulder pain is the second most common type of orthopedic pain seen by family physicians. Most shoulder problems are attributable to overuse and trauma. The shoulder is composed of one articulation, the scapulothoracic, and three true joints: the sternoclavicular, acromioclavicular, and glenohumeral.

I. **Rotator Cuff Syndrome.** The rotator cuff muscles are the supraspinatus, infraspinatus, teres minor, and subscapularis, which rotate and more importantly stabilize the humoral head.

A. **Stage I rotator cuff syndrome.**
   1. This is a rotator cuff tendinitis caused by forceful or repetitive motion, typically in those 25 years of age or younger.
   2. Pain is noted over the anterior aspect of the shoulder and is maximal when the arm is raised from 60 to 120 degrees of elevation.
   3. Treatment consists of avoiding aggravating positions and activities, applying ice packs, and taking NSAIDS.

B. **Stage II rotator cuff syndrome.**
   1. This usually occurs in patients 25 to 40 years of age with multiple previous episodes.

2. In addition to inflammation of the rotator cuff, some permanent fibrosis, thickening, or scarring is present.

3. Calcific deposits may be noted within the rotator cuff on radiographs.

4. Initial treatment is the same as that of stage I. If unsuccessful, the subacromial bursa can be injected with corticosteroids. If symptoms persist, referral to an orthopedist for a surgical consult should be considered.

C. **Stage III rotator cuff syndrome.**

1. This is a complete tear of the supraspinatus tendon and usually occurs after 40 years of age.

2. The patient may relate feeling a sudden pop in the shoulder and then suffering severe pain. The patient notes increasing weakness when trying to abduct and externally rotate his or her arm.

3. The diagnosis is confirmed by magnetic resonance imaging or a shoulder arthrogram.

4. Treatment is usually surgical repair within 6 weeks, depending on whether there is significant loss of function and other factors such as age. Many elderly patients have progressive rotator cuff loss over years as a result of the aging process.

II. **Adhesive Capsulitis (Frozen Shoulder).**

A. **Clinical features.**

1. This chronically stiff and painful shoulder may begin without any significant injury.

2. The cause is prolonged immobilization from either protracted use of a sling or disuse because of pain in the arm.

3. Shoulder motion is limited in one or more directions, with pain occurring at the limits of motion. Both passive and active range of motion are limited. Treatment involves extended, aggressive physical therapy and NSAIDs or mobilization under anesthesia. Symptoms may take 2 years to improve significantly.

III. **Tendinitis and Bursitis.** The supraspinatus and long end of the biceps are especially susceptible.

A. **Clinical features.** The primary symptom is a painful, aching shoulder of rather nondescript type. With supraspinatus tendinitis, the pain is aggravated when the shoulder is abducted and externally rotated against resistance. With bicipital tendinitis, pain is aggravated when the patient flexes forward against resistance, and pain with palpation of long head of biceps.

B. **Treatment.**

1. Overuse syndrome in the shoulder should be treated with NSAIDs, ice and rest for 5 to 7 days.

2. Most shoulder conditions can be relieved by injection of 2-5 cc of 1% bupivacaine and 40mg of triamcinolone into the effected area (e.g., subacromial bursa or tendon region).

3. Ultrasound may be useful in calcific tendonitis but is not effective for other cases. Traditional physical therapy is often of limited efficacy but mobilization is helpful.

16

ORTHOPEDICS

IV. **Acromioclavicular Injuries.** Usually result from a direct blow or fall on the tip of the shoulder.

A. **Grade I (sprain).** Partial tear of the joint capsule without joint deformity and minimal ligamentous disruption and instability. AC joint films (with and without weights) are normal. Treatment includes ice, pain medication, a sling for comfort, and early mobilization.

B. **Grade II (subluxation).** Complete tear of the acromioclavicular ligaments. The AC joint is locally tender and painful with motion. The distal end of the clavicle may protrude slightly upward. Stress radiograph of the AC joint with the patient holding a 10-pound weight in both hands reveals widening of the joint. Treatment is symptomatic in the same manner as the grade I injury but usually requires a longer period of immobilization (2 to 4 weeks).

C. **Grade III (dislocation).** Complete tear of the acromioclavicular and coracoclavicular ligaments with pain on any attempt at abduction. There is an obvious "step-off" on physical examination. Radiographs show superior displacement of the clavicle and complete dislocation of the joint with weights. Conservative treatment with a sling is appropriate, provided that the patient understands that permanent deformity may result. Patients usually return to normal function. Surgical treatment is important if symptomatic treatment fails or if it will interfere with the patient's life (as in an athlete or person who does heavy work).

V. **Glenohumeral Dislocations.**

A. **Clinical features.** 95% are anterior, most commonly subcoracoid and then subglenoid. The usual mechanism is forced abduction and external rotation. Patients complain of severe pain and usually hold the arm in tightly against their body. The shoulder appears flattened laterally and prominent anteriorly. The acromion process is prominent, and so the shoulder appears to be "squared off." The examiner must check for associated injuries, including proximal humeral fractures, avulsion of the rotator cuff, and injuries to the adjacent neurovascular structures. Axillary nerve injury is most common and is associated with decreased active contraction of the deltoid muscle and hypesthesia over deltoid.

B. **Radiographs** taken in two planes (AP and lateral scapula or axillary views) will confirm the dislocation and should be done to rule out fracture if mechanism suggestive.

C. **Treatment.** The dislocation should be reduced as soon as possible. Adequate analgesia and relaxation can be obtained by a 20ml intra-articular injection of 1% lidocaine. Narcotics (e.g., IV morphine) and muscle relaxants (e.g., diazepam) are useful as well.

1. **External rotation method** (Hennipen technique). The patient is placed supine, with the arm abducted and the elbow flexed to 90 degrees. The examiner holds the elbow in position and externally rotates the shoulder. No pressure is applied to the forearm to force external rotation. If necessary, the arm can be abducted while in

external rotation. Reduction usually occurs silently, unnoticed by the patient. This method has the lowest rate of complications.

2. **Modified Stimson reduction.**
   a. Analgesia or relaxation as noted above.
   b. The patient is placed prone on a table with the injured shoulder hanging free.
   c. Weight (up to 10-15 pounds) is suspended from the wrist, and the patient is left for 5 to 15 minutes.
   d. Further manipulation is often required consisting of gentle internal and external rotation with downward traction.

3. **Other reduction techniques** include traction-countertraction and scapular manipulation.

D. **Postreduction care.** Postreduction radiographs are obtained to ensure good relocation. Classically, the patient's arm is immobilized in a sling-and-swathe dressing for 6 weeks, although recently early mobilization as been found to be superior. However, this is not yet standard of care. Early orthopedic follow-up care is recommended. Recurrent dislocation or subluxation is common and may require surgical repair.

ELBOW

I. **Lateral Epicondylitis (tennis elbow).** A very common inflammatory process of the extensor origin of the lateral epicondyle. May be secondary to overuse/repetitive use. Pain at the lateral epicondyle, with referred pain to the extensor surface of the forearm is typical. The pain is exacerbated by resisted extension of the wrist or fingers. Treatment includes avoiding exacerbating activities, NSAIDs, and placing a constrictive "tennis elbow" band just distal from the elbow. Occasionally immobilization of the wrist in a volar splint is required. Local steroid injection or orthopedic referral may be advised in recalcitrant cases.

II. **Medial Epicondylitis.** This results from repeated flexion activities of the wrist and fingers. Pain is at the medial epicondyle and exacerbated by resistant flexion of the fingers. Treatment is the same as that of lateral epicondylitis.

III. **Radial Head Subluxation (nursemaid's elbow).**

A. The **mechanism** is a sudden pull on the extended pronated elbow of a child less than 4 years of age (for example, when one picks up a child by the forearm or swings the child). The child holds his arm in pronation and usually refuses to move it with pain on supination and palpation of the radial head.

B. Although **radiographic findings** are usually normal, one must be sure to rule out undisplaced supracondylar fracture. Frequently, the subluxation spontaneously reduces from x-ray positioning.

C. **Treatment** is firm supination of the forearm, flexing the elbow gently to 90 degrees with pressure over the radial head. Reduction is achieved with a palpable click over the radial head, and the pain is immediately relieved. The patient should resume full activity within several minutes of reduction although some are hesitant. It may take an hour or so to resume full activity.

IV. **Little Leaguer's Elbow.** Results from overuse of an adolescent's pitching elbow. On exam there is tenderness over the medial humoral epicondyle with mild swelling. An acute syndrome with sudden onset also occurs from the avulsion of a fragment of bone from the medial humeral epicondyle. Treatment includes rest for 3-6 weeks followed by rehabilitation. Loose bodies and locking elbow require referral.

V. **Olecranon Bursitis** (note: the same treatment and diagnostic modalities hold true for prepatellar bursitis as well).

A. **Clinically** there is tenderness and swelling over the olecranon bursa. Olecranon bursitis may be secondary to trauma (e.g., lying on carpet with elbows propped up while watching TV) or may be infectious (Staphylococcal). Frequently, traumatic bursitis leads to infectious bursitis.

B. **Diagnosis.** Must differentiate infectious from sterile bursitis. Tap the bursa and evaluate gram stain, cell count, crystals, and culture.

C. **Treatment** consists of repeated aspiration until fluid no longer re-accumulates. Start antistaphylococcal antibiotics (e.g., amoxicillin/clavulanate, nafcillin) if an infectious etiology is likely. May require admission for IV antibiotics the patient is toxic or there are comorbid conditions (e.g., immunosuppression, diabetes). If the etiology is not infectious, treat with NSAIDS, aspiration and compression dressings. Occasionally, an olecranon bursa must be opened surgically.

WRIST AND HAND

I. **Ganglion Cyst.** The most commonly noted nodule in the hand. Typical locations include the dorsal aspect of the lunate, radial volar aspect of the wrist, dorsal aspect of the hand, and palmar aspect of the fingers near the MCP joints. Typically accentuated with extreme flexion or extension of the wrist. If the cyst is small, aspiration of the cyst contents may be performed with an 18-gauge needle. **Steroid injection adds nothing.** About one-third will resolve with aspiration and it is unlikely that multiple aspirations will help if there is no resolution after the first aspiration. Most resolve over time but orthopedic referral may be considered for surgical removal, but even this has a limited efficacy.

II. **Carpal Tunnel Syndrome.**

A. **Clinical features.** The symptoms are a result of median nerve dysfunction because of increased pressure within the carpal tunnel. The causes include overuse, ganglion cyst, amyloid, synovial proliferation, pregnancy, rheumatoid arthritis, and hypothyroidism among others. Typical symptoms are pain, paresthesia, hypesthesia, or numbness in the median nerve distribution of the hand usually in the thumb, index, middle, and radial aspect of the ring finger. Nocturnal paresthesia is characteristic.

B. **Exam.** Tinel's sign, which is a painful sensation of the fingers induced by percussion of the median nerve at the level of the palmar wrist, may be positive, but specificity only 54% and sensitivity 50%. Phalen's sign, keeping both wrists in a palmar-flexed position may reproduce symptoms. Sensitivity varies from 10% to 88% depending on study; it has an 80% specificity.

C. **Treatment.** The patient without thenar atrophy can be treated with conservative therapy, which includes a resting splint with the wrist in *neutral* position and NSAIDs. Steroid injections of the carpal tunnel may be effective. If EMG shows impaired conduction of the median nerve at the wrist, or the carpal tunnel symptoms do not improve in 6 weeks, or if there is evidence of thenar muscle weakness or atrophy, surgical referral is indicated.

III. **Mallet Finger.**
A. Injury resulting from forced flexion of distal tip of a finger. Result is a stretching or rupture of the tendon of the extensor digitorum profundus or avulsion of part of the distal phalanx with tendon attached. Commonly occurs with basketball and baseball injuries.
B. **Exam** reveals swelling, tenderness, DIP joint held in flexion with patient unable to extend it.
C. **Treatment.**
   1. Splint finger in extension across DIP joint leaving PIP joint free to allow continued function. Splint for several weeks (6 to 12) with absolutely no flexion; longer times for injuries with delayed diagnosis.
   2. Operative repair is necessary for the minority of cases that don't respond to splinting.

IV. **Fingertip.**
A. **Paronychia.** Infection under nail fold. Treatment consists of warm soaks, antistaphylococcal antibiotics (e.g., cephalexin, amoxicillin/clavulanate) for 5-10 days and drainage using an 11 blade or 18-gauge needle guided along the nail into the site.
B. **Felon.** Infection in the digital pulp. Treatment consists of drainage and packing as well as antistaphylococcal antibiotics. Closely monitor treatment response.

V. **Interphalangeal Joint Dislocation.**
A. **Proximal interphalangeal joint.**
   1. **Mechanism** is usually a hyperextension injury with the base of the middle phalanx displaced dorsally and proximally.
   2. Reduction may be done without anesthesia or with a metacarpal block.
   3. **Reduction**
      a. Hyperextend dislocated segment and then push with thumb straight distally on the base of the dorsally displaced phalanx.
      b. As base of middle phalanx engages the joint surface the direction of force changes to an arc to follow the phalanx into slight flexion.
      c. Examiner usually feels a sense of giving way as the joint reduces.
   4. **Postreduction.**
      a. X-ray to rule out avulsion fractures.
      b. Check active extension.

    c. Splint in full extension for 3 weeks then begin exercises to restore range of motion.

HIP: BURSITIS OF THE HIP

I. **Clinically.** Bursitis of the hip largely involves the trochanteric bursa. Patients present with a history of pain with walking, running, or climbing, They may also complain of pain when lying on the affected side. There is tenderness over the greater trochanter.

II. **Treatment.** NSAIDs are frequently ineffective but are worth trying. The most effective treatment is corticosteroid injection into the bursa. Palpate the bursa and inject triamcinolone 40 mg with 5 cc of bupivacaine into the tender area. Pain is usually relieved immediately but may recur until the antiinflammatory takes effect.

KNEE PAIN

The majority of knee injuries in adults are of a ligamentous nature. In children, however, a bloody effusion after injury frequently indicates bony injury.

I. **Determination of Radiographs.** Only 5% to10% of persons with knee trauma have a fracture. Guidelines have been established to hep determine who should have a radiograph. Use clinical judgment, however.

A. **Ottawa Knee Rules.** 97% sensitive and 27% specific for fracture. X-ray those who
    1. Are age 55 or older
    2. Have tenderness at head of fibula
    3. Have isolated tenderness of patella
    4. Have inability to flex knee to 90 degrees
    5. Have inability to walk four weight-bearing steps in the ED

B. **Pittsburgh Decision Rules.** 99% sensitive and 60% specific for fracture
    1. Blunt trauma or fall as mechanism of injury plus either of the following
    2. Age >55 or <12 years old or
    3. Inability to walk four weight bearing steps in the ER

II. **Ligamentous Injuries.**

A. **Collateral ligament injury**
    1. Typically caused by direct trauma to the contralateral side of the knee, or excessive indirect force to the knee in a varus or valgus manner.
    2. Pain and a tearing sensation may have been noted by the patient at the time of injury. In case of medial collateral ligament injury, there may be tenderness along the distal femur extending to the joint line. Medial collateral ligament injuries are more commonly associated with meniscus tears.
    3. Valgus and varus tests provide assessment of the collateral ligaments. With the knee in 30 degrees of flexion, the collateral ligaments can be isolated.
    4. Grade I sprains are caused by micro-tears of the ligament and correspond to less than 5 mm of increased joint opening and no instability. Grade II sprains are a partial macro-tear of the ligament with the

presence of instability and significant increased joint opening with a point. A grade III sprain is a complete tear of the ligament with no end point distinguishable on examination.

5. **Treatment** of isolated grade I and II injuries involves conservative measures, such as ice application for 15 to 20 minutes TID and elevation for the first 24 to 72 hours, crutches with limited weight bearing, rest with an immobilizer or hinged brace for 7 to 14 days, and NSAID therapy. Lateral ligament requires 4-6 weeks of a brace. Prompt initiation of physical therapy should be included in initial treatment. Grade III injuries can be treated nonoperatively, but an orthopedic referral is recommended to assess the need for surgical intervention.

B. **Anterior cruciate ligament injury**

1. There is a history of a twisting injury accompanied by a pop or tearing feeling and a subsequent effusion. A hemarthrosis is found in 75% of cases. Frequently associated with a medial collateral ligament injury.

2. The Lachman and pivot shift tests are useful. The Lachman test is performed with the knee at 30 degrees in a supine position and involves anterior displacement of the tibia on the femur. The pivot shift test involves flexion of the knee while the lower leg is internally rotated and a valgus stress is applied with thumb on lateral knee where a palpable click is felt with extension. Treatment should be supervised by an orthopedist. Treatment of acute injuries depends on the severity. Patients without associated meniscal, collateral ligament, or posterior cruciate ligament injury should be treated by immobilization of the knee for comfort and crutches. Patients with associated ligament injury or meniscal injury should be referred immediately to an orthopedist because surgery may be necessary. Often leads to OA if untreated.

C. **Posterior cruciate ligament injury.**

1. Most injuries are the result of direct trauma to the proximal tibia when the flexed knee is decelerated rapidly, as in a dashboard injury.

2. The posterior drawer and tibial sag tests are used. In the posterior drawer test, the knee is flexed 90 degrees and posterior displacement of the tibia on the femur is attempted. In the tibial sag test, the knee is flexed to 90 degrees with hip at 45 degrees, the tibia is displaced posteriorly on the femur.

3. Isolated tears should be managed conservatively with physical therapy and quadriceps strengthening. If radiographs reveal displaced bony avulsions, posterior cruciate ligament injury may require surgical fixation. Orthopedic referral is recommended.

III. **Meniscal Tears.**

A. **Clinical features.**

1. Meniscal injuries are a common cause of knee joint pain. The median meniscus more frequently injured than is the lateral. More than one third of meniscal injuries are associated with an anterior cruciate ligament tear and possibly medial collateral ligament injuries.

16

ORTHOPEDICS

2. Patients complain of pain at the time of injury, which persists and interferes with weight-bearing activity. The most consistent physical finding is tenderness to palpation along the joint line. Patients often complain of the knee "locking," which may be attributable to pain or a physical inability to extend the knee because the torn meniscus prevents extension.

3. Several clinical tests help determine if meniscal injury is present. In the McMurray's test, the knee is fully flexed, with the leg externally rotated when one is testing for medial meniscal tears and internally rotated when testing for lateral meniscal tears. While maintaining rotation, extend the knee with a firm controlled movement. A painful click signifies a positive test. The Apley's test is performed with the patient in a prone position. The knee is flexed to 90 degrees, and an axial load is placed on the heel of the foot while the lower leg is rotated internally and externally. If pain results, the test is positive.

B. **Diagnosis.** If there are any diagnostic doubts, patients should be referred for evaluation by magnetic resonance imaging or arthroscopy.

C. **Treatment.** The knee should be immobilized if there is pain with motion. Crutches, quadriceps exercises, and NSAIDs can be used. If the knee remains locked or if symptoms of pain, giving way (a sense that the knee is going to collapse), and swelling persist, orthopedic referral should be made for surgical intervention.

IV. **Patellofemoral Pain Syndrome.**

A. **Clinical features.** Most common anterior knee problem seen by the family physician. The problem presents as anterior knee pain, which is worse after prolonged sitting with the knee flexed, or on climbing or descending stairs or slopes. Patients may complain of some snapping, popping, or crepitus about the patella.

B. Radiographs of the knee are usually negative. However, lateral displacement of the patella on a Merchant view may be present.

C. **Treatment.** NSAIDs, ice application, and appropriate exercises including those that strengthen the medial quadriceps and stretch the hamstrings are useful (such as straight leg raising with the ankle and hip externally rotated).

V. **Patellar Dislocations.**

A. **Clinical features.** Patients complain of the knee giving way or popping out. The patella may still be dislocated when patient is seen, but many spontaneously reduce. An effusion (hemarthrosis) may be present. The medial retinaculum is tender. Apprehension test: displace the patella laterally; patients feel as though the patella is going to dislocate and will be very apprehensive. Between occurrences the patella is observed to have considerable lateral mobility, particularly during active extension. The patellar ligament may be noted to angulate laterally from the axis of the quadriceps muscle.

B. **Reduction.** Encourage the patient to relax the quadriceps and push the patella medially back into place. If unable to get the patella over the lateral femoral condyle, push the patella anteriorly while passively flexing the knee (the patella usually reduces by 30 degrees of flexion). If the effusion is tense, aspiration may reduce discomfort.

C. **Postreduction care.** Adequate immobilization is obtained with the use of a knee immobilizer for 6 weeks. Have patients fully weight bearing as well as performing quadriceps isometric exercises while immobilized. After immobilization, patients are placed on partial weight bearing while quadriceps strengthening is initiated. Rehabilitation needs to include the vastus medialis, which operates only in the last 15 degrees of extension. Resume full weight bearing when flexion to 30 degrees is painless. An elastic knee support may add some patellar stability during strenuous activity. Dislocation more than three times may require surgical treatment.

VI. **Prepatellar Bursitis.** See olecranon bursitis section.

ANKLE SPRAIN

I. **Clinical features.** Sprains usually result from an inversion force; an eversion injury may result in a fracture. The most common ligament injured is the anterior talofibular ligament. A history of popping or a painful snap with ankle injury may be indicative of a significant ligament injury.

II. **Radiography.** The Ottawa ankle rules (Figure 16-1) have been developed and validated to determine who needs a radiograph. Using these rules, an occasional fracture will be missed. However, these are gener-

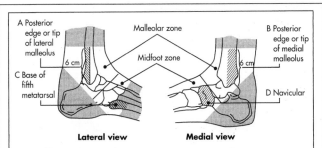

A Posterior edge or tip of lateral malleolus
6 cm
C Base of fifth metatarsal

Malleolar zone
Midfoot zone

B Posterior edge or tip of medial malleolus
6 cm
D Navicular

Lateral view   **Medial view**

An ankle radiographic series is required only if there is any pain in the malleolar zone and any of these findings is present:
(1) bone tenderness at A
(2) bone tenderness at B
(3) inability to bear weight both immediately and in the ED

A foot radiographic series is required only if there is any pain in midfoot zone and any of these findings is present:
(1) bone tenderness at C
(2) bone tenderness at D
(3) inability to bear weight both immediately and in the ED

FIGURE 16-1

Ottawa ankle rules. *From Steill IG, Greenberg GH, Wells GA, et al: JAMA 275:611-5, 1996.*

ally of no clinical significance (as with an avulsion injury). They apply only to an individual older than 17 years of age.

III. **Treatment.** In most ankle sprains, treatment includes external support such as the application of an air splint, ice application and elevation above the heart. NSAIDs or acetaminophen with or without hydrocodone or codeine can be used for pain control. The patient should be allowed partial weight bearing with crutches or a cane. Early mobilization and weight bearing hasten resolution. Patients with recurrent problems of instability or an acute grade III problem should be referred to an orthopedist for evaluation and the possibility of reconstructive surgery.

HEEL PAIN: PLANTAR FASCIITIS

I. **Clinically.** Pain over the heel on weight bearing. The pain is especially severe in the morning and after protracted sitting. Passive dorsiflexion of the toes with foot eversion may exacerbate the pain. There may be associated pes planus.

II. **Radiographs are generally not indicated.** Radiographs may show a calcaneal spur but the spur is incidental and not the cause of the fasciitis.

III. **Differential** includes subcalcaneal bursitis and herniated calcaneal fat pad. These should not worsen with toe dorsiflexion. Additionally, calcaneal fat pad pain is maximally tender over the calcaneous while plantar fasciitis is more tender distal to the heel. Finally, calcaneal bursitis should be associated with a swelling over the calcaneous.

IV. **Treatment.** Treatment for all of the above include NSAIDS, soaks, rest. For plantar fasciitis, consider orthotics to correct pes planus and a soft rubber heel cup (e.g., Tuli's heel cup). Stretching of the fascia (lean forward against wall with heel on the ground) will help as will injection of corticosteroids. Surgery is rarely indicated.

FOOT PAIN

I. **Metatarsalgia.** Pain on weight bearing in the anterior foot with tenderness over the plantar aspects of the metatarsal heads. Pain is exacerbated with wearing high heeled shoes. It is increasingly common as patient's age with loss of the normal foot fat pads. Treatment is NSAIDs and a metatarsal pad that restores the normal convex contour of the foot and takes the pressure off of the metatarsal heads. These are available at most drug stores or orthotic makers.

II. **Differentiate from** Morton's neuroma, a neurofibrillary tangle between the metatarsals, especially 2 and 3 and 3 and 4 Pain is described as burning and is exacerbated with squeezing the anterior foot to compress the metatarsals together. Treatment is avoidance of extension of the toes and pain management. Surgical therapy has a good outcome and is frequently required.

ROTATIONAL DEFORMITIES OF THE LOWER EXTREMITY

I. **In-Toeing (Pigeon-Toed).**

A. **Internal tibial torsion.** Observation of gait reveals forward facing knees with feet pointing towards the midline. To diagnose, place patient on knees and observe the foot angle, normally, the toes of either foot are pointed away from each other at an angle of 30 degrees (e.g., toes are pointed outward). With internal tibial torsion, the toes of either side are pointed inward. Also, with legs dangling over a table, the lateral malleolus will be anterior to the medical malleolus (the opposite of the normal foot). Typically resolves spontaneously by age 4. Intervention does not change outcome unless there is underlying neuromuscular pathology or the patient is older than 8 with an altered gait.

B. **Medial femoral torsion.** Most common cause of in-toeing in children. Typical child presents at age 3-4 with increasing in-toeing secondary to the alignment of the femur in the acetabulum and loss of normal lateral rotatory forces of infancy. Diagnose by placing the child prone with knees flexed 90 degrees, then internally and externally rotating the hip. Internal rotation of greater than 70 degrees with limitation of external rotation is suggestive of femoral torsion. Alternatively, observe the patient while he/she walks. If the patella faces forward, the diagnosis of femoral torsion is ruled out. No treatment generally necessary unless severely altering gait. Does not lead to increased incidence of arthritis.

C. **Metatarsus adductus.** A functional deformity where a flexible forefoot is adducted in relation to the hindfoot. The forefoot can be brought into a neutral position by gently straightening. It typically resolves by 3 months. Parents can do self-therapeutic gentle stretching with diaper changes, but there is no change in outcome. If it persists beyond 3-4 months referral should be made. **Unilateral** metatarsus adductus is related to ipsilateral hip dysplasia.

D. **Metatarsus varus.** A rigid abnormality caused by subluxation of the tarsometatarsal joint with subluxation of the metatarsals. As opposed to metatarsus adductus, in which the foot is flexible, here the defect is relatively fixed. A prominent base of the 5 the metatarsal, a convexity of the lateral border and a deep crease of the plantar surface in addition to the fixed abnormality lead to the diagnosis. Referral for serial casting should be made with the diagnosis.

II. **Out-Toeing.**

A. **Physiologic out-toeing.** An external rotational contracture of the soft tissues surrounding the hip secondary to intrauterine forces. It generally resolves spontaneously with ambulation around 18 months.

B. **Lateral tibial torsion.** Presents in the 3-5 year-old with increasing outtoeing. May lead to knee pain. Severe torsion requires referral

FRACTURES

I. **Terms.**

A. **Closed fracture.** Fracture that does not communicate with the outside.

16

ORTHOPEDICS

B. **Open fracture.** Fracture that communicates with the external environment.

C. **Comminuted fracture.** Consisting of three or more fragments.

D. **Avulsion fracture.** Fragment of bone pulled from its normal position by a muscular contraction or resistance of a ligament.

E. **Greenstick fracture.** Incomplete, angulated fracture of a long bone, particularly in children.

F. **Torus fracture.** Compression of the bone without cortical disruption. Seen especially in the forearms of children.

II. **Epiphyseal Plate Fractures.** Described using the Salter and Harris classification (Figure 16-2).

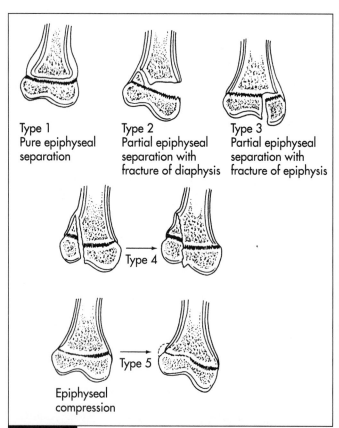

Type 1
Pure epiphyseal separation

Type 2
Partial epiphyseal separation with fracture of diaphysis

Type 3
Partial epiphyseal separation with fracture of epiphysis

Type 4

Type 5

Epiphyseal compression

FIGURE 16-2
Salter-harris classification of epiphyseal fractures.

A. **Salter I (approximately 6%).**
   1. Separation of the epiphysis from the metaphysis without evidence of a metaphyseal fragment.
   2. Usually the result of a shearing force, can be associated with birth injury.
   3. Most common in infants and young children.
   4. High index of suspicion is necessary because spontaneous reduction can occur.
   5. Prognosis is excellent because epiphyseal blood supply is usually intact and growing cells of epiphyseal plate are undisturbed.

B. **Salter II (approximately 75%).**
   1. Fracture extends transversely through the epiphyseal plate and then out through the metaphysis on the side opposite the fracture initiation resulting in a triangular metaphyseal fragment.
   2. Most frequent in children over 10 years of age.
   3. Usually treated with closed reduction.
   4. Prognosis is excellent because the blood supply is almost always intact.

C. **Salter III (8%).**
   1. Intraarticular fracture that extends from the joint surface across the epiphysis to the epiphyseal plate and out to the periphery.
   2. Commonly involves the lower tibial epiphysis.
   3. Caused by an intraarticular shearing force.
   4. Often requires open reduction.
   5. Prognosis is good if the blood supply is intact and reduction is maintained.

D. **Salter IV (10%).**
   1. Intraarticular fracture consisting of a vertical fracture through the epiphysis that crosses the epiphyseal plate and leaves through a portion of the metaphysis.
   2. Frequently involves lateral condyle of humerus.
   3. Treated with anatomic reduction and internal fixation.
   4. Prognosis is poor unless reduction is maintained.

E. **Salter V (1%).**
   1. Results from a crush injury through the epiphysis to a portion of the epiphyseal plate.
   2. Usually occurs in a joint that has only one plane of movement.
   3. Most commonly seen in the knee and ankle.
   4. Initial radiographs tend to be normal and so must suspect this fracture from the mechanism of injury.
   5. Results are poor with premature cessation of growth.
   6. Nontraumatic events causing a Salter V type of injury are metaphyseal osteomyelitis and epiphyseal aseptic necrosis.
   7. Salter V can occur in conjunction with Salter I, II, and III fractures and not be recognized until growth arrest occurs.
   8. Treat with 3 weeks of no weight bearing.

16

ORTHOPEDICS

III. **Repair.**
A. A good rule of thumb is that most bones join in 6 to 8 weeks; lower limb bones may take longer; fractures in children may take less time.
IV. **Complications.**
A. **Immediate complications,** within the first few hours, include hemorrhage, damage to arteries, and damage to surrounding soft tissues.
B. **Early complications,** within the first few weeks, include wound infection, fat embolism, shock lung, chest infection, DIC, and exacerbation of general illness. May also have compartment syndrome, with the anterior compartment of the leg most common (see Chapter 2 for details of compartment syndrome).
C. **Late complications,** months and years later, include deformity, osteoarthritis of adjacent or distant joints, aseptic necrosis, traumatic chondromalacia, and reflex sympathetic dystrophy.
D. **If a patient complains of pain after casting, assume a tight cast and possible compartment syndrome.** Bivalve the cast including all layers of cotton, stockinet, etc. and wrap with ACE wrap. Consider recasting in several days.
V. **Management of Some Specific Fractures.**
A. **Fracture of radial head.** Usually caused by a fall onto an outstretched hand. Patients are reluctant to pronate the hand or to flex the elbow beyond 90 degrees. The only roentgenographic evidence may be an anterior or posterior fat pad sign. The posterior fat pad is more specific but less sensitive. Management of nondisplaced fractures in those who can fully extend the elbow includes a sling and posterior elbow splint for 1 to 2 weeks with range-of-motion exercises after 1 week. Continue in sling for another week and do follow-up radiograph to document that no displacement has occurred with mobilization. If there is displacement of the radial head, the patient should be referred to an orthopedist for operative repair.
B. **Radial fractures.**
1. In children, the most common injury is the torus (buckle) fracture, which occurs with a fall onto an outstretched hand. Radiographic findings may show only a slight cortical disruption on the lateral film. Treatment is a short arm cast for 3 weeks.
2. In adults, the most common radial fracture is the Colles' fracture, which is extra-articular and occurs 2.5 to 3 cm proximal to the articular surface of the distal radius. This fracture occurs with the hand dorsiflexed; the distal fracture segment is angulated dorsally and causes a "silver-fork" deformity. Reduction by traction and manipulation can be performed. After reducing the fracture, a plaster short-arm cast is applied for 5 to 8 weeks. If nondisplaced, casting for 6 weeks without reduction is indicated.
C. **Metacarpal fractures.** A boxer's fracture is a fracture of the distal neck of the fifth metacarpal and is generally the result of punching something with a closed fist (generally a wall or refrigerator). Tenderness is local-

ized to the injured metacarpal bone. Radiographs reveal a fracture of the involved metacarpal or subluxation at the carpometacarpal joint. Nondisplaced fractures of the base of the metacarpals are treated with immobilization in a short arm cast. Displaced fractures are reduced by traction with local pressure over the prominent proximal end of the distal metacarpal fracture. A follow-up radiograph is necessary within 7 days. If any instability is noted after reduction or the fracture is comminuted, the patient should be referred to an orthopedist for open reduction and internal fixation.

D. **Fractured finger.**

1. **Distal tip fractures** are usually crush injuries to the tip of the finger. Protective splinting of the tip for several weeks is usually satisfactory.

2. **Middle and proximal phalangeal fractures** should be examined for evidence of angulation (by roentgenography) or rotation (by clinical examination), which require reduction. Nondisplaced extraarticular fractures can be managed by 1 to 2 weeks of immobilization followed by dynamic splinting with buddy taping to the adjacent finger. Large intra-articular or displaced fractures are usually unstable and require orthopedic referral.

3. **Small (<25%) avulsion fractures of the middle phalangeal base** occur with a hyperextension injury. These injuries are managed by 2 to 3 weeks of immobilization with up to 15 degrees of flexion at the PIP joint, followed by buddy taping for 3 to 6 weeks.

16

ORTHOPEDICS

BIBLIOGRAPHY

Libetta C et al: Validation of the Ottawa ankle rules in children, *J Accid Emerg Med* 16(9):342, September 1999.

Snider RK, editor: *Essentials of musculoskeletal care,* American Academy of Orthopedic Surgeons, 1998, Illinois.

Steill IG, Greenberg GH, Wells GA, et al: Prospective validation of a decision rule for the use of radiography in acute knee injuries, *JAMA* 275:611-5, 1996.

Tandeter HB, Shvartzman P, Stevens MA: Acute knee injuries: use of decision rules for selective radiograph ordering, *AFP* 60 (9): 2599-2608, 1999.

Wigder HN et al: Successful implementation of a guideline by peer comparisons, education, and positive physician feedback, *J Emerg Med* 17(5):807, 1999.

DERMATOLOGY

Matthew L. Lanternier
Karen Brannon

17

PRURITUS

I. **Overview.** Physiologic pruritus is a mild itch sensation due to trivial stimuli. Moderate-to-severe itchy sensations, which cause damage and interfere with well-being, are termed *pathologic pruritus.* Pruritus is mediated by histamine, prostaglandins, acetylcholine, kinins, and proteases. Common "itch spots" are located in warm areas where sweat is retained, especially the groin, foot, and scalp. Pruritus may occur spontaneously or be precipitated by the presence of chapped, dry skin, retained sweat, or psychologic factors such as anxiety or depression.

II. **Etiology.**

A. Cutaneous causes

1. **Surface causes**
   a. Most common irritants: fiberglass, wool, foreign bodies.
   b. Infestations: scabies, mites, pediculosis, jellyfish larvae
   c. Bites: mosquitoes
   d. Other: lichen planus, nodular prurigo, dermatitis herpetiformis, eczema

2. **Dermatoses:** Fungal, bacterial, viral, herpes, miliaria

B. Systemic causes

1. **Drugs**
   a. Allergic reactions (e.g., penicillin, sulfa drugs, etc.)
   b. Vasoactive drugs (e.g., nicotinic acid, caffeine, alcohol)
   c. CNS drugs (e.g., morphine, cocaine, amphetamines, codeine)

2. **Endocrinopathy** (e.g., hypothyroidism, hyperthyroidism, diabetes mellitus, diabetes insipidus, hyperparathyroidism secondary to chronic renal failure)

3. **Hepatic disease** (e.g., obstructive biliary disease, cholestasis)

4. **Malignancy** (e.g., Hodgkin's disease, polycythemia rubra vera, leukemia, mycosis fungoides, Sézary syndrome, visceral neoplasia, carcinoid syndrome, multiple myeloma)

5. **Chronic renal failure**

6. **Infection** (e.g., trichinosis, onchocerciasis, echinococcosis, focal infection)

7. **Miscellaneous** (e.g., gout, iron-deficiency anemia, primary amyloidosis, beriberi)

8. **Pregnancy**

C. **Psychogenic causes:** secondary to psychosis, anxiety, or depression.

1. Delusions of parasitosis, especially with methamphetamine abuse.

III. **Diagnosis.** History should include details about: (1) any skin lesions preceding the pruritus, (2) history of weight loss, fatigue, fever, malaise; (3) recent emotional stress; and (4) recent medications and travel. Physical with emphasis on the skin and its appendages. xerosis, excoriation, lichenification, hydration. Laboratory tests as suggested by the physical exam, which may include CBC, ESR, fasting glucose, renal and/or liver function tests, hepatitis panel, thyroid tests, stool for parasites, CXR.

IV. **Treatment.**

A. Treat any underlying systemic disorder.

B. Mild pruritus may respond to nonpharmacologic measures (e.g., avoiding irritants, using cool water compresses, trimming the nails, behavior therapy).

C. Systemic symptomatic treatment includes H1 blockers such as diphenhydramine or hydroxyzine or the nonsedating antihistamines (loratadine, cetirizine), H_2 blockers such as cimetidine or ranitidine, tricyclic antidepressants (particularly doxepin HCl and amitriptyline HCl), and as a last resort oral prednisone. Naltrexone may also be effective.

D. Topical symptomatic treatments include moisturizers, emollients, tar compounds, topical corticosteroids, topical anesthetics such as benzocaine or dibucaine, and pramoxine HCl (alone or combined with menthol, petrolatum, or benzyl alcohol). Doxepin 5% cream (Zonalon) can be used for the treatment of pruritus. It has a low potential for sensitization and is better tolerated than the oral form.

E. Other treatments include localized ultraviolet B phototherapy or intralesional injections of corticosteroid (e.g., with prurigo nodularis).

D. **For pruritus secondary to cholestasis:** consider cholestyramine, phenobarbital or naltrexone. Also consider rifampin 10mg/kg/d for those with primary biliary cirrhosis.

E. **For pruritus secondary to renal disease:** Dialysis, which may actually transiently increase pruritus, cholestyramine, or activated charcoal, 6 g/day for 6 weeks.

SKIN INFECTIONS

I. **Bacterial Infections.**

A. **Impetigo.** Usually caused by group A beta-hemolytic streptococci and/or coagulase-positive *Staphylococcus aureus.* Appear as small vesicles with yellowish crusts, or purulent-appearing bullae, which may be localized or widespread on the skin and develop over days. There is often associated adenopathy but minimal systemic signs. Itching, pain, and tenderness may occur. Moderately contagious. Treatment is with Mupirocin 2% ointment BID or systemic antibiotics (dicloxacillin 500 mg QID × 10 days, cephalexin 500 mg QID × 10 days, or erythromycin 500 mg QID × 10 day), daily bathing with antibacterial soap, and attention to personal hygiene. Need to monitor for the development of post streptococcal glomerulonephritis.

B. **Ecthyma.** Considered a deeper extension of impetigo with the same etiology except it may also be caused by *Pseudomonas.* It is characterized by a hemorrhagic crust with erythema or induration that develops over weeks. Treatment includes systemic antibiotics (see I A above) as well as debridement of the epidermis, which becomes necrotic. Scars may occur after healing. Usually occurs in debilitated patients, such as poorly controlled diabetics, but may occur in anyone.

C. **Erysipelas.** Presents as a well-demarcated tender, rapidly advancing erythematous plaque; there is pain associated with the lesion. The patient may have fever and leukocytosis. The usual organism is beta-hemolytic streptococci. Treat as per cellulitis. Patients may have multiple recurrences especially on a dependent extremity or after axillary dissection for breast carcinoma.

D. **Cellulitis.** Usually caused by Group A beta-hemolytic streptococci or *S. aureus,* it is a potentially suppurative inflammation of the dermis and subcutaneous tissue. Cellulitis usually follows trauma, a break in the skin or an underlying dermatosis. Presents with local erythema, tenderness, warmth induration, and tenderness. The border is not well defined. There may be streaks of lymphangitis with involvement of the regional lymph nodes. Systemic symptoms are common, and bacteremia and septicemia may follow. Treatment is with systemic antibiotics (if mild, dicloxacillin or cephalexin 500 mg QID × 7-10d, or if severe, nafcillin 1.5 g IV Q4h or vancomycin 1.5 g/day initially, then switch to oral). Alternative antibiotics include amoxicillin/clavulanate, erythromycin, clarithromycin, or azithromycin. The application of local heat, elevation, and immobilization can also be of benefit. For necrotizing fasciitis and synergistic gangrene, early wide surgical excision and debridement is necessary in addition to IV antibiotics.

E. **Erythrasma and related disorders.** Superficial intertriginous skin infections caused by *Corynebacteriae* organisms. It is often confused with fungal infections. Presents with skin color changes (e.g., reddish brown) and a slightly raised patch of affected skin. The bacteria produce porphyrins so the skin is coral-pink under Wood's lamp. Preferred treatment is oral erythromycin with topical clindamycin 2% as an alternative. It will respond to miconazole and clotrimazole, but the recurrence rate is high. These organisms also cause **trichomycosis axillaris** and **pitted keratolysis.** The former leads to foul axillary odor and hyperhidrosis and the latter to painful burning of the feet with pits on calloused areas. Good hygiene, antiperspirants, and topical erythromycin are used to treat both.

F. **Folliculitis** (including sycosis barbae [barber's itch], pseudofolliculitis, and "hot tub" folliculitis) is a common problem with predisposing factors such as maceration, friction, and the use of irritant chemicals. Usually caused by *S. aureus* but occasionally by *Klebsiella, Pseudomonas* (hot tub folliculitis), *Aerobacter,* or *C. albicans.* Appears as a pustule with a central hair (follicle) with surrounding erythema. The patient may notice

17

DERMATOLOGY

tenderness, pruritus, and pain. Particularly severe cases may result in scaring and the destruction of the hair follicle. Treatment includes antiseptic washes (e.g., Phisoderm or pHisoHex), which may also be used for prophylaxis. Systemic antibiotics such as dicloxacillin, cephalexin, or erythromycin 500mg QID × 7-10 days are an alternative. Mupirocin 2% ointment may be used for isolated areas. Use a fluoroquinolone to cover *Pseudomonas* (e.g., levofloxacin) for hot tub folliculitis. Complications can include cellulitis, furunculosis, and alopecia.

G. **Furuncle (boil)** is an acute, localized perifollicular abscess of the skin and subcutaneous tissue caused by coagulase-positive *S. aureus,* resulting in a red, hot, very tender inflammatory nodule that exudes pus from one opening. A carbuncle is an aggregate of connected furuncles and characteristically is painful and has a number of pustular openings. This can be an acute or chronic problem with lesions commonly on areas of friction such as buttocks, axillae, breasts, and the nape of the neck. Treatment involves systemic antibiotics (see I D above), local heat, and rest. **Incision and drainage is generally required.** Prevention is often difficult. Improved personal hygiene, use of antibacterial soaps (e.g., Phisohex, Phisoderm), frequent hand washing, daily bathing, and change of clothing are important. Elimination of carrier states in the nose and perineum by the use of topical mupirocin and systemic antibiotics is often possible.

II. **Viral Infections.**

A. **Warts (verruca vulgaris)** focal areas of epithelial hyperplasia caused by the human papilloma viruses (HPV). Lesions are most common on the hands, feet, anogenital area (condylomata), and face. They are infectious and auto-inoculable. Common in children, the elderly, or in patients with immunologic deficiencies or atopic dermatitis. Treatment is with keratolytic agents (salicylic/lactic acid/podophyllin preparations), cryotherapy, curettage, laser, or electrodesiccation. Recurrences are common and no one treatment is uniformly effective. See also Chapter 8 for treatment of condylomata accuminata. Cimetidine has been used to treat warts, but controlled trials show that there is no benefit.

B. **Herpes Simplex types I and II** are DNA viruses. The early lesions are multiple 1-2 mm diameter yellowish, clear vesicles on an erythematous base. The vesicles can ulcerate and become quite painful. Classic type I herpes occurs around the mouth and type II occurs on the genitalia, but either type I or type II can occur anywhere on the skin. Diagnosis can be made from clinical appearance, serologic antibody titers of acute and convalescent sera, Tzanck smear (Wright's stain of material obtained from the base of the lesion showing multinucleated giant cells), biopsy, and/or viral culture. A prodrome of pain, discomfort, or tingling is often reported a week to 10 days before seeing the lesions. Treatment is symptomatic with cool compresses, analgesics, and topical drying agents (i.e., Burow's solution) for the oozing, weeping stages. Antivirals (e.g., acyclovir and others) have only a modest effect on recurrent genital herpes unless used prophylactically on a daily basis (see Chapter 8 for details). If used during the prodrome, antivirals may shorten duration of lesions, reduce severity of symptoms, and shorten length of viral shedding. Discuss with patients about asymptomatic shedding of virus and the need for safer sex (e.g., use condoms). Some clinical infection syndromes are listed below:

1. **Gingivostomatitis.** Occurs periorally in children and young adults.
2. **Keratoconjunctivitis.** Ophthalmology consult is warranted. Usually heals without scarring.
3. **Vulvovaginitis**
4. **Herpes gladiatorum.** Occurs on the head, neck, or shoulder. Common in wrestlers.
5. **Eczema herpeticum.** Occurs in those with underlying skin disorders, most commonly in atopic dermatitis. Children more than adults. Consists of **disseminated** umbilicated vesicles confined to eczematous skin, which evolve into punched out erosions that may become confluent.
6. **Hepatoadrenal necrosis** and encephalitis
7. **Herpetic whitlow.** Occurs on distal portion of fingers.
8. **Cold sores** (herpes labialis)

C. **Herpes zoster (shingles).** Reactivation of latent varicella-zoster virus present in the sensory ganglia.

1. **Classic description** is that of grouped vesicles on an erythematous base in one unilateral dermatome. Thoracic nerve dermatomes are most commonly involved followed by the major branches of the trigeminal nerve.
2. **Symptoms** consist of pain, dysesthesia, and pruritus. Healing requires 2 to 3 weeks, and the afflicted persons are infectious until the lesions have crusted over (may transmit chicken pox to those who are not immune). Persons of any age can be affected, but the disease is more common and more severe in the elderly.
3. **Diagnosis** is via clinical presentation, although Tzanck smear, biopsy, and viral culture may be performed.
4. **Treatment** is oral acyclovir 800 mg 5 × a day for 7-10 days, which is effective if treatment is initiated within 2 days of the onset of the rash. Reduce the dose for all antivirals if CrCl is <60 ml/min. Alternatively, famciclovir 500 mg PO TID for 7 days can be used and may be more effective at preventing postherpetic neuralgia. Valacyclovir 1000 mg PO TID for 7 days is another alternative. Steroids are ineffective. Capsaicin creams can be used for pain relief after the lesions have healed. Amitriptyline 25-150 mg QHS may be useful in the treatment of postherpetic neuralgia. Other options include lidocaine patches (Lidoderm), carbamazepine, gabapentin, etc. For recurrent herpes zoster, if more than one dermatome is involved or bilaterally, consider malignancy or other causes of immunosuppression.

17

DERMATOLOGY

D. **Molluscum contagiosum.** Caused by a DNA pox virus. Appear as pearly papules up to 5 mm in diameter having a central dimple (umbilication). Multiple lesions are usually present. The central core (molluscum body) can be expressed with a blade. The lesions are infectious and auto-inoculation is common. Children are most commonly affected. Spontaneous resolution may occur, but there is often an eczematous reaction before to its resolution. Treatment can be limited to simple superficial curettage without anesthesia. The removal of the molluscum body, application of 50% trichloroacetic acid, or liquid nitrogen cryotherapy are equally efficacious.

III. **Fungal Infections (Dermatomycoses).**

A. **Candidiasis.** Caused by *Candida albicans*. Seen as thrush (see Chapters 11 and 12 for infants and immunosuppressed patients, respectively), diaper dermatitis, perineal infections, and intertriginous dermatitis. Diagnosis is by clinical exam, and microscopic examination of skin scraping in 10% KOH reveals yeast forms and budding hyphae. Treat with topical imidazole (miconazole, clotrimazole) creams BID to affected areas for superficial fungal infections. See Chapter 13 for vaginal candidiasis. See Chapter 11 for recurrent mucocutaneous disease. Invasive disease can be treated with fluconizole 400 mg IV QD for 7 days and then PO for 14 days after the last positive blood culture. This may be doubled in patients who deteriorate. An alternative is amphotericin B. Persons who present with recurrent infections should be investigated for an underlying illness such as diabetes mellitus, hypoparathyroidism, Addison's disease, malignancies, or HIV. Use of steroids and antibiotics are also predisposing factors.

B. **Dermatophytoses** (tinea). These fungi, belonging to the genera *Trichophyton, Microsporum, and Epidermophyton,* infect the stratum corneum of epidermis, hair, and nails. Commonly referred to by the locus of infection, i.e., tinea unguium (nails), tinea pedis (foot, "Athlete's foot"), tinea cruris (perineum, "jock itch"), tinea corporis (body, ringworm), tinea barbae (beard), tinea manus (hand), and tinea capitis (scalp and hair). Lesions can appear as grayish, scaling patches which can be quite pruritic and may lead to auto-inoculation or scalp alopecia. Skin scraping in 10% KOH will demonstrate fungal hyphae. Infected hairs when examined under black light will fluoresce a green-yellow color. Treatment of selected areas is as follows:

1. **Tinea corporis (body, ringworm), tinea cruris (perineum, jock itch), tinea pedis (foot, athlete's foot).** Topical tolnaftate (Tinactin—OTC) or clotrimazole (Lotrimin) TID until clear, and then 1 to 2 weeks longer.

2. **Tinea capitis (scalp and hair).** Micronized griseofulvin is usually used for up to 4 to 8 weeks. Itraconazole, fluconazole, and terbinafine may work also. Adjunctive therapy includes selenium sulfide shampoo Q2-3 days.

3. **Tinea unguis or onychomycosis (nails).** Griseofulvin 500 mg BID for a period of 4 to 6 months or itraconazole 200 mg BID for 4 months (1 week on, 3 weeks off), latter regimen is very expensive. An alternative is terbinafine 250 mg PO QID for 12 weeks or BID for 1 week of the month for 3 or 4 months. Success rates are about 75% but may recur. The newer nail-paint preparations are expensive and have a very poor success rate.

C. **Tinea (pityriasis) versicolor** appears as slightly pigmented, superficial, and tan scaling plaques of various sizes, primarily on the neck, trunk, and proximal arms. With sun exposure, the infected regions do not tan and appear hypopigmented. Usually caused by *Malassezia furfur.* Diagnosis is via clinical exam and KOH preparations of skin scraping. Treatment can be with topical imidazoles twice daily or washing with zinc or selenium shampoos daily for 2-3 weeks. Although not FDA approved, ketoconazole 400 mg can be given as a single dose. Have the patient exercise to a sweat and not shower for at least 4 hours afterwards. This has up to a 97% success rate in a single dose. Alternatives are ketoconazole 200 mg PO QD for 7 days or either fluconazole or itraconazole 400 mg PO QD for 7 days.

17

DERMATOLOGY

ACNE

I. **Overview.** Acne commonly begins in adolescence with stimulation of the sebaceous glands by sex hormones, primarily androgens. Can be aggravated by drugs, steroids, cosmetics, comedogenic agents, picking, and squeezing. No convincing evidence indicates diet, stress, or hygiene worsens acne. Acne has a predilection for the face, upper neck, chest, and back. In females with severe acne, consider polycystic ovarian disease (see Chapter 13), "congenital" adrenal hyperplasia, or Cushing's disease.

II. **Types of Acne and Their Treatment.**

A. **Comedones**

1. Appear as whiteheads and blackheads (closed and open comedones, respectively).

2. **Treatment** is with topical agents and takes a minimum of 2 weeks to show any improvement. Patient education is important since attempts to extrude blackheads or pustules may lead to deeper, potentially scarring lesions:

   a. **Tretinoin** (Retin A) is the treatment of choice. Begin with nightly application of 0.025% cream or 0.01% gel and increase concentration as necessary and as tolerated. Usually requires 3 to 5 months of therapy. There is now a new delivery system called Retin-A Micro (0.1% gel) is less irritating than 0.1% tretinoin cream.

   b. **Benzoyl peroxide,** available in 2.5%, 5%, and 10% strengths as lotions and gels, should be applied frequently enough (QD to BID) to produce drying and even scaling, but without significant irritation. Because it is an oxidizer, benzoyl peroxide may bleach clothing or other linens.

    c. Benzoyl peroxide in the morning can be alternated with topical tretinoin at bedtime.

    d. Scrubbing the skin is counterproductive and should be discouraged.

    e. **Azelaic acid.** First used as a treatment for hyperpigmentation. It has antibacterial and anti-keratinizing properties and is as effective as benzoyl peroxide and tretinoin. However, side effects of erythema and skin irritation are less than the other agents. Comes as 20% cream applied bid. Use with caution in darker-skinned people.

    f. **Adapalene** (Differin). Also a retinoid like tretinoin. Comes as 0.1% gel or solution and is used daily in the evening. It is at least as effective as 0.025% tretinoin gel and less irritating.

B. **Papulopustular**

  1. Have a significant inflammatory component with inflamed papules and pustules.

  2. **Treatment** is as listed above with the addition of antibiotics. As the inflammation decreases, the antibiotics can be tapered and discontinued.

    a. **For less severe cases,** use topical erythromycin 2%-4% solution, gel, or ointment applied BID; clindamycin 1% solution, gel, or lotion; or tetracycline 4% applied BID.

    b. **Moderate-to-severe cases require the use of systemic antibiotics.** Tetracycline 250 mg to 1000 mg, doxycycline 100 mg, erythromycin 500 to 1000 mg, or minocycline 50 mg QD-TID are reasonable alternatives. These should be taken for 6 weeks before efficacy can be ascertained. With improvement, the dose can be tapered gradually. NOTE: Do not administer tetracycline to pregnant women or children under 12 years of age.

C. **Nodulocystic acne**

  1. Manifested by comedones, inflammatory papules/pustules, and deep, inflamed nodules and cysts. Can result in scarring. Hypertrophic scars often form on the chest and back.

  2. **Treatment** consists of two modalities in addition to the regimens previously mentioned.

    a. **Corticosteroid.** Injection of enough corticosteroid, triamcinolone 5 mg/ml, to cause the cyst to blanch. Some recommend needle drainage of the cyst first.

    b. **Oral isotretinoin (Accutane),** 0.5-2 mg/kg/day with meals for a 4-5 month course, is usually highly effective but expensive. It is absolutely contraindicated in pregnancy; thus, a negative pregnancy test must be obtained within 2 weeks of initiating treatment, and two forms of contraception must be used from 1 month before to 1 month after therapy. Careful monitoring of liver function tests and serum lipid levels is required. Monitor for side effects as well (e.g., dry eyes, chapped lips, epistaxis, pruritus, alopecia, scaling on the palms and soles, inability to wear contacts, and pseudotumor cerebri).

    c. Other therapies include (1) estrogen with low androgenic proges-
terone (e.g., Ortho-Cept although any OCP will do) in the form
of an oral contraceptive) for girls older than age 16 years unresponsive to antibiotics and not a candidate for Accutane; (2) spironolactone for a patient with evidence of androgen excess; or
(3) comedo extraction.

III. **Other Acneform Eruptions.**
A. **Acne in the pediatric population**
    1. **Acne neonatorum**—positive family history; occurs in children less
than three months of age; usually self-limited.
    2. **Acne of infancy** occurs in infants between three months and two
years of age and there is usually a positive family history; consider
comedogenic agents, virilization, and candidiasis.
B. **Acne secondary to chemical exposure (Acne venenata, Chloracne).**
Acne caused by chemicals agent via sufficient contact in sensitive individuals. Good prognosis with avoidance. Examples are chlorinated hydro-
carbons, insoluble cutting-oils (impure paraffin-oil mixtures), and other
petroleum products (crude petroleum, heavy coal tar distillates), dioxin.
C. **Acne medicamentosa**—induction or aggravation of preexisting acne.
Agents include phenobarbital, corticosteroids, isoniazid, iodides and bro-
mides, and vitamins D and B_{12}.

17

DERMATOLOGY

PAPULOSQUAMOUS DISEASES

I. **Significant Plaque Formation.**
A. **Psoriasis.** A common skin disorder affecting over 1% of the population.
Primary lesions are erythematous papules and plaques with gray/white,
silvery scale. It usually occurs on extensor surfaces (elbows, knees, lumbosacral areas) and frequently only on the scalp (where it is difficult to
differentiate from seborrheic dermatitis). Guttate psoriasis, which presents as diffuse, small, plaques, especially on the trunk and extremities
but excluding the palms and soles, may occur after an antecedent URI
or streptococcal pharyngitis. Psoriasis may manifest the Koebner phenomenon (lesions may appear at sites of trauma, e.g., an excoriation,
tattoo, burn, etc.). Removal of the scale often causes tiny bleeding
points (Auspitz sign). Nails manifest pitting and stippling, and distal and
lateral onycholysis is common. Psoriatic arthritis can affect the DIPs and
MCPs, but rheumatoid factor is usually negative.
    1. **Treatment of psoriasis.** Topical corticosteroids can be helpful, as can
keratolytics such as salicylic acid. Keeping areas moisturized with
topical emollients or urea can be beneficial. Calcipotriene (Dovonex)
0.005% applied topically BID is a newer topical treatment for mildly
to moderately severe psoriasis (but is not used on the face or groin
where it may cause irritant dermatitis). The efficacy of calcipotriene is
comparable to mid-potency topical corticosteroids; however, it does
not cause skin atrophy or tachyphylaxis.

2. Treatment with topical crude coal tar formulas and daily exposure to UV light may also be used.

3. Severe forms of psoriasis should be referred to a dermatologist for other forms of treatment, including: etretinate (Tegison), cyclosporine (Sandimmune), isotretinoin (Accutane), methotrexate, hydroxyurea, inhibitors of EGFR kinase, CO2 resurfacing laser, electrodesiccation with curettage, or PUVA (psoralen photochemotherapy). Moreover, studies look promising using a new IL-2 fusion protein treatment.

B. **Lupus erythematosus (discoid type).** Characterized by extensive papules and plaques with adherent scaling, which later involute and scar centrally leaving an annular or polycyclic pattern with irregular borders. Primarily affects the face and scalp, but other areas include: nose, dorsa of forearms, hands, fingers, toes, and less frequently the trunk. The lupus band test (biopsy showing IgG deposits at the dermoepidermal junction) is positive in 90% of active lesions at least 6 weeks old and not recently treated with topical corticosteroids; however, the test is negative in burned-out (scarred) lesions and in normal skin. Treatment with antimalarial drugs (hydroxychloroquine 6.5 mg/kg/day), topical fluorinated corticosteroids, or intralesional corticosteroids (triamcinolone acetonide 3-5 mg/ml) helps control or clear the eruption. Only 1-5% may develop SLE. Thalidomide has been used for persistent discoid lesions in patients with SLE.

II. **Nonconfluent Papules.**

A. **Lichen planus.** A pruritic eruption in which violaceous, flat, polygonal papules occur in linear, annular, or confluent groups. Lesions of the mucous membranes appear as whitish, reticulated, lacy plaques of the buccal mucosa, which may be painful (Wickham's striae). Lichen planus exhibits the Koebner phenomenon (lesions may appear at sites of trauma, e.g., an excoriation, tattoo, burn, etc). Treatment of this chronic, idiopathic, self-limited disease is supportive with topical corticosteroids (antiinflammatory), systemic antihistamines (antipruritic), and occasionally intralesional corticosteroids (help to flatten large plaques). Short doses of alternate-day prednisone will temporarily suppress active lesions. Vulvar lichen planus can occur in isolation. It can become chronic and has malignant potential. Referral to gynecology is warranted.

B. **Pityriasis rosea.** Characterized by occurrence of a herald patch, which is larger than other lesions. The cause may be viral with recent evidence suggesting human herpes virus 7 (HHV-7), although other studies refute this. It is usually a bright red, round or oval, sharply demarcated plaque (2 to 5cm) with scaly margins and central clearing. A few days to weeks later a generalized reaction occurs, frequently in a "fir tree" pattern. Pruritus may be severe. Treatment is not indicated since the eruption is self-limited (usually clears in 4 to 10 weeks and seldom recurs). Oral antihistamines (hydroxyzine or diphenhydramine) are used to alleviate the itching and a mild hydrocortisone cream may soothe the skin. New evidence suggests that oral erythromycin used for 14 days is effective for some. Must differentiate this from secondary syphilis.

VESICULOBULLOUS LESIONS

I. **Vesicular Disease.**

A. **Dermatitis herpetiformis (DH).** Lesions consist of extremely itchy, tense, grouped herpetiform vesicles usually 3 to 6 mm in diameter and occurring in a distinctive distribution over the elbows, knees, buttocks, upper back, and posterior scalp. Because of excoriation, round crusts are often the only visible sign of the disease. The gold standard for diagnosis is biopsy with direct immunofluorescence of lesional or normal skin showing IgA deposits, usually in a granular pattern at the tips of dermal papillae. About 90% of patients will have evidence of gluten-sensitive enteropathy on small-bowel biopsy. However, fewer than 10% of patients with DH have GI symptoms suggestive of celiac disease. Both skin and bowel disease regress after several months of a gluten-free diet (see also Chapter 5). The mainstay of treatment is lifelong Dapsone 100 mg PO QD (pruritus and new lesions stop in 24 hours). CBC should be monitored every 1-2 weeks for the first 3 months to detect agranulocytosis. Liver function tests should be performed regularly to detect idiosyncratic dapsone-induced hepatitis.

II. **Bullous Diseases.**

A. **Bullous pemphigoid.** An autoimmune subepidermal disease with blisters that are tense, round, well defined, and usually occurring on a pink, edematous, inflamed base. Before the bullae form, severely itchy urticarial plaques may be present for several weeks. Flexural areas and the lower legs are the sites of predilection. Diagnosis is confirmed by biopsy of perilesional skin, which reveals many eosinophils and neutrophils in and below the bulla at the dermoepidermal junction. On electron microscopy, the split is seen at the level of the lamina lucida where the bullous pemphigoid antigen is found. Control is usually achieved with a daily dose of 60 to 80 mg of prednisone initially, followed by fairly rapid tapering to 30 to 40 mg and then slower tapering. Dapsone, cyclophosphamide, or azathioprine are often added if there is difficulty tapering the steroid. The disease often remits in 1-2 years, and steroids can be stopped. Relapse in only 10%.

B. **Pemphigus vulgaris.** Lesions begin around or in the mouth, or on the scalp, and can spread to any area. Primary lesions are flaccid, non-inflamed bullae, which break easily and leave large denuded areas, which then crust. Nikolsky's sign is positive (lateral pressure results in dramatic extension of blisters. Lesions heal with temporary hyperpigmentation but without scarring. A pemphigus-like eruption has been reported with use of certain medications: penicillamine (Cuprimine, Depen), captopril (Capoten), piroxicam (Feldene), penicillin, rifampin, phenobarbital. Diagnosis is confirmed by biopsy of the skin or oral mucosa adjacent to active blisters; in virtually 100% of pemphigus cases of all types, IgG and C3 are seen outlining the intracellular spaces of the epidermis. Therapy is with high dose steroids, which dramatically re-

17

DERMATOLOGY

duces the mortality rate; referral to a dermatologist is suggested. A common approach is to start with 80 mg of prednisone daily and increase the dose by 50% every 7 days until no new blisters form. If the dose nears 200 mg, then consider IV pulse therapy with steroids or plasmapheresis. After control is achieved, an immunosuppressive agent [most commonly azathioprine (Imuran), or cyclophosphamide (Cytoxan, Neosar)] is added to allow steroid tapering.

C. **Erythema multiforme (EM).** An acute, self-limiting vascular skin reaction with a wide variety of causes. Early lesions are pink, edematous papules; some of these evolve into hallmark target lesions (flat, dull red macules with central clearing or vesicle formation). The distribution is symmetric with lesions occurring on the palms, soles, extensor extremities, and often on oral mucosa. Herpes simplex infection causes most mild, recurrent cases. More severe, widespread cases may be caused by other infectious agents, especially Mycoplasma species and viruses, and by medications, especially penicillins, sulfonamides, anticonvulsants, nonsteroidal anti-inflammatory drugs, topical steroids, topical aminoglycosides, and allopurinol. The lesions of EM are often preceded by a prodrome of fever, malaise, myalgias, and upper respiratory symptoms. Mild cases are self limited over a 7- to 10-day period and may not require treatment. Suppressive doses of anti-herpes drug (see Chapter 8) may prevent recurrences associated with herpesvirus. For more severe or widespread disease, treatment involves prednisone (see section on treatment for EM variants).

D. **EM variants.**

1. **Stevens-Johnson syndrome.** Severe mucosal erosions (mouth, vagina, etc) accompanied by high fever and severe constitutional symptoms usually associated with extensive bullous erythema multiforme of the skin. Stevens-Johnson syndrome may be related to infections with herpesviruses or mycoplasma or a drug allergy. May require ocular steroids to prevent synechiae formation. Generally requires dermatology and/or burn unit care.

2. **Toxic epidermal necrolysis (TEN).** Almost always drug-induced (see drugs listed under EM). It is manifested by a burning or painful eruption that predominates on the trunk and proximal extremities. Painful edematous erythema of palms and soles often develops. The initial presentation is followed by epidermal necrosis and sloughing of the skin and mucous membranes. 20%-100% of total body surface area can be affected. The mortality rates are ~30%. Treatment: A short 2-3 week course of prednisone, starting at 30 to 40 mg is given. Severe cases of TEN should be treated in a burn unit. Dermatology consult should be obtained.

WHITE LESIONS

I. **White Patches And Plaques.**

A. **Vitiligo.** An idiopathic, circumscribed hypomelanosis of skin and hair. It may be an autoimmune disease and is associated with other autoimmune diseases: pernicious anemia, diabetes mellitus, and Addison's disease. Peak incidence is 10 to 30 years of age. Occurs in all races but is most cosmetically disfiguring in darker-skinned people. Affected individuals develop white macules varying in size from 1.0 mm to large areas of the body, often in a symmetrical pattern and at sites of repeated trauma, such as the bony prominences (malleoli, tip of the elbow, and necklace area). The treatment of vitiligo is most appropriately managed by a dermatologist and consists of PUVA photochemotherapy and bleaching of normally pigmented skin.

II. **White Papules.**

A. **Milia.** A 1.0 to 2.0 mm, superficial, white-to-yellow, keratin-containing epidermal cyst, occurring multiply, located on the eyelids, cheeks, and forehead in pilosebaceous follicles and at sites of trauma (often the dorsal surface of the hands and over the knees). They are usually asymptomatic. Treatment consists of incision and expression of the white keratin plug.

B. **Keratosis pilaris.** A common condition of children and young adults that consists of clustered, firm, white papules approximately 1 mm in diameter formed at a follicular orifice. The lesions have a sandpaper feel on palpation and are usually asymptomatic, though sometimes associated with mild pruritus. Lesions are most common on the lateral arms, anterior thighs, and buttocks. Topical application of alpha-hydroxy acids, such as glycolic acid and lactic acid, is quite effective.

17

DERMATOLOGY

OTHER DERMATITIDES

I. **Allergic contact dermatitis** (e.g., poison ivy, poison oak, etc.). A pruritic, inflammatory reaction that progresses from erythema and irritation to a blistering, vesiculobullous exanthem, caused by a reaction to a sensitizing chemical (not necessarily a caustic agent) via a delayed cellular (type IV) hypersensitivity mechanism. The reaction requires a prior exposure. The location of the lesion often suggests the diagnosis. The eyelids are very sensitive and may react when other skin does not. Oleoresins (poison ivy, oak and sumac) and a few chemicals (DNCB) will sensitize almost everyone. Other common agents are dyes/coloring agents, tanning chemicals, nickel, mercury, soaps, and perfumes. Common drugs include ethylenediamine, thimerosal, bacitracin, and sun-screen lotions. The patch test, in which a dilute solution of the suspected culprit is allowed to react with normal skin, is diagnostic. Treatment consists of symptomatic care with wet to dry soaks of astringent solutions (Burow's solution) and antipruritics (e.g., diphenhydramine or hydroxyzine). Acetaminophen or ibuprofen will also help with pruritus. Oral corticosteroids are effective and indicated for the treatment of severe cases with involvement of large areas of the skin, swelling of the face or genitalia, or large areas of bullae. Steroids should be tapered over several weeks. Poison ivy can be prevented by the use of Armor-All, a preexposure barrier available at drug stores. Postcontact prevention of poison ivy includes washing with soap and water and Tecnu, which neutralizes the sensitizing resin.

B. **Irritant contact dermatitis.** Caused by exposure to caustic agents. Will cause a reaction consisting of irritation progressing to erythema and inflammation. Treatment consists of thorough cleansing of the affected region with cool water, and supportive measures ranging from moisturizing lotions and antiseptic creams to systemic steroids and antibiotics depending on the insult to the skin (see also Chapter 2).

C. **Seborrheic dermatitis.** A common condition, usually first noticed as dandruff. It affects the scalp, the center of the face, the anterior portion of the chest, and/or the flexural creases of the arms, legs, and groin (i.e., areas of the body that have high concentrations of sebaceous glands). Most commonly affects infants (ages 1-3 months) and adults ages 30-60. Typically presents as a greasy scale on the scalp, with erythema and scaling of the nasolabial folds and retroauricular skin. Seborrheic dermatitis is said to be associated with: deficiencies of riboflavin, biotin, or pyridoxine; and various neurologic disorders (parkinsonism, post-CVAs, epilepsy, CNS trauma, facial nerve palsy, and syringomyelia). New onset severe seborrheic dermatitis may be associated with HIV. Treatment for infants is a mild, nonmedicated shampoo. In adults or refractory infant cases use a shampoo 2-3 times a week containing one of the following: salicylic acid (X-Seb T, Sebulex), selenium sulfide (Selsun, Exsel), coal tar (DHS Tar, Neutrogena T-Gel, Polytar), or pyrithione zinc (DHS Zinc, Danex, Sebulon). More severe cases may be treated with medicated shampoos (ketoconazole [Nizoral] 2% initially daily then tapered to once a week if possible; see Table 17-1). A new therapy is a topical form of gamma-linoleic acid, Borge oil, which is effective in infantile seborrheic dermatitis.

D. **Xerotic eczema (winter itch, asteatotic eczema).** A relatively common dermatitis that occurs in the winter and in the elderly and is characterized by dry, cracked, fissured skin and pruritus. Predisposing factors include old age; a genetic tendency for dry skin; too frequent bathing; and dry, non-humidified heated rooms. Treatment includes (1) avoidance of over-bathing with soap; (2) room humidifiers; (3) tepid water baths using bath oils with liberal application of emollients after drying; (4) medium-potency corticosteroids applied BID until eczema clears; and (5) topical alpha-hydroxy acids (e.g., glycolic acid or lactic acid).

II. **Eczema with Significant Excoriations.**

A. **Atopic dermatitis** (infantile eczema, neurodermatitis). Caused by a genetic predisposition to react to environmental allergens with the development of a pruritic, inflammatory rash. Atopic dermatitis is associated with asthma, hay fever, and urticaria. Elevated levels of IgE have been associated with atopic dermatitis. The features vary with age. Atopic dermatitis commonly begins as infantile eczema, affecting the face, scalp, and upper extremities, often associated with food consumption (cheese, egg white, wheat, legumes, nuts). This may resolve or progress to involve the neck and the upper and lower extremities, especially the popliteal and the antecubital fossae. Vesiculation, oozing, and crusting are common, and lesions are very pruritic manifesting lichenified, reddened skin due to excoriation. Stress may be a contributing factor in exacerbations. **Treatment** is directed at relieving pruritus, controlling infection, and promoting healing. Vesicals and crusting is treated with wet-to-dry dressings of cool Burow's solution and oral antihistamines to relieve the pruritus. Topical corticosteroids and emollient creams can also be used once the lesions are clean. Use of steroids and emollients under occlusion may be helpful (i.e., under gloves or a PVC body suit at night). A course of anti-staphylococcal antibiotics for 2 weeks may be helpful in acute exacerbations since there seems to be an infectious trigger to many episodes. A short course of systemic corticosteroids is not unreasonable; cyclosporine has been used in severe cases but should be prescribed under the direction of a dermatologist. **Avoidance is important,** and a trial of environmental control, elimination of specific foods, and skin testing for food and inhalant allergens might be useful.

B. **Stasis dermatitis.** Chronic dermatitis of the lower legs in people with chronic venous insufficiency. Associated with mild pruritus, pain (if an ulcer is present), aching discomfort in the limb, swelling of the ankle, and nocturnal cramps. Lesions consist of erythematous scaling plaques with exudation, crusts, and superficial ulcers particularly on the medial aspect of the ankle. Acute treatment of stasis dermatitis consists of Burow's wet dressings and cooling pastes, topical corticosteroids, and systemic antibiotics if cellulitis is present. Chronic treatment of stasis dermatitis includes: topical corticosteroids, supportive stockings (Jobst, TEDs), compressive bandages, and/or vein surgery; an Unna boot (zinc oxide impregnated gauze) can be placed for 72 hours to promote healing of skin and ulcers. If ulcers are not present, then treatment includes wet-to-dry dressings using normal saline or Dakin's solution; silver sulfadiazine applied between wet-to-dry dressings; elevation of the leg; compressive bandages; supportive stockings; and/or surgery. Becaplermin (Regranex) a platelet-growth factor has been used to promote ulcer healing but is expensive and of limited efficacy. Pentoxifylline is also beneficial in healing recalcitrant ulcers.

C. **Dyshidrotic eczema.** Presents with deep-seated, pruritic, tapioca-like vesicles on the palms, soles, or sides of the fingers. The differential diagnosis includes pustular psoriasis. Dyshidrosis may begin in childhood or adult life and may be an ID reaction to infection elsewhere, especially to tinea. **Treatment** is often unsatisfactory. Treatment of the vesicular stage includes Burow's wet dressings BID and/or "black cat" (10% crude coal tar in equal parts of acetone and flexible collodion) applied once daily. In moderate or severe disease, erythromycin or dicloxacillin 250 mg QID

17

DERMATOLOGY

should be started because bacterial infection may be present even without obvious signs (crusts, tenderness, etc.). Additional measures include the use of intermittent high-potency topical steroids or a burst of systemic steroids. Dietary restriction of certain metals (cobalt, nickel, or chromium) has been found to be successful in uncontrolled trials. PUVA is saved for severe refractory disease.

III. **Other Eczematous Eruptions.**

A. **Nummular (discoid) eczema.** A chronic, pruritic, inflammatory dermatitis occurring in the form of coin-shaped plaques (4-5 cm in diameter). Especially prevalent during the winter months and in atopic individuals. **Treatment** includes topical corticosteroids, oral dicloxacillin or erythromycin if infected, crude coal-tar pastes, and skin moisturizers.

B. **Lichen simplex chronicus (neurodermatitis).** A circumscribed area of lichenification caused by repeated physical trauma (rubbing and scratching). It occurs in the anogenital area and on the nuchal areas, arms, legs, and ankles. **Treatment.** Stop the rubbing and scratching with antiinflammatory agents (crude coal tar and topical corticosteroids) covered by continuous dry occlusive gauze dressings. Intralesional corticosteroids are effective for small, localized areas. Treatment is needed long-term and may be unsatisfactory.

URTICARIA

I. **Overview.** Urticaria is a common disorder that affect 15%-20% of the population at some time. Urticaria is characterized by a transient, pruritic, patchy eruption that consists of lightly erythematous papules or wheals with raised borders and blanched centers involving the superficial skin layers; involvement of the deeper layers and/or the submucosa is called *angioedema*. Lesions vary considerably in size, from 2 mm to over 30 cm and may be circular or irregularly shaped. The most common site for urticaria is the trunk, although lesions may occur on any part of the body. Urticaria has been divided into two major groups:

A. **Acute urticaria.** Defined as hives persisting for less than 4 to 6 weeks (usually two to three days). It occurs with a higher incidence in atopic individuals. Commonly identified causes include foods, drugs, and infections but in over half of patients there is no identifiable cause.

B. **Angioedema.** Acute attacks are manifested as large irregular areas of subcutaneous swelling. Cause is similar to urticaria but may also include hereditary angioedema (see below) or, commonly, ACE inhibitors

C. **Chronic urticaria.** Attacks which persist for six weeks or more. Patients usually are not atopic.

II. **Types Of Urticaria.**

A. **Idiopathic.** Largest category, comprising one-thirds of acute and two-thirds of chronic cases of urticaria.

B. **Physical.** Comprises approximately 15% of the cases. Consists of several types:

    1. **Dermatographism.** A reaction to firm stroking of the skin that occurs

within 1-3 minutes and lasts 5-10 minutes. It is not true urticaria, although it may be severe enough to seek medical help.

2. **Cholinergic urticaria.** Exercise and/or sweating is the provocative agent. Cause of 10% of reactions, affects young people, and may last 6-8 years. Lesions appear as 1-2 mm wheals on a confluent erythematous base and are found on the trunk and arms with sparing of the palms, soles, and the axillae.

3. **Cold urticaria.** An uncommon reaction to cold and/or rewarming after cold exposure (cold winds are an effective stimulus); can be caused by syphilis. Diagnose by exposure of the skin to an ice cube.

4. **Solar urticaria.** Rare reaction caused by exposure to light. Appears as pruritus and erythema, followed by urticaria. Sudden onset and occurs in any age group.

5. **Delayed pressure urticaria.** Rare reaction caused by sustained pressure.

6. **Aquagenic urticaria.** Rare reaction caused by contact with water.

7. **Localized heat urticaria.** Rare reaction caused by hot water.

C. **Immunologic.** Examples include anaphylaxis, serum sickness, and atopic persons with seasonal exacerbations. Some common antigens include foods (fish, nuts, berries, eggs) or insect stings (bees, wasps, hornets, yellow jackets). Drugs can induce urticaria, especially PCN and sulfonamides. Urticaria can also be caused by immune complexes seen in systemic rheumatologic diseases (systemic lupus erythematous, Sjögren's syndrome, rheumatic fever, juvenile rheumatoid arthritis, chronic hepatitis B and C, necrotizing vasculitis, and polymyositis), cryoglobulinemias, serum sickness, neoplastic disorders, transfusion reactions, Epstein-Barr virus, and streptococcal infections.

D. **Hereditary angioedema.** A potentially fatal, autosomal dominant disease caused by the functional absence of C1-esterase inhibitor. This enables vascular permeability and potentially fatal, recurrent, acute angioedema of the skin, mucosa, and airway. One retrospective survey of 58 patients found that 40% had died by asphyxiation with average age at death of 39. Occasionally, presents with acute abdominal symptoms mimicking a surgical abdomen. Serum levels of C2 are normal during asymptomatic periods but decreased during an attack. C4 and CH-50 are low all the time. Low C1-esterase inhibitor levels are diagnostic. However, there are non-functioning alleles of C1-esterase inhibitor so some individuals with the disease will have normal levels; a functional assay should be performed if clinically indicated. **Treatment.** Patients with hereditary angioedema should be pre-treated with fresh frozen plasma before painful procedures or procedures known to induce attacks. Additionally, they can be treated with fresh frozen plasma to abort an ongoing attack. C1-esterase inhibitor is currently investigational but should have FDA approval soon. Long-term therapy includes enough danazol to prevent acute attacks. (200 mg TID or less).

17

DERMATOLOGY

E. **Infections.** Urticaria is occasionally associated with acute and chronic infections including protozoan, parasitic, bacterial and viral infections. Sources such as sinusitis, dental abscesses, periodontal disease, gallbladder infection, chronic bronchitis, chronic UTIs, and low grade fungal (athlete's foot) or yeast *(Candida vaginitis)* infections should be investigated in persons with chronic urticaria.

F. **Infestations.** Most commonly due to scabies, caused by the mite *Sarcoptes scabiei.* See section on scabies in Chapter 10 for details.

G. **Urticaria pigmentosa.** An uncommon disease with focal dermal infiltration of tissue mast cells, can have infiltrates in other organs, as well with representative organ system disease. It presents as brown patches which form a wheal and flare upon stroking.

H. Miscellaneous
   1. **Neoplastic disorders.** Carcinoma (colorectal, lung, ovarian, uterine, liver), choriocarcinoma, Hodgkin's disease, lymphoma, leukemia, or myeloma.
   2. **Endocrinopathy.** Hypothyroidism or hyperthyroidism, hyperparathyroidism, diabetes mellitus, menopause.
   3. **Arthropod assault** (insect bite). A papular lesion, usually to flea/red ant bite.
   4. **Psychogenic.** A diagnosis of exclusion, but psychogenic and emotional factors are contributory/aggravating in at least one-fourth of chronic urticaria patients.

III. **Diagnostic Tests For Urticaria.**

A. **Acute urticaria.** Laboratory tests generally are not needed.

B. **Chronic urticaria.** If physical agents have been excluded as a cause, then judicious use of the following laboratory, radiographic, and pathology studies may provide clues to the diagnosis of an occult systemic illness. However, extensive work-up is expensive and rarely yields results.
   1. Routine tests
      a. **Laboratory:** CBC, chemistry profile, ESR, T_4, TSH measurements, UA and urine culture, ANA
      b. **Radiographic:** CXR, sinus films, dental films/Panorex
   2. **Selective tests:** Cryoglobulin, hepatitis and syphilis serology, rheumatoid factor, serum complement, serum IgE, IgM
   3. **Skin biopsy** (if the ESR is elevated, to exclude urticarial vasculitis).

IV. Treatment of Urticaria.

A. **Treatment as for anaphylaxis. See Chapter 2.**

B. **Hereditary angioedema** does not respond to typical therapy as outlined below. See section on hereditary angioedema for management.

C. **Eliminate or limit exposure** to the causative agent.

D. Treat any underlying disease they may be a causative factor.

E. Symptomatic care
   1. Antihistamines
      a. **Classic H_1 blockers** include chlorpheniramine (Chlor-Trimeton) 4 mg Q4-6h, cyproheptadine (Periactin) 4-8 mg Q6h, diphenhydramine (Benadryl) 25-50 mg Q6-8h, hydroxyzine (Atarax,

TABLE 17-1

POTENCY OF TOPICAL CORTICOSTEROIDS*

Group[1]	%[2]	Generic Name[3]
I	0.05	Betamethasone dipropionate
II	0.01	Amcinonide
	0.05	Fluocinonide
	0.25	Desoximetasone
III	0.5	Triamcinolone acetonide
	0.1	Betamethasone valerate
IV	0.05	Flurandrenolide
	0.025	Fluocinolone acetonide
V	0.1	Betamethasone valerate
VI	0.01	Fluocinolone acetonide
	0.03	Flumethasone pivalate
VII	0.2	Betamethasone valerate
	1-2.5	Hydrocortisone

Adapted from Habif TP: *Clinical dermatology: a color guide to diagnosis and therapy*, ed 3, St. Louis, 1993, Mosby.

*Rule of nines: For three × daily application, 9 g of cream covers 1% of skin area daily.

[1]Potencies decrease from group I (strongest) to group VII (weakest).

[2]Increasing the concentration increases the potency. At equal concentrations, potency decreases as the viscosity of the substance increases.

[3]Brand name drugs are available in a variety of strengths and vehicles (such as ointment, solution, cream, lotion).

Vistaril) 25-50 mg Q6-8h, and promethazine (Phenergan) 12.5-25 mg Q12-24h. Hydroxyzine is believed to be one of the most effective agents, while diphenhydramine and chlorpheniramine are less expensive and OTC.

b. **Nonsedating H_1 blockers** include fexofenadine (Allegra), loratadine (Claritin), and cetirizine (Zyrtec). They are equally effective compared to classic agents, less sedating, and have simpler dosing schedules.

c. **H_2 blockers** (e.g., cimetidine [Tagamet], ranitidine [Zantac], etc.) may be added in patients who do not respond to therapy with H_1 antagonists alone.

d. **Oral beta agonists,** such as terbutaline (Brethine, Bricanyl), may a useful adjunct to antihistamines in chronic urticaria.

e. **Doxepin** (Adapin, Sinequan) is a potent H1 blocker with efficacy comparable to hydroxyzine.

2. **Topical application of capsaicin** (Zostrix) or local anesthetic can suppress wheal-and-flare reactions in local heat urticaria.

3. Stress-related urticaria (adrenergic urticaria) may respond to propanolol.

4. Cold urticaria may respond to doxepin or especially cyproheptadine 4 mg PO TID.

5. **Topical or systemic corticosteroids** should be reserved for patients with refractory symptoms. Table 17-1 lists potency of topical corticosteroids. Compared to placebo, a short course (40 mg × 5 day of prednisone) is quite effective at symptom control.
6. **New therapies currently under study** in controlled trials include ketotifen (Zaditen), cyclosporine (Sandimmune), UVB phototherapy, leukotriene inhibitors, and plasmapheresis.

BIBLIOGRAPHY

Asawanonda P et al: Pendulaser carbon dioxide resurfacing laser versus electrodesiccation with curettage in the treatment of isolated, recalcitrant psoriatic plaques, *J Amer Acad Dermatol* 42(4):660-6, 2000.

Bart BJ: Annular skin eruptions: Not every ring on the skin is ringworm, *Postgrad Med* 96(1): 37-50, 1994.

Bork K et al: Asphyxiation by laryngeal edema in patients with hereditary angioedema, *Mayo Clin Proceed* 75(4):349-54, 2000.

Cohen PR: Genodermatoses with malignant potential, *Am Fam Phys* 46(5): 1479-1486, 1992.

Cribier B et al: Treatment of lichen planus. An evidence-based medicine analysis of efficacy, *Arch Dermatol* 134(12):1521-30, 1998.

Drago F et al: Human herpesvirus 7 in patients with pityriasis rosea. Electron microscopy investigations and polymerase chain reaction in mononuclear cells, plasma and skin, *Dermatology* 195(4):374-8,1997.

Fitzpatrick TB, Johnson RA, Polano MK, et al: *Color Atlas and Synopsis of Clinical Dermatology,* Second edition, New York, 1994, McGraw-Hill.

Forsman KE: Pediculosis and scabies—What to look for in patients who are crawling with clues, *Postgrad Med* 98(6): 89-100, 1995.

Gannon T: Dermatologic emergencies: When early recognition can be lifesaving. *Postgraduate Medicine,* 1994; 96(1): 67-82.

Greaves MW, Weinstein GD: Treatment of psoriasis, *N Engl J Med* 332(9): 581-588, 1995.

Healy E, Simpson N: Acne vulgaris, *Br Med J* 308: 831-833, 1994.

Holme SA et al: Latex allergy in atopic children, *Br J Dermatol* 140(5):919-21, 1999.

Janniger CK, Schwartz RA: Seborrheic dermatitis, *Am Fam Phys* 52(1): 149-155, 1995.

Kibarian MA, Hruza GJ: Nonmelanoma skin cancer—risks, treatment options, and tips on prevention, *Postgrad Med* 98(6): 39-58, 1995.

Kirsner RS: Treatment of psoriasis: Role of calcipotriene, *Am Fam Phys* 52(1): 237-240, 1995.

Klaus MV, Wieselthier JS: Contact dermatitis, *Am Fam Phys* 48(4): 629-632, 1993.

Lewis FM: Vulval lichen planus, *Br J Dermatol* 138(4):569-75, 1998.

Mahmood T: Urticaria, *Am Fam Phys* 51(4): 811-816,1995.

Metze D: Efficacy and safety of naltrexone, an oral opiate receptor antagonist, in the treatment of pruritus in internal and dermatological diseases, *J Am Acad Dermatol* 41(4):533-9, 1999.

Millikan LE: Treating pruritus: What's new in safe relief of symptoms? *Postgrad Med* 99(1): 173-184, 1996.

Millikan LE, Shrum JP: An update on common skin diseases: acne, psoriasis, contact dermatitis, and warts, *Postgrad Med* 91(6): 96-115, 1992.

O'Dell M: Skin and wound infections: An overview, *Am Fam Phys* 57(10): 2424-32, 1998.

Olson CL: Blistering disorders: Which ones can be deadly? *Postgrad Med;* 96(1): 53-64, 1994.

Phillips TJ, Dover JS: Recent advances in dermatology, *N Engl J Med* 326(3): 167-178, 1992.

Powell TJ et al: Growth inhibition of psoriatic keritinocytes by quinazoline tyrosine kinase inhibitors, *Br J Dermatol* 141(5):802-10, 1999.

Preston DS, Stern RS: Nonmelanoma cancers of the skin, *N Engl J Med;* 327(23: 1649-1662, 1992.

Reunala T: Dermatitis herpetiformis: coeliac disease of the skin, *Ann Med* 30(5):416-8, 1998.

Russell JJ: Topical therapy for acne, *Am Fam Phys* 61(2):357-365, 2000.

Shalitaar et al: Topical erythromycin vs. clindamycin therapy for acne: Multicenter, double-blind comparison, *Arch Dermatol* 120: 351, 1984

Sharma PK et al: Erythromycin in pityriasis rosea: A double-blind, placebo-controlled clinical trial, *J Am Acad Dermatol* 42(2 Pt 1):241-4, 2000.

Siddiq MA: Erythema multiforme after application of aural Gentisone HC drops, *J Laryngol Otol* 113(11):1002-3, 1999.

Strauss JS et al: Isotretinoin therapy for acne: results of a multi-center dose-response study, *J Am Acad Dermatol* 10: 490, 1984.

Van Doorn R et al: Mycosis fungoides: Disease evolution and prognosis of 309 Dutch patients, *Arch Dermatol* 136(4):504-10, 2000.

Warren KJ et al: Thalidomide for recalcitrant discoid lesions in a patient with SLE, *J Am Acad Dermatol* 39(2 Pt 1):293-5, 1998.

Winston MH, and Shalita AR: Acne vulgaris: Pathogenesis and treatment, *Pediatr Clin North Am;* 38: 899, 1991.

17

DERMATOLOGY

PSYCHIATRY

Alison C. Abreu
Julie Kay Filips

MOOD DISORDERS

I. Major Depressive Disorder (MDD).
A. **Overview.** Lifetime risk as high as 12% for men and 26% for women.
B. **Risk factors:** female gender (especially postpartum), history of depressive illness in first-degree relatives, prior episodes of major depression, prior suicide attempts, age <40 years, medical comorbidity, decreased social support, stressful life events, and current substance or alcohol abuse.
C. **Tip-offs for depression in a primary care setting.** May include fatigue, somatic complaints (such as headache, backache, chest pain, dyspepsia, and limb pain), anxiety symptoms, depressed mood, weight loss or gain, or insomnia. Diagnostic criteria are found in Box 18-1.
D. **Symptoms can be divided into:**
   1. **Emotional.** Dysphoria, irritability, anhedonia, withdrawal.
   2. **Cognitive.** Self-criticism, sense of worthlessness or guilt, hopelessness, poor concentration, memory impairment, delusions or hallucinations.
   3. **Vegetative.** Fatigue, decreased energy, insomnia, hypersomnia, anorexia, psychomotor retardation or agitation, impaired libido.
E. **Evaluation.**
   1. **History.** May use Beck Inventory (Box 18-2) or Geriatric Depression Scale (Box 18-3) to screen for high-risk patients. If

18

BOX 18-1

DIAGNOSTIC CRITERIA: DEPRESSION

DSM-IV criteria for a major depressive episode* include at least five of the following symptoms present for at least 2 weeks that represent a change from previous level of functioning.

- Depressed mood (most of day, almost daily). Note: In children and adolescents there may be an irritable mood
- Diminished interest or pleasure in all or most activities
- Significant weight loss or gain or decrease or increase in appetite nearly every day
- Insomnia or hypersomnia

- Psychomotor retardation or agitation (observable by others)
- Fatigue or decreased level of energy
- Feelings of worthlessness or inappropriate guilt
- Poor concentration or indecisiveness
- Recurrent thoughts of death or suicidal ideation

NOTE: At least one of the symptoms must be either (1) depressed mood or (2) loss of interest or pleasure.

*To be defined as a major depressive episode, the symptoms (1) must cause clinically significant distress or impairment in functioning and (2) must not be attributable to the effects of substance use, general medical condition, or bereavement.

BOX 18-2

BECK INVENTORY FOR THE SCREENING OF DEPRESSION

Name:

Date:

On this questionnaire are groups of statements. Please read each group of statements carefully. Then pick out the one statement in each group that best describes the way you have been feeling the **past week including today.** Circle the number beside the statement you picked. If several statements in the group seem to apply equally well, circle each one. Be sure to read all the statements in each group before making your choice.

1.
0   I do not feel sad.
1   I feel sad.
2   I am sad all the time and can't snap out of it.
3   I am so sad or unhappy that I can't stand it.

2.
0   I am not particularly discouraged about the future.
1   I feel discouraged about the future.
2   I feel I have nothing to look forward to.
3   I feel that the future is hopeless and that things cannot improve.

3.
0   I do not feel like a failure.
1   I feel I have failed more than the average person.
2   As I look back on my life, all I can see is a lot of failures.
3   I feel I am a complete failure as a person.

4.
0   I get as much satisfaction out of things as I used to.
1   I don't enjoy things the way I used to.
2   I don't get real satisfaction out of anything anymore.
3   I am dissatisfied and bored with everything.

5.
0   I don't feel particularly guilty.
1   I feel guilty a good part of the time.
2   I feel quite guilty most of the time.
3   I feel guilty all of the time.

6.
0   I don't feel I am being punished.
1   I feel I may be punished.
2   I expect to be punished.
3   I feel I am being punished.

7.
0   I don't feel disappointed in myself.
1   I am disappointed in myself.
2   I am disgusted with myself.
3   I hate myself.

BOX 18-2
BECK INVENTORY FOR THE SCREENING OF DEPRESSION—cont'd

8.

0   I have not lost interest in other people.
1   I am less interested in other people than I used to be.
2   I have lost most of my interest in other people.
3   I have lost all of my interest in other people.

9.

0   I make decisions about as well as I ever could.
1   I put off making decisions more than I used to.
2   I have greater difficulty in making decisions than before.
3   I can't make decisions at all anymore.

10.

0   I don't feel I look worse than I used to.
1   I am worried that I am looking old or unattractive.
2   I feel that there are permanent changes in my appearance that make me look unattractive.
3   I believe that I look ugly.

11.

0   I can work about as well as before.
1   It takes an extra effort to get started to do something.
2   I have to push myself very hard to do anything.
3   I can't do any work at all.

12.

0   I can sleep as well as usual.
1   I get tired more easily than I used to.
2   I get tired from doing almost anything.
3   I am too tired to do anything.

13.

0   I don't get tired more than usual.
1   I get tired more easily than I used to.
2   I get tired from doing almost anything.
3   I am too tired to do anything.

14.

0   My appetite is no worse than usual.
1   My appetite is not as good as it used to be.
2   My appetite is much worse now.
3   I have no appetite at all anymore.

15.

0   I don't feel I am any worse than anybody else.
1   I am critical of myself for my weaknesses or mistakes.
2   I blame myself all the time for my faults.
3   I blame myself for everything bad that happens.

Continued

18

PSYCHIATRY

BOX 18-2

BECK INVENTORY FOR THE SCREENING OF DEPRESSION—cont'd

16.

0 I don't have any thoughts of killing myself.

1 I have thoughts of killing myself but would not carry them out.

2 I would like to kill myself.

3 I would kill myself if I had the chance.

17.

0 I am no more worried about my health than usual.

1 I am worried about physical problems such as aches and pains or upset stomach or constipation.

2 I am very worried about physical problems, and it is hard to think of much else.

3 I am so worried about my physical problems that I cannot think of anything else.

18.

0 I don't cry any more than usual.

1 I cry more now than I used to.

2 I cry all the time now.

3 I used to be able to cry, but now I can't cry even though I want to.

19.

0 I have not noticed any recent change in my interest in sex.

1 I am less interested in sex than I used to be.

2 I am much less interested in sex now.

3 I have lost interest in sex completely.

20.

0 I am no more irritated now than I ever am.

1 I get annoyed or irritated more easily than I used to.

2 I feel irritated all the time now.

3 I don't get irritated at all by the things that used to irritate me.

21.

0 I haven't lost much weight, if any lately.

1 I have lost more than 5 pounds.

2 I have lost more than 10 pounds.

3 I have lost more than 15 pounds.

(I am purposely trying to lose weight by eating less. Yes _____ No _____)

Scoring:

0-9 normal

10-15 mild depressive symptoms

16-19 mild-moderate depressive symptoms

20-29 moderate-severe depressive symptoms

30 severe depressive symptoms

BOX 18-3

GERIATRIC DEPRESSION SCALE

This may be administered in oral or written format. If written, the answer sheet must have printed Yes/No after each question. The subject is instructed to circle the better response. If given orally, the question may need to be repeated to get a response of "yes" or "no." The GDS seems to work well with other age groups.

1. Are you basically satisfied with your life? N*
2. Have you dropped many of your activities and interests? Y
3. Do you feel that your life is empty? Y
4. Do you often get bored? Y
5. Are you hopeful about the future? N
6. Are you bothered by thoughts that you just cannot get out of your head? Y
7. Are you in good spirits most of the time? N
8. Are you afraid that something bad is going to happen to you? Y
9. Do you feel happy most of the time? N
10. Do you often feel helpless? Y
11. Do you often get restless and fidgety? Y
12. Do you prefer to stay home at night, rather than go out and do new things? Y
13. Do you frequently worry about the future? Y
14. Do you feel that you have more problems with memory than most? Y
15. Do you think it is wonderful to be alive now? N
16. Do you often feel downhearted and blue? Y
17. Do you feel pretty worthless the way you are now? Y
18. Do you worry a lot about the past? Y
19. Do you find life very exciting? N
20. Is it hard for you to get started on new projects? Y
21. Do you feel full of energy? N
22. Do you feel that your situation is hopeless? Y
23. Do you think that most people are better off than you are? Y
24. Do you frequently get upset over little things? Y
25. Do you frequently feel like crying? Y
26. Do you have trouble concentrating? Y
27. Do you enjoy getting up in the morning? N
28. Do you prefer to avoid social gatherings? Y
29. Is it easy for you to make decisions? N
30. Is your mind as clear as it used to be? N

*Scoring: count 1 point for each depressive answer shown after each question. 0 to 10 = normal; 11 to 20 = mild depression; 21 to 30 = moderate or severe depression.

18

PSYCHIATRY

depressive symptoms are present, determine: Time course and severity.

   a. Any prior episodes, type of treatment, and level of recovery.
   b. Any history of manic or hypomanic episodes.
   c. If other major psychiatric disorders are present.
   d. Any suicidal ideation, plan, or intent.

2. **Examination.** Evaluate for possible related medical conditions: substance abuse, medication side effects, chronic infection and endocrine dysfunction. Mental status exam, including level of alertness, orientation, mood, affect, thought content (hallucinations, delusions, suicidal/homicidal ideation, if present), thought processes, psychomotor activity, speech, insight and judgment. Folstein minimental status exam may help identify a delirium or dementia (see Chapter 9). Beck Inventory and Geriatric Depression Scales are patient-administered. Obtain an initial score, then repeat periodically to assess response to treatment.

3. **Lab tests.** Screen for medical causes of depressive symptoms (if suspected by history or physical examination). Lab tests may include complete blood count with differential, electrolytes, renal and liver functions, thyroid studies, urine drug screen, etc.

F. **Treatment**

1. **Hospitalization.** Indicated if serious suicidal ideation is present (difficult to assess because no screening tool has high sensitivity, but ask about a plan, intent, access to the means, and ability to contract for safety). Admission is also indicated if the patient is a danger to self or others, there is a complicating medical condition, or there is lack of a support system at home.

2. **Medication (Table 18-1).** Most antidepressants are believed to be equally effective in equivalent therapeutic doses. Factors to consider in selecting a particular agent include cost, side effect profile, anti-depressants previously tried, and safety in overdose. Expect a 3- to 6-week latent period before the full effect is seen at therapeutic doses. To prevent relapse, continue medication for at least 6 to 12 months after patient becomes asymptomatic. For recurrent depression, consider chronic prophylactic therapy.

   a. Second-generation, but first-line, antidepressants
      • Selective serotonin reuptake inhibitors (SSRIs). May need to start with lower doses in the elderly or others sensitive to side effects. Titrate up as needed. Side effects vary and may include nausea, anorexia, insomnia or mild sedation, sweating, headache, tremor, sexual dysfunction, and nervousness. SSRIs are considered safe for patients with cardiovascular disease. These antidepressants are favored in **post-MI depression,** as they are not associated with increased risk of ventricular arrhythmia and are thought to have antiplatelet effects. **All SSRIs are contraindicated with**

TABLE 18-1

RELATIVE COMPARISON OF ANTIDEPRESSANTS

Drug	Common Doses Range (mg/day)*	Dosage Schedule	Orthostatic Hypotension	Anticholinergic†	Sedation	Weight Gain	Therapeutic Range ng/ml
TRICYCLIC ANTIDEPRESSANTS							
Amitriptyline (Elavil)	150-200	QHS	+++++	+++++	+++++	++	>120
Desipramine (Norpramin)	50-300	QHS	++++	++	+++	+	>125
Imipramine (Tofranil)	150-200	QHS	+++++	++++	++++	++	>225
Nortriptyline (Pamelor)	50-150	QHS	++	++	++	+	50-150
SEROTONIN-SPECIFIC REUPTAKE INHIBITORS (SSRIS)							
Fluoxetine‡ (Prozac)	20-40	QAM	Minimal to neutral with regards to sedative, anticholinergic, and orthostatic hypotensive side effects; may cause mild weight loss in some individuals. May cause akathisia if titrated up too rapidly. Also, GI side effects, anorgasmia, decreased libido.				
Paroxetine (Paxil)	20-40	QAM or QHS					
Fluvoxamine (Luvox)	120-200	QHS or BID					
Citalopram (Celexa)	20-40	QAM or QHS					
Sertraline (Zoloft)	75-150	QAM or QHS					

Adapted from Knesper DJ et al: *Primary care psychiatry*, Philadelphia, 1997, WB Saunders.

*Doses should be lowered in the elderly.

†Blurred vision, constipation, dry mouth, urinary retention.

‡Fluoxetine can be dosed 60mg PO q week for those stable on 20 mg/day.

Continued

18

PSYCHIATRY

TABLE 18-1

RELATIVE COMPARISON OF ANTIDEPRESSANTS—cont'd

Drug	Common Doses Range (mg/day)*	Dosage Schedule	Orthostatic Hypotension	Anticholinergic†	Sedation	Weight Gain	Therapeutic Range ng/ml
SEROTONIN–NONSELECTIVE REUPTAKE INHIBITORS							
Venlafaxine (Effexor)	75–225	QD-TID	0	±	+	0	NE
DOPAMINE ACTIVE							
Bupropion (Wellbutrin)	150–450	BID-TID	0	+	+	–	NE
(Wellbutrin SR)	300–400	QD-BID					
OTHER							
Nefazodone (Serzone)	300–500	BID	±	±	++	0	NE
Mirtazapine (Remeron)	15–60	QHS	±	0	+++	++	NE
Trazodone (Desyrel)	50–400	QHS-TID	+++	++	+++++	+	NE
Reboxatine (Vestra)	NA						

Adapted from Knesper DJ et al: *Primary care psychiatry,* Philadelphia, 1997, WB Saunders.
NA, Not available; *NE,* not established.
*Doses should be lowered in the elderly.
†Blurred vision, constipation, dry mouth, urinary retention.
‡Fluoxetine can be dosed 60mg PO q week for those stable on 20 mg/day.

MAOIs. If switching from an SSRI to a MAOI, need a drug-free period of 14 days for paroxetine, sertraline or fluvoxamine or 5 weeks for fluoxetine (it has a longer half-life). Taper short-acting SSRIs over several days to avoid flu-like symptoms. More expensive per pill than generic TCAs.

- **Bupropion (Wellbutrin)** a norepinephrine-dopamine reuptake inhibitor. Very low incidence of sexual dysfunction. Safe in patients with history of cardiac disease. It may be especially useful in those with prominent apathy. SR formulation improves compliance with BID dosing instead of TID. Contraindicated in patients with seizure disorder (lowers seizure threshold, risk of seizures 0.4%) or history of bulimia or anorexia nervosa. Also used for smoking cessation (Zyban).

- **Venlafaxine (Effexor).** Monitor for blood pressure elevation. Demonstrated effective for patients with melancholic depression. Consider using it in patients with resistant depression.

- **Nefazodone (Serzone).** Consider for patients experiencing either poor response or intolerable side effects from other antidepressants. Especially good in those with insomnia. Safe for patients with heart disease.

- **Mirtazepine (Remeron).** Well tolerated, sexual side effect rate equal to placebo. Sedating, useful for patients with comorbid sleep disturbance (give at bedtime). Also good in those with anorexia.

- **Trazodone (Desyrel).** Can be quite sedating at therapeutic doses. Some but not all studies have shown it to be as effective as SSRIs in those who tolerate it. Patients with cardiac arrhythmias or mitral valve prolapse should be closely monitored. Because it is highly sedating, low doses (50-200 mg) are often used as monotherapy or adjunct to certain antidepressants as a sleep aid at bedtime. Risk of priapism 1:6000.

- **Reboxetine (Vestra).** A newer agent in the class of Selective Norepinephrine Reuptake Inhibitors (SNRIs). Studies show it to be as effective as SSRIs and TCAs. May particularly benefit depressed patients with atomisation and anhedonia.

b. **Tricyclic antidepressants (TCAs).** Although no longer first-line, this class of antidepressants is useful in certain circumstances. They are generally less expensive than the newer agents, they are often sedating and can aid in sleep restoration, and they are also useful in management of chronic or neuropathic pain. They are a poor choice in patients who may take an overdose. May be fatal in overdoses around 2000 mg or more in adults. In selecting a TCA consider the patient's sedation requirements as well as ability

18

PSYCHIATRY

to tolerate orthostatic hypotension, weight gain, and anticholinergic adverse effects (see Table 18-1). TCAs are usually given QHS to take advantage of sedating effects. All TCAs may cause slowing of cardiac conduction. They are contraindicated in the first 6 weeks after a myocardial infarction because of increased risk of ventricular arrhythmia. In patients with pre-existing first degree AV block, blood levels and ECG monitoring are recommended. A therapeutic trial usually is considered >100 mg/day of amitriptyline or its equivalent for at least 3 weeks. There are therapeutic window plasma levels for nortriptyline, desipramine, and imipramine. **Note: Nortriptyline (Pamelor) has the lowest risk for orthostatic hypotension of all TCAs making it a safer choice in the geriatric patient.**

c. **Monoamine oxidase inhibitors (MAOIs).** Sometimes used in depression refractory to the other treatments. Consider consulting a psychiatrist before starting because of the serious adverse effect potential and dietary restrictions.

d. **Psychostimulants** (e.g., methylphenidate). Consider for use in the hospitalized medically or surgically ill patient with prominent apathy. This allows for a more immediate effect while the traditional antidepressant takes effect. These drugs can be very useful in a post-stroke patient failing rehabilitation.

3. **Psychotherapy.** Supportive therapy is always part of depression treatment. Other types of psychotherapy have been shown to be helpful in mild, moderate, and severe depression, alone or with medication. Referral to a counselor or therapist is often a beneficial supplement to pharmacologic treatment.

4. **Electroconvulsive therapy** (ECT) is the most effective and rapid method of treating severe MDD. Indicated for patients with poor response to medications, poor tolerance of usual antidepressants, severe vegetative symptoms, or psychotic features. It is considered very safe and has few contraindications. The decision to administer ECT should be made by a psychiatrist.

II. Bipolar Affective Disorder (BPAD).

A. **Overview.**

1. **Lifetime prevalence ~1%.** Affects males and females equally. Age of onset usually late teens to mid-30s.

2. **Bipolar I disorder.** Characterized by **one or more manic episodes, or mixed (manic and depressive) episodes.** Individuals affected often have a history of one or more episodes of depression. More than 90% of individuals with a manic episode have future episodes of depression or mania.

B. **DSM-IV criteria for manic episode.** A distinct period of abnormally and persistently elevated, expansive, or irritable mood lasting at least 1 week (or any duration if hospitalized). During this period, the patient must exhibit at least three of the following (four if mood is only irritable):

- Grandiosity
- Decreased need for sleep
- Pressured speech or unusually talkative
- Racing thoughts or flight of ideas
- Distractibility
- Psychomotor agitation or increased goal-directed activity (social, work, school, or sexual)
- Excessive involvement in pleasurable activities with a high potential for painful consequences (such as unrestrained buying sprees, sexual indiscretions).
- Symptoms are not better accounted for by another general medical, mental, or substance abuse disorder.
- Symptoms cause pronounced impairment of functioning, require hospitalization, or are associated with psychotic features.

C. **Evaluation.**
  1. **History.** Interviews with family or friends are essential. Often a family history of affective disorders and alcoholism is present in first-degree relatives. If patient is >40 years of age and has first manic episode, look for medical causes.
  2. **Examination.** Evaluate for medical cause, such as drug abuse or intoxication.
  3. **Laboratory tests.** Tests are needed before starting lithium carbonate, carbamazepine, or valproate (see below under specific medications). They should also be performed to rule out certain causes of secondary mania, such as substance abuse, megaloblastic anemia, hyperglycemia and hypoglycemia, hyperthyroidism and hypothyroidism, systemic lupus erythematosus, syphilis, HIV, and liver disease induced by alcohol or other substances.

D. **Treatment.** Hospitalization is usually indicated for full manic syndromes, since the patient's well-being is at risk because of impaired judgment. This includes a risk of death from exhaustion. Consider ECT in medication nonresponders and pregnant women.

E. **Medications.**
  1. **Antipsychotics.** Often required initially for sedation, control of behavior, or psychotic symptoms. Consider atypical antipsychotics (e.g., olanzapine, risperidone) if the patient will take oral medications. Injectable forms of typical antipsychotics such as haloperidol are available for acute agitation and patients unable to take oral medications. Benzodiazepines are a useful adjunct for sedation.
  2. **Antimanic drugs (mood stabilizers).**
    a. **Lithium carbonate.** Best studied and usually the drug of choice for mania with response rates of 80%. Up to 3 weeks generally needed at therapeutic blood levels before clinical effects noted.

Also beneficial for prophylaxis of depressive episodes associated with bipolar illness.

- Dose is 600 to 2400 mg/day. Give with food and initially in divided doses to minimize GI side effects. Then change to a single dose QHS (if less than or equal to 1800 mg/day) or BID (if less than or equal to 3000 mg/day) to minimize potential tremor, polyuria, and kidney damage.
- Monitor serum trough levels (12 hours after last dose) at least twice weekly initially and then Q2-3 months for maintenance. In acute mania, 0.9 to 1.4 mEq/L levels needed. Maintenance levels range from 0.4 to 0.8 mEq/L (with elderly requiring the higher range).
- Side effects. Polyuria and polydipsia, muscle weakness, tremor, GI upset or diarrhea, hypothyroidism, and sedation. Psoriasis also possible.
- Toxicity may occur at serum levels just over the therapeutic range. Mild toxicity symptoms are exacerbations of side effects listed above. More severe toxicity includes primarily neurologic manifestations (lethargy, confusion, coma, seizures, ataxia, dysarthria, nystagmus) and nephropathy. Nephrogenic diabetes insipidus and chronic renal failure may result. Over-dose not responsive to charcoal but may respond to polystyrene resins and dialysis.
- Lab monitoring. Baseline tests before starting lithium include BUN and creatinine, pregnancy test, THS/free T4 (lithium may induce hypothyroidism), ECG for patient >40 years of age and consider a CBC. During the first 6 months of lithium treatment, monitor BUN and Creatinine every 2 to 3 months and thyroid function tests 1 or 2 times. Subsequently check creatinine and thyroid functions (Q6-12 months) while patient is receiving maintenance lithium treatment.
- Warnings. Avoid use in pregnancy (especially first trimester) unless benefits outweigh risks. Dehydration and sodium-restricted diets may increase lithium levels and risk for toxicity.
- Drug interactions. Any medication that can decrease renal clearance (such as NSAIDs); sodium-depleting diuretics should be used with caution.

3. **Carbamazepine (Tegretol).** Along with valproic acid, carbamazepine is a second-line treatment to lithium for treatment of mania. Dosage 600 to 2000 mg/day for acute mania. Onset of action 1 to 2 weeks; therapeutic trial 3 weeks. No established therapeutic blood levels for treatment of mania. Monitor for leukopenia and liver dysfunction. Avoid use in pregnancy unless benefits outweigh risks.

4. **Valproic acid (Depakene, Depakote).** Along with carbamazepine, valproic acid is a second line treatment for mania. **However, it is the pre-**

ferred choice in rapid cycling and mixed mania. Usual starting dose is 15 mg/kg/day in 2 or more divided doses. Therapeutic blood level not established for mania. Increase dose until therapeutic response or adverse effects occur. Obtain baseline hematologic and hepatic tests. Instruct patients about potential symptoms of leukopenia and liver disease. Depakote may be less likely to produce GI side effects than Depakene. Avoid use in pregnancy unless benefits outweigh risks.

5. **Gabapentin (Neurontin).** Another anticonvulsant with mood stabilizing properties. Well tolerated, few adverse effects. No blood monitoring required. Start 300 mg/day, increase by 300 mg daily up to 300 mg TID. Max dose 1200 mg TID.

6. **Lamotrigine (Lamictal).** An anticonvulsant shown in one placebo-controlled trial to be more effective than placebo in treatment of mania. Not enough data to be considered first-line treatment, however.

7. **Olanzapine (Zyprexa).** One of the atypical antipsychotics. May have some mood stabilizing effect in mania, but not FDA approved for this use. Start 5-10 mg/day, increase daily by 5 mg. Max dose 20 mg/day.

8. **Verapamil (Calan).** A consideration for treatment of mania in patients who have failed all other medications. Efficacy compared to other agents not well delineated. Antimanic dosages range from 160 to 480 mg/day.

18

PSYCHIATRY

ANXIETY DISORDERS

I. **Overview**

A. **Definition of anxiety.** Unpleasant and unwarranted feelings of apprehension sometimes accompanied by physiologic symptoms.

B. **Types of anxiety disorders:** Generalized anxiety disorder, panic disorder, agoraphobia, social or simple phobias, obsessive compulsive disorder, posttraumatic stress disorder

C. **Differential diagnosis of anxiety disorders**
1. **Psychiatric:** Anxious depression, drug abuse or withdrawal (alcohol, benzodiazepines), stimulant use (caffeine, amphetamines), some personality disorders, akathisia in patients on antipsychotic medications,
2. **Medical**
   a. Cardiovascular (such as angina, cardiac arrhythmias, MI, CHF, HTN, mitral valve prolapse).
   b. Respiratory (such as asthma, COPD, hyperventilation, hypoxia, PE).
   c. Endocrine (such as hypoglycemia, hyperthyroidism, menopause, pheochromocytoma, Cushing's syndrome).
   d. Neurologic (such as delirium, multiple sclerosis, partial complex seizures, postconcussion syndrome, vestibular dysfunction).
   e. Drugs (such as theophylline, bronchodilators, steroids, calcium-channel blockers, neuroleptics, anticholinergics).
   f. Gastroesophageal reflux.

II. **Generalized Anxiety Disorder (GAD).**

A. **Overview.** Probably the most common anxiety disorder in primary care with lifetime prevalence of 5%. Gradual onset with peak onset in the teen years. High risk for other comorbid psychiatric disorders

B. **DSM-IV diagnosis.**

1. Excessive anxiety and worry on most days for at least 6 months, about a number of issues.

2. Difficulty controlling the worry.

3. The anxiety and worry are associated with at least 3 of the following 6 symptoms for the past 6 months:
   - Restlessness or feeling on edge
   - Irritability
   - Being easily fatigued
   - Difficulty concentrating
   - Muscle tension
   - Sleep disturbance

4. Focus of the anxiety and worry does not relate to another major emotional disorder (for example, worry is **not** about having a panic attack as in panic disorder).

5. Anxiety causes significant distress or impairment in functioning.

6. The symptoms are not attributable to substance use or a medical condition and are not present only during the course of a mood, psychotic, or developmental disorder.

C. **Treatment.**

1. **Therapy.**

   a. **Psychotherapy.** Most patients with mild symptoms can be treated with supportive counseling and education without need for medication.

   b. **Other therapies.** Relaxation training and cognitive therapy.

2. **General measures.** Regular exercise, adequate amounts of sleep, avoidance of caffeine and alcohol.

3. **Medications.**

   a. **SSRIs.** Several have received FDA approval for treatment of GAD, all are probably effective. Use in doses similar to those for panic disorder (see below). In select patients may add a benzodiazepine for first several weeks of treatment, since it has a quicker onset of action and avoids potential initial side effect of increased anxiety with SSRIs.

   b. **Benzodiazepines.** Usually of short-term use with no long-term efficacy proved. Use lowest dose that alleviates anxiety. Longer half-life drugs may be easier to taper and reduce incidence of dependence. May cause rebound anxiety with taper or withdrawal.
   Examples: clonazepam, alprazolam (Xanax), diazepam (Valium), lorazepam (Ativan).

   c. **Venlafaxine (Effexor).** FDA approved for GAD, considered as an alternative to SSRIs.

d. **TCAs.** Imipramine 25 to 150 mg/day. Does not become effective for 2 to 3 weeks. Most beneficial in patients with comorbid depression or sleep disturbance.

e. **Beta-blockers.** Propranolol (Inderal) may help physical symptoms such as racing heart, akathisia (not FDA approved) but has no effect on psychic component of anxiety. Can also be used for performance anxiety.

f. **Antihistamines.** Hydroxyzine (Atarax, Vistaril) 50 to 100 mg QID may be used PRN, as an adjunct to other medications, or as an alternative therapy for patients with addiction potential.

g. **Buspirone.** Clinically appears **less effective than other agents.** Start 5 mg PO TID and increase to typical dose of 20 to 30 mg/day. Takes 2 weeks to be effective. Non-sedating with little abuse potential.

III. **Panic Disorder**
A. **Overview.** Estimated lifetime prevalence is greater than 3%.
B. **DSM-IV diagnosis.** Recurrent unexplained panic attacks (discrete periods of intense fear) (Box 18-4).
   1. At least one of the attacks has been followed by 1 month (or more) of one (or more) of the following:
      a. Concern about having future attacks
      b. Worry about consequences of the attack
      c. Change in behavior related to the attacks
   2. Panic attacks are not substance induced, related to a general medical condition, or better accounted for by another mental illness.
   3. During the attack at least 4 of the following symptoms develop quickly and peak within 10 minutes:
C. **Treatment.**
   1. **Medications.**
      a. **SSRIs** are the drugs of choice (Zoloft and Paxil are FDA-approved for this indication). **Recommended dosage ranges:** Zoloft (sertraline) 50 to 100 mg/day, Paxil (paroxetine) 20 to 50 mg/day, Celexa (citalopram) 20 to 40 mg/day, Luvox (fluvoxamine) 50 to 300 mg/day, and Prozac (fluoxetine) 10 to 60 mg/day. Start at

18

PSYCHIATRY

BOX 18-4
SYMPTOMS OF PANIC ATTACKS

Palpitations or tachycardia	Depersonalization (feeling detached from oneself)
Trembling or shaking	
Feelings of choking	Sweating
Nausea or abdominal discomfort	Feelings of dyspnea
Feeling dizzy, unsteady, or faint	Chest pain or discomfort
Fear of losing control or going crazy	Fear of dying
	Paresthesias
Derealization (feelings of unreality) **or**	Flushing or chilling

lowest dose and may increase after first week as tolerated (such as Prozac 10 mg PO QOD for week 1, 10 mg QD for week 2, and then 20 mg QD for week 3). Monitor for initial paradoxical anxiety secondary to drug side effect, which usually resolves with time.

b. **Tricyclic antidepressants.** For example, start imipramine at 10 to 25 mg QHS and increase by 10 to 25 mg Q3 or 4 days until effective, side effects predominate, or initial target dose of 150 to 200 mg QHS is reached. If no response after 4 to 6 weeks at target dose, may increase to maximum dose of 300 to 400 mg QHS as tolerated. Clinical experience has shown that serotonergic TCAs are more effective than noradrenergic TCAs.

c. **Benzodiazepines** have a quicker onset of action than other drugs; may use as a short-term adjunct to SSRIs if initial paradoxical anxiety arises. They may be used long term if patients fail treatment or are unable to tolerate SSRIs or TCAs.

d. **MAOIs** are reserved for patients who do not respond to SSRIs or TCAs because of serious adverse drug reactions. Before starting, consider consulting a psychiatrist.

e. **Propanolol** is not a first-line agent for panic disorder but is very effective for physical symptoms of panic attacks associated with performance anxiety.

f. **Buspirone (Buspar)** has demonstrated **little** efficacy in patients with panic disorders.

2. **Psychotherapy.**

a. Supportive therapy is always included.

b. Addition of cognitive therapy may be beneficial.

IV. **Agoraphobia**

A. **Overview.** Age of onset most often in 20s and 30s. More common in women. Often occurs with panic disorders.

B. **DSM-IV diagnosis criteria require:**

1. Fear of being in place or situations from which escape might be difficult or embarrassing in the event of suddenly developing a panic attack or panic-like symptoms.

2. The situations are avoided, or else endured with considerable anxiety about having panic-attacks symptoms, or require a companion.

3. Anxiety and avoidance are not better accounted for by another mental disorder.

C. **Treatment**

1. **Agoraphobia with panic attacks.** Choices include SSRIs, TCAs, benzodiazepines, or MAOIs. See section on panic disorder above. Medications in combination with behavioral therapy most beneficial.

2. **Agoraphobia alone.** Systematic desensitization with exposure to real-life feared situations is the treatment of choice. Consult a psychologist.

V. **Social Phobias and Other Phobias**

A. **Overview.** Social phobia has a lifetime prevalence of 13% with onset most common in the mid-teens. Other specific phobias are more common in females, and impairment is usually minimal.

B. **DSM-IV criteria.**

1. Persistent fear of humiliation or embarrassment in certain social situations (social phobia) or irrational fear of other circumscribed stimuli (specific phobia).

2. Exposure to the particular stimulus provokes anxiety, which may include a situationally bound panic attack.

3. The person usually realizes that the fear is excessive.

4. The fear results in avoidance of the stimulus that interferes with patient's social environment or produces significant distress.

5. The fear or avoidance is not attributable to substance use, a general medical condition, or another mental disorder.

C. **Treatment.**

1. Systematic desensitization and exposure (for specific phobias) and cognitive behavioral therapy (for social phobias).

2. Beta-blockers may be effective in treating performance-anxiety symptoms.

3. Drugs used in generalized social phobias include SSRIs (only Paxil currently has the FDA-approved indication, start at 20 mg/day, increase up to 60 mg/day) **or** an MAOI (such as phenelzine).

VI. **Obsessive-Compulsive Disorder (OCD)**

A. **Overview.** Lifetime prevalence of 2.5%. Onset usually in adolescence or early adulthood.

B. **DSM-IV diagnosis.** Obsessions or compulsions that significantly interfere with daily functioning because of distress or time consumption.

1. **Obsessions.** Recurrent, persistent thoughts that are experienced as intrusive and inappropriate. Examples include fear of contamination, constant worry about performing inappropriate or dangerous acts. The person recognizes the thoughts as a product of his or her own mind and attempts to ignore or suppress them.

2. **Compulsions.** Repetitive, purposeful behaviors performed in response to an obsession or according to certain rules. Includes repetitive handwashing, checking rituals, organization rituals, ritualistic counting. These are designed to neutralize or prevent discomfort. In general, recognized by the patient as unreasonable.

C. **Treatment.** Generally not curative but can obtain significant improvement.

1. **Behavior therapy** uses exposure and response prevention to limit the dysfunction that results from the obsessions or compulsions.

2. **Medications.**

a. **SSRIs.** Start at low dose and titrate to doses higher than those used for depression (such as fluoxetine [Prozac] start 20 mg daily; usual daily dose 40 to 80 mg). If a therapeutic trial with one SSRI fails, another one may be efficacious.

18

PSYCHIATRY

b. **Clomipramine (Anafranil).** Start with 25 mg, and titrate up to 150 to 250 mg daily. Give in divided doses with meals to minimize GI side effects, or at bedtime to minimize sedation.

3. **Cingulotomy.** A last resort for severe treatment-resistant patients. May benefit up to 80% of patients receiving the surgery, but results may be inconsistent.

VII. **Posttraumatic Stress Disorder (PTSD)**

A. **Overview.** Lifetime prevalence 1% to 14%. PTSD can occur at any age. Symptoms usually begin within 3 months after the inciting trauma.

B. **DSM-IV diagnosis criteria.** PTSD occurs in individuals who experienced an extraordinarily distressing event (combat, sexual abuse or rape, natural disasters) involving self or others. In addition, the person's response includes intense fear or helplessness.

1. Characterized by persistent re-experiencing of the event in at least one of the following ways:
   - Intrusive, recurrent recollections of the event
   - Recurrent distressing dreams of the event
   - Sudden sense of reliving the experience (flashbacks, hallucinations)
   - Intense distress with exposure to symbols or representations of the event (such as anniversaries)

2. Results in avoidant behavior of stimuli associated with the trauma or decreased responsiveness to the external world (psychic numbing).

3. Associated with 2 or more symptoms of increased arousal (insomnia, irritability, anger, poor, concentration, hypervigilance, or exaggerated startle).

4. The disturbance lasts more than 1 month and causes significant distress or functional impairment.

C. **Treatment.**

1. Supportive therapy that is appropriate for grief reaction.

2. Group therapy may be helpful.

3. Individuals may benefit from medical treatment (such as treating depressive or anxiety symptoms). Zoloft (sertraline) has FDA approval for this indication, any of the SSRIs may be beneficial.

4. Some evidence indicates that the use of beta-blockers soon after the event may prevent the disorder by blocking the negative physical response but this is still preliminary.

SUBSTANCE-USE DISORDERS

I. **Overview** (Tables 18-2 to 18-4).

A. **Epidemiology.** Marijuana is the most commonly used illicit drug with 10 million current users. One-third of the US population has tried marijuana at least one time in their lifetimes. Cocaine is used by 2 million Americans. Substance use rates are highest in ages 18 to 25 years. Substance use is involved in 50% of all highway deaths and over 50% of domestic violence.

TABLE 18-2
DRUGS OF ABUSE

Opioids	Hallucinogens	Depressants	Stimulants	Cannabinoids
Heroin	Phencyclidine (PCP)	Alcohol	Cocaine	Marijuana
Hydromorphone	Lysergic acid diethylamide (LSD)	Benzodiazepines	Amphetamines	Hashish
Oxycodone	Mescaline	Barbiturates		
Methadone	Psilocybin	Methaqualone		
Meperidine	MDMA (3,4-methylenedioxy-methamphetamine, "ecstasy")	Meprobamate		
		Glutethimide		
		Ethchlorvynol		

Adapted from Hyman SE, Tesar GE: *Manual of psychiatric emergencies*, ed 3, Boston, 1994, Little, Brown & Co.

TABLE 18-3

INTOXICATION AND OVERDOSE

Signs or Symptoms	Opioids	Depressants	Stimulants	Hallucinogens	Phencyclidine (PCP)
Anxiety	−	+	+	+	+
Arrhythmia	−	−		−	−
Coma	+	+	−	+	+
Delirium	+	+	−	+	+
Diaphoresis	−	−	+	+	+
Euphoria	+	+	+	+	+
Hallucinations	−	−	+	+	+
Hypertension	+	−	+	+	+
Hypotension	+	−	−	−	−
Hyperthermia	−	−	+	+	+
Nausea and vomiting	+	−	+	+	+
Nystagmus	−	+	−	−	+
Pupils, dilated	−	−	+	+	−
Pupils, pinpoint	+	−	−	−	−
Reflexes increased	−	−	+	+	+
Respiratory depression	+	+	+	−	±
Seizures	−	−	+	−	+
Tachycardia	−	−	+	+	+
Tremor	−	−	+	+	+
Violent or bizarre behavior	−	+	+	+	+

Compiled from Hyman SE, Tesar GE: *Manual of psychiatric emergencies*, ed 3, Boston, 1994, Little, Brown & Co.

B. **Substance-dependence DSM-IV criteria.** Maladaptive pattern of substance use leading to significant impairment or distress with at least 3 of the following occurring within a 12-month period:
   1. Tolerance (increased amount of substance required to produce desired effect).
   2. Withdrawal syndrome, or using a substance to relieve withdrawal symptoms.
   3. Substance taken in larger amounts or over longer periods than intended.
   4. Persistent desire or unsuccessful attempts to cut down use.
   5. Significant amount of time spent in obtaining, consuming, or recovering from the substance.

TABLE 18-4

WITHDRAWAL

Signs or Symptoms	Opioids	Depressants	Stimulants
Anxiety	+	+	−
Depression	−	+	+
Fatigue	−	−	+
Hallucinations	−	+	+
Hypertension	+	+	−
Hypotension (orthostatic)	−	+	−
Insomnia	+	+	−
Nausea and vomiting	+	+	−
Pupils, dilated	+	−	−
Reflexes, hyperactive	−	+	−
Seizures	−	+	−
Tachycardia	+	+	−

Compiled from Hyman SE, Tesar GE: *Manual of psychiatric emergencies*, ed 3, Boston, 1994, Little, Brown & Co.

18

PSYCHIATRY

6. Important social or occupational activities reduced because of substance use.
7. Persistent use despite knowledge of social, psychologic, or physical problems caused by its use.

C. **Substance-abuse DSM-IV criteria.**
   1. Maladaptive pattern of use leading to a significant impairment or distress with at least one of the following within a 12-month period:
      a. Recurrent substance use resulting in a failure to fulfill major role obligations at work, school, or home.
      b. Recurrent use in situations where use is physically hazardous (driving while intoxicated).
      c. Recurrent substance abuse-related legal problems.
      d. Continued use despite knowledge of having a persistent/recurring social or interpersonal problem that is caused or worsened by the substance use.
   2. Symptoms have never met criteria for substance dependence for this class of substance.

II. **Alcohol**
A. **Prevalence.** Lifetime prevalence of alcohol abuse or dependence at 15% to 20% in males. Males outnumber females 5:1.
B. **Suspect alcohol abuse if any of the complaints in Box 18-5 are present.**
C. **Complications of alcohol abuse (Box 18-6)**
D. **Alcohol-withdrawal syndromes.**
   1. **Uncomplicated alcohol withdrawal.** Begins 12 to 18 hours after cessation of drinking. Peaks between 24 to 48 hours. Untreated,

---

BOX 18-5

SYMPTOMS AND SIGNS SUGGESTIVE OF ALCOHOL ABUSE

Chronic anxiety or tension   Chronic depression
Legal or marital problems   Insomnia
Headaches or blackouts   Seizures
Frequent falls or minor injuries   Vague GI problems

BOX 18-6

COMPLICATIONS OF ALCOHOL ABUSE

Gastritis or peptic ulcer disease   Pancreatitis
Hypertension   Insomnia
Liver disease (cirrhosis, ascites) Erectile dysfunction
Depression   Cardiomyopathy
Myopathy   Peripheral neuropathy
Nutritional deficiencies   Dementia

---

shakes subside within 7 days. Characterized by tremors, nausea, vomiting, tachycardia, and hypertension.

2. **Alcohol seizures.** Occur 7 to 38 hours after cessation of alcohol and peak at 24 to 48 hours. Phenytoin is not useful in preventing seizures. However, lorazepam 2 mg IV given after a first seizure will reliably prevent the majority of recurrent seizures.

3. **Alcohol-induced psychotic disorder, with hallucinations.** Onset within 48 hours of cessation and may last 1 week or more. Characterized by unpleasant auditory hallucinations without evidence of delirium.

4. **Alcohol-withdrawal delirium (delirium tremens [DTs]).** May begin 2 or 3 days after cessation and peak in 4 or 5 days. Typically lasts 3 days but can persist for weeks. Symptoms include mild fever, autonomic hyperarousal, and delirium. Important to monitor closely in the hospital as risk for mortality if untreated.

E. **Evaluation.**

1. Screening with **CAGE** questions. One positive answer to any of the following questions may be significant:

   • Have you ever felt you should **cut down** on your drinking?
   • Have people **annoyed** you by criticizing your drinking?
   • Have you ever felt bad or **guilty** about your drinking?
   • Have you ever had a drink first thing in the morning to steady your nerves or get rid of a hangover (**eye-opener**)?

2. **History.** Ask about previous alcohol problems, prior treatment for detoxification or in a rehabilitation program. History of DWI (driving while in-

toxicated). History of public intoxication charges, fights while intoxicated, or other legal complications. Family history of alcohol abuse.

3. **Physical exam.** Early findings may include hepatomegaly, tremor, or mild peripheral neuropathy. In later stages, sequelae such as pneumonia, hypertension, Wernicke's syndrome (ophthalmoplegia, ataxia, and confusion), Korsakoff's syndrome (amnesia, disorientation, impairment of recent memory, and confabulation), gynecomastia, and spider angiomas may occur.

4. **Laboratory tests.** Blood alcohol level, CBC, liver enzymes, PT/PTT, general screen. Consider other tests: hepatitis B and C, RPR, vitamin B_{12}, folate, Mg, amylase, UA, urine drug screen, stool guaiac, CRX, TB skin test, and HIV based on risk factors and clinical situation.

F. **Management.**

1. **Psychotherapy.** Includes cognitive behavioral therapy that stresses goal setting, self-monitoring, identifying antecedents to drinking, learning alternative coping skills, and social skills training. Total abstinence and relapse prevention are the goals.

2. **Alcoholics Anonymous.** Encourage patient to attend AA meetings.

3. **Detoxification.** May be required if tolerance or withdrawal present.

   a. **Vitamins**
      (1) To prevent Wernicke-Korsakoff syndrome give thiamine 50 to 100 mg IV or IM immediately and then 100 mg PO QD.
      (2) Folate 1 mg PO daily.
      (3) Multivitamin daily.

   b. **Benzodiazepines** should be used to decrease withdrawal symptoms in medically unstable patients and as prophylaxis in patients with history of DTs.
      (1) In medically stable patients, benzodiazepine treatment is necessary only if 3 of 7 signs or symptoms of withdrawal occur: temperature >38.3° C, pulse >110 bpm, SBP >160 mm Hg, DBP >100 mm Hg, nausea, vomiting, or tremors.
      (2) Chlordiazepoxide (Librium) or diazepam (Valium) taper may be used, such as chlordiazepoxide 50 mg PO Q4h × 24 hours, then 50 mg Q6h × 24 hours, then 25 mg Q4h × 24 hours, and then 25 mg Q6h × 24 hours. Hold dose if any of the following occur: nystagmus, sedation, ataxia, slurred speech, or the patient is asleep.
      (3) An alternative regimen involves treating the patient with a benzodiazepine **only when the patient has symptoms** as opposed to scheduled doses. Use PRN IV diazepam or lorazepam. This may reduce total dose of benzodiazepines needed.

   c. **Beta-blockers** are sometimes used with benzodiazepines to reduce autonomic nervous system hyperactivity. Masks symptoms of withdrawal, however, which complicates assessment.

   d. **Haloperidol** PO or IM for patients with alcohol-induced psychotic disorder and agitation associated with DTs.

e. **For DTs,** supplement benzodiazepine as necessary for agitation. Seclusion and restraints as necessary. Adequate hydration and nutrition.

4. **Disulfiram (Antabuse). Controlled trials have not demonstrated benefits over placebo in achieving total abstinence or delaying relapse.** May benefit some individuals who remain employed, socially stable, and motivated. Advise patient to avoid all forms of alcohol (24 hours before starting disulfiram to 14 days after last dose) to prevent toxic and potentially fatal reaction. Dosage range 125 to 500 mg PO QHS.

5. **Naltrexone (Revia).** FDA approved for alcohol dependence to decrease risk for relapse. No disulfiram-like reactions as a result of ethanol ingestion. Average dose is 50 mg PO QD for 12 weeks. Revia proved superior to placebo in measures of drinking including abstention rates (51% versus 23%), number of drinking days, and relapse (31% versus 60%). Patients must be highly motivated to discontinue alcohol. Liver function tests prior to initiation then again at one month after initiation and periodically thereafter are recommended. Naltrexone should be avoided in those patients with severe liver disease or hepatitis before consulting a liver specialist.

ACUTE PSYCHOSIS

I. **Definition.** Significant impairment of sense of reality (incoherence, looseness of associations, delusions, hallucinations, catatonic or disorganized behavior) that results in impairment of ability to communicate, emotional turmoil, and impaired cognitive abilities.

II. **Differential Diagnosis**

A. **Substance-induced (intoxication or withdrawal).** For example, hallucinogens, amphetamines, cocaine, alcohol withdrawal, anticholinergic drugs, corticosteroids, and L-dopa.

B. **Acute exacerbation or initial episode of chronic psychotic disorder (schizophrenia).**

C. **Major affective syndrome,** anxiety disorder, manic episode in bipolar disorder, or personality disorder (cluster A).

D. **Secondary to general medical condition.** For example, temporal lobe epilepsy, CNS tumors, stroke, trauma, endocrine or metabolic disorders, infections autoimmune disorders, vitamin deficiency, and toxins. Suspect psychosis caused by a medical condition if:

1. Delirium is present (clouding of the sensorium, see chapter 9, neurology).
2. No personal or family history of psychotic disorder
3. Age over 35 years
4. Rapid development of psychosis in a previously functioning individual

III. **Laboratory Tests**

A. May include CBC, UA, liver enzymes, electrolytes, calcium, BUN, Cr, TSH/free T4, VDRL, and HIV. Also urine drug screen and occasionally heavy-metal screen and ceruloplasmin (Wilson's disease), urine for porphobilinogen (acute intermittent porphyria). Also perform head CT or MRI in selected patients.

IV. **Treatment**

A. **General.** Antipsychotics initially used to control behavior, including rapid tranquilization. Long-term treatment will depend on the cause. Further history may need to be obtained from family or friends to evaluate baseline functioning. Hospitalization may be indicated for patient safety.

B. **Rapid tranquilization (Table 18-5).** Used to treat violent, assaultive, or extremely agitated patients. It is very useful in the emergency department as well as for inpatients. It is effective for treatment of symptoms regardless of the cause of the aggression that is, it works for schizophrenia, mania, dementia, delirium, etc.).

C. **Medications used in rapid tranquilization.** *Patients who have been tranquilized must have vital signs closely monitored.*

   1. **For rapid sedation. Droperidol (Inapsine).** Used for the short-term symptomatic treatment of acute violence or agitation, especially in young, healthy patients. **Produces much more rapid sedation than haloperidol when given IM.** Usual dosage 2.5 to 10 mg IM or IV (dose should be individualized, based on weight, age, and clinical situation). Increased risk of hypotension, sedation, and cardiovascular effects (ECG changes, dysrhythmias in doses >25 mg). Do not use in those with underlying cardiac disease. **Haloperidol 5-10 mg plus lorazepam 2-4 mg** is another option for rapid chemical control.

   2. **Extrapyramidal or dystonic reactions** (such as Parkinsonism, dystonic reactions [torticollis, facial grimacing, or oculogyric crisis], or akathisia [restlessness, pacing]) can be treated with diphenhydramine 25-50 mg IM or IV or benztropine (Cogentin) 1-2 mg IV or IM. Long term, these medications can be given PO. Vitamin E, 1000 mg PO BID may help prevent the development of tardive dyskinesia, etc.

TABLE 18-5

RECOMMENDED ANTIPSYCHOTIC DOSE FOR RAPID TRANQUILIZATION

Drug	IM (mg)	Oral Concentrate (mg)
HIGH POTENCY		
Haloperidol (Haldol)	5	10
Fluphenazine (Prolixin)	5	10
Thiothixene (Navane)	10	20
Trifluoperazine (Stelazine)	10	20
LOW POTENCY		
Chlorpromazine (Thorazine)	50	100
Thioridazine (Mellaril)	NA	100
OTHER		
Droperidol (Inapsine)	2.5-10	NA

NA, Not applicable.

3. **Atypical antipsychotics.** Consider using atypicals for acute management if patient is able and willing to take oral medications. For example, risperidone 1-2 mg PO q4-6 hours, up to 8 mg/day, or olanzapine 5-10 mg PO q4-8 hours up to 30 mg/day. Start with lower doses in the elderly (risperidone 0.5 mg PO BID or olanzapine 5 mg PO QHS). These agents have fewer adverse effects, particularly with long-term use. These are not yet available in injectable forms. Ziprasidone (Zeldox) is a newer atypical (available in both oral and intramuscular formulations). It has shown good efficacy in both rapid neuroleptization and long-term maintenance therapy. It appears well-tolerated and may have low risk for extrapyramidal symptoms. **Atypical antipsychotics have been associated with the development of diabetes so patients should be monitored.** This may be a metabolic effect that reduces glucose tolerance.

4. **Benzodiazepines.** Drug of choice for alcohol or benzodiazepine withdrawal (see previous alcohol abuse section). May be used as an adjunct to antipsychotics for sedative effect, such as lorazepam (Ativan) 2 to 4 mg IM Q30 min to 2 hours up to 120 mg/24 hours, offering more rapid and complete IM absorption than other benzodiazepines. Watch for respiratory depression.

SCHIZOPHRENIA AND OTHER PSYCHOTIC DISORDERS

I. Schizophrenia

A. **Prevalence.** The most common psychotic disorder, affecting 1% of the world population, and having a strong familial tendency. Between one third and one half of homeless Americans have schizophrenia.

B. **DSM-IV criteria.**

1. **Characteristic symptoms.** Two (or more) of the following, each present for a significant time during a 1-month period (or less if treated successfully):
   - Delusions
   - Hallucinations
   - Disorganized or catatonic behavior
   - Disorganized speech
   - Negative symptoms (such as, affective flattening, alogia [poverty of speech or thought content], or avolition [inability to initiate and persist in goal-directed activities])

2. **Social or occupational dysfunction.** Significant impairment in work, relationships, or self-care since onset of illness.

3. **Continuous signs of the disturbance** persist for at least six months.

4. **Exclusions.** Symptoms not attributable to a mood disorder or to the effects of a general medical condition or psychoactive substance.

C. **Differential diagnosis.** Any condition that can produce acute psychosis (see previous section on acute psychosis).

D. **Treatment.**
  1. **First psychotic episode.** Consider atypical antipsychotics such as risperidone, olanzapine, and quetiapine as first choice. These medications have little extrapyramidal side effects which improve compliance with medication. **Clozapine should be considered second line** because of the frequent blood monitoring needed and is not recommended. The patient needs 6-8 weeks at a therapeutic dose for adequate trial. If no response consider switching to another atypical antipsychotic. If two fail then consider the typical antipsychotics. Typical antipsychotics are chosen based on the side effects the patient will tolerate best (see examples in Table 18-6). If medication noncompliance is an issue consider administration of medications under supervision or change medication to decanoate injections which are currently available in typical antipsychotics (haloperidol and fluphenazine (Prolixin)) only. Patients should be maintained on their medications for one to two years. The above is usually done in consultation with a psychiatrist. **The atypical antipsychotics can lead to the development of diabetes mellitus.**
  2. **Relapsing psychosis.** Requires long-term treatment with antipsychotics (Table 18-6). Minimize dose of medication to help prevent long-term side effects such as tardive dyskinesia with typical agents and weight gain and anticholinergic effects with atypical agents.
     a. **Supportive psychotherapy.** Individual or family counseling may be a helpful adjunct to reduce risk for relapse.
     b. **Community programs.** Beneficial in providing support, social skills training, and vocational rehabilitation. May also be able to provide support services to help improve medication compliance.
E. **Special Antipsychotic Adverse Reactions**
  1. **Neuroleptic malignant syndrome.** May occur at any point during the course of treatment, seen with atypical and typical antipsychotics. Includes symptoms of autonomic instability, altered mental status, which may progress to hyperthermia, stupor, and muscle hypertonicity. Death may occur. See section on neuroleptic malignant syndrome in chapter 2, emergency medicine, for treatment.
  2. **Tardive dyskinesia.** Involuntary movements of the tongue, face, mouth, or jaw associated with long-term administration of antipsychotics. Elderly females at highest risk. May be irreversible. Patients should be made aware of this possible side effect, which is thought to occur less when atypical antipsychotics are used. Benztropine and diphenhydramine can be used to reduce extrapyramidal symptoms. Vitamin E, 1000u BID may help prevent the development of extrapyramidal symptoms.
  3. **Diabetes mellitus** with the atypical antipsychotics.

18

PSYCHIATRY

TABLE 18-6

ANTIPSYCHOTIC DOSES AND SIDE EFFECTS FOR CHRONIC USE

Drug	Relative Potency (mgm equivalents)	Dose (mg/day)	Anticholinergic*	EPS†	Sedation	Orthostatic Hypotension
TYPICAL ANTIPSYCHOTICS						
Chlorpromazine (Thorazine)	100	100-2000	+++	++	+++++	++++
Thioridazine (Mellaril)	100	100-600	+++++	+	++++	+++++
Trifluoperazine (Stelazine)	5	5-60	++	+++	+	++
Thiothixene (Navane)	5	5-60	++	+++	++	++
Fluphenazine (Prolixin)	4	5-30	++	+++++	++	++
Haloperidol (Haldol)	4	2-100	+	+++++	++	+
ATYPICAL ANTIPSYCHOTICS						
Risperidone (Risperdal)	1	1-6	±	+	+	++
Clozapine (Clozaril)‡	50	25-900	+++++	±	+++++	+++++
Olanzapine (Zyprexa)	2	5-20	±	±	++	+
Quetiapine (Seraquil)		75-800	±	±	++	++
Ziprasidone (Zeldox)	N/A					

Adapted from Bernstein JG: *Handbook of drug therapy in psychiatry*, ed 3, St. Louis, 1995, Mosby.

*Dry mouth, constipation, blurred vision, urinary retention.

†Extrapyramidal side effects (dystonia, parkinsonism, akathisia, tardive dyskinesia).

‡Requires weekly WBC because of risk of agranulocytosis.

EATING DISORDERS

I. **Anorexia Nervosa (AN).**

A. **Overview.** Onset is usually in adolescence and affects females 10:1 over males. Prevalence in young women is up to 3.7%. Some will also have episodes of binge eating or purging. Anorexia is a life-threatening disorder, with mortality over 10%.

B. **Diagnosis.**
1. **Early signs** may include withdrawal from family and friends, increased sensitivity to criticism, sudden increased interest in physical activity, anxiety or depressive symptoms.
2. **DSM-IV criteria.**
   a. Refusal to maintain body weight over a minimal normal weight for age and height (such as weight less than 85% of expected).
   b. Intense fear of becoming fat even though underweight.
   c. Disturbed body image or denial of seriousness of current low body weight.
   d. Absence of 3 consecutive menstrual periods.

C. **Laboratory tests.** No single lab test helps with the diagnosis; however, a battery of tests should be performed to rule out medical complications of starvation. CBC, general screen (to include electrolytes, glucose, calcium, phosphate, BUN, and Cr), Mg, liver and thyroid function tests, amylase, carotene, UA, ECG. Other useful tests include CK with isoenzymes if an ipecac abuser; or bone densitometry if amenorrheic for >6 months.

D. **Potential medical complications.** Dry skin, hypothermia, bradycardia, hypotension, dependent edema, anemia, lanugo, infertility, osteoporosis, cardiac failure, and death (most commonly results from starvation, suicide, or electrolyte imbalances).

E. **Treatment.**
1. **Indications for hospitalization** may include any of the following:
   a. Patient's weight less than or equal to 70% of ideal body weight.
   b. Persistent suicidal ideation.
   c. Need for withdrawal from laxatives, diet pills, or diuretics.
   d. Failure of outpatient treatment.

F. **Outpatient.**
   a. Treat the medical complications of starvation.
   b. Nutritional counseling to establish a balanced diet, an expected rate of weight gain (up to 2 lbs per week), and a final goal weight.
   c. Use behavioral techniques to reward weight gain.
   d. Individual and group cognitive therapy to alter attitude towards food, enhance autonomy, and improve self-esteem.
   e. Family therapy may also be useful.
   f. Treat any associated mood disorder. Antidepressants have not been shown to improve weight restoration but may help maintain weight after it has been restored.

18

PSYCHIATRY

II. **Bulimia Nervosa (BN).**
A. **Overview.** Onset is usually in late adolescence or early adulthood and is more prevalent in females than in males. As many as 17% of college-aged women engage in bulimic behaviors. Bulimics tend to be of normal weight to slightly overweight. Associated dysphoria or depression is common. 30% to 80% of bulimics have a history of anorexia nervosa.
B. **DSM-IV criteria.**
  1. **Recurrent episodes of binge eating** characterized by:
    a. Eating large amounts of food in a discrete period of time.
    b. Lack of control over eating behavior.
  2. **Regular inappropriate compensatory behavior** to prevent weight gain (such as use of self-inducing vomiting, laxatives, diuretics, fasting, or excessive exercise).
  3. Binge episodes and compensatory behaviors both occur on average twice a week for at least 3 months.
  4. Persistent over concern with body shape and weight.
C. **Laboratory tests.** No single lab test helps with the diagnosis; however, to check for complications, several tests should be performed: general screen (to include electrolytes, glucose, calcium, phosphate, BUN, and Cr), Mg, and amylase.
D. **Potential medical complications.** Erosion of dental enamel, dental caries, parotitis, menstrual irregularity, laxative dependence, electrolyte disturbances, gastric rupture, cardiac arrhythmias, and chronic pancreatitis.
E. **Treatment.** Should include medical stabilization, routine monitoring of serum K^+ and Mg^{++}, education about medical complications, supportive and cognitive behavioral therapy and nutritional counseling. Prozac 60 mg PO QAM has been shown to reduce the number of binge episodes and associated vomiting (start at 20 mg PO QD and titrate up) (it is the only medication FDA approved for treatment of bulimia). Hospitalization in a minority of patients (admission criteria similar to those of anorexia nervosa except for weight loss).

ATTENTION DEFICIT DISORDER

I. **Overview:** The prevalence of ADHD in school-age children is 3%-6% with males outnumbering females. Onset is in childhood with symptoms first being apparent in early grade school (by definition by age 7). Contrary to previously held beliefs, approximately 65% will have symptoms that persist into adulthood. Patients can have primarily mixed, inattentive, or hyperactive subtypes. Many patients with ADHD have a co-morbid psychiatric disorder.
II. **Diagnosis of ADHD** (Box 18-7).
III. **Diagnostic Tools.**
A. Interview with child's caregivers
B. Mental status exam of the child
C. Physical exam for general and neurologic health with a hematocrit drawn if the patient has a history of lead exposure, hearing and vision testing.

BOX 18-7

CRITERIA FOR THE DIAGNOSIS OF ADHD

1. Some of the symptoms must be present before 7 years of age.
2. There is clear evidence of significant impairment in functioning that is present in two or more settings such as work, school, and home, for example.
3. The symptoms are not better accounted for by another disorder.

Attention. At least 6 of the below must be present for at least 6 months and evident in at least two situations (e.g., home, school, play, etc.)

- Fails to give close attention to detail
- Fails to sustain attention
- Seems to not listen when spoken to
- Often doesn't follow through with instructions on work
- Has difficulty organizing
- Avoids/dislikes work requiring sustained mental effort
- Loses things
- Is easily distracted
- Is often forgetful

Hyperactivity/Impulsivity. At least 4 of the below must be present for 6 months.

- Fidgets
- Leaves seat in situations where seating is expected
- Often runs about in inappropriate settings
- Has difficulty playing quietly
- Is often "on the go"
- Talks excessively
- Blurts out answers to questions
- Has difficulty awaiting one's turn
- Intrudes on others

18

PSYCHIATRY

D. Cognitive ability screen
E. ADHD rating scales to be filled out by teacher and parent
F. School reports on the patient.

IV. **Pharmacologic Treatment.**

A. **Stimulants** such as methylphenidate, dextroamphetamine, and pemoline are first line treatment. Response rate is 70-90 per cent. REMINDER: favorable response does not confirm the diagnosis of ADHD. Side effects include decreased appetite, headache, insomnia, jitteriness, stomachache, and occasional mood dysphoria. There have been rare cases of amphetamine abuse reported. Pemoline is associated with infrequent hepatotoxic effects and should be considered for use only after methylphenidate and dextroamphetamine have failed. Dosage range for regular release methylphenidate is 0.3-0.6 mg/kg/dose and is given as BID or TID dosing. Dosage range for dextroamphetamine is 0.15-0.3 mg/kg/dose and is given twice daily. Both medications come in sustained release formulations along with regular release.

B. **Antidepressants** such as imipramine are used in patients with ADHD and tic disorders. Side effects are anticholinergic in nature. Tricyclic medications are known to be associated with prolongation of the QT interval and as such EKG monitoring is recommended.

C. **Alpha-adrenergic agents** such as clonidine and guanfacine are helpful for hyperactivity. The primary side effects are sedation and hypotension.

TABLE 18-7

SYNOPSIS OF PERSONALITY DISORDERS

Personality Disorders	Characteristics	Complications
CLUSTER A: ODD OR ECCENTRIC		
Paranoid	Unwarranted mistrust and suspicion manifested by jealousy, questioning loyalty, tendency to be easily slighted, and bearing grudges.	Delusions
Schizoid	Indifference to social relationships, few or no friends, emotional constriction, and preference for solitary activities.	None
Schizotypal	Peculiar thoughts, appearance, perceptions, and behavior plus deficits in interpersonal relations.	Transient psychosis under stress
CLUSTER B DRAMATIC, EMOTIONAL, OR ERRATIC		
Antisocial	Chronic antisocial and irresponsible behavior starting before age 15 with conduct disturbance.	Premature violent death, substance abuse
Borderline	Unstable relationships, impulsiveness, emotional instability, identity disturbance, inappropriate anger and self-mutilating behavior.	Depression, substance abuse psychosis, suicide
Histrionic	Attention-seeking, seductive, immature, overreactive, and excitable self-dramatizing behavior.	Conversion, somatization
Narcissistic	Grandiose sense of self importance, exhibitionistic, lack of empathy, hypersensitivity to evaluation by others, high sense of entitlement, and preoccupation with success.	Depression, psychosis
CLUSTER C ANXIOUS OR FEARFUL		
Avoidant	Low self-esteem, timidity, hypersensitivity to rejection, and social withdrawal but desire for acceptance.	Social phobia
Dependent	Submissive to others, low self-confidence, indecisiveness, fears abandonment, and dislikes solitude.	Depression
Obsessive-Compulsive	Rigid, perfectionistic, overconscientious, restricted affect, preoccupation with details, and inflexibility	OCD, hypochondriasis, depression

Adapted from Fuller AK, LeRoy JB: *Southern Med J* 86 (4): 431-432, 1993.

Doses should be titrated slowly from 0.05 mg TID as a starting dose for clonidine. Avoid use in children with cardiovascular disease.

V. **Nonpharmacologic Therapies.**

A. Includes parental and patient psychoeducation, behavioral therapy, and supportive therapy. Multimodal therapy is most recommended.

PERSONALITY DISORDERS

I. **Overview.**

A. **DSM-IV definition of personality disorder** (PD) is an enduring pattern of inner experience and behavior that deviates markedly from the expectations of the individual's culture, is inflexible and pervasive, has an onset in early adulthood or adolescence, is stable over time, and leads to distress or impairment. The clinical manifestations of a PD should not be better accounted for as a consequence of another mental disorder.

B. PDs occur in at least 10% of the population.

C. Many people with personality disorders do not seek treatment on their own and may minimize their personality problems.

D. A brief description of PDs and their consequences is found in Table 18-7.

II. **Treatment.**

A. **General.** Treatment is guided by a patient's symptoms and may include psychotherapy (psychodynamic, interpersonal, cognitive, and behavioral) and/or pharmacologic therapy. Establish safeguards to protect patients from dangerous impulsive behavior (e.g., limit medication supply) Periods of hospitalization may be needed.

B. **Cluster A Personality Disorders:** (1) Maintain honest, courteous relationship; (2) acknowledge understanding of patient's inner feelings and need for privacy; (3) avoid expressing too much warmth; (4) outline plan for care to reassure.

C. **Cluster B Personality Disorders:** (1) Develop sympathetic understanding relationship; (2) be calm and firm; (3) establish limits and define professional boundaries; 4) communicate understanding of patient's strengths, vulnerabilities, and fears; 5) avoid repetitive exams when findings are negative.

D. **Cluster C Personality Disorders:** (1) Build an undemanding, trusting relationship; (2) involve the patient in decision making; (3) balance necessary restrictions with minor concessions.

BIBLIOGRAPHY

American Psychiatric Association: *Diagnostic and statistical manual of mental disorders,* ed 4, Washington, DC, 1994, American Psychiatric Association.

American Psychiatric Association: *Diagnostic and statistical manual of mental disorders,* ed 4, primary care version, ed 1, Washington, DC, 1995, American Psychiatric Association.

American Psychiatric Association: Practice guideline for the treatment of patients with eating disorders (revision), *Am J Psychiatry* 157 (1):1-39, 2000.

American Psychiatric Association: Practice guideline for the treatment of patients with major depressive disorder (Revision), *Am J Psychiatry* 157(4):1-45, 2000.

18

PSYCHIATRY

American Psychiatric Association: Practice guideline for the treatment of patients with substance use disorders: alcohol, cocaine, and opioids, *Am J Psychiatry* 152(11): 5-80, 1995.

Andreasen NC, Black DW: *Introductory textbook of psychiatry,* ed 2, Washington, DC, 1995, American Psychiatric Press.

Andreasen NC: Symptoms, signs, and diagnosis of schizophrenia, *Lancet* 346:477-481, 1995.

Aquila R et al: Compliance and the rehabilitation alliance, *J Clin Psychiatr* 60 suppl 19:23-27, 1999.

Blumenreich PE, Lippmann SB: Phobias: how to help patients overcome irrational fears, *Postgrad Med* 96(1):125-134, 1994.

Boyer W: Serotonin uptake inhibitors are superior to imipramine and alprazolam in alleviating panic attacks: a meta-analysis, *Int Clin Psychopharmacol* 10(1):45-49, 1995.

Bruce TJ et al: Social anxiety disorder: A common, underrecognized mental disorder, *Am Fam Phys* 60(8)2311-2320, 1999.

Bustillo JR et al: Schizophrenia: Improving outcome, *Harvard Rev Psychiatr* 6(5): 229-240, 1999.

Eddy MF et al: Recognition and treatment of obsessive-compulsive disorder, *Am Fam Phys* 57(7)1623-1630, 1998.

Goldman HH, editor: *Review of general psychiatry,* ed 4, East Norwalk, Conn., 1995, Appleton & Lange.

Goldman LS et al: Diagnosis and treatment of attention-deficit/hyperactivity disorder in children and adolescents. Council on Scientific Affairs, American Medical Association, *JAMA* 279(14): 1100-7,1998.

Guze B et al: *The psychiatric drug handbook,* ed 2, St. Louis, 1995, Mosby.

Jibson MD, Tandon R: New atypical antipsychotic medications, *J Psychiatr Res* 32:215-228, 1998.

Kaplan HI, Sadock BJ: *Pocket handbook of clinical psychiatry,* ed 2, Baltimore, 1996, Williams & Wilkins.

Miller NS et al: *Manual of therapeutics for addictions,* New York, 1997, Wiley-Liss.

Noyes R, Hoehn-Saric R: *Anxiety disorders,* New York, 1996, Cambridge University Press.

Perry P et al: *Psychotropic drug handbook,* ed 7, Washington DC, 1997, American Psychiatric Press.

Peterson CB, Mitchell JE: Psychosocial and pharmacological treatment of eating disorders: a review of research findings, *J Clin Psychol* 55(6):685-97, 1999.

Pliszka SR: The use of psychostimulants in the pediatric patient, *Pediatr Clin North Am* 45(5):1085-1097, 1998

Sadock BJ, Sadock VA: *Kaplan and Sadock's comprehensive textbook of psychiatry,* ed 7, Philadelphia, 2000, Lippincott-Williams & Wilkins.

Thase ME: Do we really need all these antidepressants? Weighing the options, *J Practical Psychiatr Behavior Health* 3(1):3-17, 1997.

Weiden PJ: Olanzapine: a new "atypical" antipsychotic, *J Practic Psychiatr Behav Health* 3(1):49-53, 1997.

OPHTHALMOLOGY

Matthew L. Lanternier

EYE EXAMINATION

I. **Miosis** = constricted pupil(s); **mydriasis** = dilated pupil(s).

II. **Assess pupil size, shape, reactivity, and accommodation (i.e., constriction when eyes cross nasally).** *Anisocoria* refers to pupils of different size. This is normal in a proportion of the population, and baseline pupil size should be established before one looks for a cause. Causes include cranial nerve III palsy (as from diabetes mellitus, multiple sclerosis), uncal herniation (patient comatose, other CNS signs and symptoms), Horner's syndrome (interruption of sympathetic innervation of eye causing miosis, ptosis, ipsilateral decreased sweating (anhidrosis); may be secondary to lung cancer, etc.), Adie's syndrome (parasympathetic dysfunction at or distal to the ciliary ganglion from trauma, etc., leading to unilateral dilated pupil), ocular trauma or inflammation, prescription or OTC eye drops, or Argyll-Robertson pupil (pupils may be small, accommodating to near vision but not reacting to light or painful stimuli; seen with neurosyphilis or Lyme disease). Common causes of weak reactivity include the problems aforementioned plus optic nerve and retinal disease. A dilated pupil is not indicative of pending herniation unless the patient is comatose.

A. **Swinging flashlight test.** Normal is constriction on direct light and constriction when the contralateral eye is stimulated (consensual reflex). **A consensual constriction of a pupil with absent direct response indicates** an afferent pupillary defect (that is visual loss at the eye with preserved brain function allowing consensual reflex). May be caused by optic neuritis, ischemic optic neuropathy, chiasmal tumors, retinal artery or vein occlusion, retinal detachment, acute angle-closure glaucoma, etc.

III. **Ocular Motility.** Check six cardinal positions of gaze, corneal light reflection, and the cover test. Common causes of motility and alignment abnormalities include congenital and childhood-onset strabismus, cranial nerve palsies (e.g., from diabetes), orbital trauma, Graves' disease, myasthenia gravis, stroke, or brain tumor.

IV. **Fluorescein Staining.** Moisten fluorescein paper and gently touch to inner surface of lower lid. Disrupted corneal epithelium will fluoresce under Wood's lamp or cobalt blue slitlamp. However, this may miss up to 21% of defects. A dendritic defect will be highlighted in herpes simplex keratitis. Don't forget the usefulness of the slit lamp, if available.

V. Always check visual acuity and evert upper and lower lids to look for foreign body.

VI. **Topical Anesthetic.** Can be used to differentiate topical problems such as foreign body and corneal abrasions from deeper problems such as iritis and glaucoma. If pain resolves with topical anesthetic, this finding is suggestive of, but does not prove, a superficial cause.

VI. **Some Useful Drugs.**

A. **Mydriasis.** Cyclopentolate: maximal dilatation at 25 to 75 minutes, lasting 6 to 24 hours; homatropine: maximal dilatation is rapid, must be used TID or QID to maintain mydriasis; scopolamine: dilatation at about 1 hour, must be used TID to QID.

B. **Miosis.** Pilocarpine in 0.25%, 0.5%, and 1.0%. Generally needed only once per day. See section on acute glaucoma for exception.

C. **Anesthesia.** Tetracaine 1%, proparacaine 0.5%. These cause corneal toxicity with repeated use—NEVER prescribe for home use.

THE RED EYE (TABLE 19-1)

I. **Conjunctivitis.** Conjunctival erythema/injection caused by hyperemia of superficial vessels. Etiology includes infection, allergies, chemicals, and tear deficiency. May be accompanied by itching, burning, or foreign-body sensation. Often discharge or drainage is present, and crusting of the eyelids may occur while sleeping. Vision is generally not affected. If particularly severe symptoms, consider gonococcal disease. If seen in a neonate, *Chlamydia* may be the culprit (usually 3 weeks of age).

A. **Viral.** The so-called "pink eye." Usually adenoviruses. Acute redness, watery discharge with foreign-body sensation and preauricular lymphadenopathy. Usually self-limited but may last up to 2 weeks.

   1. **Treatment.** Antibiotics are not helpful and are not indicated. Boric acid washes, which can be obtained over the counter, often provide excellent symptomatic relief. Patients should throw away eyeliner, etc., which may be a reservoir for infection. OTC drops (e.g., artificial tears, Oxymetazoline) may help as well. Oxymetazoline should not be used in children because of risk of toxicity.

B. **Bacterial.** Acute redness with copious purulent discharge. Usually *Staphylococci* spp., *Streptococcus pneumoniae,* and *Haemophilus* spp. **Treatment:** Ttreat with topical agents for 2-3 days **EXCEPT** gonococcal and chlamydial. Examples include sulfacetamide sodium, erythromycin, fluoroquinolone, bacitracin or gentamicin drops or ointment. Avoid a neomycin because of a higher chance of hypersensitivity. If no corneal destruction, gonococcal is treated with 1g IM ceftriaxone. Refer if any evidence of corneal ulceration is noted. Treat chlamydia with oral tetracycline, doxycycline, or erythromycin for 2 weeks. May use topicals concomitantly with the latter two organisms.

C. **Allergic.** Often a history of atopic problems—allergic rhinitis, asthma, and eczema. Watery, red, itchy eyes, without purulent drainage, but can see stringy mucoid discharge. May also see "chemosis," which is boggy edema of conjuctivae that gives the sclera a jelly-like appearance. Usually seen in late childhood/early adulthood and may be seasonal or perennial.

   1. **Treatment.** Systemic treatment with antihistamines will help and are indicated if the patient has other allergic symptoms. If symptoms are isolated to the eye or not responsive to oral therapy, topical mast cell stabilizers (e.g., cromolyn, lodoxamide) are recommended for mild to

TABLE 19-1
THE RED EYE

	Conjunctivitis			Corneal Injury or Infection	Iritis	Glaucoma
	Bacterial	Viral	Allergic			
Vision	NL	NL	NL	< or <<	<	<<
Pain	—	—	—	+	+	+++
Photophobia	—	±	±	+	++	—
Foreign-body sensation	—	±	++	+	—	—
Itch	±	±	++	—	—	—
Tearing	+	++	Clear	++	+	—
Discharge	Mucopurulent	Mucoid	—	—	—	—
Preauricular adenopathy	—	+	—	—	—	—
Pupils	NL	NL	NL	NL or small	Small	Mid-dilated and fixed
Conjunctival hyperemia	Diffuse	Diffuse	Diffuse	Diffuse and ciliary flush	Ciliary flush	Diffuse and ciliary flush
Cornea	Clear	Sometimes faint punctate staining or infiltrates	Clear	Depends on disorder	Clear or lightly cloudy	Cloudy
Intraocular pressure	NL	NL	NL	NL	<, NL, or >	>>

NL, Normal; <, Decreased; >, Increased; —, negative or absent.

19

OPHTHALMOLOGY

moderate cases. Topical antihistamines can be used (e.g., levocabastine), NSAIDs (e.g., ketorolac) may also be useful. Topical vasoconstrictor/antihistamine combinations (e.g., Vasocon-A or Naphcon-A) work well and are now OTC. However, they may cause rebound hyperemia with prolonged use.

II. **Iritis.**

A. **Symptoms.** Photophobia and ciliary injection of straight deep vessels radiating from the limbus. The pupil is small and poorly reactive because of inflammation and distant vision may be impaired. On slitlamp examination, white precipitates can be visualized on the posterior surface of the cornea, and inflammatory cells in the anterior chamber appear as "dust particles". Topical anesthetic will not relieve pain.

B. **Etiology.** Most common etiology is posttraumatic, but history should include questions about the presence of collagen vascular and autoimmune diseases. Diseases commonly associated with iritis include ankylosing spondylitis, sarcoidosis, juvenile rheumatoid arthritis, lupus, Reiter's syndrome, Wegener's granulomatosis, brucellosis, leptospirosis, and Behçet's syndrome, among others.

C. **Treatment.** Blocking pupillary sphincter and ciliary body action with a cycloplegic agent (such as 0.25% scopolamine, 2% homatropine, or 1% cyclopentolate) will reduce pain and photophobia. Topical corticosteroids are indicated to suppress inflammation, **but patients should be seen by an ophthalmologist if this diagnosis is considered.**

III. **Acute Closed-Angle Glaucoma.**

A. **General. This is an ocular emergency requiring immediate diagnosis and treatment.** Caused by the closure of an already narrow anterior chamber angle. It is more common in Asians, hypermetropia, and elderly (physiologically enlarged lens).

B. **Symptoms.** Expect greatly decreased visual acuity with peripheral-field losses, orbital pain, headache, mid-dilated fixed pupil, diffuse conjunctival hyperemia, steamy cornea, and elevated intraocular pressures. Precipitants include being in a dark room (dilates pupil), stress, and certain drugs (e.g., sympathomimetics or anticholinergics). **Acute glaucoma may present as abdominal pain, nausea and vomiting, and this diagnosis should not be overlooked in those with a GI presentation. An ophthalmologist should be consulted immediately upon making the diagnosis.**

C. **Diagnosis.** Is clinical along with the demonstration of an elevated intraocular pressure.

D. **Treatment.** Treat with acetazolamide 500 mg PO or IV followed by 250 mg Q6h with or without topical beta-adrenergic antagonists (timolol maleate 0.5% one dose) to decrease aqueous humor production. Constrict pupil with topical pilocarpine 2% one drop every 5 minutes for the first 2 hours. Vitreous humor volume can be decreased with systemic hyperosmotic agents such as mannitol 1 g/kg IV. Sedate the patient, provide adequate analgesia, and **refer immediately to an ophthal-**

mologist. Definitive treatment involves laser iridotomy or peripheral iridectomy.

IV. **Corneal Abrasion.**

A. **General.** A localized loss of epithelium from the cornea typically caused by foreign bodies, fingernails, or contact lenses (i.e., direct trauma).

B. **Symptoms.** Sudden pain and foreign-body sensation in the eye; this is relieved by topical anesthetics. There may be associated injection of the conjunctival vessels, tearing, and photophobia.

C. **Diagnosis.** Made by fluorescein staining. Carefully search for any remaining foreign bodies using the slitlamp and everting the lids. Foreign bodies can be removed using a Q-tip or needle. Always evaluate for a rust ring when the foreign body is metallic.

D. **Treatment.** Most heal in 24-48 hours. Topical antibiotics may reduce the risk of infection. However, aminoglycosides may reduce the rate of reepithelialization. Avoid prescribing topical anesthetics as they retard healing and may lead to corneal epithelial breakdown. Topical steroids also retard healing and increase infection risk. Tetanus status should be ascertained and updated, if needed. Patching abrasions not related to contact lens use is traditional. However, recent evidence indicates that patching may increase discomfort and decrease rate of healing. Patients should be advised to avoid reading, watching TV, and other "eye-intensive" activities. Short-acting cycloplegic agents (e.g., 0.25% scopolamine, 2% homatropine, or 1% cyclopentolate) decrease severe pain by helping to reduce ciliary spasm. Close, daily follow-up care is required.

E. **Contact lens-related and "dirty" abrasions (as from dogs, contaminated foreign body) should never be patched and should be treated with an aminoglycoside antibiotic because of increased risk of Pseudomonas infection. Patients with corneal ulcers should have an ophthalmologic consultation.**

V. **Subconjunctival Hemorrhage.** Sharply demarcated area of injection resulting from the rupture of small subconjunctival vessels. Hemorrhages can result from trauma, bleeding diathesis, coughing, vomiting, straining, or viral hemorrhagic conjunctivitis (adenovirus, enterovirus, and coxsackievirus). Excessive rubbing from dry eyes may contribute. Subconjunctival hemorrhage alone is self-limited and requires no treatment. **The presence of blood in the anterior chamber indicates a hyphema and requires immediate ophthalmologic referral.**

VI. **Hyperthyroidism May Cause Conjunctival Injection.**

TRAUMA

I. **Blunt Trauma.**

A. **Orbital wall fracture** should be considered after any blunt eye trauma. Signs and symptoms may include diplopia, epistaxis, ecchymosis, crepitus, hypesthesia in the infraorbital nerve distribution, and restricted upward gaze secondary to inferior rectus entrapment. A CT scan with axial

19

OPHTHALMOLOGY

and coronal cuts is necessary for definitive diagnosis. Plain facial films are frequently inadequate although fluid in the sinus or fat protruding from the orbital floor are presumptive evidence of a fracture. Visual impairment or globe injury warrants immediate referral.

B. **Hyphema** is the presence of blood in the anterior chamber and is typically easily visualized. Symptoms include pain, photophobia, and blurring of vision. Elevated intraocular pressure is a possible side effect and should be treated like acute angle closure glaucoma. Bed rest with elevation of the head and patching of the affected eye may prevent the frequent complication of rebleeding, but the data are unclear. Immediate ophthalmologic consultation should be obtained to determine need for surgical evacuation.

C. **Periorbital contusions** are treated with ice, head elevation, and reassurance that symptoms will resolve in 2 to 3 weeks.

D. **Air Bag Trauma.** Most common injuries are to the eyelids, conjunctiva, and cornea. Hyphemas frequently occur. Less commonly seen are retinal detachment, scleral rupture, and lens dislocation. Injuries are bilateral in 27%. All patients should get complete ophthalmologic exam because of this high-velocity trauma. Can also get alkaline chemical keratitis from the NaOH produced during the chemical reaction that inflates the bag.

II. **Penetrating Trauma.**

A. **Corneal laceration, scleral laceration, intraocular foreign body, or globe rupture.** Treatment includes placement of a shield (an inverted paper or Styrofoam cup will do) **without applying pressure to the globe,** initiation of systemic antibiotics to cover both gram-positive and gram-negative organisms (such as vancomycin and gentamicin), tetanus prophylaxis, sedation, analgesia, and urgent referral.

B. **Chemical exposure (especially alkali).** Expect to find lacrimation, blepharospasm, painful red sclera, and photophobia. Direct lavage should be done at the scene for at least 15 minutes with any water or saline solution available. To irrigate in the emergency department, instill a topical anesthetic (Pontocaine, tetracaine and others). Sweep under lids and in conjunctival cul-de-sacs to remove particulate matter. Hang IV solution bags of normal saline connected through IV tubing to an 18-gauge plastic IV catheter or a continuous-flow contact lens. For patients who cannot tolerate saline, balanced salt solution is a good, although expensive, alternative. **Lavage should be continued for at least 20 minutes by the clock.** When adequately lavaged use litmus paper to ensure that eye pH is neutral immediately after the lavage is completed and again 10 minutes later. This is especially crucial to document in alkali injuries. Continue to irrigate until the pH is neutral (pH = 7.4 to 7.6). Once pH is normal, use fluorescein stain to evaluate for damage or residual abrasions. Reapply ophthalmic anesthetic and apply two drops of 0.25% scopolamine, 2% homatropine, or 1% cyclopentolate for cycloplegia into the affected eye or eyes if indicated by severity of injury. This will prevent spasm of the pupil, which can cause pain. Use an antibiotic ointment. Erythromycin is a good choice. Gentamicin and other aminoglycosides inhibit corneal repair. Provide adequate oral analgesia and follow-up within 24 hours. Contact lenses should not be worn for 2 weeks. Refer immediately for any of the following: (1) acid or alkali burn of significance (that is, corneal epithelial damage, any haziness of cornea), or (2) subnormal visual acuity, severe conjunctival swelling. See all others back in 24 hours. Prescribe oral pain medications, since these are often painful injuries.

ORBIT, EYELIDS, AND LACRIMAL APPARATUS

19

OPHTHALMOLOGY

I. **Orbital Cellulitis.** Infection of tissues posterior to the orbital septum. Rarely seen, it is typically caused by extension of sinusitis (usually maxillary and ethmoid) or periorbital cellulitis. It is more likely to be seen in children than adults. Presentation includes dull aching periorbital pain, conjunctival injection, fever, URI symptoms, violaceous swelling, and tenderness of upper and lower lids, impaired vision, and limited ocular movement. CT or MRI is necessary for diagnosis and to rule out orbital subperiosteal abscess and tumor. Complications include orbital abscess, cavernous sinus thrombosis, brain abscess, and meningitis. *S. aureus, Strep.* spp., *Enterobacteriaceae,* and rarely *H. influenzae* are bacterial pathogens. Consider viruses, fungi, and parasites in the immunocompromised. In diabetics, think of mucormycosis. Treatment includes IV antibiotics (e.g., ampicillin/sulbactam $\pm$ vancomycin). Other options include second- or third-generation cephalosporins (e.g., IV cefuroxime, cefoxitin, or cefotetan). Appropriate surgical consultation is necessary.
II. **Periorbital Cellulitis.** Infection confined to structures anterior to orbital septum. The possibility of orbital extension must always be considered. Vision is normal, and ocular movements are intact. Adults may be managed as outpatients with penicillinase-resistant antibiotics (such as amoxicillin-clavulanate) and daily examinations. Children should be hospitalized because of a strong association with bacteremia, septicemia, and meningitis.
III. **Dacryocystitis and Dacryostenosis.** Inflammation of the lacrimal sac, which is usually unilateral and secondary to nasolacrimal duct obstruction.
A. **Congenital.** Usually presents by 3 to 12 weeks of age and generally resolves by 6 months. It can be treated by BID massaging of the lacrimal duct area, although this is of questionable efficacy. Antibiotics are used if infection develops (see below). Occasionally requires surgical probing to open the duct.
B. **Infectious.** Mucopurulent discharge, excessive tearing, erythema, and tender swelling of the medial lower lid are seen. Culturing of the purulent material expressed from the lacrimal punctum should be performed to aid in antibiotic choice. Usual organisms include *S. pneumocystis, S. aureus, H. influenzae,* and *S. pyogenes.* Use oral first generation cephalosporin, erythromycin, or penicillinase-resistant penicillin. Daily examinations are necessary because orbital cellulitis is a possible

complication. Adults may warrant referral for dacryocystorhinostomy. Surgery may be indicated if abscess develops.

IV. **Hordeolum** (acute infection of anterior lid margin usually related to staphylococci).

A. **Acute external hordeolum (stye).** A stye is an infection of Moll's glands along the lash line. Exam reveals a tender **focal mounding** of one eyelid that develops over days, often with pustule formation. Treatment includes warm compresses BID to QID as well as topical or oral antibiotics depending on severity. Pulling the affected lash may promote drainage. Expect spontaneous drainage within one week. Rarely, if the stye does not drain, I&D is required along with systemic antibiotics. Frequently, can be done in the office with an 18-g needle once the abscess is "pointing."

B. **Acute internal hordeolum (chalazion).** A chalazion is a chronic granulomatous inflammation in the meibomian gland. It can become secondarily infected resulting in an acute internal hordeolum. Acute chalazion is treated with oral antibiotics and warm compresses. The chronic chalazion will continue to grow, and excision or steroid injection is required for cosmetic reasons or when vision is affected.

V. **Blepharitis** (eyelid inflammation caused by chemicals, seborrhea, rosacea, or staphylococci)

A. **Anterior blepharitis.** Chronic bilateral inflammation of the skin, cilium follicles, or accessory glands of the eyelids. Recurrent conjunctivitis, burning, and itching of the eyelids are common complaints. The lid margins are erythematous with dry crusted areas. Treatment involves removing crusts and cleaning the lid margins with diluted baby shampoo daily. Antistaphylococcal antibiotic ointment (i.e., bacitracin or erythromycin) should be applied to the lid margins BID to QID for two weeks, then nightly.

B. **Posterior blepharitis.** Chronic bilateral inflammation of the eyelids caused by inflammation and plugging of the meibomian glands. Individuals with rosacea or seborrheic dermatitis of the scalp and face are especially vulnerable to this posterior form. Treatment involves warm compresses, expression of the meibomian gland secretions, and long-term systemic antibiotic therapy (tetracycline 0.5 to 1 g/day in four divided doses or doxycycline 50 to 100 mg once or twice daily.

CORNEA AND LENS

I. **Corneal Ulcers.** The result of an epithelial defect with stromal infiltration. Ulcers of the cornea appear as whitish, infiltrated areas surrounding a corneal epithelial defect. It is usually a complication of conjunctivitis, contact lens use, or of a corneal abrasion. Soft contact and extended-wear lenses are up to 19 times more likely than daily-wear lenses to cause ulceration. Fluorescein examination will reveal the lesion. Apply topical gentamicin or tobramycin hourly and obtain immediate ophthalmology consultation.

II. **Optic Photalgia (Flash Burns, "Welder's Burns").** Occurs as a result of exposure to ultraviolet radiation (welders, sun exposure, snow blindness) and generally presents several hours after the insult. Fluorecin will show a epithelial keratitis with diffuse uptake in the cornea. Patch both eyes, bed rest, strong oral analgesia, and sedation if necessary. If no reduction of symptoms is noted after 24 hours, refer. Topical analgesics produce slow healing and may lead to additional injury.

III. **Corneal Abrasions. See section on Red Eye.**

IV. **Corneal Transplantation.** Successful procedure for restoring sight in corneal disease. Most common indication is edema after cataract extraction. Rejection is a life-long risk and topical steroids are used to reduce risk.

V. **Cataracts.** Most common cause of blindness worldwide. Common cause of vision loss in elderly. Can be congenital but most are acquired. Some medications (e.g., steroids, including inhaled) and systemic diseases (e.g., diabetes) can contribute. Prevalence increases with age: <5% prior to age 65 to up to 50% >75 years old. UV light may accelerate progression but generally progress over months to years. Symptoms include blurred vision, glare, and monocular diplopia. Treatment is surgical and done only when vision loss interferes with everyday life. Most common technique is phacoemulsification (ultrasound fragmentation of lens with aspiration). Artificial lens implants are placed. Posterior lens capsule opacification occurs in up to 50% within 3-5 years. Treat with laser capsulotomy. Overall, >90% derive visual improvement with surgery. Potential complications include glaucoma, vitreous loss, retinal detachment and loss of vision, but complications occur in less than 1%.

19

OPHTHALMOLOGY

RETINA

I. **Retinal Detachment.** The separation of the neurosensory retinal layer from its underlying pigmented epithelium. Patients will experience some degree of visual loss and may complain of cloudy vision, floaters, flashes of light, or a black curtain across their vision. Risk factors include aging, myopia, eye surgery, inflammation, trauma, a prior retinal detachment, or a family history of retinal detachment. Funduscopic exam reveals a gray or opaque retina instead of the normal pink color. The arterioles and venules may appear dark, and floaters may be visualized. Retinal detachment is an ocular emergency, and prompt surgical intervention is necessary.

II. **Retinal Vascular Occlusion.** May involve either retinal arterial occlusions (resulting from embolism or thrombosis), or venous occlusions (resulting from thrombosis). Both present as painless monocular vision loss, with arterial occlusion occurring suddenly and venous occlusion causing vision to decrease over hours. The patient may experience transient episodes of blindness before the final event.

III. **Retinal Arterial Occlusion.** On ophthalmoscopic exam, a small occlusion produces a flame-shaped hemorrhage or a cotton-wool spot; a large occlusion produces a pale retina and a "cherry red spot" in the area of the macula. Intermittent digital pressure should be applied to the globe in an attempt to dislodge the embolus. Increasing the $pCO2$ to dilate the artery can be attempted if one has the patient breathe into a paper bag or inhale carbogen. Urgent consultation should be obtained.

IV. **Retinal Vein Occlusion.** Ophthalmoscopic exam reveals a "blood-and-thunder optic fundus" - massive hemorrhage covering the retinal surface and dilated veins. There is no immediate treatment for retinal vein occlusion, and the deficits are often reversible. Look for a cause including hyperviscosity, hypertension, glaucoma, and diabetes. These patients need to be followed by an ophthalmologist, since many will develop neovascularization of the iris or retina.

V. **Diabetic Retinopathy.** Most common cause of blindness in middle adulthood. Prevalence increases with duration of diabetes. Symptoms include blurred vision, floaters, field loss, and poor night vision. **Nonproliferative** includes microaneurysms, hemorrhages, cotton-wool spots, lipid exudate, and macular edema. **Proliferative** refers to neovascularization from optic disc, retina, or iris secondary to retinal ischemia. These new vessels require laser photocoagulation. Tight glucose control reduces the development and progression of this problem. Early detection/treatment are best to reduce vision loss: all diabetics should see an ophthalmologist at least annually **and** at the time of initial diagnosis.

VI. **Age-Related Macular Degeneration** (ARMD). Most common cause of vision loss over age 65. Prevalence increases with age: 11% ages 65-74 and 28% age over 75. Macula serves central vision but symptoms can include blurred vision, image distortion (metamorphopsia), central scotoma, and trouble reading. Risk factors: age, family history, cardiovascular disease, smoking, UV light, blue eyes, and antioxidant vitamin deficiency. Two types exist: **nonexudative** or "dry" and **exudative** or "wet". 90% have the dry form but this accounts for only 10-20% of severe vision loss. Dry is characterized by drusen (deposits of extracellular debris that appear yellow on exam) and geographic atrophy (patches of dead retinal layers). Wet is characterized by choroidal neovascularization secondary to retinal injury. These vessels leak fluid and blood. Fibrosis develops months to years later leaving a macular scar. Laser photocoagulation in can reduce severe vision loss in wet ARMD but only 10-13% of patients are candidates. Recurrence is high and laser can worsen vision. Low vision aids help. Verteporfin, a light activated drug which is administered IV, concentrates in new vessels sclerosing them. Experimental treatments include: surgery, radiation, and antiangiogenic drugs (e.g., interferon alpha-2a and thalidomide). Antioxidant supplements may help prevent ARMD but are controversial. Patients above age 65 should see an eye doctor annually and use an Amsler grid periodically to self check for vision problems.

OPTIC NERVE AND VISUAL PATHWAY

I. **Strabismus and Esotropia.** Ocular misalignment, affecting 4% of children, causing amblyopia (a vision loss that is uncorrectable by refractive lenses), reduced stereo vision, and a deformed appearance. It is described according to the direction of the misalignment: **esotropia** refers to an inturning of the eye; **extropia,** an outward turning of the eye; and **hypertropia,** an upturning of the eye. It may also be categorized as paralytic or nonparalytic depending on whether the involved eye moves at all. Paralytic strabismus is suggestive of the possibility of a brainstem lesion. Amblyopia secondary to strabismus is correctable if treatment is begun by 3-4 years of age. Once 6 to 7 years is reached, vision loss is generally permanent.

A. **Predominant causes** in adulthood include cranial-nerve palsies, ocular myopathies, and myasthenia gravis. Consider MS, diabetes, etc.

B. **To determine misalignment,** look at the corneal light reflex when the patient looks in all directions. The light should be reflected on the same portion of the cornea bilaterally (that is, light reflects off center of cornea bilaterally when child looks forward). Alternatively, use the cover test. Cover each eye in turn as child looks at an object about 20 feet away. When the eye is covered, the uncovered eye should not move in a normal individual. In those with strabismus, the uncovered eye will move to focus properly on the object being looked at.

C. The four common childhood forms are:

1. **Strabismus of visual deprivation.** Often develops when clear vision is interrupted in one or both eyes. The most serious underlying causes are retinoblastoma and optic nerve or chiasmal tumors. **Any strabismus in which there is visual loss at the onset of strabismus must be investigated immediately.**

2. **Pseudostrabismus.** Eyes are functioning well, but infant appears to have strabismus because of exaggerated nasal skin and lids.

3. **Esotropia.**

    a. **Infantile esotropia (also known as congenital esotropia) (nonparalytic) - 20%.** An idiopathic form that is present at birth or develops in the first months of life. If it is intermittent, it should resolve by 6 months of age and does not need to be investigated before this age. Generally no systemic findings. If it is constant, it should be investigated immediately, since it is suggestive of a paralytic cause. Treat by patching the normal eye. Permanent visual loss may occur if not treated by 4 years of age.

    b. **Accommodative esotropia: 45% to 50%.** Occurs in children who have a hyperopic refractive error and must therefore accommodate to see clearly. Begins as intermittent and then becomes permanent as vision gets worse. As part of this accommodative effort, convergence is triggered, and esotropia may develop. This usually first appears between 6 months to 7 years of age (2 years

19

OPHTHALMOLOGY

average) but may appear as early as 2 month of age. Treat with the use of refractive lenses.

c. **Nonaccommodative esotropia.** Results as a defect of vision in one eye generally as a result of unequal refractive errors. May also be attributable to cataract formation or corneal scars.

4. Treatment may be surgical for muscle imbalance, use of refractive lenses, or patching the normal eye to allow the affected eye to regain strength and vision.

BIBLIOGRAPHY

Cheng KH et al: Incidence of contact-lens-associated microbial keratitis and its related morbidity, *Lancet* 354:181-184, 1999.

Cumming RG et al: Inhaled corticosteroids and cataract: prevalence, prevention, and management, *Drug Safety* 20(1): 77-84, 1999.

Handler JA, Ghezzi KT: Emergency treatment of the eye, *Emerg Med Clin North Am* 13:521-699, 1995.

Hara JH: The red eye: diagnosis and treatment, *Am Fam Phys* 54(8): 2423-2430, 1996.

Hulbert MFG: Efficacy of eyepad in corneal healing after corneal foreign body removal, *Lancet* 337(8742):643, 1991.

Jampel HD: Questions and answers: patching for corneal abrasions, *JAMA* 274:1504, 1995.

Janda AM: Ocular trauma: triage and treatment, *Postgrad Med* 90:51-60, 1991.

Kaiser PK: A comparison of pressure patching versus no patching for corneal abrasions due to trauma or foreign body removal. Corneal Abrasion Patching Study Group, *Ophthalmology* 102:1936-1942, 1995.

Kirkpatrick JNP et al: No eye pad for corneal abrasion, *Eye* 7:468, 1993.

Klein BR, Sears ML: Consultation with the specialist: eye injury, *Pediatr Rev* 13:127-128, 1992.

Pederson JE: Glaucoma: a primer for primary care physicians, *Postgrad Med* 90:41-48, 1991.

Quillen DA: Common causes of vision loss in elderly patients, *Am Fam Phys* 60(1): 99-107, 1999.

Silverman H et al: Treatment of common eye emergencies, *Am Fam Phys* 45:2279-2287, 1992.

Tintinalli JE et al: *Emergency medicine: a comprehensive study guide,* New York, 2000, McGraw-Hill.

Weinstock FJ, Weinstock MB: Common eye disorders: six patients to refer, *Postgrad Med* 99(4):107-117, 1996.

Weinstock FJ, Weinstock MB: Common eye disorders: six patients to treat, pitfalls to avoid, *Postgrad Med* 99(4):107-117, 1996.

Weston BC, White GL: Corneal transplantation, *Am Fam Phys* 54(6): 1945-1948, 1996.

OTOLARYNGOLOGY

Matthew L. Lanternier

HEARING LOSS

I. **General.** Hearing loss may develop over time or acutely.

A. **Chronic hearing loss** has a prevalence of about 46% in adults aged 48-92 years and is more commonly in men.

B. **Conductive hearing loss.** Ossicle disruption from trauma, tympanic-membrane perforation from cotton-tipped applicator or from noise, etc., cerumen in the canal, otitis media, barotrauma,

C. **Sensorineural hearing loss.** CVA (including sickle cell ds, polycythemia, hypercoagulable states, thrombocytosis) , tumor, Ménière's disease, infection (syphilis, CMV, influenza, Herpes zoster [may see vesicles, etc.] collagen-vascular disease, ototoxic drugs (e.g., salicylates, aminoglycosides). An isolated vascular event causing unilateral hearing loss is not uncommon in young adults.

II. **Presentation.** Decrease in auditory acuity. Audiometry can be especially useful if readily available.

III. **To Differentiate between Conductive and Sensorineural Hearing Loss.**

A. **Rinne** test measures air conduction versus bone conduction. In a conductive hearing loss (e.g., otosclerosis, perforated TM), bone conduction will be greater than air conduction. The opposite is true for sensineural.

B. **Weber** tests lateralization of sound. The sound will be **louder** on the side with a **conductive** problem. The sound will be softer on the side with a sensineural problem.

C. Use these two tests together to determine the type of hearing loss present.

IV. **Approach.** Treat cause if found. If no obvious cause is found and serious illness has been ruled out by a complete history and physical (especially neurologic exam ± CT scan), patient may be discharged with a follow-up appointment with ENT or audiology for further evaluation.

V. **Neonatal Screening.** Universal screening with automated auditory brainstem response can optimize language development in those with hearing loss. Test failure rate is about 4% and incidence of bilateral loss needing aids is 1.4/1000. False positive rate was 3.5%. However, there is not enough evidence to recommend routine screening of the normal newborn at this time.

TRAUMA

I. Box 20-1 lists the differential diagnosis of earache (otalgia).

II. **Auricular Trauma.** The exposed and prominent auricle makes it susceptible to trauma.

A. **Auricular hematoma** is a subperichondral collection of blood typically caused by blunt trauma to the pinna. The hematoma separates the perichondrium from the cartilage predisposing the cartilage to avascular necrosis, infection, and "cauliflower-ear" deformity (blood stimulates overlying perichondrium causing asymmetric new cartilage formation resulting in a deformed auricle). **The hematoma must be evacuated by needle or an incision.** A compressive dressing (e.g., a dental roll trimmed to fit over undermined skin on both sides of ear and held in place with a through-and-through suture) is then placed to prevent recollection of the hematoma. The ear should be examined daily for signs of infection or recurrence of the hematoma. Use oral prophylactic antibiotics in immunocompromised patients or diabetics. If patient presents 10 days or more post injury the ear usually has fibrosis and needs open otoplasty.

B. **Lacerations** involving cartilage should be thoroughly cleaned, sutured (carefully realign to maintain auricular contour), covered with antibiotic ointment, and reevaluated daily for signs of infection or hematoma collection.

C. **Thermal Injuries.** See Chapter 2.

NASAL TRAUMA

I. **Septal Hematoma.** Diagnosis requires a high index of suspicion and direct inspection of the septum after any nasal trauma. The main symptom is progressive posttraumatic nasal obstruction. The nostril may be obstructed by a large, soft, red, or bluish mass. Its appearance can be confused with a polyp, a deviated septum, or enlarged turbinates. Septal hematomas can be easily missed unless the entire septum is observed visually and palpated with a blunt instrument.

A. **Evacuation of the hematoma** as soon as possible to avoid avascular necrosis of the cartilage, abscess formation, or saddle deformity of the nose. Any finding of a boggy, fluctuant septum that is tender out of proportion to other findings warrants treatment.

II. **Nasal Fracture.** Palpate dorsum of nose for deformity, instability, crepitus, and tenderness after any blunt injury causing bleeding from the nose. Diagnosis is confirmed by radiographs. However, treatment is based on the presence of deformity when swelling is resolved, and so deferring radiographs until swelling is resolved is acceptable; this should be discussed with the patient. **Initial bleeding should be controlled and septal hematoma ruled out.** Early reduction is possible if the injury is acute and swelling insignificant. Closed reduction should occur within 3 to 7 days for children and 5 to 10 days for adults.

EAR PATHOLOGY

I. Box 20-1 lists the differential diagnosis of earache (otalgia).

II. **Otitis Externa (OE).** Inflammation or infection of external auditory canal and auricle.

A. **Examination.** Expect to find canal maceration, purulent otorrhea, erythema, edema (may cause hearing loss or aural fullness), perhaps fungal colonization, ulceration, and pain with manipulation of the pinna or with mastication. Fever and lymphadenitis may be seen in severe cases.

BOX 20-1

DIFFERENTIAL DIAGNOSIS OF EARACHE (OTALGIA)

AURICULAR DISEASE	REFERRED PAIN

AURICULAR DISEASE

CANAL DISEASE
- Otitis externa
- Foreign body (including wax)
- Trauma (such as from Q-tip)
- Ear eczema

MIDDLE EAR DISEASE
- Otitis media
- Mastoiditis
- Other middle ear disease
- Meniere's disease (pressure sensation)

REFERRED PAIN
- Dental problems, including abscess, impacted molar, and caries
- TMJ syndrome
- Pharyngeal disorders, including pharyngitis, malignancy, foreign body, etc.
- Carotidynia
- Cervical spine problems, including osteoarthritis and spondylolysis
- Neurologic problems, including herpes zoster, glossopharyngeal neuralgia, trigeminal neuralgia
- Bell's palsy (frequently starts with retroauricular headache)
- Any **cranial** nerve 5, 7, 9, or 10 lesion
- Upper **cervical** nerve lesions

20

OTOLARYNGOLOGY

B. **Predisposing conditions include** lack of cerumen, which is antimicrobial, and active removal of cerumen that causes breaks in the skin and exposure to water, which macerates the skin and raises pH allowing growth of pathogens. *Pseudomonas aeruginosa* and *Staphylococcus aureus* are the most common pathogens in acute OE.

C. **Treatment.**
   1. The canal can be anesthetized with 4 drops of ophthalmic tetracaine for 5 minutes. Lidocaine aerosol 10% and lidocaine 4% topical suspension have also been shown to be very effective at providing local analgesia, but lidocaine 5% solution has not.
   2. Clean debris from the canal. Depending on severity of disease, insert a wick (cotton or Merocel sponge packs) into the canal and then moisten the wick with 4 to 5 drops of either polymyxin B-neomycin otic suspension (Cortisporin otic suspension and others) or a drying, acidic agent (Vosol and others) every four hours for 2 or 3 days. Other options such as ciprofloxacin drops, etc. are more expensive but can be used in the patient allergic to neomycin.
   3. If cotton-like fibers of otomycosis are seen (especially in warm, moist climates), add topical clotrimazole 1% solution. *Aspergillus* accounts for 80%-90% and *Candida* 10%-20%. Frequent removal of debris from the ear is crucial; the wick will help. Alternatives include amphotericin B (Fungizone), nystatin (Mycostatin), acetic acid (otic Domeboro), or gentian violet (2% in 95% alcohol).

4. Change the wick or wicks daily in all cases. Use oral antibiotics if auricular/facial cellulitis or lymphadenitis is present. Generally, use antistaphylococcal drugs or extend spectrum fluoroquinolones such as levofloxacin. **Note: This is not for malignant external otitis. See below for the treatment and diagnosis of malignant external otitis.**

D. **Preventive measures** include waterproof earplugs for swimming. Do not use Q-tips—dry the canal with a blow dryer on cool or use 70% ethanol mixed 50/50 with vinegar following swimming or other water exposure.

III. **Malignant Otitis Externa.** A progressive, necrotizing *Pseudomonas* infection typically occurring in elderly diabetic patients. The infection may extend to involve the parotid gland, cartilage, bone, nerves, and blood vessels. Potential complications include osteomyelitis of the temporal bone, facial nerve paralysis, meningitis, and brain abscess. Prolonged IV antibiotics with an aminoglycoside and third-generation cephalosporin may result in complete resolution. CT scan is necessary to evaluate bony involvement. Hyperbaric oxygen and surgical débridement may be necessary for more advanced cases.

IV. **Otitis Media (OM).**

A. **General.** OM is the most common reason for the prescription of outpatient antibiotics and accounts for more than 25 million office visits per year. Many episodes are viral in origin with recent research suggesting RSV as the primary virus invading the middle ear during OM. The most common bacterial pathogens are *Pneumococcus* (40%-50% and least likely to resolve without treatment), *Haemophilus influenzae* (20%-30%), and *Moraxella catarrhalis* (10%-15%). To reduce antibiotic resistance, it is critical to distinguish acute OM (AOM) from OM with effusion (OME) and defer antibiotics for the latter. This would avoid up to 8 million unnecessary antibiotic courses per year.

B. **Definitions.**

1. **Otitis media (OM).** Fluid in the middle ear demonstrated by insufflation or tympanometry with systemic or local signs and symptoms including otalgia, fever and irritability.

2. **Otitis media with effusion (OME).** Fluid in the middle ear without evidence of infection (e.g., lack of systemic manifestations). Antibiotics are not recommended for this group. This may be present in 10% of patients for up to 3 months after an episode of acute otitis media or a URI.

C. **Diagnosis.** Over-diagnosis and unnecessary prescribing has contributed to spread of antimicrobial resistance. Hyperemia of the TM is an early sign of otitis media, but "red ear" alone does not establish the diagnosis. OM must meet the criteria listed above and requires documented middle ear effusion (MEE) by insufflation or tympanometry.

D. **Treatment of otitis media.** Treatment with antibiotics is standard of care in the United States but the effect of antibiotics is small. It is necessary to treat 7 patients to affect the outcome in 1 patient. 80% untreated have clinical resolution in 1-2 weeks versus 95% treated. It is difficult if not impossible to demonstrate the superiority of one antibiotic over another. Few controlled data support the traditional 10-day course. Much research suggests that a 5-day course is effective. However, the shortened course should be reserved for those older than 2 years and those not at high risk for failure (e.g., no history of chronic and recurrent OM). If there is evidence of TM rupture, add Cortisporin otic **suspension** QID. The solution is acidic and tends to sting when administered.

1. **The most cost-effective, first line agents.**
   a. Amoxicillin 40 mg/kg/day divided TID (125 mg/5 ml or 250 mg/5 ml suspensions) for 10 days. Use 80-90 mg/kg/day in children at high risk for drug-resistant *Streptococcus pneumoniae* (DRSP), recent antibiotic exposure, age <2, attends daycare. This is safe and delivers a higher concentration of drug to the middle ear but is not officially FDA approved.
   b. Trimethoprim-sulfamethoxazole oral suspension 1 ml/kg/day divided BID (8 mg/kg trimethoprim and 40 mg/kg sulfamethoxazole per day) for 10 days. Avoid in children less than 2 months of age. Some evidence suggests that if the pathogen is resistant to amoxicillin then it is more likely resistant to TMP/SMX, as well as macrolides. So the usefulness of these two agents may be more limited in an era of DRSP.
2. **The "second-line" drugs, which are more expensive.**
   a. The second line drugs of choice are cefuroxime axetil and amoxicillin/clavulanate.
   b. Amoxicillin-clavulanate dosed as 40 mg amoxicillin/kg/day divided TID for 10 days.
   c. Cefuroxime. Children >2 years of age 250 mg PO BID,. Children 3 months to 2 years of age, 125 mg PO BID, otherwise, 30 mg/kg PO divided BID with maximum dose of 1000 mg.
   d. Erythromycin-sulfisoxazole dosed as 50 mg of erythromycin per kilogram per day divided QID (suspension is 200 mg of erythromycin per 5 ml) for 10 days [$47]. See above note in 1b.
   e. Clarithromycin 500 mg PO BID or 7.5 mg/kg PO BID for children.
   f. Ceftriaxone 50 mg/kg IM has been shown to be almost as effective as a traditional 10-day course of antibiotics. However, it is expensive and, because of emerging resistant bacteria, should be reserved for cases in which compliance is questionable or as an alternative when treatment failure is apparent at 3 days of therapy.
3. **When to change antibiotics.** If treatment failure occurs in 3 days, consider changing antibiotic to amoxicillin-clavulanate, cefuroxime axetil, or IM ceftriaxone. Many of the other 13 FDA-approved antibiotics lack good evidence for efficacy against DRSP.

D. **Treatment of OME.** Persistent middle ear effusion is expected at the end of AOM. 70% at 2 weeks, 50% at 1 month, 20% at 2 months, and 10% at 3 months. Overall, the benefit of antibiotics is marginal and increases the chance of drug-resistant *Streptococcus pneumoniae* car-

20

OTOLARYNGOLOGY

riage. **See below for criteria for antibiotic prophylaxis and tympanostomy tubes.**

E. **Follow-up.** Although traditional, a follow-up exam is not necessary in the asymptomatic patient who is older than a range of 15 months to 2 years of age. If, however, the patient is still symptomatic or the parent does not believe the otitis is resolved, follow-up exam can be done at 2 weeks.

   1. In adults, complete resolution of symptoms such as ear fullness may take 6 weeks.
   2. Decongestants play no role in the resolution of acute otitis media though they may be needed for associated conditions.
   3. Pain control with topical solutions (such as Auralgan) or systemic agents such as acetaminophen, ibuprofen, or acetaminophen with codeine or hydrocodone may be required from patient comfort.

F. **For recurrent AOM**

   1. **Antibiotic prophylaxis** (use erythromycin, amoxicillin, TMP/SMX qd) use should be based on strict criteria. Prophylaxis should be reserved for those with >3 episodes of AOM in 6 months or >4 in 12 months. High-risk patients are those <2 years old and day care attendees. Don't use for more than 6 months since longer courses are less effective and resistance is more likely. TMP/SMX is the most effective first line drug.
   2. **Tympanostomy tubes.** Referral for discussion of tympanostomy tube placement should be considered if there is chronic bilateral effusions of more than 3 months in duration **with** bilateral hearing loss, language-development delay, hearing loss of >20 dB, or failure of antibiotic prophylaxis to prevent recurrent OM.
   3. Other preventive measures include xylitol gum or syrup, avoiding smoke, reducing day care attendance and the use of pacifiers, giving influenza/pneumococcal vaccines, and encouraging breast feeding.

FACIAL NERVE PARALYSIS

I. **Bell's palsy** (idiopathic) is the most frequent diagnosis but is a diagnosis of exclusion. Bell's palsy (a peripheral seventh cranial nerve lesion) can be differentiated from a central seventh nerve lesion by exam. In Bell's palsy, the motor fibers of all three branches are involved including the ophthalmic branch (forehead weakness). In a central seventh nerve lesion, the forehead is partially spared because of crossed nerve fibers.

II. **Symptoms include** preceding retroauricular headache, numbness of middle and lower areas or the face (which may not be demonstrable on exam) otalgia, hyperacusis, decreased tearing, altered taste (anterior ⅔ of tongue), and facial weakness with equal weakness in all branches of the seventh cranial nerve. Annual incidence is about 25 per 100,000 per year.

III. **Onset is rapid** over 24-48 hours with maximum paralysis within 5 days. Up to 16% develop sequelae after Bell's palsy.

IV. **Differential and possible causes.** Lyme disease (bilateral in 30%), *Mycoplasma*, sarcoid (Heerford syndrome), vasculitis, diabetes, rickettsial disease, intracranial pathologic condition (e.g., acoustic neuroma), complication of otologic surgery, HIV, otitis media, multiple sclerosis, and trauma. Herpes zoster oticus (Ramsay-Hunt syndrome) will present with vesicular eruptions. There is some evidence that herpes simplex virus may be an inciting factor in at least some cases of Bell's palsy. Intracranial pathology (tumor, meningitis, CVA) should be ruled out by history, physical exam, and testing as indicated. History of facial twitching, slowly progressing weakness, hearing loss, or additional cranial nerve involvement is suggestive of tumor and should be evaluated with CT or an MRI.

V. **Treatment.** Characterized by a high rate of spontaneous recovery, up to 86% in two weeks.

A. If the patient is unable to close the eye, tape or patch the eye with lubricating ointment (such as Lacri-Lube at night and artificial tears during the day) to prevent corneal drying and injury. In severe cases surgery can be done to put a gold weight in the upper eyelid or do a tarsorrhaphy.

B. Although steroids continue to be widely used, their use is controversial, and there is no good evidence that they change the course of the illness. If you choose to use steroids, a reasonable course is 60 mg PO QD for 5 days with a tapering off over 7 to 10 days. It will certainly be of no benefit if started over 72 hours after onset of symptoms. Over 85% will resolve without treatment within 3 weeks. Many others will improve up to 6 months out.

C. Acyclovir has been used but again there is no evidence that it is helpful.

D. Those with a dense paralysis or with evidence of complete muscle denervation by EMG have a worse prognosis. **An EMG can be checked during the second week of disease if there is no evidence of improvement.** Some recommend surgical decompression of the nerve at this point.

E. Some evidence suggests a benefit with prednisone/acyclovir combination but this needs further trials to confirm.

F. Influenza-like symptoms and erythema chronicum migrans should be suggestive of Lyme disease. See Chapter 10 for further information.

20

OTOLARYNGOLOGY

NOSE

I. **Rhinitis**

A. **General.** Rhinitis is inflammation of the nasal membranes resulting in sneezing, itching, rhinorrhea, post-nasal drip, and nasal congestion. **Examination of a smear of nasal mucus stained with Wright's stain can often make the diagnosis.**

1. **The presence of eosinophils** is suggestive of an allergic rhinitis or, in the absence of other allergic symptoms, a nonallergic eosinophilic rhinitis. Risk factors for allergic rhinitis include a family history of atopy, higher socioeconomic class, and exposure to indoor allergens.

2. **The presence of many PMNs** is suggestive of an infectious cause (e.g., bacterial or viral).

3. If cells area not present, it indicates vasomotor rhinitis.

B. **Allergic rhinitis.** Affects 20-40 million people. Often has a seasonal component or specific inciting agents such as animals or dust. Exam often reveals excessive tearing, pale mucous membranes, and allergic facies (long face, dark color beneath eyes, arched palate).

1. **Antihistamines** help itching, sneezing and rhinorrhea but have little effect on nasal congestion. For the latter symptom use decongestants like pseudoephedrine or phenylpropanolamine. Antihistamines also help the commonly associated allergic conjunctivitis. Chlorpheniramine is the most cost effective. Other options include the non-sedating antihistamines such as cetirizine (Zyrtec), loratadine (Claritin) and fexofenadine (Allegra). **Antihistamines have class characteristics. If a patient does not respond to an antihistamine in one class, consider changing classes.**

2. Nasal steroids such as aqueous beclomethasone or flunisolide are more effective than oral antihistamines for isolated nasal symptoms. Cromolyn (Nasalcrom) can is another alternative as is ipratropium nasal spray.

3. Consider a short course of oral steroids for very severe symptoms or for those with concomitant nasal polyps.

4. Some evidence suggests that oral leukotriene inhibitors may help, but their role needs to be further studied and they should not be used for this indication at this time.

5. Consider referral to allergy or ENT if symptoms are recalcitrant since allergen immunotherapy or surgery (e.g., for septal deviation) may be useful.

C. **Vasomotor rhinitis.** Characterized by nasal mucosal swelling and rhinorrhea secondary to nonspecific, nonallergic causes such as recumbency, cold, and humidity. Oral decongestants, topical decongestants (such as Afrin), as well as nasal steroids and ipratropium nasal spray (0.06%) may be helpful. Don't use Afrin more than 3-4 days because of the risk of rhinitis medicamentosa.

D. **Nonspecific eosinophilic rhinitis.** May respond to the same measures as vasomotor rhinitis, especially the topical steroids.

E. **Hormonal rhinitis.** Seen mainly in hypothyroidism and pregnancy (second month to term). Treatment is the same as for allergic rhinitis.

II. **Acute Sinusitis.**

A. **General.** Accounts for 16 million visits annually. Data suggest that this is the fifth most common diagnosis for which antibiotics are used. However, only 0.5% of URIs in adults develop into this. Sinusitis can occur in any age group and will frequently involve the maxillary and ethmoid sinuses in children. Children can have 6-12 URIs per year and about 5%-10% are sinusitis. A CT scan or MRI can radiographically evaluate the sinuses. However, abnormal radiographic findings are seen in most children and adults with URI and in many asymptomatic children (i.e., high false positive rate) so a positive CT does not always indicate sinusitis. Children are also prone to mucopurulent rhinitis. *Pneumococcus* and *H. influenzae* are responsible for 70% of cases with most other cases being secondary to *M. catarrhalis*. *Staphylococcus* and anaerobes may be involved in those with chronic and recurrent disease. Fungi (usually *Aspergillus*) can be causative in diabetes and the immunocompromised. Some evidence suggests fungi may be involved in severe/chronic cases. Risk factors for sinusitis include URI, allergic rhinitis, abnormal nasal anatomy, iatrogenic issues (e.g., NG tube), and immunocompromise.

B. **Clinically.** A history of a recent URI where the symptoms are biphasic—initial improvement followed by worsening, facial fullness, purulent nasal drainage, dental pain (especially with maxillary infection), and failure of OTC preparations to resolve the symptoms are all predictive of sinusitis. Other clinical findings may include fever, facial headache with pain worsened with bending over, malaise, and failure of the sinus to be transilluminated (indicating a fluid-filled sinus).

C. **Positive history and clinical findings are sufficient to treat.** Although many cases of sinusitis will resolve spontaneously (self-limited in 40%-50%), antibiotics do shorten the time course and provide symptomatic relief.

D. **Treatment.** Topical decongestants (oxymetazoline [Afrin] two inhalations each nostril BID for 3 days or phenylephrine nasal spray 2 sprays Q4h), with rinsing of the nose several times a day with saline solution, oral decongestants, increased clear liquid intake with occasional shower or sauna steamy air inhalation, and finally antibiotics. Antihistamines dry the mucous membranes and may cause crusts that block the sinus ostia. Traditionally, a 10- to 14-day course of antibiotics has been prescribed for initial episodes though a 3-day course of TMP/SMX given with a topical decongestant (oxymetazoline [Afrin] or phenylephrine) may be effective in acute uncomplicated sinusitis. Those who fail a 3-day course can be treated with a 10- to 14-day course. Multiple studies suggest that broad-spectrum antibiotics have no superior outcome. For recurrent disease, 4 to 6 weeks of antibiotics may be needed.

1. **"First line" regimen (by far the most cost effective).**
   a. Amoxicillin 500 mg PO TID
   b. Trimethoprim-sulfamethoxazole DS PO BID

2. **"Second line" if initial treatment fails to reduce symptoms.**
   a. Amoxicillin-clavulanate 500 mg PO TID
   b. Cefuroxime axetil 500 mg PO BID
   c. Cefixime 400 mg PO QD
   d. Clarithromycin 500 mg PO BID
   e. Clindamycin 300 mg PO TID

E. If a "second-line" regimen is deemed necessary to treat a **refractory acute sinusitis**, it is often necessary to treat for 4 to 6 weeks with antibiotics.

20

OTOLARYNGOLOGY

Refer for possible surgical intervention if pathologic condition is discovered or sinusitis becomes recurrent, chronic, or refractory to treatment. Sinus CT may be helpful prior to referral. Functional endoscopic sinus surgery (FESS) restores normal sinus ventilation and improves symptoms in up to 90% and may be more effective than adenoidectomy.

III. **Epistaxis.**

A. **Causes.** Nose picking, external trauma, dry nasal mucosa with vascular fragility, foreign bodies, blood dyscrasias, neoplasms, infections, vitamin deficiencies, toxic metal exposures, septal deformities, telangiectasias, angiofibromas, and aneurysm ruptures.

B. **Determining the source of bleeding** is often the most difficult part of the examination. The posterior area of the nose is supplied by the ethmoid arteries (from the superior internal carotids) and the sphenopalatine arteries (from the external carotids); bleeding from these vessels is often difficult to control. Kiesselbach's arterial plexus supplies the anterior nasal mucosa, and is easier to tamponade with a pack.

C. If the bleeding has been prolonged, check the patient's Hgb and Hct. A PT/INR, PTT, and platelet count may also be indicated depending on the clinical situation.

1. If bleeding is easily seen and is coming from the septum, direct pressure to the site after generously spraying of the area with the vasoconstrictor-anesthetic solution may be sufficient (pinch nose for 10 to 15 minutes).

2. If this doesn't work, try silver nitrate for small bleeders or electrocautery for the larger vessels on a well-anesthetized septum. Although there is no clear advantage to electrocautery, it may be effective in a patient who fails chemical cautery.

3. If this is ineffective, or if the bleeding is from under the turbinates, insert the dry Merocel pack entirely into the nostril (using a lubricant such as K-Y Jelly) and moisten it with phenylephrine or saline until it has completely formed to the convoluted nasal passage, leaving it in for at least 24 hours. Alternatively, pack with Vaseline gauze soaked with phenylephrine.

4. Prescribe broad-spectrum antibiotics to all patients requiring nasal packing while they are packed, since there is a high risk of sinusitis; TMP/SMX, amoxicillin-clavulanate, or clarithromycin are good choices.

5. Examine the uvula. If it's still dripping blood, hemostasis is inadequate and posterior packing may be required. Temporizing measures include the use of one of several commercially available posterior nasal packs or the use of a Foley catheter inserted into the posterior nasal area and inflated. Anyone requiring posterior packing should also have an anterior pack placed. Obtain an otolaryngologic consultation and hospitalize any patient with a posterior nose bleed for observation or vascular intervention.

6. Surgical treatment includes arterial ligation, endoscopic cauterization, and angiographic embolization.

TONGUE AND MOUTH

I. **Aphthous Ulcers, "Canker Sores."**

A. **General.** Aphthous ulcers are recurrent painful lesions of non-keratinized mucosa that vary in size and may appear as solitary lesions or in clusters (herpetiform ulcerations). The typical appearance is of an erythematous periphery with a white or yellow depressed center. Healing within 10 to 14 days is the rule.

B. **Causes.** Viral (coxsackievirus, herpesvirus), systemic illness (Crohn's disease, lupus, Behçet's disease, erythema multiforme), toothpaste (sodium lauryl sulfate), stress, and smoking. Dental trauma, vitamin B_{12}, folate, and iron deficiency have also been implicated in some cases.

C. **Treatment.** Symptomatic relief can be obtained by the use of diphenhydramine elixir as a mouth rinse that is not swallowed. Alternatively, viscous lidocaine 2% can be used in the adult. This may suppress the gag reflex, however, and may result in systemic toxicity in children. The application of a topical steroid (triamcinolone as 0.1% in Orabase) or steroid mouth rinse (betamethasone syrup) may accelerate recovery. Herpetiform ulcerations may respond to tetracycline syrup, which is used as a mouth rinse and then swallowed. A burst of oral prednisone may be required in some cases. The use of multiple other drugs including cyclosporin A, colchicine, thalidomide, and dapsone attest to the stubborn nature of these lesions. A mixture of nystatin 12,500 U, diphenhydramine 1.25 mg, and hydrocortisone 0.25 mg/ml has been used as a "shotgun" solution. Some also include tetracycline syrup in the mixture. A new product called amlexanox (Aphthasol) 5% oral paste came on the market in 1999. In one study, healing at 3 days was 21% versus 8% with placebo. Complete resolution of pain after 3 days was reported for 44% and 20% of patients, respectively.

D. **Prevention.** Using a toothpaste free of sodium lauryl sulfate or changing toothpaste has been shown to be helpful in some cases. Topical use of steroids, mouth rinses, may decrease recurrence. Avoid smoking and make sure there are no nutritional deficiencies.

E. **Herpes simplex virus** infrequently causes recurrent intraoral herpes. The lesions occur as a cluster of vesicles that rupture leaving superficial ulcerations that remain for 3 to 10 days. Keratinized tissues, attached gingiva, and the hard palate are often involved, and such features distinguish herpes from aphthous ulcers. Treatment with acyclovir may decrease healing time.

II. **Xerostomia (Dry Mouth).**

A. **Causes.** Sjögren's syndrome, anticholinergics, radiation changes, dehydration, surgical changes, infection (as by CMV), mouth breathing diabetes mellitus (lack of saliva can increase risk of infection—thrush—and

20

OTOLARYNGOLOGY

cavities). Leads to problems with eating, speaking, swallowing, dentures, and sometimes taste.

B. **Treatment.** Artificial saliva, mouth washes, hard candy, pilocarpine (saliva stimulant) tablets 5 mg PO TID, pilocarpine solution 15 gtt 1% in 4 oz of water and swish and spit. This can also be swallowed and will provide 5 mg of pilocarpine. Another option is cevimeline (Evoxac) or pilocarpine pills. However, swish and spit pilocarpine has fewer cholinergic side effects.

THROAT

I. **Pharyngitis and Tonsillitis.**

A. **General.** Most sore throats are caused by viruses and thus don't require antibiotics. Acute tonsillitis and pharyngitis present with throat pain that may radiate to the ears and dysphagia. Fever is more commonly associated with group A beta-hemolytic streptococci *(Streptococcus pyogenes),* which accounts for about 15% of all cases. The proportion of pharyngitis and tonsillitis that is cause by group A streptococci is related to the patient's age. In children 6 to 15 years of age, approximately 50% of the pharyngitis that presents for care is caused by streptococci. The primary reason to diagnose and treat strep is to decrease acute renal failure (incidence 0.2-2 per 100,000).

1. **Classic strep symptoms** include sore throat, dysphagia, fever, malaise, and headache **in the absence of other URI symptoms.** Occasional patients will have abdominal pain and vomiting. Signs include exudative erythema, palatal petechiae, and tender anterior cervical adenopathy.

2. **Other causes of exudative pharyngitis** include *Mycoplasma,* Epstein-Barr virus, adenovirus, influenza virus, *Arcanobacterium hemolyticum,* gonococcal pharyngitis, etc.

3. **Noninfectious causes of pharyngitis** include mouth-breathing secondary to nasal obstruction (as with a URI). Mouth breathing classically presents as a sore throat that is worst in the morning and abates as the day progresses. **Viral thyroiditis** may present as a "sore throat" as may **carotidynia,** an ill-defined entity characterized by tenderness over the carotid artery, painful swallowing, and pain radiating to the ears. Carotidynia will respond to NSAIDs; antibiotic treatment is not indicated. Consider adult epiglottitis in the febrile adult with severe sore throat, trouble in swallowing and anterior neck tenderness. Also consider peritonsillar abscess. See Table 20-1.

B. **Testing for streptococci.** Rapid streptococcal tests demonstrate a sensitivity of approximately 95%. Avoid false negatives with proper sampling technique (i.e., vigorous samples of both tonsils and posterior pharynx while avoiding the uvula and soft palate as they dilute the sample). The newer tests have a concordance of 91% to 95% with those of a culture.

C. **Who to treat.** The central question in pharyngitis is deciding which patients require antibiotics and doing so in a cost-effective manner keeping

TABLE 20-1

PARTIAL DIFFERENTIAL OF "SORE THROAT" WITH SOME DISTINGUISHING FEATURES

Cause	Oral Examination	Skin Examination	Systemic Symptoms	Adenopathy	Age Group
Streptococcalpharyngitis	Beefy red pharynx, palatal petechiae	Sandpaper-like rash with scarlet fever only	Fever, absent URI symptoms	Tender anterior cervical adenopathy	Children
Mononucleosis-like illnesses (EBV, CMV)	Injected pharynx exudate	Rash in response to amoxicillin	Fatigue, fever	Posterior cervical adenopathy, axillary adenopathy, perhaps splenomegaly	Young adults
Arcanobacterium hemolyticus	Injected pharynx with exudate	May have morbilliform rash			Young adults
Viral pharyngitis	Mild injection, pain out of proportion to exam	No rash	URI symptoms may be present	Rare	All
Adenovirus	Exudative pharyngitis	No rash	Conjunctivitis, cough, bronchitis		Primarily children but also adults
Carotidynia	Throat exam normal	No rash	None	Tender over carotid, no adenopathy	Adults

20

OTOLARYNGOLOGY

in mind antibiotic resistance. The treatment and approach to pharyngitis is mired in controversy.

1. **Adults.** A reasonable approach in adults is to treat all patients with fever, systemic symptoms, and tonsillar exudate with antibiotics because they are likely to have streptococcal pharyngitis. Patients exhibiting little or no evidence suggestive of bacterial pharyngitis (those with concurrent URI symptoms, obvious cause such as mouth breathing, little or no visual evidence of pharyngitis, absent adenopathy) may be reassured and treated symptomatically with lozenges or addressing the underlying problem (humidity, nasal congestion, etc.). Streptococcal cultures or quick streptococcal tests can be reserved for those patients in whom the diagnosis is not clear or has an intermediate probability. Testing for mononucleosis can be reserved for those with appropriate adenopathy (see Table 20-1) and those who do not respond to conservative treatment.

2. **Children.** Most authors recommend a quick streptococcal test followed by a pharyngeal culture for group A beta-hemolytic streptococci if the quick streptococcal test is negative. This recommendation is based on the increased incidence of streptococcal pharyngitis and sequelae in pediatric patients as well as the frequently limited reliability of the physical examination in this age group. Many clinicians advocate empiric therapy with antibiotics and systemic analgesia while awaiting culture results. However, antibiotics should NOT be given in the absence of a definite diagnosis. This selects for resistance, carries a risk of allergy, and creates unnecessary cost. Antibiotics started within 9 days of onset are effective in preventing renal failure.

D. **Treatment.** Treat for entire 10-day course. Clinical/bacteriologic cure >90% (shorter courses less effective).

1. There are no isolates of group A beta-hemolytic streptococci that are penicillin resistant in the United States. However, there are some isolates resistant to macrolides (<3.5% with higher rates in Japan)

2. Some resistance to treatment may be noted if the patient is simultaneously colonized with *H. influenzae* that is beta-lactamase producing.

3. The first drugs of choice are penicillin (that is, Pen-VK 500 mg PO BID or TID or Penicillin G Benzathine 1.2 million U IM in adults, 600,000 U IM in children) and erythromycin 250 to 500 mg PO Q6h for 10 days. Consider amoxicillin for young children since it is more palatable and just as inexpensive. If these fail, a first-generation cephalosporin (such as cephalexin 250 mg PO QID or 500 mg PO BID) may be used. Alternatives include amoxicillin/clavulanate, azithromycin, clarithromycin, cefixime, cefuroxime and clindamycin.

4. **Children may return to school** after 24 hours of therapy. Suggest that patients obtain a new toothbrush since strep can be harbored on toothbrushes and lead to recurrent disease. Treating other family members empirically is controversial and a matter of personal judgment.

E. **Indications for tonsillectomy.** History of peritonsillar abscess, history of airway obstruction (sleep apnea) secondary to tonsil hypertrophy; some would suggest 4 or 5 episodes of streptococcal pharyngitis in a 1-year period or "chronic sore throat" with adenopathy for 6 months that is unresponsive to treatment. However, there is little data to support this and it is only a relative indication. Tonsillectomy **will not** prevent recurrent otitis media although adenoidectomy may.

F. **Scarlet fever.** Scarlet fever is a self-limited systemic manifestation of streptococcal pharyngitis. Symptoms include "strawberry tongue" (a red tongue with red or whitish papillae), a fine "sandpaper" rash that appears as a diffuse erythema beginning and concentrating in the skin folds (especially axillary) but spares the palms and soles. Frequently, there is circumoral pallor. A fine desquamation that begins on the fingers and toes may occur. The differential diagnosis includes Kawasaki's disease.

G. **For recurrent disease streptococcal disease,** attempt to identify carrier in family with throat and nasal cultures. Treat any identified carriers. Consider IM treatment to rule out noncompliance as a reason for treatment failure. Change all toothbrushes.

II. **Peritonsillar Abscess (Quinsy).**

A. **General.** A localized abscess that is typically unilateral and occurs in patients with tonsillitis.

B. **Cause.** Depending on the series, the most common organism is *Streptococcus* followed by anaerobes.

C. **Clinically.** Symptoms include severe throat pain with radiation to the ear, drooling from inability to swallow saliva, trismus, and fever. Almost pathognomonic of a peritonsillar abscess is a muffled, "hot potato," voice. On exam there is unilateral swelling of the palate and anterior pillar with displacement of the tonsil downward and medially and deviation of the uvula away from the involved side.

D. **Treatment.** IV or IM penicillin and tonsillectomy. Several series have documented good results using oral antibiotics and needle drainage, which may need to be done many times. The major concern is the possibility of airway obstruction though this is a very rare event. ENT consultation is recommended.

III. **Mononucleosis.**

A. **General.** Classically, the term *mononucleosis* has referred to the syndrome caused by the Epstein-Barr virus, which is characterized by an exudative pharyngitis, diffuse lymphadenopathy (including splenomegaly in 50%), malaise, fever, and fatigue. So-called heterophil negative mononucleosis with the same symptoms may be caused by other organisms including CMV, *Toxoplasma,* acute HIV infection, or leptospirosis. Mononucleosis is most common in young adults, and most of the adult population has had clinically inapparent EBV disease as evidenced by antibody titers. If patients with mononucleosis are treated with ampicillin or similar drug, they will almost uniformly develop a morbilliform rash. Rarely EBV may cause genital ulcerations.

20

OTOLARYNGOLOGY

B. **Diagnosis.** Diagnosis is by CBC revealing a lymphocytosis with atypical lymphocytes. This will be present in most of the mono syndromes. A positive heterophil antibody (monospot test) may or may not be present in the early stages of the disease (only 60% by 2 weeks) but will eventually become positive in 90% of young adults. The heterophil test rarely becomes positive in those <5 years of age. If there is any doubt, an EBV antibody titer can be performed. Liver enzymes are almost uniformly elevated.

C. **Complications.** CNS complications including encephalitis and aseptic meningitis, hematologic complications including hemolytic anemia and splenic rupture, hepatitis as well as airway obstruction secondary to paratracheal lymphadenopathy. Rarely, there may be acute renal failure secondary to interstitial nephritis.

D. **Treatment** is symptomatic, and the illness generally resolves within 2 weeks. However, prednisone has been shown to reduce the length of the illness. A steroid burst of 30 to 60 mg of prednisone PO per day for 3 days or 4 mg of methylprednisolone PO TID for a week may be used but should be reserved for treating the complications of mononucleosis, including respiratory obstruction, myocarditis-pericarditis, aseptic meningitis, and hemolysis-thrombocytopenia. Contact sports or activities producing other forms of trauma should be avoided because of the risk of splenic rupture. Spontaneous rupture can occur in 0.1%-0.5% of documented mononucleosis.

IV. **Hoarseness (Dysphonia).**

A. **Hoarseness.** A descriptive term used when the quality of a voice changes. This results from various pathological processes affecting the vocal cords. Voice quality may be described as breathy, weak, strained, or tremorous. Descriptions can suggest certain diagnoses (see Box 20-2).

B. **Causes.** Infectious laryngitis is the most likely cause in primary care practice. However, history should elicit information regarding smoking and alcohol (risk factors for laryngeal cancer), voice abuse (risk factors for singers' nodules), and trauma. Hypothyroidism may cause a gradual and progressive hoarseness that will resolve with treatment. Gastroesophageal reflux disease and tumor should also be considered (including HPV papillomatosis). Other causes include neurologic disease (stroke, Eaton-Lambert syndrome, Myasthenia gravis, Parkinson's, essential tremor), lung malignancy, and other pulmonary processes (Wegener's granulomatosis, sarcoid), especially with hilar involvement, inhalation injury (smoke etc.). Also consider recurrent laryngeal nerve injury from surgery or trauma.

C. **Hydration and voice rest** are the primary therapy of suspected infectious laryngitis. Address the underlying cause. May include vocal hygiene, voice therapy, GERD treatment, speech therapy, surgery, or radiation. If symptoms persist beyond 2 or more weeks in the absence of URI refer preform nasopharyngoscopy or refer for evaluation.

BOX 20-2

DIFFERENTIAL DIAGNOSIS OF HOARSENESS

Breathy: Vocal cord paralysis, abductor spasmodic dysphonia, functional dysphonia

Hoarse: Vocal cord lesion, muscle tension dysphonia, reflux laryngitis

Low-pitched: Reinke's edema, vocal abuse, reflux laryngitis, vocal cord paralysis, muscle tension dysphonia

Strained: Adductor spasmodic dysphonia, muscle tension dysphonia, reflux laryngitis

Tremor: Parkinson's disease, essential tremor of the head and neck, spasmodic dysphonia, muscle tension dysphonia

Vocal fatigue: Muscle tension dysphonia, vocal cord paralysis, reflux laryngitis, vocal abuse

From Rosen CA et al: *AAFP* June, 1998.

TEMPOROMANDIBULAR JOINT

I. Temporomandibular Joint (TMJ) Disorders

A. **General.** TMJ disorders include arthritis of the joint, anterior cartilage (meniscus) displacement, and pain in the muscles of mastication (myofascial pain dysfunction).

B. **Symptoms.** May include ear pain, headache, pain on chewing or opening the mouth wide with pain radiating to the ear, limited jaw mobility, clicking or crepitance, and tenderness on palpation of the joint.

C. **Treatment.** The balance of the data does not favor one treatment as best for initial management. True efficacy of most therapies for TMJ are unknown since they have not been adequately evaluated in long-term studies. Avoiding clenching and grinding the teeth (bruxism). Eat a soft diet, use moist heat, massage, and NSAIDs. Avoid gum chewing. Some patients may benefit from the use of muscle relaxants, bite appliances worn at night, or physical therapy. Relaxation and cognitive behavioral therapy are effective for chronic pain. Referral to otolaryngology, oral surgery, or TMJ centers should be considered for refractory pain.

BIBLIOGRAPHY

Albino JE et al: Management of temporomandibular disorders, *J Am Dent Assoc* 127(11):1595-1606, 1996.

Asgari MM et al: Spontaneous splenic rupture in infectious mononucleosis: a review, *Yale J Biol Med* 70(2):175-182, 1997.

Cruickshanks KJ et al: Prevalence of hearing loss in older adults in Beaver Dam, Wisconsin. The epidemiology of hearing loss study, *Am J Epidemiol* 148(9):879-886, 1998.

Crump J et al: Pharyngitis, University of Michigan Health System Pharyngitis Guideline Team, 1996.

Desmond, J. Bell's palsy and prednisolone, *J Accid Emerg Med* 16(6):445, November 1999

Dowell SF et al: Acute otitis media: management and surveillance in an era of pneumococcal resistance—a report from the Drug-resistant *Streptococcus pneumoniae* Therapeutic Working Group, *Pediatr Infect Dis J* 18(1):1-9, 1999.

Dowell SF et al: Otitis media—principles of judicious use of antimicrobial agents, *Pediatrics* 101(1): 165-171, 1998.

Dykewicz MS et al: Diagnosis and management of rhinitis, *Ann Aller Asthma Immunol* 81(5):478-518, 1998.

Fagnan LJ: Acute sinusitis: A cost-effective approach to diagnosis and treatment, *Am Fam Phys* 58(8):1795-1801, 1998.

Greenspan D: Xerostomia: diagnosis and management, *Oncology* 10(3 suppl):7-11, 1996.

Heikkinen T et al: Prevalence of various respiratory viruses in the middle ear during acute otitis media, *New Engl J Med* 340(4), 1999.

Hudson LB et al: Necrotizing genital ulcerations in a premenarcheal female with mononucleosis, *Obstet Gynecol* 92(2):642-644, 1998.

Khandwala A et al: 5% Amlexanox oral paste, a new treatment for recurrent minor aphthous ulcers, *Oral Surg Oral Med Oral Pathol* 83(2):222-230, 1997.

Lee D et al: Initial management of auricular trauma, *Am Fam Phys* 53(7):2339-2344, 1996.

Lee KJ: *Essential otolaryngology: head and neck surgery,* East Norwalk, Conn, 1995, Appleton & Lange.

Lobbezoo F et al: Do bruxism and TMJ disorders have a cause-and-effect relationship? *J Orofacial Pain* 11(1):15-23, 1997.

Logan M et al: The utility of nasal bone radiographs in nasal trauma, *Clin Radiol* 49(3): 192, 1994.

Mason JA et al: Universal infant hearing screening by automated auditory brainstem response measurement, *Pediatrics* 101(2):221-228, 1998.

Maximum access to diagnosis and therapy, Electronic Library of Medicine, Boston, 2000, Little, Brown & Co.

Mayer HB et al: Epstein-barr virus-induced infectious mononucleosis complicated by acute renal failure:case report and review, *Clin Infect Dis* 22(6):1009-1018, 1996.

Roob G et al: Peripheral facial palsy: etiology, diagnosis and treatment, *European Neurol* 41:3-9, 1999.

Rosen CA et al: Evaluating hoarseness: keeping your patient's voice healthy, *Am Fam Phys* 57(11):2775-2780, 1998.

Schwartz B et al: Pharyngitis—principles of judicious use of antimicrobial agents, *Pediatrics* 101(1): 171-174, 1998.

Sharp JF et al: Routine X-rays in nasal trauma: the influence of audit on clinical practice, *J Royal Soc Med* 87(3):153, 1994.

Slack R et al: Functional endoscopic sinus surgery, *Am Fam Phys* 58(3):707-718, 1998.

Spector SL et al: Parameters for the diagnosis and management of sinusitis, *Ann Aller, Asthma, Immunol* 102(6):s107-s1044, 1998.

Tintinalli JE et al: *Emergency medicine: a comprehensive study guide,* New York, 2000, McGraw-Hill.

Williams JW et al: Does this patient have sinusitis: diagnosing acute sinusitis by history and physical examination, *JAMA* 270(10):1242, 1993.

Williams JW et al: Randomized controlled trial of 3 vs. 10 days of trimethoprim-sulfamethoxazole for acute maxillary sinusitis, *JAMA* 273(13):1015, 1995.

OFFICE/HOSPITAL PROCEDURES

Sarah Thomas

TYMPANOMETRY

I. **Indications.** Useful in detecting fluid in the middle ear, negative middle ear pressure, tympanic membrane perforation, ossicular chain disruption, or the patency of ventilation tubes.

II. **Procedures.**

A. Examine the ear canal and remove any occluding cerumen or exudate. Inspect tympanic membrane. Select the appropriate tip for the tympanometer.

B. Grasp the helix and straighten the ear canal. Position the probe. When the probe is positioned properly, the automatic recording device will be triggered.

C. Leave the probe in position until the tympanometer signals the conclusion of the test. Repeat in the contralateral ear. (See Figure 21-1 for interpretation.)

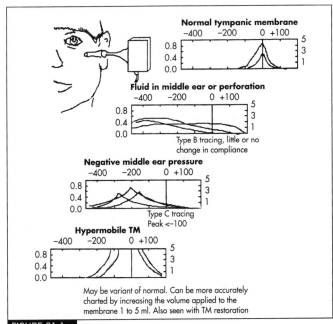

FIGURE 21-1

Tympanometry.

CHEST TUBE PLACEMENT

I. **Indications.**

A. Pneumothorax.

B. Hemothorax.

C. Drainage of pleural effusion.

II. **Contraindications.**

A. There are no contraindications to chest tube placement in patients symptomatic from the above listed indications. However, care should be used in patients with a potential for serious bleeding.

III. **Materials**

A. Materials needed:

Iodine & alcohol swabs for skin prep
Sterile drapes & gloves
#11 scalpel blade & handle
Mayo clamp
Kelly clamp
Silk suture (size 0)
Needle holder
Petrolatum-impregnated gauze

Sterile gauze
Tape
Suction apparatus
Chest tube (size 32 to 40 Fr, depending on clinical setting)
1% lidocaine with epinephrine, 10 cc syringe, 25- & 22-g needles

IV. **Technique (Figure 21-2).**

A. Position patient with affected side up. Identify the insertion site, which is generally at the anterior axillary line just behind the lateral edge of the pectoralis major at the level of the nipple. Prep and drape the insertion site. Generously anesthetize the insertion site along the insertion tract to the pleura. Appropriate position can be checked by aspirating through the needle used for instilling the local anesthetic.

B. The skin should be incised directly over the body of the rib, the incision length being 1½ times the diameter of the chest tube to be used. The Kelly or Mayo clamp is then used to bluntly dissect superiorly over the superior margin of the next higher rib. The Mayo clamp is then pushed through the parietal pleura with tips closed and with slow steady pressure. Once the pleura has been penetrated, the clamps are opened wide to enlarge the insertion tract and removed. Operator's index finger can also be inserted along the tract to further enlarge the opening if needed.

C. The chest tube is grasped near the end to be inserted with the Mayo clamp (jaws of the clamp parallel to the length of the tube), and advanced into the pleural space. Once the tube is inserted so that all drainage ports are inside the thoracic cavity, the tube is connected to suction and sutured in place with silk suture by closing the skin edges of the incision around the tube and tying the suture ends up around the tube. The area should be dressed with petrolatum-impregnated gauze and sterile gauze sponges. Chest x-ray should be obtained to confirm proper placement.

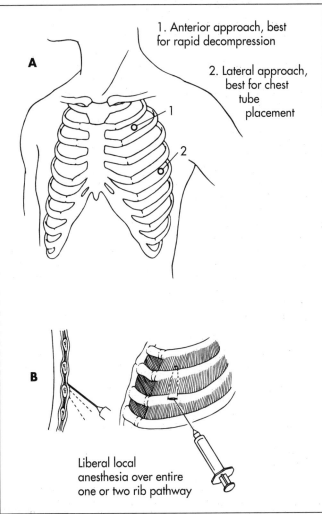

FIGURE 21-2

A to D, Chest tube placement.

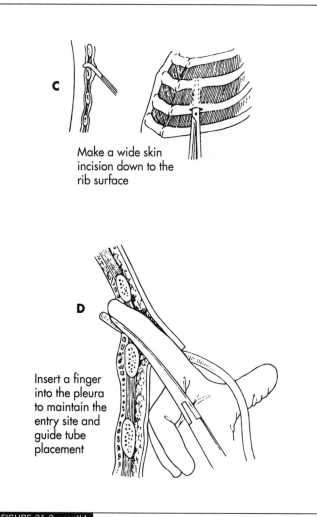

C

Make a wide skin incision down to the rib surface

D

Insert a finger into the pleura to maintain the entry site and guide tube placement

FIGURE 21-2—cont'd

A to D, Chest tube placement.

D. Removal is accomplished by having the patient inhale fully, hold his/her breath, and pulling the tube out swiftly. Cover with antibiotic impregnated gauze.

IV. **Complications**

A. Potential complications include:

Hemorrhage at the site of insertion	Lung laceration
Infection	Laceration of intraabdominal organs if tube
Hematoma	is inadvertently inserted into the
	abdominal cavity

INTRAOSSEOUS INFUSION

Intraosseous infusion can provide a very rapid and dependable route of vascular access in children age 3 or less (where vascular access is likely to be difficult in settings where it is most urgent). Almost any infusate can be instilled at a rapid rate through an intraosseous line, including blood and blood products, Plasmanate, glucose, crystalloids, pressor agents including epinephrine, dopamine and dobutamine, and atropine.

I. **Indications.**

A. Emergency fluid infusion, especially in setting of circulatory collapse where rapid IV access is essential.

B. Difficult IV access.

C. Burn or other injury preventing access to the venous system at other sites.

II. **Contraindications.**

A. Overlying cellulitis.

B. Bony lesion at site.

C. Osteomyelitis.

III. **Technique (Figure 21-3).**

A. Identify landmarks and prepare the insertion site with iodine or alcohol solution. Sites for insertion:
   1. Proximal tibia 2-5 cm below the tibial tuberosity in the midline in children.
   2. Distal tibia in the midline 2-5 cm above medial malleolus in adults.

B. Infiltrate the overlying skin to the periosteum if the patient is sensitive to pain.

C. For insertion in the proximal tibia, the spinal needle is directed inferiorly at a 45-degree angle from the perpendicular. If the insertion site is the distal tibia, the needle should be angled 45 degrees superiorly. In both instances the goal is to angle away from the region of the growth plate and/or joint.

D. Advance needle (with stylet in place) through skin, subcutaneous tissue and cortex of bone into the marrow space using a rotary motion.

E. Remove stylet and confirm placement by aspirating back marrow. Try infusing 5 cc of saline with a syringe.

21

OFFICE/HOSPITAL PROCEDURES

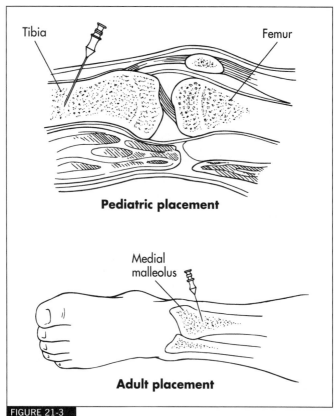

Tibia   Femur

Pediatric placement

Medial
malleolus

Adult placement

FIGURE 21-3

Intraosseous infusion.

F. Detach syringe and connect IV tubing to begin infusion. Secure in position with tape.
IV. **Complications.**
A. Local abscess or cellulitis.
B. Osteomyelitis.
C. Injury to growth plate has not been identified as a complication that occurs with any significant frequency.

REGIONAL BLOCKS

I. **Prep Skin and Draw Up Anesthetic.** Always raise skin wheal before advancing the needle, and always inject slowly and aspirate to avoid intravascular administration.

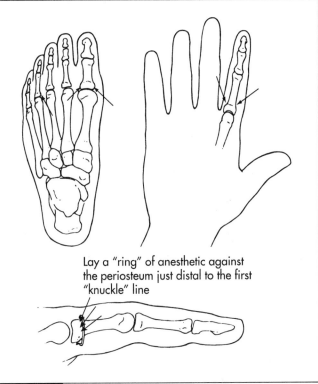

Lay a "ring" of anesthetic against
the periosteum just distal to the first
"knuckle" line

FIGURE 21-4

Digital nerve block techniques.

II. **Digital Blocks** for complete finger anesthesia for reductions or repair of lacerations (Figure 21-4).

A. Raise skin wheal using 1% lidocaine without epinephrine at base of digit at the level of the interphalangeal skin creases.

B. Angle ⅝-inch 25-gauge needle 45 degrees from finger in the horizontal and vertical planes and advance until the bone is reached.

C. While butting the needle tip against the bone of the proximal phalanx and aspirating-for-blood/injecting local anesthetic periodically, "walk" the needle through the same puncture site over the dorsal and volar aspects of the phalanx to leave a complete "half-ring" of anesthetized tissues on both sides of the digit. Use no more than 1 to 2 cc through either puncture site and set the syringe aside for further use if needed. Gently massage the zone of anesthesia to ensure that an adequate block occurs after 5-10 minutes. If distal pinprick sensation is still

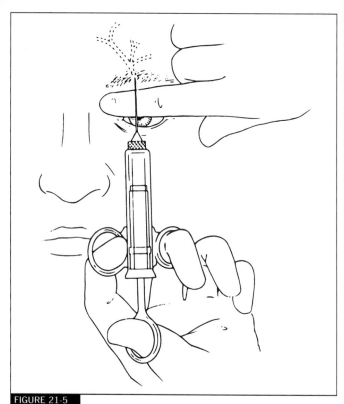

FIGURE 21-5

Supraorbital nerve block.

present by 10 minutes, you may repeat the procedure through the same puncture sites using another 1cc of lidocaine on either side.

III. **Supraorbital Nerve Block.** Anesthesia for upper eyelid to scalp line from midline to lambdoid suture (Figure 21-5).

A. With the patient looking directly ahead, palpate the supraorbital notch above the midline pupil in the mid-to-lower eyebrow.

B. Advance needle superiorly until paresthesias are noted. Apply pressure to the upper lid, and inject 2 cc of 1% lidocaine without epinephrine.

IV. **Infraorbital Nerve Block.** Anesthesia of the upper lip, nose, lower eyelid, and maxillary portion of the face.

A. Palpate infraorbital foramen immediately below midline pupil. Raise skin wheal at this site.

B. Advance the needle until paresthesias are elicited, and inject 2 cc of 1% lidocaine without epinephrine while applying pressure above the infraorbital rim.

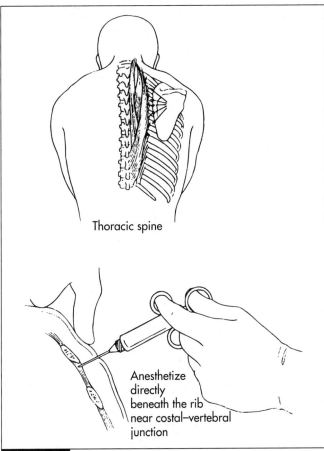

Thoracic spine

Anesthetize
directly
beneath the rib
near costal–vertebral
junction

FIGURE 21-6

Intercostal nerve block.

V. **Mental Nerve Block.** Anesthesia of the chin and lower lip.
A. Identify the mental foramen, which is palpable subcutaneously halfway between the upper and lower border of the mandible. A line drawn connecting the supraorbital and infraorbital foramina and the corner of the mouth would pass through the mental foramen. Prep the skin with providone-iodine. Raise a skin wheal at the injection site.
B. Advance the 25-gauge needle to but not into the foramen and inject 3 cc of 1% lidocaine without epinephrine.
VI. **Intercostal Nerve Block.** Relieve chest wall pain caused by rib fractures. (Figure 21-6).

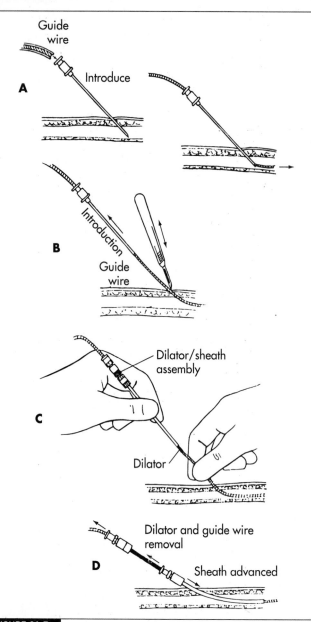

Guide
wire

Introduce

A

Introduction

B

Guide
wire

Dilator/sheath
assembly

C

Dilator

Dilator and guide wire
removal

D

Sheath advanced

FIGURE 21-7

A to D, Seldinger catheter-over-wire technique.

A. Have patient sit, leaning forward onto a Mayo tray. Identify affected rib and the angle formed by the rib and paraspinous muscle. Raise skin wheal at this angle, over the inferior border of the rib.

B. Advance the needle to just under the inferior border of the rib, aspirate, and inject 5 cc of 1% lidocaine with epinephrine. Marcaine may also be used for prolonged effect.

CENTRAL VENOUS LINES (FIGURE 21-7)

THORACENTESIS

I. **Indications.** Evaluation of a pulmonary effusion or relieve respiratory distress caused by large effusion.

II. **Contraindications.**

A. Severe coagulopathies.

B. Small stable effusions.

C. Patients who are unable to cooperate.

D. Patients responding to medical therapy.

III. **Technique.**

A. Determine puncture site by CXR and percussion. Have patient sit leaning forward. Put on sterile gloves. Prep and drape area.

B. Choose entry site below air-fluid interface and at the upper edge of the rib. Raise skin wheal with 25-gauge needle and carry anesthesia down through the chest wall. Use 21-gauge 2-inch needle to anesthetize the pleural surface. "Pop" the needle into the pleural space and confirm location with aspiration of fluid.

C. Remove needle, and attach it to the 3 way stopcock and 50 cc syringe. Reinsert and withdraw enough fluid to fill the specimen tubes.

D. To remove a large volume of fluid, fill 50 cc syringe and turn the stopcock to permit emptying. Repeat if necessary. If you will be emptying up to 1 liter of fluid, attach a vacuum bottle by rubber tubing to a 15-gauge needle clamp tubing, and insert needle in clamp and allow vacuum to aspirate the fluid.

E. When finished aspirating, withdraw needle and apply pressure over site for a few minutes and dress with pressure dressing. Observe for dyspnea. Send fluid for cell count and differential, protein, glucose, LDH, culture, gram stain, specific gravity, cytology, AFB, fungal cultures. Obtain post-tap CXR.

V. **Interpretation.** See Chapter 4.

VI. **Complications.**

A. Pneumothorax.

B. Hematoma.

C. Hemothorax.

D. Infection.

NASAL FOREIGN BODY REMOVAL

I. **Indications.**

Common in young children and mentally retarded adults. Suspect nasal foreign body with sudden onset respiratory distress, nasal flaring, unilateral mucopurulent discharge, and foul smell.

II. **Contraindications.**

Few contraindications exist. ABC's take precedence over any procedures.

III. **Materials.**

None.

IV. **Technique.**

A. Reassure and calm the patient and instruct the caregiver or parent to give the patient a breath "mouth-to-mouth" while occluding the unobstructed naris.

B. Place the child supine in Trendelenburg position. Then place the child's head in a "sniffing position" with his or her mouth open widely.

C. The parent may obtain full cooperation by telling the child that he or she is going to give the child a big kiss. Then the parent delivers a breath with a tight seal. Subsequently, the obstructing object is dislodged, often onto the cheek of the caregiver.

D. Re-attempts may be required with minor adjustments. Alternatively, an Ambu bag may be used to deliver a "breath." A drop of local vasoconstrictor may also be used prior to the procedure to minimize mucosal edema.

V. **Complications.**

Recommend ENT referral for objects that are sharp or not dislodged with this technique. Other techniques, using a Foley catheter or Fogarty biliary balloon catheter, positive pressure ventilation or high frequency ventilation, and bronchoscopic removal will not be discussed here.

BIBLIOGRAPHY

Driscoll CE et al, eds: *Handbook of family practice,* Chicago, 1986,Year Book Medical Publishers.

Driscoll CE, Rakel RE, eds: *Procedures for your practice,* Oradell, New Jersey, 1988, Medical Economics.

Pfenninger JL, Fowler GC: *Procedures for primary care physicians,* 1994, St. Louis, Mosby.

Roberts JR, Hedges JR: *Clinical procedures in emergency medicine,* Philadelphia, 1985, WB Saunders.

Weiner HL, Levitt LP: *Neurology for the House Officer,* fourth edition, Baltimore, 1989, Williams & Wilkins.

HERBAL FORMULARY

Teresa Bailey Klepser
Michael W. Kelly

TABLE 22-1

UNSAFE HERBAL PREPARATIONS

Carcinogens	Hepatotoxicity	Miscellaneous Toxicity
Borage	Chaparral	Licorice
Calamus	Germander	Ma Huang
Coltsfoot	Life root	Pokeroot
Comfrey		
Life root		
Sassafras		

22

TABLE 22-2

HERBAL FORMULARY

Indication	Efficacy	Contraindication
BLACK COHOSH		
PMS symptoms, painful or difficult menstruation, and neurovegetative symptoms (hot flashes) caused by menopause.	Proven in double-blind control trial and 3 open label trials. Shown to be superior to placebo and comparable to estriol, conjugated estrogens, and estrogen-progesterone therapy.	Pregnancy. Unknown if suitable where HRT is contraindicated such as estrogen-receptor positive breast cancer. German Commission E recommends length of use should not exceed 6 months.
CHASE TREE BERRY *(VITEX AGNUS-CASTUS)*		
Disorders of the menstrual cycle, PMS, and mastodynia.	Proven in open-label trial and one double-blind trial. Efficacy is mild.	Pregnancy, lactation, and women receiving HRT. Contains progestins, and long-term effects of "natural hormones" on development of various hormone-mediated neoplasms is unknown.

Drug Interactions	Side Effects	Dose
None known	Occasional intestinal problems may occur; weight gain possible. Large doses may cause dizziness, nausea, severe headaches, stiffness, and trembling limbs.	Remifemin: standardized product that contains 40 mg black cohosh to be taken BID. Standardized to 1 mg of 27-deoxyacteine per tablet.
No drug interactions reported; however, dopamine-receptor antagonists, such as haloperidol, may weaken or block effects.	Reported in a few patients: GI and lower abdominal complaints, allergic reactions (i.e., itching and rash), headache, increased menstrual flow. Early menstruation after delivery rare side effect.	Available as aqueous-alcoholic extracts (50%-70% V/V) from crushed fruit, tinctures, tea, or capsules. Some preparations formulated to give average daily dose 20-40 mg of berries. Daily dose of crushed fruit may be divided and administered BID or TID. Extract contains 175-225 mg; recommended to be standardized to contain 0.5% agnuside. Unknown why preparations are standardized to 0.5% agnuside since agnuside is an inactive ingredient in Vitex. Herbalists recommend 1-2 ml of tincture TID or 40 drops standardized tincture daily. To make tea, add cup boiling water onto 1 t ripe berries and infuse 10-15 min. Ingest tea TID. Results as early as 4 months or as long as 18 months.

22

HERBAL FORMULARY

Continued

TABLE 22-2

HERBAL FORMULARY—cont'd

Indication	Efficacy	Contraindication
CHONDROITIN		
Nonapproved for visco-elastic agent in ophthalmic procedures and osteoarthritis.	Efficacy studies included glucosamine, which may be the active agent.	Previous hypersensitivity to chondroitin sulfate.
COENZYME Q10		
Nonapproved for CHF, hypertension, stable angina, ventricular arrhythmias, cancer, heart surgery, and periodontal disease.	Effective for CHF in double-blind, placebo-controlled trial. Efficacy for angina, etc., not yet proven, although studies suggestive	Biliary obstruction, diabetes mellitus (hypoglycemia), hepatic insufficiency, renal insufficiency
DONG QUAI		
Menstrual disorders, anemia, constipation, insomnia, rheumatism, neuralgia, and hypertension.	Negative results in placebo-controlled trial.	Pregnancy (uterine stimulant), lactation, diarrhea, hemorrhagic disease, hypermenorrhea, during colds or flus. Allergy to parsley.
ECHINACAEA		
Internal use: Supportive therapy for URIs (colds) and lower urinary tract. External use: Local application for treatment of hard-to-heal superficial wounds and ulcers.	Melchart et al reviewed 26 controlled clinical trials evaluating echinacaea's ability to strengthen body's own defense mechanisms. Thirty of 34 echinacaea therapies were more effective compared to controls.	Infectious and autoimmune diseases (tuberculosis, leukosis, collagenosis, multiple sclerosis, AIDS, HIV, and lupus). Caution should be used in patients who are allergic to members of sunflower family. Effects of echinacaea in pregnancy, lactation, and children are unknown.

Drug Interactions	Side Effects	Dose
None reported	Nausea and epigastric pain	400 mg TID.
Hypolipidemic agents lower plasma concentrations of CoQ10. Oral hypoglycemic agents potentially inhibit affects of exogenous administration.	Rash and GI disturbances (nausea, anorexia, epigastric pain, diarrhea). Elevations of serum aminotransferases occurred with relatively high oral doses.	100 mg daily, up to 600 mg daily.
Unknown if interacts with anticoagulants, such as warfarin, other cardiovascular drugs such as procainamide.	Photodermatitis may occur in persons collecting plant. Safrole, found in oil of Dong Quai, is carcinogenic and not recommended for ingestion.	Variety of doses are suggested. No standardized produce available. Most common dose is powdered root 3-4 g divided BID-TID (5.4-12 g/day).
None known.	None known.	Variety of doses is recommended. Most common dose is dried powder, 1 g or two 500 mg capsules orally TID. Therapy should not exceed 8 weeks. Some evidence shows that prolonged use of echinacaea may depress the immune system possibly through overstimulation.

22

HERBAL FORMULARY

Continued

TABLE 22-2

HERBAL FORMULARY—cont'd

Indication	Efficacy	Contraindication
FEVERFEW		
Prophylaxis of migraine headaches.	Proven effective in a double blind, placebo controlled trial.	Feverfew should be avoided in pregnancy, lactation, and children under 2 years old.
GARLIC		
Support dietary measures for treatment of hyperlipoproteinemia and prevent age-related changes in blood vessels (arteriosclerosis).	Proven to reduce blood pressure and cholesterol, but data not the best.	Caution in diabetics and pregnancy (emmenagogue and abortifacient).

Drug Interactions	Side Effects	Dose
Feverfew may interact with anticoagulants, increasing the risk of bleeding	Gastric discomfort. Minor ulcerations of oral mucosa, irritation of tongue, and swelling of lips may occur when fresh leaves are chewed. Heart rate increased by 26 beats/min in two patients. Canadian Health Protection Branch advises consumers not to take feverfew continuously for more than 4 months without medical advice. Discontinuation may produce muscle/joint stiffness and cluster of CNS reactions (rebound of migraines, anxiety, and poor sleep patterns).	Usual dose is 125 mg daily. Product containing at least 0.2% parthenolide is recommended.
Anticoagulants (increased bleeding). Antiretrovirals (decreased levels).	GI discomfort (heartburn, flatulence), sweating, lightheadedness, allergic reactions, and menorrhagia.	0.6-1.2 g dried powder (2-5 mg of allicin) daily or 2-4 g fresh garlic. Alliinase (enzyme that converts alliin to allicin) inactivated by acids. Enteric-coated tablets or capsules allow more absorption because they pass through the stomach and release their contents in alkaline medium of small intestine.

Continued

22

TABLE 22-2

HERBAL FORMULARY—cont'd

Indication	Efficacy	Contraindication
GINGKO		
Treatment for cerebral circulatory disturbances resulting in reduced functional capacity and vigilance (vertigo, tinnitus, weakened memory, and mood swings accompanied by anxiety). Treatment of peripheral arterial circulatory disturbance such as intermittent claudication.	7 of 8 well-done trials show positive effect on CNS function (including in Alzheimer's disease). Two well-done trials suggest benefit in claudication.	None known.
GINGER		
Dyspepsia and prophylaxis of symptoms of travel sickness.	No benefit overall for motion sickness.	Avoid for postoperative nausea because it may prolong bleeding time and delay immunologic changes. Contraindicated for gallstone pain. Recommended in pregnancy only on advice of physician (uterine relaxant [low doses]; uterine stimulant [high doses]).

Drug Interactions	Side Effects	Dose
Antiplatelets—a case report of spontaneous hyphema (bleeding from iris into anterior chamber) from ginkgo and aspirin.	Gastric disturbances, headache, dizziness, and vertigo. Toxic ingestion may produce tonic-clonic seizures and loss of consciousness.	Recommended dose is 40 mg TID with meals for at least 4-6 weeks. Standardized preparations containing 6% terpene lactones and 24% ginkgo flavone glycosides are recommended.
None known.	None reported.	For travel sickness: Daily dose is 2-4 g. Two 500-mg capsules taken 30 min before travel, then 1-2 more capsule(s) Q4hr as needed.

Continued

22

HERBAL FORMULARY

TABLE 22-2

HERBAL FORMULARY—cont'd

Indication	Efficacy	Contraindication
GINSENG (ASIAN)		
Tonic to combat feelings of lassitude and debility, lack of energy and ability to concentrate, and during convalescence.	Shown to be of benefit in randomized, double-blind, controlled study for fatigue.	Pregnancy, children, and patients with hypertension, emotional/psychologic imbalances, headaches, heart palpitations, insomnia, asthma, inflammation, or infections with high fever.
GINSENG (SIBERIAN)		
Tonic for fatigue, convalescence, decreased work capacity, or difficulty in concentration.	No benefit in randomized, placebo controlled study.	Avoid in hypertension. Not recommended in patients in febrile states, hypertonic crisis, or MI.
GLUCOSAMINE		
Nonapproved for osteoarthritis.	Superior to ibuprofen in a double-blind study. Spared and repaired cartilage.	Hypersensitivity to glucosamine. Diabetics may have impaired insulin secretion.

Drug Interactions	Side Effects	Dose
May interact with phenelzine, producing hallucinations and psychosis. May decrease INR of warfarin.	Nervousness and excitation first 4 days. Inability to concentrate with long-term use. Diffuse mammary nodularity and vaginal bleeding may be due to estrogen-like effect in women. Hypertension, euphoria, restlessness, nervousness, insomnia, skin eruptions, edema, and diarrhea reported with long-term use with average dose of 3 g ginseng root daily.	1-2 g crude herb daily or 100-300 mg of ginseng extract TID. Standardized products that contain at least 4%-5% ginsenosides are recommended
Serum levels of digoxin may increase when taken with Siberian ginseng. Hexobarbital and Siberian ginseng increase sleep latency and duration.	Mild, transient diarrhea and insomnia. May lower blood glucose.	2 capsules (each capsule containing 400-500 mg of powdered root) TID. Total of 2-3 g daily. Solid concentrated extract standardized on eleutherosides B and E 300-400 mg daily recommended.
Fluoxetine may increase glucosamine serum concentrations.	GI side effects such as epigastric pain and tenderness, heartburn, diarrhea, nausea. CNS side effects such as drowsiness, headache, and insomnia. Long-term side effects unknown.	500 mg TID.

Continued

TABLE 22-2

HERBAL FORMULARY—cont'd

Indication	Efficacy	Contraindication
HAWTHORN		
Mild cardiac conditions such as CHF NYHA stages I or II, uneasiness and oppressed feeling of the heart, not yet digitalized heart, and light forms of bradycardic arrhythmia.	Proven effective in two double-blind, placebo-controlled studies for symptomatic relief of CHF.	Pregnancy, lactation. Note for self-treatment.
HORSE CHESTNUT SEED		
Venous conditions, eczema, leg pains, hemorrhoids, phlebitis, menstruation.	Shows benefit in double-blind, placebo-controlled studies.	Renal and hepatic insufficiency.
KAVA		
Insomnia, nervousness.	Proven effective in open-label study (weaker evidence than double-blind, placebo-controlled).	Depression (increased risk of suicide), operating machinery or motor vehicles. Pregnancy, lactation, children. Should not be taken longer than 3 months without doctor's supervision.

Drug Interactions	Side Effects	Dose
Unknown with other cardiovascular drugs such as digoxin, calcium channel blockers, beta-blockers, and antiarrhythmics.	Large doses may induce hypotension, arrhythmias, and sedation.	160-900 mg/day divided into BID-TID.
Anticoagulants.	GI irritation, pruritus, giddiness.	Aescin 30-150 mg daily. Venastat 300 mg (standardized aescin 50 mg).
Sedatives, anxiolytics, monoamine oxidase inhibitors, alcohol, antidepressants. Antiplatelets. Levodopa (decreased levels).	Yellowing skin, nails, hair. Allergic skin reactions; "Kava dermopathy" (dry, scaly skin rash on palms of hands, soles of feet, forearms, back, and shins, swollen face, blood-shot eyes); GI complaints; pupil dilation; disorders of oculomotor equilibrium; morning fatigue, neurologic choreoathetosis, dystonic reactions; dyskinesia. Tolerance: not reported Toxicity: ataxia, muscle weakness, ascending paralysis without loss of consciousness.	200-250 mg of kava lactones divided into two or three doses.

Continued

22

HERBAL FORMULARY

TABLE 22-2

HERBAL FORMULARY—cont'd

Indication	Efficacy	Contraindication
LICORICE		
Expectorant and the treatment of ulcers.	Negative human evidence.	German Commission E stipulates that duration of use be no longer than 4-6 weeks. Liver cirrhosis, cholestatic liver disorders, hypertonia, kidney diseases, cardiovascular diseases, especially hypertension, hypokalemia, and pregnancy.
MA HUANG		
Derivative of ephedrine; CNS stimulant	Dangerous; should not be used.	Patients with heart conditions, hypertension, diabetes, or thyroid disease.
MELATONIN		
Orphan Drug Status. Treatment of circadian rhythm sleep disorders in blind people with no light perception. Nonapproved Indications. Jet lag, insomnia, depression, and cancer.	Shown effective in jet lag and insomnia but ineffective in preventing fatigue in shift workers.	Melatonin may aggravate depressive symptoms.
MILK THISTLE		
Supportive treatment for chronic inflammatory liver conditions and cirrhosis.	Seems to be effective in controlled trials.	Safety not established in pregnancy.

Drug Interactions	Side Effects	Dose
Potassium loss may be increased in the presence of other drugs, e.g., thiazide and loop diuretics. With loss of potassium, sensitivity to digitalis glycosides increases.	Prolongation of P-R and Q-T intervals. With long-term use or acute toxic ingestion, pseudoaldosteronism (headache, lethargy, sodium and water retention, hypokalemia, high blood pressure, heart failure and cardiac arrest).	1-2 g licorice root TID or 200-800 mg glycyrrhizin per day.
Similar to drug interactions of ephedrine/pseudoephedrine. Avoid consumption with caffeine.	Nervousness, headache, insomnia, dizziness, palpitations, skin flushing, tingling, vomiting, hypertension, and MI.	Ephedra herb contains small concentrations of ephedrine (~1%). Maximum ephedrine dose = 100 mg/24 hrs.
Vitamin B12 influences melatonin secretion. Low levels of vitamin B12 will produce low levels of melatonin. MAOI may increase melatonin serum concentrations. SSRIs may increase melatonin serum concentrations. Beta-blockers may decrease nocturnal secretion of melatonin.	Heavy head, headache, and transient depression. Long-term side effects are unknown.	3 mg HS.
None reported.	Rare: Mild transient diarrhea and rash.	Daily dose is 200-400 mg per day of silymarin.

Continued

	TABLE 22-2	

HERBAL FORMULARY—cont'd

Indication	Efficacy	Contraindication
SAW PALMETTO		
Treatment of micturition difficulties associated with benign prostatic hyperplasia.	No difference between saw palmetto and finsateride at 6 months in randomized study. (Draw your own conclusions: Does finasteride work?).	Pregnancy, children.
ST JOHN'S WORT		
Anxiety and depression.	Proven as effective as low dose tricyclics in placebo-controlled studies.	Caution in fair-skinned persons when exposed to bright sunlight. Caution in pregnancy (emmenagogic and abortifacient). No negative influence on general performance or the ability to drive a car or operate heavy machinery has been reported.
VALERIAN		
Restlessness and nervous disturbance of sleep	Proven double-blind, placebo-controlled studies trial to improve sleep (450 mg dose).	Caution while driving or performing other tasks requiring alertness and coordination is recommended.

Drug Interactions	Side Effects	Dose
None reported.	Headache, stomach upset.	1-2 g saw palmetto or 320 mg lipophilic extract daily, usually given 160 mg BID. Take with food. Standardized products containing 90% free and 7% esterified fatty acids are recommended.
DRUGS: Antidepressants (serotonin syndrome); antiretrovirals (decreased effect); oral contraceptives (decreased effect); digoxin (decreased levels); theophylline (decreased levels); cyclosporine (decreased levels). FOOD: May be similar to MAOIs (tyramine-containing foods: cheeses, beer, wine, herring, and yeast).	Photodermatitis, GI irritations, allergic reactions, fatigue, restlessness.	2-4 g daily of herb. Standardized products containing 0.4-2.7 mg hypericin/day or 0.3% hypericin are recommended. Metabolized via cytochrome P450.
May potentiate sedative effect of barbiturates, benzodiazepines, opiates, or alcohol.	Headaches, hangover, excitability, insomnia, uneasiness and cardiac disturbances. Toxicity: ataxia, decreased sensibility, hypothermia, hallucinations, and increased muscle relaxation.	Dried herb or extract: 2-3 g daily, up to TID.

REFERENCE MATERIALS

Mark A. Graber

PEDIATRIC SEDATION

I. **Sedation can facilitate procedures in the ED** and minimize the psychologic trauma to the child as well as to the ED staff and the parents.

II. **Sedation requirements.**

A. Need good monitoring including O_2 saturation, pulse, BP if possible, level of consciousness and respirations. The child should be closely monitored until he or she has returned to functional baseline value.

B. **Sedation does not equal pain relief.** Give medications that relax the child and medications that provide pain relief.

C. The traditional DPT (demerol, phenergan, and thorazine) or Kiddy Cocktail/Lytic Cocktail is fraught with problems and cannot be recommended.

D. Benzodiazepines have the advantage of causing amnesia, especially midazolam.

E. Despite drug company marketing, there is no significant difference in the recovery times of diazepam and midazolam when used as a single dose for sedation in the ED. In fact, the recovery time was faster with diazepam in most studies.

F. Postsedation discharge requires a return to baseline verbal skills if appropriate, baseline muscular control, baseline mental status, and a parent or responsible person who can understand instructions.

III. Drugs for sedation and pain control in children are found in Table 23-1. Note: **Sedative doses are for conscious sedation, which requires constant monitoring. Be familiar with these agents and their side effects before using!**

23

TABLE 23-1

MEDICATIONS FOR SEDATION AND PAIN CONTROL IN CHILDREN

Medication	Route	Dose (mg/kg)	Maximum Dose	Side Effects and Comments
PAIN MEDICATIONS				
Fentanyl	IV	2-3 µg/kg	0.05 mg	Rapidly effective IV (1-2min) and short-acting (20-30 min). Causes respiratory depression.
Meperidine (Demerol)	IV/IM	0.5 to 1.0 mg/kg	100 mg	Reversible with naloxone (watch for respiratory depression). May cause hypotension.
Morphine	IV/IM	0.1 to 0.2 mg/kg	10 mg	Same as above
Codeine	PO	1.0 mg/kg	60 mg	Same as above
SEDATIVES				
Diazepam (Valium and others)	IV	0.05 to 0.2 mg/kg	10 mg	Watch for respiratory depression. Reversible with flumazenil.
	PR	0.5 mg/kg		
Midazolam (Versed)	IV/IM	0.01 to 0.08 mg/kg (some have used up to 0.2 mg/kg	4 mg	Titrate to effect; precautions as above.
	PO/IN/PR	0.3 to 0.7 mg/kg		As above

Chloral hydrate	PR	25 to 100 mg/kg PO or PR	1000 mg, although some will go to 2000 mg	Cannot reverse. Less likely to be effective in head injured or neurologically impaired patients.
DISSOCIATIVE AGENTS				
Ketamine	IV	0.5-2.0 mg/kg IV up to 4 mg/kg IM	100 mg IV	Onset 1 min with duration of 15 min. IM use prolongs ED stay. Excellent drug, few adverse reactions (but raises ICP and IOP). Airway reactivity and respirations generally maintained. Do not use if <3 mon of age or respiratory infection. Administer with atropine 0.01 mg/kg, maximum 0.5 mg.
	IM	2-4 mg/kg IM (4 mg generally produces optimal effect)	—	
TO REVERSE				
Naloxone (Narcan)	IV or IM	0.01 mg/kg/dose	2 mg/dose but may repeat	Watch for narcotic withdrawal.
Flumazenil (Romazicon)	IV or IM	0.01 mg/kg/dose	1 mg but may repeat	(Do not use flumazanil for those with chronic benzodiazepine use!)

IM, Intramuscular; *IN,* intranasal; *IV,* intravenous; *PO,* by mouth; *PR,* per rectum.

23

REFERENCE MATERIALS

TABLE 23-2

PEDIATRIC VITAL SIGNS

Age	Heart Rate		Blood Pressure		Respiratory Rate
	Awake	Sleeping	Systolic	Diastolic	
Neonate	100-180	80-160	70-100	50-65	30-60
6 months	120-160	80-180	87-105	53-66	25-50
2 years	80-150	70-120	90-106	55-67	18-35
5 years	80-110	60-90	94-109	56-69	17-27
10 years	70-110	60-90	102-117	62-75	15-23
>10 years	55-100	50-90	105-128	66-80	10-23

TABLE 23-3

FAHRENHEIT/CELSIUS CONVERSION

Fahrenheit	Celsius	Fahrenheit	Celsius
104	40	100.2	37.9
103.8	39.9	100	37.8
103.6	39.8	99.9	37.7
103.5	39.7	99.7	37.6
103.3	39.6	99.5	37.5
103.1	39.5	99.3	37.4
102.8	39.4	99.1	37.3
102.7	39.3	99	37.2
102.6	39.2	98.8	37.1
102.4	39.1	98.6	37
102.2	39	98.4	36.9
102	38.9	98.2	36.8
101.8	38.8	98	36.7
101.6	38.7	97.9	36.6
101.5	38.6	97.7	36.5
101.3	38.5	97.5	36.4
101.1	38.4	97.3	36.3
100.9	38.3	97.2	36.2
100.8	38.2	97	36.1
100.6	38.1	96.8	36
100.4	38		

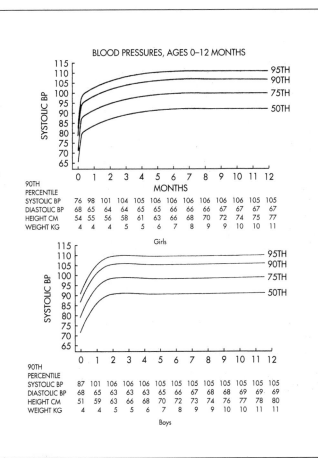

23

REFERENCE MATERIALS

FIGURE 23-1

Blood pressures, ages from birth to 12 months. *From Horan MJ:* Pediatrics *79:1, 1987.*

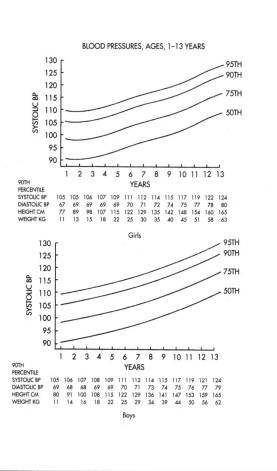

BLOOD PRESSURES, AGES, 1-13 YEARS

Girls

90TH PERCENTILE													
SYSTOLIC BP	105	105	106	107	109	111	112	114	115	117	119	122	124
DIASTOLIC BP	67	69	69	69	69	70	71	72	74	75	77	78	80
HEIGHT CM	77	89	98	107	115	122	129	135	142	148	154	160	165
WEIGHT KG	11	13	15	18	22	25	30	35	40	45	51	58	63

Boys

90TH PERCENTILE													
SYSTOLIC BP	105	106	107	108	109	111	112	114	115	117	119	121	124
DIASTOLIC BP	69	68	68	69	69	70	71	73	74	75	76	77	79
HEIGHT CM	80	91	100	108	115	122	129	136	141	147	153	159	165
WEIGHT KG	11	14	16	18	22	25	29	34	39	44	50	56	62

FIGURE 23-2

Blood pressures, ages from 1 to 13 years. *From Horan MJ: Pediatrics 79:1, 1987.*

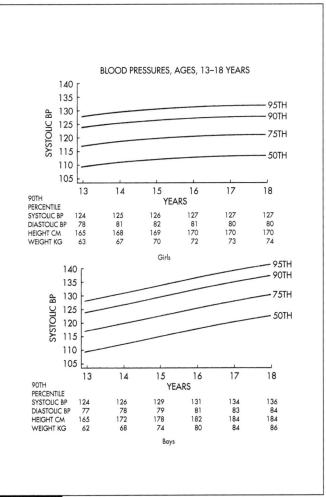

FIGURE 23-3

Blood pressures, ages from 13 to 18 years. *From Horan MJ: Pediatrics 79:1, 1987.*

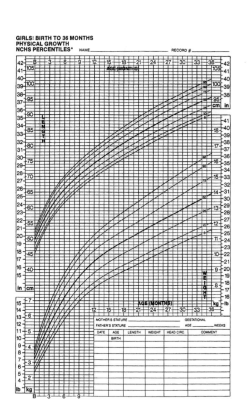

FIGURE 23-4

Length and weight of girls from birth to 23 months. *Adapted from Hamill PVV et al: Am J Clin Nutr 32:607-629, 1979. Data from the Fels Longitudinal Study, Wright State University School of Medicine, Yellow Springs, Ohio.*

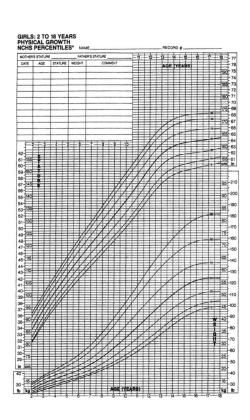

FIGURE 23-5

Stature and weight of girls from 2 to 18 years. *Adapted from Hamill PVV et al:* Am J Clin Nutr *32:607-629, 1979. Data from the Fels Longitudinal Study, Wright State University School of Medicine, Yellow Springs, Ohio.*

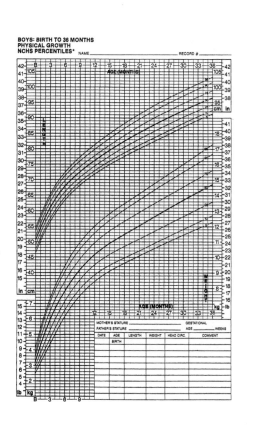

FIGURE 23-6
Length and weight of boys from birth to 36 months. *Adapted from Hamill PVV et al: Am J Clin Nutr 32:607-629, 1979. Data from the Fels Longitudinal Study, Wright State University School of Medicine, Yellow Springs, Ohio.*

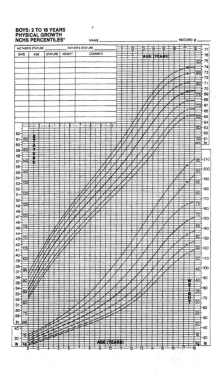

FIGURE 23-7

Stature and weight of boys from 2 to 18 years. *Adapted from Hamill PVV et al:* Am J Clin Nutr *32:607-629, 1979. Data from the Fels Longitudinal Study, Wright State University School of Medicine, Yellow Springs, Ohio.*

TABLE 23-4

DEVELOPMENTAL MILESTONES/LANGUAGE SKILLS

AGE	Gross Motor	Visual Motor	Language	Social
1 mon	Raises head slightly from prone, makes crawling movements, lifts chin up	Has tight grasp, follows to midline	Alert to sound (e.g., by blinking, moving, startling)	Regards face
2 mon	Holds head in midline, lifts chest off table	No longer clenches fist tightly, follows object past midline	Smiles after being stroked or talked to	Recognizes parent
3 mon	Supports on forearms in prone, hold head up steadily	Holds hands open at rest, follows in circular fashion	Coos (produces long vowel sounds in musical fashion)	Reaches for familiar people or objects, anticipates feeding
4-5 mon	Rolls front to back, back to front, sits well when propped, supports on wrists and shifts weight	Moves arms in unison to grasp, touches cube placed on table	Orients to voice; 5 mo: orients to bell (localized laterally), says "ahgoo," razzes	Enjoys looking around environment
6 mon	Sits well unsupported, puts feet in mouth in supine position	Reaches with either hand, transfers, uses raking grasp	Babbles; 7 mo: orients to bell (localizes indirectly); 8 mo: "dada/mama" indiscriminately	Recognizes strangers
9 mon	Creeps, crawls, cruises, pulls to stand, pivots when sitting	Uses pincer grasp, probes with forefinger, holds bottle, finger-feeds	Understands "no," waves bye-bye; 10 mo: "dada/mama" discriminantly; 11 mo: one word other than "dada/mama"	Starts to explore environment, plays pat-a-cake
12 mon	Walks alone	Throws objects, lets go of toys, hand release, uses mature pincer grasp	Follows one-step command with gesture, uses 2 words other than "dada/mama"; 14 mo: uses 3 words	Imitates actions, comes when called, cooperates with dressing

15 mon	Creeps upstairs, walks backward	Builds tower of 2 blocks in imitation of examiner, scribbles in imitation	Follows one-step command without gesture, uses 4 to 6 words and immature jargon (runs several unintelligible words together)	
18 mon	Runs, throws toy from standing without falling	Turns 2 or 3 pages at a time, fills spoon and feeds self	Knows 7 to 20 words, knows 1 body part, uses mature jargon (includes intelligible words in jargon)	Copies parent in tasks (e.g., sweeping, dusting), plays in company of other children
21 mon	Squats in play, goes up steps	Builds tower of 5 blocks, drinks well from cup	Points to 3 body parts, uses 2-word combinations, has 2-word vocabulary	Asks to have food and to go to toilet
24 mon	Walks up and down steps without help	Turns pages one at a time, removes shoes, pants, etc., imitates stroke	Uses 50 words, 2-word sentences, uses pronouns (I, you, me) inappropriately, points to 5 body parts, understands 2-step command	Parallel play

Continued

TABLE 23-4

DEVELOPMENTAL MILESTONES/LANGUAGE SKILLS—cont'd

AGE	Gross Motor	Visual Motor	Language	Social
30 mon	Jumps with both feet off floor, throws ball overhand	Unbuttons, holds pencil in adult fashion, differentiates horizontal and vertical line	Uses pronouns (I, you, me) appropriately, understands concept of "one," "repeats 2 digits forward	Tells first and last names when asked, gets drink without help
3 yr	Pedals tricycle, can alternate feet when going up steps	Dresses and undresses partially, dries hands if reminded, draws a circle	Uses 3-word sentences, plurals, and past tense. Knows all pronouns. Minimum of 250 words, understands concept of "two"	Group play, shares toys, takes turns, plays well with others, knows full name, age, sex
4 yr	Hops, skips, alternates feet going downstairs	Buttons clothing fully, catches ball	Knows colors, says song or poem from memory, asks questions	Tells "tall tales," plays cooperatively with a group of children
5 yr	Skips, alternating feet, jumps over low obstacles	Ties shoes, spreads with knife	Prints first name, asks what a word means	Plays competitive games, abides by rules, likes to help in household tasks

TABLE 23-5
DENTAL DEVELOPMENT*

| | Deciduous Teeth | | | | | | Permanent Teeth | |
| | Eruption | | Shedding | | | | Eruption | |
	Maxillary	Mandibular		Maxillary	Mandibular		Maxillary	Mandibular
Central incisors	6-8 mon	5-7 mon		7-8 yr	6-7 yr		7-8 yr	6-7 yr
Lateral incisors	8-11 mon	7-10 mon		8-9 yr	7-8 yr		8-9 yr	7-8 yr
Cuspids	16-20 mon	16-20 mon		11-12 yr	9-11 yr		11-12 yr	9-11 yr
1st premolar	—	—		—	—		10-11 yr	10-12 yr
2nd premolar	—	—		—	—		10-12 yr	11-13 yr
1st molars	10-16 mon	10-16 mon		10-11 yr	10-12 yr		6-7 yr	6-7 yr
2nd molars	20-30 mon	20-30 mon		10-12 yr	11-13 yr		12-13 yr	12-13 yr
3rd molars	—	—		—	—		17-22 yr	12-22 yr

Adapted from Driscoll CE et al: The family practice desk reference, ed 3, St. Louis, 1996, Mosby.
*Sexes are combined, although girls tend to be slightly more advanced than boys. Averages are approximate values derived from various studies.

23

REFERENCE MATERIALS

TABLE 23-6

NORMAL VALUES—HEMATOLOGY

Age	Hb (g/dl), mean (−2 SD)	HCT (%), mean (−2 SD)	MCV (fl), mean (−2 SD)	MCHC, mean (−2 SD)	Reticulocytes (%)	WBC/mm² × 100, mean (−2 SD)	Platelets 10³/mm³, mean ± SD
GESTION*							
26-30 wks	13.4 (11)	41.5 (34.9)	118.2 (106.7)	37.9 (30.6)	—	4.4 (2.7)	254 (180-327)
26 wks	14.5	45	120	31	(5-10)	—	275
32 wks	15.0	47	118	32	(3-10)	—	290
TERM†							
Cord	16.5 (13.5)	51 (42)	108 (98)	33 (30)	(3-7)	18.19-30‡	290
1-3 days	18.5 (14.5)	56 (45)	108 (95)	33 (30)	(3-7)	18.19-30‡	290
2 wks	16.6 (13.4)	53 (41)	105 (88)	31.4 (28.1)		11.4 (5-20)	252
1 mo	13.9 (10.7)	44 (33)	101 (91)	31.8 (28.1)	(0.1-1.7)	10.8 (5-19.5)	
2 mo	11.2 (9.4)	34 (28)	95 (84)	31.8 (28.3)			

Age							
6 mo	12.6 (11.1)	36 (31)	76 (68)	35 (32.7)	(0.7-2.3)	11.9 (6-17.5)	
6 mo-2 yr	12 (10.5)	36 (33)	78 (70)	33 (30)		10.6 (6-17)	(150-350)
2-6 yr	12.5 (11.5)	37 (34)	81 (75)	34 (31)	(0.5-1.0)	8.5 (5-15.5)	(150-350)
6-12 yr	13.5 (11.5)	40 (35)	86 (77)	34 (31)	(0.5-1.0)	8.1 (4.5-13.5)	(150-350)
12-18 YR							
Male	14.5 (13)	43 (36)	88 (78)	34 (31)	(0.5-1.0)	7.8 (4.5-13.5)	(150-350)
Female	13 (12)	41 (37)	90 (78)	34 (31)	(0.5-1.0)	7.8 (4.5-13.5)	(150-350)
ADULT							
Male	15.5 (13.5)	47 (41)	90 (80)	34 (31)	(0.8-2.5)	7.4 (4.5-11)	(150-350)
Female	14 (12)	41 (36)	90 (80)	34 (31)	(0.8-4.1)	7.4 (4.5-11)	(150-350)

MCHC, Mean corpuscular hemoglobin concentration; *MCV,* mean corpuscular volume.

*Values are from fetal samplings.

†Under 1 month, capillary hemoglobin exceeds venous: 1 hour, 3.6 g difference; 5 days, 2.2 g difference; 3 weeks, 1 g difference.

‡Mean (95%) confidence limits).

TABLE 23-7

CEREBROSPINAL FLUID

Component	Normal Values
Cell count (WBCs/mm^3)	
Preterm mean	9.0 (0-25.4), 57% PMNS
Term mean	8.2 (0-22.4), 61% PMNS
>1 mon	0-7, 0% PMNS
Glucose (mg/dl)	
Preterm	24-63 (mean, 50)
Term	34-119 (mean, 52)
Child	40-80
CSF glucose/blood glucose (%)	
Preterm	55-105
Term	44-128
Child	50
Lactic acid dehydrogenase: mean, 20 units/ml (range, 5-30 units/ml)	
Myelin basic protein: <4 ng/ml	
Pressure: initial LP (mm H$_2$O)	
Newborn	80-110 (<110)
Infant/child	<200 (lateral recumbent position)
Respiratory movements	5-10
Protein (mg/dl)	
Preterm	65-150 (mean, 115)
Term	20-170 (mean, 90)
Children	5-15, ventricular 5-25, cisternal 5-40, lumbar

TABLE 23-8

RECCOMENDATIONS FOR PARTICIPATION IN COMPETITIVE SPORTS

	Contact/ Collision	Limited Contact/ Impact	Noncontact		
			S	MS	NS
ATLANTOAXIAL INSTABILITY					
Swimming: no butterfly, breaststroke, or diving starts*	No	No	Yes	Yes	Yes
ACUTE ILLNESS					
Needs individual assessment such as contagiousness to others, risk of worsening illness	2	2	2	2	2
CARDIOVASCULAR					
Carditis	No	No	No	No	No
HYPERTENSION					
Mild	Yes	Yes	Yes	Yes	Yes
Moderate	2	2	2	2	2
Severe	2	2	2	2	2
Congenital heart disease	3	3	3	3	3
EYES					
Absence or loss of function of one eye	2	2	2	2	2
Detached retina	3	3	3	3	3
Availability of ASTM-approved eye guards may allow a competitor to participate in most sports, but this must be judged on an individual basis. Consult an ophthalmologist.					
NEUROLOGIC					
History of serious head or spine trauma, repeated concussion, or craniotomy	2	2	Yes	Yes	Yes
CONVULSIVE DISORDER					
Webb controlled	Yes	Yes	Yes	Yes	Yes
Poorly controlled	No	No	Yes	Yes	Yes
No swimming or weight lifting; no archery or riflery.					
RESPIRATORY					
Pulmonary insufficiency	2	2	2	2	2
Asthma	Yes	Yes	Yes	Yes	Yes
May be allowed to compete if oxygenation remains satisfactory during a graded stress test.					

Continued

23

REFERENCE MATERIALS

TABLE 23-8

RECCOMENDATIONS FOR PARTICIPATION IN COMPETITIVE SPORTS—cont'd

| | Contact/ Collision | Limited Contact/ Impact | Noncontact | | |
			S	MS	NS
MISCELLANEOUS					
Inguinal hernia	Yes	Yes	Yes	Yes	Yes
Kidney: absence of one	No	Yes	Yes	Yes	Yes
Liver: enlarged	No	No	Yes	Yes	Yes
Ovary: absence of one	Yes	Yes	Yes	2	Yes
Musculoskeletal disorders	2	2	2	Yes	2
Sickle cell trait	Yes	Yes	Yes	Yes	Yes
Skin: boils, herpes, impetigo, scabies	2	2	Yes		Yes
No gymnastics with mats, martial arts, wrestling, or contact sports until not contagious.					
Spleen: enlarged	No	No	No	Yes	Yes
Testicle: absent or undescended	Yes	Yes	Yes	Yes	Yes

Adapted from American Academy of Pediatrics: *Sports medicine: health care for young athletes,* Elk Grove Village, Ill., 1991 American Academy of Pediatrics.

S, Strenuous; *MS,* moderately strenuous; *NS,* nonstrenuous; *1,* certain sports may require a protective cup. *2,* needs individual assessment. *3,* patients with mild forms can be allowed a full range of activities; patients with moderate or severe forms or those who are postoperative need evaluation by a cardiologist before athletic participation; *ASTM,* American Society for Testing and Materials.

*Certain sports may require a protective cup.

PEAK FLOW RATES

TABLE 23-9

NORMAL PREDICTED AVERAGE PEAK EXPIRATORY FLOW
FOR CHILDREN IN L/MIN

Height (inches)	Peak Flow	Height (inches)	Peak Flow	Height (inches)	Peak Flow
43	147	51	254	59	360
44	160	52	267	60	373
45	173	53	280	61	387
46	187	54	293	62	400
47	200	55	307	63	413
48	214	56	320	64	427
49	227	57	334	65	440
50	240	58	347	66	454

From www.parentsplace.com.
Normal (green zone): 80%-100% of patient's best or normal value (above).
Caution (yellow zone): 60%-80% of patient's best or normal. Patient should institute written plan and closely follow peak-flow.
Danger (red zone): <60% of patient's best or normal. Institute written plan **and** contact health care provider.

23

REFERENCE MATERIALS

TABLE 23-10

NORMAL PREDICTED AVERAGE PEAK EXPIRATORY FLOW
IN L/MIN (POSTPUBERTAL)

Height (inches)	Peak Expiratory Flow (L/min)
MALES	
60"	554
65"	602
70"	649
75"	936
80"	740
FEMALES	
55"	390
60"	423
65"	460
70"	496
75"	529

From www.parentsplace.com.
Normal (green zone): 80%-100% of patient's best or normal value (above).
Caution (yellow zone): 60%-80% of patient's best or normal. Patient should institute written plan and closely follow peak-flow.
Danger (red zone): <60% of patient's best or normal. Institute written plan **and** contact health care provider.

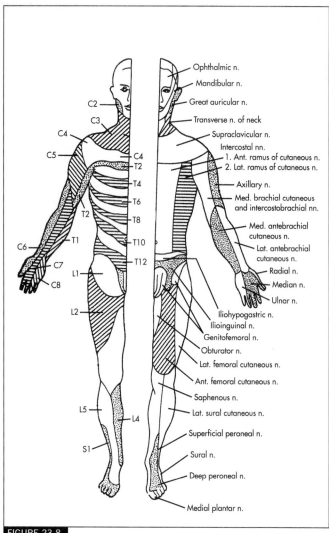

FIGURE 23-8

Anterior view of dermatomes *(left)* and cutaneous areas supplied by individual peripheral nerves *(right)*. *(Modified from Carpenter MB, Sutin J: Human neuroanatomy, Baltimore, 1983, Williams & Wilkins: Isselbacher KJ et al, editors: Harrison's principles of internal medicine, ed 13, New York, 1994, McGraw-Hill.)*

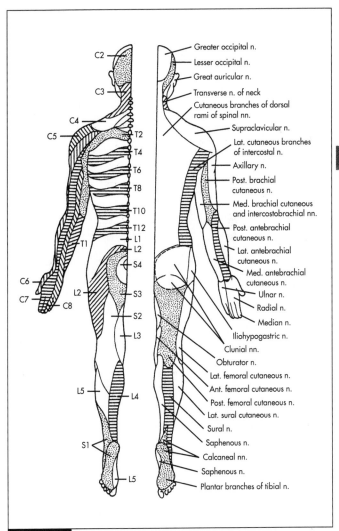

FIGURE 23-9

Posterior view of dermatomes *(left)* and cutaneous areas supplied by individual peripheral nerves *(right)*. *(Modified from Carpenter MB, Sutin J:* Human neuroanatomy, *Baltimore, 1983, Williams & Wilkins: Isselbacher KJ et al, editors:* Harrison's principles of internal medicine, *ed 13, New York, 1994, McGraw-Hill.)*

23

REFERENCE MATERIALS

RECOMMENDED CHILDHOOD IMMUNIZATION SCHEDULE*—UNITED STATES, JANUARY–DECEMBER 2001

Vaccine	Birth	1 mo	2 mos	4 mos	6 mos	12 mos	15 mos	18 mos	24 mos	4-6 yrs	11-12 yrs	14-18 yrs
Hepatitis B[†]		Hep B #1									Hep B	
			Hep B #2			Hep B #3						
Diphtheria and tetanus toxoids and pertussis[§]			DTaP	DTaP	DTaP		DTaP	DTaP		DTaP	Td	
H. influenzae type b[¶]			Hib	Hib	Hib	Hib						
Inactivated Polio[**]			IPV	IPV	IPV	IPV				IPV		
Pneumococcal conjugate[††]			PCV	PCV	PCV	PCV						
Measles-mumps-rubella[§]						MMR	MMR			MMR	MMR	
Varicella[¶¶]						Var	Var				Var	
Hepatitis A[•••]									Hep A in selected areas			

☐ Range of recommended ages for vaccination.

⬭ Vaccines to be given if previously recommended doses were missed or were given earlier than the recommended minimum age.

▨ Recommended in selected states and/or regions.

*This schedule indicates the recommended ages for routine administration of currently licensed childhood vaccines as of November 1, 2000, for children through age 18 years. **Additional vaccines may be licensed and recommended during the year.** Licensed combination vaccines may be used whenever any components of the combination are indicated and the vaccine's other components are not contraindicated. **Providers should consult the manufacturer's package inserts for detailed recommendations.**

†**Infants born to hepatitis B surface antigen (HBsAg)-negative mothers** should receive the first dose of hepatitis B vaccine (Hep B) by age 2 months. The second dose should be administered at least 1 month after the first dose. The third dose should be administered at least 4 months after the first dose and at least 2 months after the second dose, but not before age 6 months. **Infants born to HBsAg-positive mothers** should receive Hep B and 0.5 mL hepatitis B immune globulin (HBIG) within 12 hours of birth at separate sites. The second dose is recommended at age 1–2 months and the third dose at age 6 months. **Infants born to mothers whose HBsAg status is unknown** should receive Hep B within 12 hours of birth. Maternal blood should be drawn at delivery to determine the mother's HBsAg status; if the HBsAg test is positive, the infant should receive HBIG as soon as possible (no later than age 1 week). **All children and adolescents (through age 18 years)** who have not been immunized against hepatitis B should begin the series during any visit. Providers should make special efforts to immunize children who were born in or whose parents were born in areas of the world where hepatitis B virus infection is moderately or highly endemic.

§The fourth dose of diphtheria and tetanus toxoids and acellular pertussis vaccine (DTaP) may be administered as early as age 12 months, provided 6 months have elapsed since the third dose and the child is unlikely to return at age 15–18 months. Tetanus and diphtheria toxoids (Td) is recommended at age 11–12 years if at least 5 years have elapsed since the last dose of diphtheria and tetanus toxoids and pertussis vaccine (DTP), DTaP, or diphtheria and tetanus toxoids (DT). Subsequent routine Td boosters are recommended every 10 years.

¶Three *Haemophilus influenzae* type b (Hib) conjugate vaccines are licensed for infant use. If Hib conjugate vaccine (PRP-OMP) (PedvaxHIB or ComVax [Merck]) is administered at ages 2 and 4 months, a dose at age 6 months is not required. Because clinical studies in infants have demonstrated that using some combination products may induce a lower immune response to the Hib vaccine component, DTaP/Hib combination products should not be used for primary immunization in infants at ages 2, 4 or 6 months unless approved by the Food and Drug Administration for these ages.

**An all-activated poliovirus vaccine (IPV) schedule is recommended for routine childhood polio vaccination in the United States. All children should receive four doses of IPV at age 2 months, age 4 months, between ages 6 and 18 months, and between ages 4 and 6 years. Oral poliovirus vaccine should be used only in selected circumstances (1).

‡‡**The heptavalent pneumococcal conjugate vaccine (PCV) is recommended for all children age 2–23 months. It is also recommended for certain children age 24–59 months (2).**

§§The second dose of measles, mumps, and rubella vaccine (MMR) is recommended routinely at age 4–6 years but may be administered during any visit, provided at least 4 weeks have elapsed since receipt of the first dose and that both doses are administered beginning at or after age 12 months. Those who have not received the second dose should complete the schedule no later than the routine visit to a health-care provider at age 11–12 years.

¶¶Varicella vaccine (Var) is recommended at any visit on or after the first birthday for susceptible children, i.e., those who lack a reliable history of chickenpox (as judged by a health-care provider) and who have not been immunized. Susceptible persons aged ≥13 years should receive two doses given at least 4 weeks apart.

***Hepatitis A vaccine (Hep A) is recommended for use in selected states and/or regions, and for certain high-risk groups. Information is available from local public health authorities (3). Additional information about the immunization schedule is available on the National Immunization Program World-Wide Web site, http://www.cdc.gov/nip, or by telephone, (800)232-2522 (English) or (800)232-0233 (Spanish).

FIGURE 23-10

Recommended childhood immunization schedule—United States (January to December 2000). *From MMWR 50(1):7-10, 19, January 12, 2001.*

METABOLIC FORMULAS

$$\text{Estimated creatinine clearance} = \frac{(140 - \text{Age [yr]})(\text{Body weight [kg]})}{72\ (\text{Serum creatinine [mg/dl]})}$$

I. For women, multiply this figure by 0.85. May not reflect early renal damage because of compensatory hypertrophy of remaining glomeruli.
II. Normal for healthy adult is 94 to 140 ml/min for men and 72 to 110 ml/min for women.
III. The creatinine clearance normally decreases with age.

ELECTROLYTE FORMULAS

I. **Hyperglycemia Effect on Serum Na^+.**

Correct serum Na^+ = Measured sodium + 1.6 × [([Measured serum glucose − 100] / 100)] for serum glucose over 100 mg/dl

Note: Correction may be up to 2.4 mg/dl.

II. **Hyperlipidemia or Hyperproteinemia Effect on Na^+.**

Correct serum Na^+ = Measured sodium × (93/% serum H_2O) % serum H_2O = 99 − 1.03 (lipids in g/L) − 0.73(protein in g/dl)

III. Fractional Excretion of Na^+ (FE_{Na}).

% FE_{Na} = [(Urine Na/Serum Na)]/ [(Urine Cr/Serum Cr) × 100]

IV. Serum Na^+ Requirement in Hyponatremia.

Desired Na^+ mEq/L = (Desired serum Na − Measured Na) × TBW
TBW (total body water in liters) = 0.6 × Body weight in kg

V. **Body Water Deficit in Hypernatremia.**

Deficit = Desired TBW − Current TBW
[Desired TBW = Measured Na × (Current TBW/normal serum Na)
Current TBW = 0.6 × Current body weight in kg
or
Deficit = 0.6 (Current weight in kg) × ([Serum Na/140] − 1)

VI. **Serum osmolarity.**

$$2(Na + K) + BUN/2.8 + Glucose/18 = serum\ omolarity$$

A. Normal value 280 to 296 mOsm/kg of water
B. A difference between the measured and calculated osmolarity (osmolar gap) can indicate a circulating osmotically active substance such as ethanol, methanol, or ethylene glycol (antifreeze).

VII. **Anion Gap.**

$$Na - (Cl + Bicarbonate) = anion\ gap$$

A. Normal is up to 15. Greater than this in presence of acidosis indicates an anion gap acidosis (see Chapter 6 for discussion).

VIII. **A/a gradient.**

$$A\text{-}a\ gradient = PaO_2\ (alveolar) - PaO_2\ (arterial)$$
$$PAO_2\ (alveolar) = 150 -$$
$$1.2(PaCO_2),\ assuming\ patient\ breathing\ room\ air\ (FIO_2\ 21\%).$$

Normal A-a gradient is 5-20 and increases with age.

IX. **Mean arterial pressure (MAP).**

$$MAP = [systolic\ pressure + (2*diastolic\ pressure)]/3$$

X. **Relationship between pco_2 and pH.**
If uncompensated, a change in pCO_2 of 10 results in a pH change of 0.08.

INDEX

A

N